CELESTIAL LANCETS

鍼灸史略和麻醉理論

鲁桂珍
李约瑟 著

張香桐題

CELESTIAL LANCETS
A HISTORY AND RATIONALE OF ACUPUNCTURE AND MOXA

Lu Gwei-djen
and
Joseph Needham

With a new introduction by
Vivienne Lo

Routledge
Taylor & Francis Group
LONDON AND NEW YORK

First Published by
Cambridge University Press in 1980
by Routledge
2 Park Square, Milton Park, Abingdon, Oxfordshire OX14 4RN

Simultaneously published in the USA and Canada
by Routledge
711 Third Avenue, New York, NY 10017

Routledge is an imprint of the Taylor and Francis Group, an informa business

First issued in hardback 2015

British Library Cataloguing in Publication Data
A catalogue record for this book is available from the British Library

Library of Congress Cataloging in Publication Data
A catalog record for this book has been requested

ISBN 978-0-7007-1458-2 (pbk)
ISBN 978-1-138-13716-5 (hbk)

Publisher's Note

The publisher has gone to great lengths to ensure the quality of this reprint but points out that some imperfections in the original may be apparent.

CONTENTS

LIST OF ILLUSTRATIONS

LIST OF TABLES

LIST OF ABBREVIATIONS

The following abbreviations are used in the text and footnotes. For abbreviations used for journals and similar publications in the bibliographies, see pp. 320 ff.

B Bretschneider, E. (*1*), *Botanicon Sinicum.*

CC Chia Tsu-Chang & Chia Tsu-Shan (1), *Chung-Kuo Chih-Wu Thu Chien* (Illustrated Dictionary of Chinese Flora), 1958.

CCCY Kao Wu, *Chen Chiu Chü Ying* (*Fa Hui*) (A Collection of Gems in Acupuncture and Moxibustion), +1537.

CCIF Sun Ssu-Mo, *Chhien Chin I Fang* (Supplement to the Thousand Golden Remedies), between +660 and +680.

CCTC Yang Chi-Chou, *Chen Chiu Ta Chhêng* (Principles of Acupuncture and Moxibustion), +1601.

CCYF Sun Ssu-Mo, *Chhien Chin Yao Fang* (Thousand Golden Remedies), between +650 and +659.

CHS Pan Ku (and Pan Chao), *Chhien Han Shu* (History of the Former Han Dynasty), *c.* +100.

CIC Huangfu Mi, *Chen Chiu Chia I Ching* (Treatise on Acupuncture and Moxibustion), between +256 and +282.

CLPT Thang Shen-Wei *et al.* (ed.), *Chêng Lei Pên Tshao* (Reorganised Pharmacopoeia), ed. of +1249.

CSHK Yen Kho-Chün (ed.), *Chhüan Shang-Ku San-Tai Chhin Han San-Kuo Liu Chhao Wên* (Complete Collection of prose literature (including fragments) from remote antiquity through the Chhin and Han Dynasties, the Three Kingdoms, and the Six Dynasties), 1836.

HFT Han Fei, *Han Fei Tzu* (Book of Master Han Fei), early −3rd cent.

HHS Fan Yeh & Ssuma Piao, *Hou Han Shu* (History of the Later Han Dynasty), +450.

HNT Liu An *et al.*, *Huai Nan Tzu* (Book of the Prince of Huai-Nan), −120.

ICK Taki Mototane, *I Chi Khao* (*Iseki-kō*) (Comprehensive Annotated Bibliography of Chinese Medical Literature [Lost or Still Existing]), finished *c.* 1825, pr. 1831; repr. Tokyo, 1933, Shanghai, 1936.

ITCM Wang Khên-Thang & Chu Wên-Chen (ed.), *I Thung Chêng Mo Chhüan Shu* (Complete Collection of Works on Medicine and Sphygmology), +1601.

K Karlgren, B. (1), *Grammata Serica* (dictionary giving the ancient forms and phonetic values of Chinese characters).

KHTT Chang Yü-Shu (ed.), *Khang-Hsi Tzu Tien* (Imperial Dictionary of the Khang-Hsi reign-period), +1716.

LPC Lung Po-Chien (*1*), *Hsien Tshun Pên Tshao Shu Lu* (Bibliographical Study of Extant Pharmacopoeias and Treatises on Natural History from all Periods).

MCPT Shen Kua, *Mêng Chhi Pi Than* (Dream Pool Essays), +1089.

NC *Nan Ching* (Manual of (Explanations concerning Eighty-one) Difficult Passages in the Yellow Emperor's Manual of Corporeal Medicine), −1st cent. or +1st cent. In *ITCM* pên 19–20, and in *TSCC*, I shu tien, chs. 89–90; repr. Jen-min Wei-shêng, Peking, 1959, as *I Pu Chhüan Lu*, vol. 2. Both these texts have Hua Shou's commentary (+1361), *Nan Ching Pên I*.

NC/PH Chhen Pi-Liu (*1*), *Nan Ching Pai Hua Chieh* (The 'Manual of...Difficult (Passages)...' expressed in Modern Colloquial Language).

NCCC Wang Wei-I, Wang Chiu-Ssu *et al.* (ed.), *Nan Ching Chi Chu* (Collected Commentaries on the Manual of Difficult Passages). In *Shou Shan Ko Tshung Shu* and *I Tshun Tshung Shu* collections.

NCCS Hsü Kuang-Chhi, *Nung Chêng Chhüan Shu* (Complete Treatise on Agriculture), +1639.

NCLS *Huang Ti Nei Ching, Ling Shu* (The Yellow Emperor's Manual of Corporeal (Medicine); the Vital Axis [or, the Mysteriously Effective Controllers]), prob. −1st cent. Repr. of the Chao Fu Chü Ching Thang ed. from the original Ming blocks kept at Han Fên Lou in Shanghai, under title *Huang Ti Su Wên Ling Shu Ching*.

NCLS/MC *Huang Ti Nei Ching, Ling Shu* (The Yellow Emperor's Manual of Corporeal (Medicine); the Vital Axis [or, the Mysteriously Effective Controllers]), prob. −1st cent. With the commentaries of Ma Shih (+1586) and Chang Chih-Tshung (+1672).
In *TSCC*, I shu tien, chs. 67–88; repr. Jen-min Wei-shêng, Peking, 1959 as *I Pu Chhüan Lu*, vol. 2 [Anon. (*76*)].

NCLS/PH Chhen Pi-Liu & Chêng Cho-Jen (*1*), *Huang Ti Nei Ching, Ling Shu, Pai Hua Chieh* (The 'Yellow Emperor's Manual of Corporeal (Medicine); the Vital Axis [or, the Mysteriously Effective Controllers]' expressed in Modern Colloquial Language).

NCNA *New China News Agency Bulletin.*

NCSW *Huang Ti Nei Ching, Su Wên* (The Yellow Emperor's Manual of Corporeal (Medicine); Questions (and Answers) on Living Matter), −2nd cent. Wang Ping's edition in *I Thung Chêng Mo Chhuan Shu* Collection (Peking, 1923). Mod. ed., Com. Press, Shanghai, 1931, repr. 1955.

NCSW/C *Huang Ti Nei Ching, Su Wên* (The Yellow Emperor's Manual of Corporeal (Medicine); Questions (and Answers) on Living Matter), −2nd cent.
With Chang Chih-Tshung's commentary, +1672, ed. 1890.

NCSW/PH Chou Fêng-Wu, Wang Wan-Chieh & Hsü Kuo-Chhien (*1*), *Huang Ti Nei Ching, Su Wên, Pai Hua Chieh* (The 'Yellow Emperor's Manual of Corporeal (Medicine); Questions (and Answers) about Living Matter' expressed in Modern Colloquial Language).

NCSW/WMC *Huang Ti Nei Ching, Su Wên* (The Yellow Emperor's Manual of Corporeal (Medicine); Questions (and Answers) on Living Matter), −2nd cent. With the commentaries of Wang Ping (+762), Ma Shih (+1586) and Chang Chih-Tshung (+1672). In *TSCC*, I shu tien, chs. 21–66; repr. Jen-min Wei-shêng, Peking, 1959 as *I Pu Chhüan Lu*, vol. 1 [Anon. (76)].

NCTS Yang Shang-Shan (ed. & comm.), *Huang Ti Nei Ching, Thai Su* (The Yellow Emperor's Manual of Corporeal (Medicine); the Great Innocence [i.e. the fully formed body and mind of man, and what can then happen to it]), i.e. the *Nei Ching* re-arranged in a supposed original form, *c.* +615.

PTKM Li Shih-Chen, *Pên Tshao Kang Mu* (The Great Pharmacopoeia), +1596.

PWYF Chang Yü-Shu (ed.), *Phei Wên Yün Fu* (encyclopaedia), +1711.

R Read, Bernard E. *et al.*, Indexes, translations and précis of certain chapters of the *Pên Tshao Kang Mu* of Li Shih-Chen. If the reference is to a plant see Read (1); if to a mammal see Read (2); if to a bird see Read (3); if to a reptile see Read (4 or 5); if to a mollusc see Read (5); if to a fish see Read (6); if to an insect see Read (7).

RP Read & Pak (1), Index, translation and précis of the mineralogical chapters in the *Pên Tshao Kang Mu.*

SC Ssuma Chhien, *Shih Chi* (Historical Records), *c.* −90.

SCC Needham, Joseph; with the collaboration of Wang Ling, Lu Gwei-Djen, Ho Ping-Yü, Lo Jung-Pang, K. Robinson, N. Sivin, *et al.*: *Science and Civilisation in China*, 7 vols. in *c.* 20 parts, Cambridge, 1954–.

SF Thao Tsung-I (ed.), *Shuo Fu* (Florilegium of (Unofficial) Literature), *c.* +1368.

SHC *Shan Hai Ching* (Classic of the Mountains and Rivers), Chou and C/Han.

SIC Okanishi Tameto, *Sung I-Chhien I Chi Khao* (Comprehensive Annotated Bibliography of Chinese Medical Literatutre in and before the Sung Period). Jen-min Wei-shêng, Peking, 1958.

SKCS *Ssu Khu Chhüan Shu* (Complete Library of the Four Categories), +1782; here the reference is to the *tshung-shu* collection printed as a selection from one of the seven imperially commissioned MSS.

SKCS/TMTY Chi Yün (ed.), *Ssu Khu Chhüan Shu Tsung Mu Thi Yao* (Analytical Catalogue of the *Complete Library of the Four Categories*), +1782; the great bibliographical catalogue of the imperial MS. collection ordered by the Chhien-Lung emperor in +1772.

SNPTC *Shen Nung Pên Tshao Ching* (Classical Pharmacopoeia of the Heavenly Husbandman), C/Han.

SSIW Toktaga (Tho-Tho) *et al.*; Huang Yü-Chi *et al.* & Hsü Sung *et al.* *Sung Shih I Wên Chih, Pu, Fu Phien* (A Conflation of the Bibliography and Appended Supplementary Bibliographies of the History of the Sung Dynasty). Com. Press, Shanghai, 1957.

SYEY	Mei Piao, *Shih Yao Erh Ya* (The Literary Expositor of Chemical Physic; or, Synonymic Dictionary of Minerals and Drugs), +806.
TCTC	Ssuma Kuang, *Tzu Chih Thung Chien* (Comprehensive Mirror (of History) for Aid in Government), +1084.
TKKW	Sung Ying-Hsing, *Thien Kung Khai Wu* (The Exploitation of the Works of Nature), +1637.
TPHMF	*Thai-Phing Hui Min Ho Chi Chü Fang* (Standard Formularies of the (Government) Great Peace People's Welfare Pharmacies), +1151.
TPYL	Li Fang (ed.), *Thai-Phing Yü Lan* (the Thai-Phing reign-period (Sung) Imperial Encyclopaedia), +983.
TSCC	Chhen Mêng-Lei *et al.* (ed.), *Thu Shu Chi Chhêng* (the Imperial Encyclopaedia of +1726). Index by Giles, L. (2). References to 1884 ed. given by chapter (*chüan*) and page. References to 1934 photolitho reproduction given by *tshê* (vol.) and page.
TSCCIW	Liu Hsü *et al.* & Ouyang Hsiu *et al.*; *Thang Shu Ching Chi I Wên Ho Chih.* A conflation of the Bibliographies of the *Chiu Thang Shu* by Liu Hsü (H/Chin, +945) and the *Hsin Thang Shu* by Ouyang Hsiu & Sung Chhi (Sung, +1061). Com. Press, Shanghai, 1956.
TT	Wieger, L. (6), *Taoisme*, vol. 1, Bibliographie Générale (catalogue of the works contained in the Taoist Patrology, *Tao Tsang*).
WTPY	Wang Thao, *Wai Thai Pi Yao* (Important Medical Formulae and Prescriptions revealed by the Governor of a Distant Province), +752.
YHSF	Ma Kuo-Han (ed.), *Yü Han Shan Fang Chi I Shu* (Jade-Box Mountain Studio collection of (reconstituted and sometimes fragmentary) Lost Books), 1853.

AUTHORS' FOREWORD

This book is primarily about acupuncture, one of the oldest and most deeply characteristic of the techniques of traditional-Chinese medicine. For some two thousand five hundred years, perhaps three thousand, the implantation of needles into the subcutaneous connective tissue and muscles at a great number of different points on the body's surface has been used to heal a wide variety of illnesses and malfunctions. That the needles stimulate many kinds of nerve-endings and nociceptors is today undoubted, with all that this may imply of further repercussions in the central and autonomic nervous systems. The relief of pain was one of the keynotes of the procedure, so it was not altogether surprising that in the course of time the trial was made of acupuncture as a possible technique for achieving a painlessness or analgesia adequate for the interventions of modern major surgery. During the past twenty years or so a million or more successful operations of this kind have been performed. So striking have the results been that almost for the first time modern-Western medical scientists have felt obliged to take seriously an aspect of traditional-Chinese medicine; and naturally this has led to a reconsideration of the older system of acupuncture therapy. To some extent also the parallel practice of moxibustion, i.e. the use of *Artemisia* tinder for cautery and heat treatments of varying intensities, has shared in such a reconsideration.

Our discussion in this monograph really belongs to Vol. 6 of the *Science and Civilisation in China* series, but so widespread is the current interest in acupuncture throughout the world that it has seemed advisable to issue our account in separate form without waiting for its appearance in the cadre of a discussion of the history of Chinese medicine as a whole. The subject has presented us with a case quite different from most of our concerns in the earlier volumes of that series. Chapters there were primarily historical, and they dealt with subjects in which East and West were integrated long ago—for example, astronomy, mechanical engineering or chemistry. They did not therefore involve us with the task of summarising a large and rapidly growing body of contemporary scientific research literature, directed to the understanding of an age-old Chinese procedure in terms of modern science. We present therefore not only a history of acupuncture and moxa but an attempt to sketch a rationale of it in terms of modern knowledge. One could think of this as a contribution to that oecumenical medicine which will combine all the true powers discovered both in China and Europe, a medicine still *in statu nascendi*. What we are not offering is another clinical manual similar to the many that already exist in several Western languages.

Rationality evokes another feature of classical Chinese medicine which it is important to be clear about. There was in China a counterpart of the Hippocratic Corpus, the *Huang Ti Nei Ching*, *Su Wên* and *Ling Shu*, not quite so old, but not very much younger; and no less rational than the best medical thought of the Greek and Hellenistic worlds. As readers will have the opportunity of seeing, it was in some ways more advanced than that, for example in its circulation-mindedness (which led already in the Han to a doctrine of the blood-circulation only sixty times slower than the speed of the Harveian one today accepted); and later, in the Sung, its appreciation of those diurnal or circadian rhythms, both physiological and pathological, which modern science has only recently recognised. Or again, one could instance the module system, starting in the Thang, whereby acu-points could be identified with precision in persons of widely different size and build.

Of course the body of theory which was developed by Chinese medical thinkers during the ancient and medieval centuries was essentially of its time, an interplay of the Yin and Yang forces and the Five Elements, a conviction of the circulation of *chhi* (*pneuma*) through the channels of the body (as well as blood), and a technical vocabulary of many terms such as plerosis and asthenia, patefact and subdite, agmen and vexilla, calid and algid, humid heat and dry heat, etc. The theoretical structure of traditional-Chinese medicine is indeed medieval, but at the same time remarkably subtle and sophisticated; it never lost sight of the psycho-physical organism as a whole, and its grand design was the restoration of natural harmony, a balanced *krasis* of the body. Explanations of the effects of acupuncture today tend to be in terms of modern neuro-physiology, neuro-biochemistry, endocrinology and immunology, sciences of which the old Chinese physicians necessarily knew nothing. We are consequently faced with the profoundly difficult problem of translating the medieval theories into terms of modern science, a process which may well prove impossible, yet traditional physicians used them for some two and a half millennia for organising their vast clinical experience. There is a paradox here not yet resolved.

The problem is just as acute in China as anywhere else, and it was there compounded by the urgent necessity of providing medical services to nine hundred million people. By good fortune conditions facilitated the integration of the traditional-Chinese physicians with those trained in modern-Western medicine, but for a period the shortening of medical education to three years was a necessity, and the training of large numbers of paramedical personnel (the 'barefoot doctors') enabled emergency medical care to be extended to the remotest villages. But one of the casualties of this successful campaign was the patient study of the theoretical system of traditional-Chinese medicine, which formerly, in the good old days of personal apprenticeship, could take a couple of decades before proficiency was attained.

An even worse truncation has attended the practical literature on acupuncture in Western languages. Even when these works are based on translations of Chinese handbooks for professional acupuncturists, they usually tend to approach the Western reader with the assumption that all he needs is a set of charts, a list of illnesses, and a case of needles with instructions as to where to stick them in, then hope for the best. The Western enthusiast, unlike the 'barefoot doctor', does not have a deeply skilled specialist at his base hospital to whom reference can be made. In the hands of real experts, acupuncture can, in our belief, be very effective, both for therapy and analgesia, but when performed by amateurs, cranks or under-educated practitioners, it can have ill effects. Indeed, as the reader will find, acupuncture has been prohibited at times, both in China and Japan, for just such reasons.

As for its history, from the times of I Huan, Pien Chhio and Shunyü I onwards, this in its unfolding has been a veritable epic. Many conclusions which had formerly to be based on philological arguments about the dating of texts, have now received dazzling confirmation from archaeological discoveries, as for example the four manuscripts on silk which contain descriptions of the acu-tracts and were recovered only very recently from the Han tombs of the −2nd century at Ma-wang-tui. These scrolls reveal a development of acupuncture a good deal earlier than the *Nei Ching*. And from that same −2nd century there are the acupuncture needles found among the grave-goods of the Prince of Chung-shan, Liu Shêng. Or one could instance the acupuncture texts intended to accompany those life-size bronze figures demonstrating acu-points which were introduced first in the +11th century, texts which were later discovered inscribed on stone tablets that had been buried in the gate bastions of a city wall. It is to be expected that future archaeological finds will throw much further light on the development of Chinese medicine as a whole.

Lastly we must be allowed to voice a few votes of thanks. First as by right, we acknowledge with much gratitude our conversations with many physicians, surgeons and historians of medicine in China over the years, notably Dr Wang Chi-Min and Dr Chhen Pang-Hsien. Dr Chang Hsiang-Thung helped us greatly with neurophysiological interpretations. Dr Hu Tao-Ching and Dr Sung Ta-Jen were especially generous to us regarding the collection of essential literature. All these things and many others, including studies in hospitals and clinics, were made possible by the ever-welcoming support of the Chinese Academy of Sciences. Secondly, we have to thank the collaborators in our own group, notably Mrs Diana Brodie, our faithful and unerring secretary, and Miss Muriel Moyle, our indefatigable indexer. Professor Nathan Sivin, now of Philadelphia, kindly read and commented upon our typescript. Next there are many medical and physiological colleagues too numerous to name, though we cannot fail to thank Professor Peter Lisowski and his staff at Hongkong, Professor Ronald Melzack of Montreal, Dr Raymond Evans of Toronto and Professor Patrick Wall of London. Last, but not least, there come the members of the British Medical Acupuncture Society, presided over by Dr Felix Mann, who also helped us with literature. And never can we cast up such reckonings as these without thinking of the kind staff of the Cambridge University Press and our friend Mr Peter Burbidge, author of a thousand benefits and Chairman of our East Asian History of Science Trust. Owls perch, we think, from time to time, on the top of the Pitt Press tower, so that we can say, borrowing a tag from a famous bibliopole: *Tute sub aegide Pallas*.

LU GWEI-DJEN
JOSEPH NEEDHAM

EDITORIAL PREFACE TO THE REPRINTED EDITION

Celestial Lancets was first published in 1980. For anybody else but Lu Gwei-djen and Joseph Needham a single work of such broad sweep and deep learning would have been sufficient to establish a lifetime's reputation as researchers in the highly recondite field of Chinese medical theory and practice. But as we know, they were both more ambitious, and for them *Celestial Lancets* was just one more landmark in their explorations of vast areas of China's cultural roots.

At the time it was published, this book led the field as the most scholarly as well as one of the clearest and most accessible studies of any area of Chinese medicine in any Western language. Over the last twenty years the field has continued to advance – not least because of the stimulus given by Lu and Needham's work, but also because of the impact of several important finds of ancient manuscripts. However, as Dr Vivienne Lo notes in her introduction, it is striking how far *Celestial Lancets* is still the best available place to start reading. It still has the power to communicate a unique range of insights, and as Dr Lo herself has experienced, to suggest new and fruitful directions for research. This is an indispensable book.

Given the continuing importance of this book, it was something of a surprise to me as Chair of the Needham Research Institute Publications Board to learn that the original publishers of *Celestial Lancets* had taken an irrevocable decision to let it go out of print – and this only a short time before the impending publication of other medical writings by Joseph Needham and Lu Gwei-djen in Volume 6 part 6 of *Science and Civilisation in China* (Cambridge 2000). But fortunately owing to the enterprise and initiative of Jonathan Price and Curzon Press, the situation was saved, and a fresh generation of readers – students of Chinese culture and of acupuncture alike – can enjoy and profit from this important study.

It would have done no justice to Lu and Needham's enterprise to have reprinted their book without giving the reader a helping hand in making the link between their own ground-breaking work and the advances in the field in recent years. Fortunately Dr Lo's lively and very well informed introduction does that job superbly well, as well as constituting a valuable 'state of the field' review in its own right. She is a representative of the rising generation of researchers in the field of acumoxa as well as Chinese medicine in its wider sense, and has the immense advantage of being a professional acupuncturist as well as an academic historian and sinologist in full control of all the materials that 21st century scholars must master. The reader who turns to her writing while using Lu and Needham will be in expert hands, and will certainly be in no doubt that the torch of scholarship lit by the original authors in 1980 is still burning brightly.

Christopher Cullen

Department of History, School of Oriental and African Studies,
University of London, March 2001

INTRODUCTION

Vivienne Lo

SURVEY OF RESEARCH INTO THE HISTORY AND RATIONALE OF ACUPUNCTURE AND MOXA SINCE 1980

IT was with great pleasure that I accepted the invitation to write an introduction to this edition of *Celestial Lancets*. I never met Lu Gwei-djen and only came across Joseph Needham in his last and least vigorous year. Naturally, in the early years of reading the history of Chinese medicine for my PhD, *Celestial Lancets* was a foundational text. And I have come to think of them both as personal benefactors, especially when I have the opportunity to use the elegant library and home of the *Science and Civilisation* project at the Needham Research Institute.

It is not just the relative comfort that their lives' work bequeathed to the next generation of scholars that makes me think fondly of them. We need no introduction to Needham's monumental scholarly achievement in the on-going *Science and Civilisation in China series. Celestial Lancets* should be seen as a minor excursion from the great enterprise, which is a history of science, technology and medicine in China, embedded in the fullest possible social and intellectual context and delivered with a deep empathy for both cultures, Chinese and European.

Lu Gwei-djen 魯桂珍, Needham's life-long collaborator and, latterly, his wife, brought to the partnership a knowledge of Chinese medicine that was her professional inheritance. Lu Mou-Thing, Gwei-djen's father, was a progressive pharmacist trained in the dispensing of modern Western medicine as well as the *materia medica* of ancient China. He nurtured his daughter's education in the sciences. She trained in chemical pathology at Peking Union medical college before leaving for England. Lu Gwei-djen's life was spent in the service of science, nutrition and medicine as well as in bridging China, Europe and America in academic life. She achieved an internationalism quite remarkable in an oriental woman of her era. In a poem written by Joseph Needham and read at Lu Gwei-djen's funeral service, their spirit of internationalism, at once religious, political, social and scientific, finds its roots in a quotation from Liji 禮記, the classic *Book of Rites, 'Tianxia Da Tong'* 天下大同 *(All under Heaven shall be One Community)*. As the principal author of this monograph on Chinese medicine, Lu Gwei-djen leaves her imprint on *Celestial Lancets* in those same themes that bridge modern science and traditional therapeutics, East and West. Her influence is on-going. A conference organised in 1995 to celebrate Lu Gwei-djen's life and work brought together an international community of American and European scholars working on different areas in the history of Chinese medicine. The proceedings of the conference are published in the volume *Innovation in Chinese Medicine*, edited by Elisabeth Hsu.[1]

Together, Lu and Needham's efforts to offer access to and general awareness of that history have almost single-handedly made the history of Chinese science,

1 Elisabeth Hsu ed. *Innovation in Chinese Medicine* (Cambridge: CUP, 2001).

medicine and technology a part of the common cultural heritage of us all. Through their writings they have radically changed the ways in which scholars and scientists evaluate the history of Chinese medical culture. For my own part, whenever I conceive of a new direction in my own research into the history of acupuncture and moxibustion, I still begin by scanning through *Celestial Lancets* to see what they read and said on the subject. Certainly, thanks to the breadth of their reading, there will be many references to help me begin gathering evidence. Very often they have already anticipated my most original conception in a simple throwaway comment, or I stumble across a passing thought which stimulates the research for my next paper.

Poring over the Venn diagrams that illustrate a crossover of social/activity spheres in early China, all of which shared a "lore of vital spots" for controlling, harming or healing the body, gave me confidence to frame my PhD topic. Where they illustrate speculation about the dynamics between Daoist respiratory exercises, medical gymnastics, unarmed combat and the development of medical acupuncture and moxibustion, I had observed evidence of similar relationships in newly excavated medical manuscripts from the Western Han period. These earlier manuscripts, unavailable in the 1970s, clearly demonstrate the influence of the self-cultivation culture of the southern Chinese élite in the formative period of classical Chinese medicine. Building on their work I added sexual cultivation to the spheres of related activity and managed to establish the importance of late Warring States and Western Han hygienic practices in stimulating medical discourse about the nature of the inner body, its physiological basis and methods of stimulation and therapeutic intervention.

At that early phase of my research into the history of Chinese acupuncture and moxibustion, being rather blinded by the science of *Celestial Lancets*, I did not scour the volume cover to cover. If I had I might have come to my recent research topic more quickly. On page 128 (fig. 26) is a photograph of the so-called *jiufa tu* 灸法圖, one of the scroll manuscripts in the Dunhuang collection with a one-paragraph summary of Professor Ma Jixing's introductory article. They state rather laconically, 'it is not at all a systematic text but seems rather to record the personal experiences and practice of a plebeian physician'. And so it does. This manuscript bears the earliest image of the moxibustion points, and a rare testimony to the nature of popular moxibustion practice in mediaeval times. It pre-dates the well-known Song bronzes that set out the acupuncture points by some two or three centuries. Part of a collection of 83 medical manuscripts taken from the Buddhist caves at Dunhuang on the Silk Roads of Northwest China, it is now housed at the British Library.[2] For the last twenty years, despite a handful of articles in Chinese, little more has surfaced in the English language about the moxibustion charts, despite their convenient location in the heart of London. But now, following an international project and conference aimed at promoting awareness of the manuscripts and their content, the proceedings, including a full set of manuscript abstracts, will soon be published.[3]

2 S6168 and S6262. A complete transcript of the medical manuscripts including copies of the charts is in Ma Jixing ed., *Dunhuang yiyao wenxian jijiao* 敦煌醫藥文獻輯校, (Jiangsu: Jiangsu guji, 1998).

3 Lo and Cullen, *Mediaeval Chinese Medicine: The Dunhuang Medical Manuscripts* (forthcoming).

From whatever perspective we view *Celestial Lancets*, it remains a unique contribution to the history of acupuncture, and one that, for the reasons that I will outline below, is unlikely to be superseded. To begin with, both Lu Gwei-djen and Joseph Needham were scientists before they became historians, and inevitably applied biomedical research perspectives to their historical findings as well as to the evaluation of the efficacy of the medicine they studied. Needham was also both a Christian and a Socialist, legendary for his subversion of eurocentric and colonial histories of science and technology. *Celestial Lancets* was published at a time when public awareness of and eagerness for access to China was developing momentum. Their success in opening people's eyes to innovations in the history of Chinese sciences and technology was revolutionary then and remains compelling for generations taught to be suspicious of swallowing received wisdom whole.

As a product of a very particular research environment at the forefront of their field, it is inevitable that some of Lu and Needham's methodology and findings remain the gold standard for histories of acupuncture and moxibustion while others, through twenty years of shifting research paradigms, have themselves become the object of study. For example, *Celestial Lancets* remains the only English-language source which traces the growth of the number of acupoints through early acupuncture literature. The authors also scan received literature for evidence of the practice of acupuncture and moxibustion at acupoints, and although there have been more comprehensive treatments of the subject in Chinese and Japanese, and some of the information has now been reinterpreted, theirs remains the best treatment available in English. *Celestial Lancets* has an unparalleled treatment of the transmission of ideas about acupuncture and moxibustion outside of China. Beginning with the earliest evidence for the exchange of ideas in Korea they refer to the dissemination of medical thought and substances to Japan and south towards Vietnam, Yunan and Annam. It is only in the last year that Roberta Bivins's *Acupuncture Expertise and Cross-Cultural Medicine* (Palgrave, 2000) has extended their treatment of European impressions of acupuncture and moxibustion in the 17th to 19th centuries. Bivins pulls together the records into an insightful account of therapeutic needling as the subject of European medical debates, demonstrating both the process of innovation and the cultural specificity of medical knowledge. Trade, and the Dutch East India Company in particular, rather than political embassies provided the point of contact for medical practitioners, writers and naturalists to begin to convey their observations of Chinese and Japanese practice.

Most of the developments in the field have been stimulated by newly discovered source material. But we will also see, in the course of this introduction, that many of the areas just touched upon in *Celestial Lancets* have now been substantially elaborated. Other areas, particularly those involving popular practice, which were given little value by Lu and Needham, have now become the subject of more serious academic attention. Sivin gives a well-balanced review of Needham's work in his introduction to the *Medicine* volume of *Science and Civilisation*.[4] He also examines a number of Needham's assumptions in an essay which reviews the evidence for a relationship between science and Daoism.[5]

Given the generosity of spirit that floods through their work I suspect that Lu and Needham would have been the first to promote and appreciate the role of *Celestial Lancets* as a springboard for the next generation of research, regardless of how it might challenge their own findings. Part of the aim of this introduction is then to guide the reader through research into the history of acupuncture and moxibustion since 1980, when *Celestial Lancets* was first published, concentrating on areas that contrast with, complement or extend Lu and Needham's approach. I have divided the discussion into two parts, the first concerned with topics in the history of acupuncture and moxibustion and the second with the rationale and evaluation of acupuncture therapy.

History

Two-thirds of *Celestial Lancets* is dedicated to a history of acupuncture and moxibustion beginning in the middle Zhou period (6th century B.C.) and ending in the twentieth century. Together Lu and Needham set out a vast amount of primary text in translation with an impressive array of tables and illustrations. They researched the book through the 1970's, and since then there have been some major changes in the field of research into early Chinese medicine. The first arises from another field of research, that of Chinese archaeology, where recently excavated texts and artefacts with medical significance have forced medical historians to reconsider the traditional datings for the development of acupuncture theory and practice. Many thousands of tombs dating from the late Warring States and Han period still await excavation and always threaten to yield new evidence to overturn the latest theories. Professor Ma Jixing of the Academy of Research into Chinese Medicine has been writing and re-writing the history of acupuncture for over fifty years and still feels he has to embrace the latest excavated materials before his work is complete. At present his handwritten volumes fill a bookcase six feet high.

Secondly, methodology is in a constant state of evolution and the boundaries of different academic disciplines have become less rigid. With interesting new perspectives derived from the work of social historians, medical anthropologists, art historians and archaeologists, the question of reassessing the origins and development of a technique begins to look like an ever more complex task. Historians now aim to look further than establishing a particular dynamic between theory and technology that is consistent with a normative view of acumoxa; the new sources afford us a better understanding of the changing nature of medical practice

4 Joseph Needham, with the collaboration of Lu Gwei-djen, *Science and Civilisation in China* Vol. 6 Biology and Biological Technology Part VI: Medicine, edited and with introduction by Nathan Sivin (Cambridge: CUP, 2000), 1–37. Also see Nathan Sivin, "Science and Medicine in Imperial China – The State of the Field", *Journal of Asian Studies* 47, 1 (February 1988), 41–90.

5 Nathan Sivin, "Taoism and Science", in *Medicine, Philosophy and Religion in Ancient China, Researches and Reflections*, (Variorum, 1995), 10–49.

and the many agencies at work in the specific cultures within which ideas about acupuncture and moxibustion first began to emerge.

Popular histories still tend to date the origins of acupuncture to the mythological Yellow Emperor, an anachronism which is no doubt perpetuated by the title of the most famous corpus of early medical writings, the *Huangdi neijing* 黃帝內經, "The Yellow Emperor's Inner Canon". Originally the habit of attributing authorship to a cult hero, divinity or revered historical figure served to confer authority and status on the writing. There is no longer any excuse for this kind of historiography. From the work of philologists involved in reconstructing ancient texts we now know that the four works (*Huangdi neijing lingshu* 靈樞, *suwen* 素問, *taisu* 太素 and *mingtang* 明堂 hereafter simply Lingshu, Suwen etc.) which have *Huangdi neijing* in their titles are compilations of many different treatises. Each treatise may reflect the work of a different teaching lineage or, alternatively, an individual's collection of small units of medical texts.[6] It seems that there was a pool of these texts circulating amongst physicians and literati. There is therefore no "original" text, but simply different collections of similar material. Any one collection therefore represents the end of one lineage of collecting, as if frozen in time. The effective transmission of any one collection may be due to the prominence of its compilers or, alternatively, it might be accidental. For this and other reasons we cannot assume that the content of any one collection is representative of the medicine of its time.[7]

Until the 1970s, the work of historians attempting to date the origins of acupuncture was centred on dating the received canon of medical literature. It is still widely held to this day in China, that the *Huangdi neijing* corpus was largely a Warring States compilation. In the 1970's Lu and Needham brought that date forward to the first century B.C., equating the *Lingshu* (Numinous Pivot) with the *Zhenjing* (Needle Canon) 針經 of Han bibliographies, and attributing the *Suwen* to the previous century. (New evidence, set out below, indicates an earliest dating of the first century B.C. for any of the compilations). However they also cite rather cryptic passages in the *Zuo Zhuan* 左傳 and refer to the existence of needles to justify the assertion that acumoxa therapy was already practised during the middle Zhou period (ca. 600 B.C.). Manuscripts and artefacts from the late Warring States and early imperial period, excavated in the last three decades, have forced historians to review the evidence. While some of the tombs had already been excavated when *Celestial*

6 See Yamada Keiji 山天慶兒, "The Formation of the Huang-ti Nei-ching", 67–89. Yamada compares the structure and content of the Mawangdui texts *Yinyang jiujing* and the *Zubi jiujing* with the "Jingmai" treatise of the *Huangdi neijing taisu* 黃帝內經太素, the version of the text which he considers the closest to the original *Huangdi neijing*. He also discusses the various schools of thought represented in the treatises of *Huangdi neijing*. See also David Keegan, "The 'Huang-ti Nei-ching': The Structure of the Compilations; The Significance of the Structure", (PhD. diss., University of California, Berkeley, 1988). Keegan compares the Mawangdui editions of *Yinyang jiujing* and *Zubi jiujing* to *Lingshu*, 10 "Jingmai".

7 To what extent the combined treatises of the *Huangdi neijing* reflect medical orthodoxy of the Han dynasty is questioned by Akira Akahori 赤倔昭 who compares the *Huangdi neijing* material with medical ideas in the work of the contemporary author Wang Chong 王充. See Akira Akahori, "Go-kan shoki no igaku no ichi danmen" 後漢初期の醫學の一斷面, in *Toyo no kagaku to gijutsu*. 東洋の科學と技術 (Kyoto: Dohasha, 1982), 171–89.

Lancets was in preparation, difficult working conditions in China meant that it took a decade or more for site reports, collation, transcription and, in some cases, the photographic record to become available to historians. Those finds that have already had a significant bearing on the history of medicine include Han burial sites at Zhangjiashan 張家山 (tomb closed ca 186 B.C.), Mawangdui 馬王堆 (tomb closed ca 168 B.C.), Wuwei 武威 (ca 1st century A.D.) and Mianyang 綿陽 (before 118 B.C.).[8]

Much essential philological work, collating and annotating excavated medical texts, is carried out in the history departments of the Beijing *Zhongyi yanjiu yuan* 中醫研究院 Academy of Research into Chinese Medicine under the direction of Professor Ma Jixing and *Zhongguo shehui kexueyuan* 中國社會科學院 Chinese Academy of Social Sciences under Professor Li Xueqin. We are badly in need of scholarly, annotated translations of both the newly excavated texts and the received canons. The current spate of poorly translated and virtually unannotated editions of pre-modern texts produced in East and West does little to help and much to hinder in-depth research. Fortunately a handful of scholars are working in this area, notably Professor Paul Unschuld, whose translation of *Suwen* is eagerly awaited.[9] An excellent annotated English translation of the entire collection of medical manuscripts excavated from the Mawangdui burial site, the first ever into any language, is in Donald Harper's *Early Chinese Medical Literature: The Mawangdui Medical Manuscripts*.[10] His prolegomena to the translation gives a comprehensive introduction to the world of medical people, ideas and practice as it was developing through the few centuries before and after the establishment of the first empire (221 B.C.). These were the years of rapid political, social, intellectual and technical change when the theories and practices at the foundation of acupuncture, moxibustion and Chinese pharmacology were first set out. It is here in the marriage of all these factors that we must make a reassessment of the origins of the medicine.

Of the newly excavated sources, important medical manuscripts discovered at the burial sites of Mawangdui and Zhangjiashan now show medical theory of the channel system at a relatively primitive stage.[11] Anatomical pathways of *mai* "channels", some bearing such titles as *tai yang mai* 太陽脈 (Great Yang Channel) or *shao yang*

8 A survey of early Chinese excavated texts related to medicine can be found in Paul U. Unschuld and Zheng Jinsheng, 'Manuscripts as Sources in the History of Chinese Medicine' in Lo and Cullen, *Mediaeval Chinese Medicine: The Dunhuang Medical Manuscripts* (forthcoming), previously published in German in *Monumenta Serica*, 48 (2000).

9 See also Unschuld's translation of *Nanjing* 難經 (Canon of difficulties; first or second century A.D.). Paul U. Unschuld, *Nan-Ching: The Classic of Difficult Issues*, (Berkeley: University of California Press, 1986).

10 Donald Harper, *Early Chinese Medical Literature: The Mawangdui Medical Manuscripts* (London: The Sir Henry Wellcome Asian Series, KPI, 1998).

11 Transcriptions of the Zhangjiashan medical manuscripts are in Jiangling Zhangjiashan Hanjian zhengli xiaozu, 'Jiangling Zhangjiashan Hanjian (*Maishu*) shiwen' 江陵張家山漢簡脈書釋文, in *Wenwu* 文物 1989. 7, 72–74 and Zhangjiashan Hanjian zhengli zu, "Zhangjiashan Hanjian *Yinshu* shiwen" 張家山漢簡引書釋文, in *Wenwu* 1990.10, 82–86. See also Gao Dalun 高大倫 who has published two annotated transcripts complete with modern Chinese translations. Gao Dalun, *Zhangjiashan Hanjian Maishu Jiaoshi* 張家山漢簡脈書校釋 (Chengdu: Chengdu chubanshe, 1992). Gao Dalun, *Zhangjiashan Hanjian Yinshu Yanjiu* 張家山漢簡引書研究 (Chengdu: Bashu shushe chuban faxing, 1995).

mai 少陽脈 (Lesser Yang Channel), share similar nomenclature to the *jingmai* 經脈 or *jingluo* 經絡 of later acumoxa theory.[12] But other information about the channels provided by the various excavated sources is far from consistent and, however similar they may first appear, we must be particularly circumspect in how we relate these early sources with later works as well as how closely we associate the different excavated sources themselves.

The newly excavated Western Han textual sources have already altered our perception of the early development of channel theory. They do not reveal a network of channels systematically associated with the internal organs[13] or with an acupoint system. Their channels proceed in more parallel fashion along the limbs to the torso and head. They sometimes cross but do not "join" at the ends in a continuous ring. The practice of lancing the body is mainly associated in these texts with abscess bursting, and the principles of practice related to the channels are extremely basic. Despite this juxtaposition of medical innovation with surgical procedures, it is not possible to identify a monolinear development from petty surgery with stones to the modern acupuncture needle and this is a point stressed by both Yamada Keiji and Paul Unschuld. We can identify many influences at work in that process, from bloodletting to deep heat treatments and a range of self-cultivation practices common to elite circles in early imperial times.

The early texts document a first systematic attempt at physiological speculation. In them we can see evidence of a movement away from the view of disease as a hostile entity, external to the body, towards an emphasis on interpreting signs of illness as the breakdown of a state of harmony within the body. By the time of the compilation of the "Jingmai" treatise of the *Lingshu* each anatomical plane associated with a channel has been linked to the organs or bowels, such as the liver or large intestine. The body is described, not in terms of its anatomical mass, but rather as a series of functional units with prescribed spheres of influence. Such physiological ideas became central to theories of pathological physiology and illness that survived throughout the imperial era and remain current in the modern practice of Chinese medicine.

12 The word *mai* is difficult to translate. Harper translates "vessel," which draws out the early association with the arteriovenous system. See Donald Harper, *Early Chinese Medical Literature: The Mawangdui Medical Manuscripts*, 82–83. I prefer to follow the contemporary analogy with *du* 瀆 "channel" or "canal" found in the *Maishu* 脈書 (Channel document). See Jiangling Zhangjiashan Hanjian zhengli xiaozu, 1989. 7, 74. The translation "channel" also serves to emphasize the relationship of the *mai* to the superficial anatomical channels as defined by muscle and bone, as they were understood before the more elaborate theories of the *jingluo* 經絡 and *jingmai* 經脈 found in the *Huangdi neijing*). *Jingluo* or *jingmai* has been variously translated as "conduit," "meridian," "circulation tract," etc. See Nathan Sivin, *Traditional Medicine in Contemporary China* (Ann Arbor: Center for Chinese Studies, The University of Michigan, 1987), 34, 122 n. 11; and Paul Unschuld, *Medicine in China: A History of Ideas* (Berkeley: University of California Press, 1985), 75, 81–83.

13 Several Yin channels recorded in the newly excavated Western Han texts are connected to the *zang* 臟 "internal organs," but the organs are not integral to the classification system of the channels, nor do we know much about how they were conceived. By the time of *Lingshu* 10 the organs form part of the name of each channel. Nominal Western correlates would be *xin* 心 "heart," *pi* 脾 "spleen/pancreas," *fei* 肺 "lungs," *shen* 腎 "kidneys", *gan* 肝 "liver." For a more detailed discussion of the concept and translation of *zang* see Unschuld, *Medicine in China: A History of Ideas*, 77–83; and Sivin, *Traditional Medicine in Contemporary China* 121–33.

Western medical historians agree that an essential fusion of the technical and theoretical elements at the foundation of acumoxa therapy could not have happened much before the first century B.C and may have been a century later. This now also appears to be the earliest period during which the *Huangdi* corpus could have been compiled.[14] At least, as Sivin points out, 'the burden of proof is now taken to fall upon those who insist that the great gaps between the two manuscripts (channel texts from the Mawangdui site) and the *Huangdi neijing* were bridged in much less than two centuries, i.e., that any significant part of the latter text was set down before the mid-first century B.C.'[15]

The section entitled "Historical Growth" in *Celestial Lancets* begins with an extensive discussion of the development of the concept of the *jingluo* and the *jingmai*, the system of tracts/vessels or channels, main and subsidiary, through which *qi* and blood were thought to flow. Here we can find the best and most comprehensive of early attempts to describe the problems in translation of various terms and graphs that refer to the different elements of the system. From the *Huangdi* corpus Lu and Needham also identify a large number of locations for acupuncture needling. They quantify those that are recorded directly by name, and others that are deduced from description.

In recent years much thought has been devoted to whether the tracts/channels/vessels preceded the moxibustion or acupuncture points or vice versa. It is interesting that many of the acupuncture locations in the *Huangdi* corpus are not given by name, but by their anatomical location. *Maishu* 脈書 or parallel texts at Mawangdui make no mention of specific acupoints. Neither, as we shall see below, are there any acupoints definitively revealed in Chunyu Yi or Bian Que's treatments. In the intervening centuries between the composition of the *Suwen* and *Lingshu* and the *Zhenjiu jiayi jing* 針灸甲乙經, written by Huangfu mi 皇甫謐 (d. 282) we find a massive increase in the recording of acupuncture points by name. The gradual systematisation of knowledge during this period is consistent with what we know about intellectual activity in other technical fields such as mathematics.

The Mianyang figurine, a lacquered wood carving of the human body excavated from a Western Han tomb provides us with fascinating new evidence. It is covered with lines that bear some similarity to the channels described in Zhangjiashan and Mawangdui channel texts.[16] But it does not reveal the kind of holes, all systematically engraved with individual names, that we are familiar with from the cast bronze acupuncture models of the Northern Song period. So we can only conclude that so far there is no evidence to

14 See Paul Unschuld, *Medicine in China: A History of Ideas*, 92–99; and Sivin, Nathan. "Huang ti nei ching", in *Early Chinese Texts: A Bibliographical Guide*, ed. Michael Loewe (Berkeley: SSEC and IEAS, University of California, 1993), 197.

15 Sivin, Nathan. "Huang ti nei ching", in *Early Chinese Texts: A Bibliographical Guide*, 201.

16 See He Zhiguo & Lo, 'The channels: a preliminary examination of a lacquered figurine from the Western Han period' in *Early China* 21 (1996), 81–123 for an extensive discussion of the figurine. See He Zhiguo 何志國, "Woguo zuizao de renti jingmai qidiao" 我國最早的人體經脈漆雕, *Zhongguo wenwubao* 中國文物報 1994, 15 (April 17), 4 for the first description of the discovery of the figurine. A detailed discussion of the figurine can be found in He Zhiguo, "Xi Han renti jingmai qidiao kao",西漢人體經脈漆雕考, *Daziran tansuo* 大自然探索 1995.3, 116–20.

show that stimulating the channel network via a mature acupoint system with metal needles was a feature of therapy before the first century B.C. at the earliest.[17]

Claims for evidence of acupuncture needling at acupoints have often relied on *Shiji juan* 105 when Bian Que "扁鵲, treating the Crown Prince of Guo 虢, sent his disciple Ziyang 子陽, to "sharpen needles and needling stone to *qu* 取 (select and stimulate?) the *waisanyang wuhui* 外三陽五會 "outer three Yang and five meetings".[18] If we understand this term to be the alternative to *baihui* 百會 "hundred meetings", an acupoint on the top of the head, as it is listed in *Zhenjiu jiayi jing*, we could then say that Bian Que's treatment is the earliest explicit reference to acupuncture at an acupoint.[19] But Huangfu Mi may well have based his opinion on Sima Qian's account in *Shiji*. And we cannot know for sure what Sima Qian was referring to.[20]

The Mianyang figurine offers us a new and, I believe, a most satisfactory explanation for the term, since it does not reveal either one acupoint or one anatomical location on the top of the head. If we compare the figurine and the descriptions of the channels in the excavated texts we can find two bilateral and one medial red lines. These lines are all, arguably, *yang* in nature since they traverse the superior and posterior (and therefore *yang*) surfaces of the body, including the crown of the figurine's head. These five lines are intersected by one of the extensions of the arm lines which splits the crown horizontally. Here there are the three Yang and five meetings, with the "outer *sanyang wuhui*" being the intersections furthest away from the centre of the head.

In summary, evidence from the figurine helps to identify the location of *sanyang wuhui* as five different places on the top of the head where the lines meet. I doubt, therefore, that the *Shiji* reference is to a single acupoint. One reproduction of a set of stone reliefs discovered at Liangcheng shan 兩城山, Weishan 微山 county that are illustrated in *Celestial Lancets*, also seems to support the theory that early acupuncture involved multiple needling. The relief depicts a half-bird/half-man physician (probably the physician Bian Que) brandishing a stone lancet. Of a collection of eight reliefs, two show two women and a child. The women, according

17 The acupoints which seem to exist in the excavated texts that describe sexual-cultivation are in fact simply anatomical locations. *Quepen* 缺盆 "Broken Bowl" is a term used in pre-coital massage to refer to the area of the clavicle, and *zhongji* 中極 Middle Extremity is a significant anatomical location where *qi* transforms, without yet being the name and location for the acupuncture point *Ren* 3 that it eventually becomes.

18 *Shiji* 史記 105 (Beijing: Zhonghua, 1972), 2792.

19 *Zhenjiu jiayi jing* 針灸甲乙經 3 (Beijing: Renminweisheng, 1979), 331. See also *Zhenjiu Dacheng* 針灸大成 7 (Tianjin: Tianjin kexue jishu, 1992), 367.

20 Yamada Keiji examines a number of different theories on the matter. His problem centres around whether *sanyang wuhui* is one or two terms (the *wuhui* of the *sanyang* or the *sanyang* and *wuhui*), and how the term relates to the *sanyang wushu* 三陽五輸 found in a similar account in the earlier *Hanshi waizhuan* (ca. 2nd century B.C.). In summary, *sanyang* might refer to one of two locations – either the three Yang channels that we meet in the excavated texts, yang *ming*, *shao* yang or *tai* yang or it might refer to the third Yang, just one of these channels. But are they the three Yang of the arm or the leg? Yamada believes that the two terms *wushu* and *wuhui* are identical and refer to the *jing* 井, *rong* 榮, *jing* 經 and *he* 合 locations that we know from later acumoxa theory. He rejects the idea that they are the *wushu* 五輸, also of later theory, that is acupoints on the *tai* Yang channel that connect to the inner Yin organs. If they were to form a part of or belonged to the *san* Yang, he argues, then it is unlikely that they would refer, as the *wushu* do, to the Yin organs. Yamada Keiji in "Hen Shaku densetsu" 扁鵲傳說, *Toho gakuho* 東方學報 60, 1988, 130–132.

to an interpretation by Ye Youxin have short fine (and therefore probably metal) needles placed in a line between the hair line and the skin of the face as well as all along the woman's arm.[21] Since the needles are not equally visible on all the rubbings we must suspend judgment pending closer examination of the original reliefs. Similarly, when Chunyu Yi, the physician whose biography is contained in the official Han history, treats a case of hot sore feet, he pierces the channels at three different places on the sole of the foot and on the *yangming* 陽明 channel.[22]

The existence among the Mawangdui and Zhangjiashan medical treaties of a genre of medical literature which describes channels without acupoints has been taken to suggest that the channels came first. However, as Li Jianmin points out, there is evidence in the excavated texts that terms thought to be the names of channels actually refer to single locations.[23] Mediaeval moxibustion texts such as the Dunhuang *Jiufa tu* (Chart of moxibustion techniques), described above, also give testimony to this tradition. Lu and Needham point out that Yufu 俞跗, an eminent physician cited by Bian Que in Sima Qian's *Shiji* biography, does not use stone needles, but diagnoses the condition of the viscera through a knowledge of *shu* 輸. *Shu* becomes the term referring to acupoints, but in Chunyu Yi's time it may simply refer to trigger points on the surface of the skin.[24] Individual locations, they point out, may well have been 'recognised long before their assembly into constellations'. Their view is corroborated by the separate development of erogenous zones evident in Western Han sexual cultivation literature. The zones are referred to in lyrical terms similar to the names of acupoints found in later medical literature.[25]

Earlier medical literature often refers to stone or stone needling, but it does not follow that this is the application of stone or needle to strategic locations on the channels known as *zhenxue* 針穴 "acupoints".[26] Yamada Keiji gives the best review of early references to medical utensils in *The Origins of Acupuncture, Moxibustion and Decoction*.[27] What we do know is that there are increasing references to acupuncture with needles from the first century A.D. Medical texts excavated from a tomb at Wuwei 武威 (ca 1st century A.D.) provide us with the earliest datable detail of acupoints by name and the site of needle insertion and manipulation technique.[28]

21 See Ye Youxin 葉又新, "Shishi Dong Han huaxiangshi shang kehua de yizhen" 試釋東漢畫象石上刻劃的醫針 in Shandong zhongyi xueyuan xuebao 山東中醫學院 1981.3, 60–68. It should be noted that other reproductions of the stone relief do not show the same number of needles so clearly.

22 *Shiji*, 105.2804.

23 Li Jianmin, *Sisheng zhi yu* 死生之域 (Institute of History and Philology, Academia Sinica, 2000).

24 *Shiji*, 105.2804.

25 See Vivienne Lo, 'The influence of nurturing life culture on early Chinese medical theory' in *Innovation in Chinese Medicine*. (Cambridge: CUP, 2001) 19–50.

26 See Vivienne Lo 'Spirit of Stone: Technical Considerations in the Treatment of the Jade Body', *SOAS Bulletin* 2001 (65/1 forthcoming).

27 Yamada Keiji, *The Origins of Acupuncture, Moxibustion and Decoction*, (Kyoto: International Research Centre for Japanese Studies, 1998).

28 Zhang Yanchang 張延昌 and Zhu Jianping 朱建平 eds., *Wuwei Handai yijian yanjiu*. 武威漢代醫簡研究, (Beijing: Yuanzineng chubanshe, 1996), 21–23.

> When there is cold *qi* in the stomach, where in the abdominal duct, the intestines are swollen XXXXX the patient who is being needled breathes out forty or fifty times before taking out the needle. Next, pierce in the space between five *cun* below the knee to the depth of three *fen* into the flesh; leave the needle for as long as it takes to steam a *sheng* of rice; take the needle out; this is called three *li* 里 "miles". Next pierce the nape of the neck, from upper to lower, on either side of the eleventh vertebrae, to the depth of four *fen* into the flesh; leave the needle for 120 breaths; take out the needle; this is the lung *shu* 輸 "transporter".

Here the prescription for cold in the stomach is to needle two places *sanli* (three li "miles") 三里 and *feishu* "lung transporter" 肺輸, (now names of acupoints that are familiar to modern acupuncturists), at given depths for a given period of time. Even though the exact location does not entirely accord with later theory they are in the same general vicinity and the language and process are classical.[29] The Wuwei site is contemporary with or just subsequent to currently favoured dates for the *Huangdi* compilation. We can therefore be reasonably certain that significant and rapid changes had taken place in both theory and technology around the time of, or shortly after, the closure of the Mawangdui (168 B.C.) and Zhangjiashan (ca. 186 – 154 B.C.?) tombs and before the time of the closure of the Wuwei tomb.

Where the first treatise of *Lingshu* suggests manipulating *qi* by piercing the body with fine needles a distinction is made between the crude quality of stone lancets and small, metal needles. Modern acupuncture needles are made from finely tempered steel of a quality that was not available to the authors of *Lingshu*. Most tools and weapons in the late Warring States and Han period were made of cast iron which, due to foundry production, allowed for cheap mass production. But cast iron, with its high carbon content, would have been brittle and dangerous when fashioned as finely as a "mosquito proboscis", a description of the *hao zhen* 毫鍼.[30] Iron with a low carbon content was difficult to cast and had to be wrought with smithy methods.

Technically it would have been possible to smith a fine iron or steel needle from before the third century B. C., but excavations have not unearthed any examples from this period and Lu and Needham's speculation that there were acupuncture needles at that time remains unproven.[31] Many swords made from wrought iron and mild steel survive from Qin and Han times. A number of sewing cases containing fine iron and steel sewing needles have also been recovered from Han tombs.[32] An object described as a *gang zhen* 鋼針 was excavated from a Chu tomb in Baoshan, Hubei,

29 See the discussion in Zhang Yanchang and Zhu Jianping eds., *Wuwei Handai yijian yanjiu*, 86–90.

30 *Lingshu juan* 1, *pian* 1. *Sibu beiyao* 四部備要, vol. 205, fasc. 1, 1.

31 Donald Wagner discusses the development of wrought iron and steel working in Han times in *Iron and Steel in Ancient China* (Leiden, New York, Koln: EJ Brill, 1993), 267–288. Also see Donald Wagner. *The State and the Iron Industry in Han China*, (forthcoming).

32 Vivi Sylwan, "Investigation of silk from Edsen-gol and Lop-nor," Reports from the Scientific Expedition to the north-western provinces of China under the leadership of Dr Sven Hedin, Stockholm 1949, 85. The finds are summarised in Hayashi Minao 林巳奈夫, *Kandai no bunbutsu*

but archaeologists have not published sufficient evidence to determine whether it is iron or steel.[33] Copper, bronze, tin, gold or silver could also be beaten quite thin, but these would still make clumsy, fragile instruments. Besides, gold and silver were expensive and tools of this quality would not have been widespread.

The *hao zhen*,would have to have been more sophisticated than those nine silver and gold needles excavated at the Mancheng burial site.[34] They are all much finer and sharper than needles recovered from the Zhou period, but they are still a long way from steel needles and especially from those described as *hao zhen*. The holes in the handle shaft also suggest that the needles might have been hung, or more likely that they had a threading function – especially in this particular tomb which contained the two suits made of jade pieces sewn together with gold wire. It seems certain that these are sewing needles (despite the suggestion of medical use made by a nearby bowl in the grave site inscribed with the words *yigongpan* 醫工盤 "bowl for medical use").

The failure of archaeologists to discover steel medical needles in Han tombs should not distress us. Changes in burial culture after the 1st century B.C. meant that the wealthy were no longer buried along with their medical treatises and the content of their medical cabinets. Excavations are also, in a sense, random and we cannot draw definitive conclusions from what they do not contain. But the burden of proof falls to those who would state that acupuncture to move *qi* with fine metal needles pre-dates the second century B.C.

With the subsuming of the separate practices of acupuncture and moxibustion into the single category *zhenjiu* "acumoxa" there has been a tendency to attribute to them a common history in which the importance of *zhen* "needles" in the canonical literature rather eclipses the practice of *jiu* 'moxibustion'. *Celestial Lancets* gives us useful background for understanding the separate development of moxibustion, highlighting the number of moxibustion manuals in the Sui official bibliography and physicians' preferences for one or other therapy. Archaeologically recovered texts discovered during the last century, combined with a fresh review of received medical literature elevates the importance of moxibustion therapy. Treatment with needles and with moxibustion were sometimes opposed and we can also identify different traditions within the history of moxibustion alone: where the Mawangdui channel texts link moxibustion to a system of channels, the Dunhuang charts reveal a way of practice which has no explicit relationship to a concept of circulating *qi* through an integrated network of channels.

漢代 文物 (Tokyo: Jinban Kagaku kenkyusho,1976), 27 and figs 1–42, 1–43. There are also a number of examples in Sun Ji 孫极, *Handai wuzhi wenhua ziliao tushuo* 漢代物質文化資料圖説 (Beijing: Zhongguo lishi bowuguan, 1991).

33 Hubeisheng Jingzhou tielu kaogudui Baoshan mudi zhengli xiaozu, "Jingmenshi Baoshan Chumu fajue jianbao, 荊門包山楚墓發掘報" *Wenwu* 1988.5, 10, fig 23.

34 Of those needles, five were intact with long, thin squared handles pierced with one or two holes; two are 6.6 cm long, gold needles with a very sharp 7 degree angle on the conical tip; one is a 6.5 cm gold needle with a three faceted 50 degree angle on the tip and two are 6.9 cm round and sharp tipped needles – one of gold, the other of silver. See *Mancheng Hanmu fajue baogao* 滿成漢墓墓發掘報, (Beijing: Wenwu, 1980), 116.

Yamada Keiji in *The Origins of Acupuncture, Moxibustion and Decoction* gives good evidence that the development of moxibustion with mugwort was related to an earlier use of mugwort to ward off inauspicious elements and drive away demons.[35] The people of Chu in particular wore mugwort dolls at their waist. He also describes the use of a related plant *xiao* 蕭, as a form of incense to attract the gods, concluding that "mugwort must originally have been more than just a medicinal herb. *Ai* and *xiao* belong to the same mugwort genus, but one was used as incense to beckon the gods, whereas the other was used to drive away demons that caused illness." These represent two contrasting approaches to ensuring that the body only played host to benign entities. Yamada raises the possibility that the channel system was discovered by those using moxibustion for "magical therapies" because "the routes or areas of illness caused by gods of illness invading the body is highly compatible theoretically with the concept of the vessels (channels).[36]

Social history

When a core technology changes rapidly, that change is usually linked with transforming social or cultural boundaries and involves complex interactions between many individuals and their environment in the broadest sense. A thorough examination of early Chinese society is a huge task which has barely begun. Lu and Needham were among the first to suggest systematically that a study of sociopolitical, economic and religious factors is essential in any history of medicine. In *Celestial Lancets* they referred to research into Bao Gu 鮑姑 (3rd century A.D.) , the wife of Ge Hong 葛洪, author of *Bao Puzi* 保璞子, who was apparently expert in moxa and needle. I am not aware of any further studies of her work in the English language. They also record details of the life and work of a number of different medical practitioners and theorists such as Hua Tuo 華佗 and Zhang Zhongjing 張仲景, as well as the four great scholar-physicians of the Jin and Yuan period.

Individual scholar physicians sometimes influenced the development of Chinese medical theory, but research into the history of medical care in China reveals a complex society of competing and complementary practitioners: at any one time religious healers, scholar physicians, wise women or healing programmes run by mass millenarian cults may all have coexisted. Literature, and especially novels from the Ming and Qing (1644–1911) period, provide us with a colourful impression of the complex medical worlds that interact around their characters.[37] Naturally we are confined to

35 Yamada Keiji, *The Origins of Acupuncture, Moxibustion and Decoction*, 66–78. Yamada compares the stages in one *Wushier bingfang* prescription for hernia which involve minor surgery, the applications of paste and alcohol and fumigation, to the stages in a ritual ceremony described in *Li Ji*. The fumigation, he believes, was intended to drive away the god of sickness and prevent it from entering the wound. Here we have a repetition of that theme where openings in the body, here a wound but elsewhere the orifices, are both vulnerable to malevolent activity as well as pivotal in methods to support and protect the body.

36 Harper, *Early Chinese Medical Literature*, 244 and Yamada 1985a: 58–63.

37 Christopher Cullen, 'Patients and Healers in Late Imperial China: Evidence from the *Jinpingmei*' in *History of Science* 31, 1993.

that information that the author selects as useful to the narrative and are subject to fictional stereotypes. But it is arguable that the images of every day life gathered from novels are no more distorted than physicians' own accounts of their work.

Despite their commitment to the social history of acupuncture *Celestial Lancets* shows little enthusiasm for reading classical and canonical medical sources as a key to the many dimensions of more popular or religious practice. A number of studies have attempted to examine both received and excavated literature for evidence of the dynamic between different technicians, religious healers, professional physicians and home care self-help medicine. With a deeper foundation in the nature of the early Chinese social groups involved in health care we will also be able to reinterpret many of the concepts in the canonical acupuncture literature. In *Medicine in China a History of Ideas* Unschuld first attempts to redress the balance with a lively treatment of the provenance of demonological and religious healing at different times in Chinese society, a trend which continues to be fulfilled in recent histories such as Ma Boying's *Zhongguo yixue wenhuashi* 中國醫學文化史.[38] Unschuld was also the first to introduce to many European and American practitioners of Chinese medicine the evolution of medical ideas in their relationship to the changing sociopolitical scene.

Medical manuscripts excavated from Warring States and Western Han tombs suggest a range of magical, religious and divinatory practices many of which assume the involvement in illness of various forms of spirits, ancestors or divinities. Harper's chapter 'Magic' in *Early Chinese Medical Literature* gives a good introduction to this type of medicine. Many aspects of magico-religious medicine shaped physiological concepts retained in canonical Chinese medicine.[39] Notions of attack and invasion by malign entities, for example, ultimately became abstracted into forms of *xie qi* 邪氣 'evil or perverse *qi*'. Wind, for example, originally personified as a demon, came to be viewed as part of a more naturalistic model where the body was subject to attack from the elements, including heat, cold or damp.[40]

Lu and Needham described how the upper middle and lower parts of the human body accord to the cosmological triad of heaven, earth and man. New primary sources from the formative period of classical Chinese medicine, have shown that 'numbers' techniques, including those employing divination methods, were as important in the formation of classical Chinese medicine as they were in post Tang times. Until recently these sources have remained relatively unexplored, in part due to post 1949 Chinese tendencies, perhaps shared with Lu and Needham, to avoid material that might portray Chinese medicine as 'superstitious.' Recent research into technical literature, untrammelled by such sensibility, has begun to build a deeper view of those aspects of intellectual history that pervade all layers of early Chinese

38 Ma Boying 馬伯英 ed., *Zhongguo yixue wenhua shi* (Shanghai: Shanghai Renmin, 1994), 138-174. See also Ngo Van Xuyet, *Divination Magie et Politique* (Paris: Presses Universitaires de France, 1976). DeWoskin, Kenneth J. *Doctors, Diviners and Magicians of Ancient China: Biographies of Fang-shih* (New York: Columbia University Press, 1981).

39 Harper, *Early Chinese Medical Literature*, 148–183.

40 See the chapter 'Wind and Self' in Shigehisa Kuriyama's *The Expressiveness of the Body: and the Divergence of Greek and Chinese Medicine*, (New York: Zone Books, 1999), 233–270.

society.[41] The application of certain astrological and calendrical calculations to a wide variety of practices gives us a better idea of how medicine, and in this case acupuncture, integrated into more pervasive systems of knowledge. An in depth study of numerological techniques as they emerge in the mediaeval period is in process under Marc Kalinowski at the École des Hautes Études in Paris and includes Donald Harper and Liu Lexian, who have both published on 'numbers techniques' in early and mediaeval Chinese medicine.

A relatively new area of research in Chinese medical history is in the genre of case histories.[42] *Celestial Lancets* describes Sima Qian's account of the physician Chunyu Yi. Yi was arraigned on an unknown charge and called to account for his education, professional competence and therapeutic successes. In his defence he listed his teachers and methods of learning, his medical skills and the books he owned. He then cited more than twenty-five case histories from his, mostly well-to-do, clientele, wherein we learn a great deal of the social history of medicine as well as its theory and practice in second century B.C. China.[43]

Rapid expansion of the printing industry, of commerce and merchant culture during the Ming period (1368–1644) brought a popularisation of medical knowledge. Direct contact between master physician and disciple became less important as essential texts were distributed more widely than before. New publishing initiatives included reprints of classical works and medical prescriptions written in verse form as an aid to memory. Collections of case histories also became increasingly popular. In families of hereditary physicians, the later generations would publish the writings of their forefathers, no doubt to recount successful treatments, prove theoretical points, demonstrate new techniques and thereby advertise the lineage in general. Case history collections give us some impression of how medical theory was put into practice. They inevitably take us a little closer to the process of interpretation and synthesis in practice undertaken by individual and lineages of medical physicians.

New trends in the history of the body

New trends in the field of medical anthropology, which take an interest in the body as both subject and object of cultural diversity have much to offer historians of medicine.[44] Certainly, we can now accept the wisdom of cultural specificity in histories of the body, of seeing the body as a passive object upon which each culture,

41 See for example Marc Kalinowski, 'The Xingde Texts from Mawangdui' in Early China 23–24 (1988–99) 125–202. See also Donald Harper. "Iatromancy, Prognosis, and Diagnosis, in Early Chinese Medicine", in *Innovation in Chinese Medicine*.

42 Christopher Cullen, 'Yi'an 醫案: the origins of a genre of Chinese medical literature' in *Innovation in Chinese Medicine*. (Cambridge: CUP, 297–323).

43 Bridgman, Robert F. "'La médicine dans la Chine antique d'apr"es les biographies de Pien-ts'io et de Chouen-yu Yi', *Melanges chinois et bouddhiques* 10, (1955), 1–213.

44 A collection of essays in *Embodiment and Experience* represent this approach in the field of medical anthropology. They describe a move away from a position which understands the body as "the biological raw material upon which culture operates" and generally acknowledge that our bodies play an active role in the process through which we perceive things. Each of the essays

indeed each individual, constructs different religious, social and political realities. At the same time we can take a body centred perspective and move towards an understanding how the body itself participates in culture.[45]

Lu and Needham began to explore the metaphorical body of early Chinese medicine. They quoted early treatises which show how Chinese perceptions of the body mirrored its philosophical, political and religious realities, replicating every aspect of the natural and human worlds in anatomical and physiological form. At its most extreme the body contained the entire universe: the sun and moon, stars and constellations, mountain ranges, waterways, animals and plants all find emblematic representation. Patterns of human organisation, administrative and architecture plans were also reflected in the structures and relationships of the body. In their quotation from the *Yantie lun* 鹽鐵論 (*Treatise of Salt and Iron*) of 81 B.C. we can see how the removal of obstacles and blockages with acupuncture was mixed with metaphors for the state distribution of resources.

Recent research offers a move away from writing histories of the body based on its representations towards exploring the way in which those representations were constructed. We can approach the construction of early Chinese medical bodies in many ways. In *Sisheng zhi yu* 死生之域 (*The Territory between Life and Death*), Li Jianmin highlights a plurality of factors that come to bear in the development of the concept of *mai* 脈 'channels' of acupuncture. The *mai*, he finds are "a field of temporal spaces" that act as a pivot of many different worlds. They are at once analogous to the rivers of China, to astronomical movements, to rivers of blood and channels of communication, a pattern upon which human disharmony with the environments could be judged. He finds geographical variation in the interpretation of the mai as well as three different states in the development which correspond to the movement of heavenly bodies, self-cultivation and the development of the neurological body.[46]

Shigehisa Kuriyama contrasts the different sensual modalities through which Chinese and European perceptions of the body formed. Ways of knowing the body are conditioned by forms of language and communication unique to individual cultures. On the one hand he argues that a "interest in the muscularity of the body was inseparable from a preoccupation with the agency of the self". He sees the potential for voluntary, and therefore individual, action (as distinct from the autonomic physiology of digestion), epitomised in the unnaturally defined musculo-skeletal patterns common to classical European art and sculpture. The training of the eye to pick out these patterns was then reinforced by anatomical advances that made visible the full structure of the muscles.[47]

takes a very different position. As Csordas drily notes that "if there is an essential characteristic of embodiment, it is indeterminacy". Csordas, Thomas. *Embodiment and Experience* (Cambridge: Cambridge University Press, 1994), 1–12.

45 Michel Feher summarises this perspective on histories of the body in his introduction to a collection of essays by historians and anthropologists. See *Fragments for a History of the Human Body*, Feher et al., (New York: Zone, 1989) part 1, 11–17.

46 Li Jianmin, *Sisheng zhi yu*.

47 Shigehisa Kuriyama, *The Expressiveness of the Body: and the Divergence of Greek and Chinese Medicine*.

To emphasise the contrast with Chinese ways of knowing the body Kuriyama describes how they privileged different styles of seeing. He argues that complexion diagnosis, the art of seeing disharmony in the aura of the face was rooted in botanical metaphors long established in the language and culture of early China. The complexion, like the blossom of a flower, was the visible expression of the strength or weakness of the underlying organism. Similarly Kuriyama distinguishes differences between haptic knowledge in the different traditions. Contrasting palpation of the *mai* and the knowledge of the pulse that begun in the Greek medical tradition, he emphasises how the most immediate experience of the body is constantly subject to a relationship with theoretical preconceptions distinctive to a particular culture.

At the intersection between where political, sociological and technological change impacts upon the body and where the body, as subject, begins to assert its own phenomenologically perceived realities another field of research opens out. To what extent can we see the agency of the body itself operating within the text? Adding to Li Jianmin's analysis of the channels as a reflection of the known universe in Han times, an examination of the role that recording pain played in laying out their exact pathways and layout has shed light on how medical theorists observed the body. Equally the provenance of many canonical medical ideas can be found in the expressiveness and animation of the body in early self-cultivation literature as distinct from the 'objectified' body of professional medical literature. The pervasive influence of self-cultivation in early Chinese medicine permanently shaped holistic elements in Chinese medical discourse.[48]

The next generation of researchers into the history of Chinese medicine inevitably face the challenge of participating in the reform of research methodology in their field. It is an exciting time. But they can rest assured that they will not be asked to take on the vast archive of transmitted Chinese medical texts single handed. Lu and Needham set out to write a diachronic history of those elements of acupuncture and moxibustion theory and practice that seemed, retrospectively, to define the art. They began with the development of the channels, the acupoints, the idea of circulating *qi*, with technological developments, texts and teaching aids. In doing so they sowed the seeds for many of the trends in contemporary research. They not only sketched a diachronic history of these elements, but touched upon social history, boundaries with other technologies and ideas about the construction of the body in early China. In the intervening twenty years the revolution in research methodology has been driven largely by the excavation of early Chinese medical objects and texts which tell a different story. The task of writing a diachronic history has become too enormous for lesser scholars than Lu and Needham to contemplate, when there are more pressing imperatives concerned with the explication of the texts and artifacts with reference to the cultures of their own time. On the one hand this current and on-going paradigm shift reflects wider intellectual trends emerging in the field of anthropology that favour a finer focus on regional and temporal variation in the characteristics of culture. At the

48 Vivienne Lo, 'The influence of *yangsheng* culture on early Chinese medical theory', 240–267 and 'Tracking the Pain', *Suddoffs Archiv* 83 (1999), 191–211.

same time it is unlikely that there will be a return to the particular marriage of history and science embodied by Lu and Needham, and at the heart of *Celestial Lancets.* Their explicit research agenda set out in the subtitle 'A History and Rationale of Acupuncture & Moxa' is a subject deserving of more detailed attention given in the next section.

Rationale

The juxtapositioning of history and rationale in *Celestial Lancets* had the effect of structuring information in a unique manner. One recent book, Filshie and White's *Medical Acupuncture – A Scientific Approach*, an edited volume, takes a similar approach, but the very superficial historical treatment is relegated to one article that attempts to reinterpret traditional concepts according to their 'scientific' (empirical) value.[49] In the grand sweep of their own project, an insistence on the unitary nature of scientific knowledge led Lu and Needham to justifications of acupuncture and moxibustion which "consider the whole acupuncture complex in terms of modern scientific knowledge", built on the assumption "that the scientific rationale of acupuncture will in due course be established". Thus we are given the overall impetus behind the structure of the book.

Diversions from the diachronic narrative, for example, are often taken to demonstrate how Chinese knowledge might match the Western equivalents in anticipating scientific truths as they are understood in biomedicine today. Seventeen pages are thus devoted to understanding the Chinese concept of 'circulation' of blood and *qi* and in particular a magnification of those elements that accord with a modern understanding. To emphasise comparative sophistication on the part of the Chinese, there is a long discussion about William Harvey's own inaccuracies in measurement and his appeals to contemporary astrological thought. One recurring theme charts the causes of decline in acupuncture and moxibustion. Lu and Needham, followed by François Beyens in *Medical Acupuncture – A Scientific Approach*, repeatedly posit a golden age of 'empirical' medical activity at the foundation of classical theory, a scientific spirit that was ultimately stifled after the Tang period when "abstraction trampled over empiricism" in the hands of those more learned in astrological calculation than practical medicine.[50] The best that they can say about these systematisers is that, as a result of their obsession with cycles, they recognised the importance of diurnal and circadian rhythms in the body and therefore anticipated modern knowledge of a 'biological clock' where health and illness was governed by subtle rhythms. As a corollary of this view, for Lu and Needham Chinese medical philosophy simply provided a "trellis work to long clinical experience". As apologists for an apparently anti-rational system they reasoned that its "correlative linkages probably originate in the attempts of the ancient physicians to systematise their vast fund of clinical

49 Jacqueline Filshie and Adrian White ed., *Medical Acupuncture* (Edinburgh, London etc.: Churchill Livingstone, 1998).

50 F Beyens, 'Reinterpretation of traditional concepts in acupuncture' in Filshie and White ed., *Medical Acupuncture*, 391–408.

observations". But their treatment of the subject, indeed their very title, *Celestial Lancets*, gives as yet unparalleled space to the astrological foundations of early Chinese medicine. In retrospect their treatment of the subject is strangely prophetic.

Ironically, one of the biggest growth areas in research into the history of acupuncture and moxibustion is exactly those arbitrary correlative linkages of astrological calculation. Where Lu and Needham refer to a "characteristic noise or redundance" which always accompanies the growth of systematic classifications in all cultures, modern historians may concentrate their attention on the elements of medical practice that did not succeed in becoming become part of a canonised tradition. Engagement with this kind of detail will reveal the power of understanding medicine as a key to knowledge in broader intellectual and social traditions. Ideas about the body are surely the most essential reflection of contemporary sociopolitical prejudices, assumptions and conflicts. And for history's sake, and without denying many stunning elements of medical progress, we must be wary of privileging what Porter calls the 'winners' story', the canonical account, whether of Eastern or Western medical traditions.[51] Investment in transcribing, translating and describing the sources as we find them is critical to understanding the human condition past and present.

Broadly speaking, the project to find a scientific rationale for acupuncture can be divided into two fields. Firstly there are the attempts to define a physiological process through which acupuncture stimulation and effect are mediated in biomedical terms and secondly there is a ever increasing literature concerned with evaluating the efficacy of acupuncture. Lu and Needham generally defend the classical tradition of the system of tracts and channels, while regarding it as a useful construct without material substrate. They refer to various attempts at establishing an equivalent substratum that matches them to corpuscles and thin ducts, intra and extra vascular conduits and set out early research claiming evidence of a relationship to nerve endings as well as electrical methods for testing skin resistance as a method of confirming point and channel locations.

Sadly, given the wide range of applications for acupuncture and moxibustion, research into the way the effect of the acumoxa traditions is mediated has been predominantly confined to the short term treatment of pain by needle insertion. For most involved in the general practice of acupuncture the field of research remains so narrow that it has little bearing on their own perception of personal clinical efficacy. Acupuncturists claiming to work with traditional models tend to treat a wide range of symptoms and expect a long term effect.

Research that focuses on establishing a structure that matches the channels and acupoints as they are classically represented has now virtually been abandoned. More recent attempts are discussed in an article by Bensoussan.[52] The favoured approach in mainstream biomedical research remains that of studying elements of the

51 Roy Porter, *The Greatest Benefit to Mankind: A Medical History of Humanity from Antiquity to the Present* (London: Fontana Press, 1999), 12.

52 A Bensoussan 'Part: 1 Acupuncture meridians – myth or reality? *Complementary Therapies in Medicine* 2(1), 21–6 and 'Part 2: Acupuncture meridians – myth or reality?' in *Complementary Therapies in Medicine* 2(2), 80–85.

segmental and non-segmental effects of acupuncture in their relationship to the structures involved in the central and autonomic nervous conduction – in other words the differentiation of local and distal effect according to whether the response is mediated through local or central nervous systems.[53]

In the latter enterprise *Celestial Lancets* was one of the first places to review the Xi'an research on dermatomes, a structure thought to explain the phenomenon of referred pain and the complex relationship of visceral pathology and pain on the surface of the body. The first and enduring proposition was that the channels in some way correspond to cutaneous areas supplied by the different sections of the spinal cord. Associated research centred on trigger point acupuncture where dry needling or injections of anaesthetic are injected into sites of small circumscribed tender points in muscles in order to resolve referred muscular pain.[54]

Neurophysiological mediation of the non-segmental effect of acupuncture has centred on "gating theories" where it has been posited that the pre-emptive stimulation of non-pain receptors inhibits neural exchange, preventing pain making its way up to the cerebral cortex. Where distal pain relief has been established through a pain suppressing system activated by needle stimulation at sites, regardless of whether they are acupuncture points or not, this is currently labelled DNIC (diffuse noxious inhibitory controls).[55] DNIC is a non specific neurophysiological mechanism described by Le Bars whereby any noxious stimulant triggers a natural opioid system in both humans and animals.[56] Decreased DNIC is consistent with decreased firing rates in the convergent interneurons in the affected segments of the spinal cord – compared with increases elsewhere.

Lu and Needham reported on the body's own ability to produce chemicals which combat stress and reduce inflammatory responses. Particularly attractive to them were the measurable effects of acupuncture as it stimulated the naturally occurring morphine analogues, corticosteroids and antibodies as a correlate of reported pain. Acupuncture and moxibustion, it seems, may trigger events in the hypothalmus, stimulating both pituitary and suprarenal cortex. That acupuncture operates largely through an endorphin-related mechanism is supported in the context of acute pain within an animal model demonstrates conclusively that acupuncture's effects are sometimes related to the release of a variety of natural opioids and that this opioid-based effect is naloxone reversible. Pain relief by trigger point injection with bupicane is also reversed by naloxone.[57] Equally impressive was the

53 See the chapters by AJR Macdonald, R Bekkering and R van Bussel in Section 3 'Theory and basic science', *Medical Acupuncture*, 67–150.

54 See P Baldry, 'Trigger point acupuncture' in *Medical Acupuncture*, 33–61.

55 S Marchand and J Li, 'The effect of electro-acupuncture on perceived heat pain at different body locations' in Proceedings of the 7th World Conference on Pain, 427.

56 D Le Bars, AH Dickenson and JM Besson, "Diffuse noxious inhibitory controls (DNIC). I Effects on dorsal horn convergent neurones in the rat; II – Lack of effect on non-convergent neurones, supraspinal involvement and theoretical implications' in *Pain* 6, 283–327.

57 VL Clement-Jones, S Tomlin, LH Rees, L McLouglin, GM Besser and Hl Wen, 'Increased beta-endorphin but not met-enkephalin levels in human cerebrospinal fluid after acupuncture for current pain' in *Lancet* ii, 946–8. Cheng and Pomeranz first demonstrated that low-frequency (not high frequency) electroacupuncture could produce analgesic effects in mice and

generation of antibodies through the reticulo enothelial system, which was likened to the stress mechanism insomuch that it created a stage of increased resistance and reduced inflammatory response. Thus there were reports of a four-fold increase in typhoid and para-typhoid antibodies after acupuncture, increasing with electro-acupuncture.

During the '70's any European/American observer interested in acupuncture and moxibustion could not fail to be impressed with the reportage of acupuncture analgesia during major surgery. What could be more incontestable than the images of fully conscious, conversing patient in mid-operation? Subsequent research has shown that although electro-acupuncture has a definite analgesic effect, the results are less universally applicable than originally hoped. The optimum indications for applying the technique as part of a health-care programme have yet to be established and are not simply attributable to a greater tolerance of pain in the Chinese race or a greater susceptibility to hypnotism.[58] Thirty years on, acupuncture analgesia barely survives in Chinese hospitals. Recent studies have equated the promotion of acupuncture analgesia with the Chinese nationalist desire to demonstrate the superiority of tradition in the face of Western scientific scrutiny.[59] Nevertheless, acupuncture treatment of musculo-skeletal pain and headache remains a significant area of research with encouraging research results emerging in the treatment of lower back pain, nausea and equivocal results for migraine.[60]

One-third of *Celestial Lancets* is devoted to the explanation and evaluation of the clinical effect of acupuncture in biomedical terms. In the '70's this was an ambitious task and it remains so. To put the enterprise into perspective we should consider that rigorous controlled trials of biomedical interventions are not necessarily standard. The work of Professor David Eddy suggests that only 15% of biomedical interventions are supported by solid scientific evidence and only 1% of articles in medical journals, despite their bias, stand up to scrutiny – many treatments have never been assessed at all.[61] A double-blind controlled trial for by-pass surgery proved the surgery ineffective, yet it remains a popular form of treatment for arteriosclerosis. The weakness and inconsistency of scientific evidence for many clinical interventions made by GPs fosters diversity and individuality in practice. To reduce choice to treatments of 'proven' effect would be inconsistent with mainstream biomedical practice and of dubious ethical standing in any health care system.

In the absence of adequately monitored clinically controlled experiments, attempts to evaluate acupuncture, or to establish a biomedical/physiological explanation for its

that this was naloxone reversible. RSS Cheng and B Pomeranz, Electroacupuncture analgesia could be mediated by at least two pain-relieving mechanisms:endorphin and non-endorphin systems. *Life Sciences* 25, 1957–1962.

58 Adrian White, 'Electroacupuncture and acupuncture analgesia' in *Medical Acupuncture*, 153–173. VJ Knox, K Shum and DM Mclaughlin, 'Response to cold pressor pain and to acupuncture analgesia in Oriental and Occidental subjects' in *Pain* 4(1): 49–57.

59 Elisabeth Hsu, 'Innovations in acumoxa: acupuncture analgesia, scalp and ear acupuncture in the people's republic of China' in *Social Science and Medicine* vol. 42, 421–430.

60 Section 5 'Clinical usage and evidence' in *Medical Acupuncture* 203–389.

61 Summarised in R Smith, 'Where is the wisdom ...?' in *British Medical Journal* 303 (6806), 155–6.

efficacy are largely anecdotal. In 1980 the studies that Lu and Needham reported seemed to confirm the positive effect of acupuncture in the treatment of sub-acute appendicitis, as well as conditions customarily associated with acupuncture, such as asthma, herpes, erythema nodosum, colitis and chronic skin disease. Improvement noted in other conditions included ulcerating varicose veins, lumbago, Paget's disease, Parkinson's disease, infantile convulsions and diarrhoea. One of the few studies showing incontestably positive results has begun to corroborate the relationship of one acupoint to its well known effect of reducing nausea.[62] But there are no hypotheses about the mechanisms involved in acupuncture for the digestive system not to speak of any other internal diseases.

By 2000 current attempts at evaluation have made faltering progress in framing the issues of efficacy. Problems encountered can be classified as belonging to a number of categories including the theoretical issues of control, the single or double-blind trial, ethical problems experienced by acupuncturists in providing placebo acupuncture, standardisation of treatment by individual or by the tradition(s) of acupuncture. Distortion of information by the bias of researcher/patient is a common occurrence. It is also not possible to remove the results of any one trial from the context of its funding. The need to write research proposals to suit the board who ratify them will inevitably reflect in the way the hypothesis is framed, which in turn will influence researcher bias and the patients expectation.

Much progress has been made by psychologists in explaining the complex phenomena known as placebo. Many variables have been tested in attempts to characterise the typical placebo responders, but neither sociodemographic characteristics or intelligence and psychological profiling has yielded conclusive evidence. While Lu and Needham were wont to dismiss the placebo effect in the same terms as 'susceptibility to hypnosis', a number of different elements now add new dimensions to that analysis. Patient gratitude to the therapist, coupled with an eagerness to respond to the therapist's expectation is thought to have significant effect. Where the practitioner demonstrates greater interest or confidence in the therapy, is of a higher status or uses higher technology intervention the therapy gives a demonstrably better effect. The more radical the procedure, the greater the effect. Adherence to treatment procedure has been shown to be a significant indicator of effect. Remarkably, in one study, risk of death from myocardial infarction was greater in patients who took less than 75% of their prescribed medication whether the medication was a beta blocker or a placebo.[63]

The importance of understanding a specific client or practitioner group is critical to the success of evaluation. There is apparently no evidence of an identifiable group equivalent to those that might be 'susceptible to hypnosis'. On the contrary, a survey of people in Britain shows that those who chose to visit complementary therapists tend to be 67% female of I and II social class, and demonstrated better biological

62 J W Dundee and C McMillan, 'Positive evidence for P6 acupuncture antiemesis' in *Postgraduate Medical journal* 67, 417–422.

63 Charles Vincent and Adrian Furnham, *Complementary Medicine: a Research Perspective*, (Chichester: Wiley, 1997), 133–145.

knowledge and a relatively greater consciousness of health and environmental, dietary issues.[64] Acupuncture patients in one survey demonstrated relatively higher degrees of practitioner loyalty and placed more importance on a healthy state of mind. Perhaps as a corollary to these findings acupuncture dealt with more psychologically based patients than did equivalent local GP practitioners – and this is an area of significant growth in current research into efficacy.[65]

On the question of controlled trials we can develop our analysis from two directions. Firstly if it is valid to try to define the elements of acupuncture therapy that link to a desired therapeutic outcome, then it is theoretically possible to design trials that isolate and evaluate those elements. Secondly we must consider whether that assumption is valid, either in theory or practice.

Those involved in designing acupuncture trials still debate whether single or double blind trials are appropriate. Recently it has also been deemed necessary to establish a no treatment control, such as a wait list group to eliminate spontaneous symptom fluctuation and remission. In *Complementary Medicine, A Research Perspective*, Furnham and Vincent point out that double blind trials are not appropriate to any skilled intervention. They cite surgery as a parallel; at some point during the clinical encounter the practitioner , if they are a skilled professional, will become aware that they are giving a sham treatment. If they do not, then their skill must be called into question as well as their ability to participate properly in the trial i.e. either it is not truly blind or the practitioner is insufficiently trained to create the conditions necessary to simulate the treatment. Such conditions are bound to result in inadequate information.[66]

Methods of control used to theoretically isolate the elements of 'true' acupuncture, all discussed in *Celestial Lancets*, continue to include mock TENS, a form of transcutaneous nerve stimulation administered without the usual electrical current. Minimal acupuncture, where the patient is needled very superficially at sites where no classical acupoints exist, is a favoured option. The latter seems to mimic the conditions of acupuncture most effectively while isolating the specific choice of needling and acupuncture points for the real treatment. However superficial needling only gives information about effective sites of needling and does not exclude the important and pervasive *ah shi* 呵是 "ah that's the place" techniques when a needle is inserted into the locus of pain. Nor does it account for Japanese styles of acupuncture which require minimal stimulation and sometimes no insertion at all.

Undoubtedly there is value in continuing the search for repeatable acupuncture prescriptions, regardless of context. More standardised acupuncture treatments will be

64 SJ Fulder and RE Munro, 'Complementary Medicine in the United Kingdom; patients, practitioners, and consultations' in *Lancet* 2 (84554), 542–5 and KJ Thomas, J Carr, L Westlake and BT Williams, 'Use of non-orthodox and conventional health care in Great Britain' in *British Medical Journal* 302 (6770), 207–10.

65 A Furnham, C Vincent and R Wood, 'The health beliefs and behaviours of three groups of complementary medicine and a general practice group of patients' in *Journal of Alternative and Complementary Medicine* 1, 347–59.

66 Charles Vincent and Adrian Furnham, *Complementary Medicine: a Research Perspective*, 164–166.

linked with specific effects and consequently made amenable to hospital practice. The treatment of addiction with ear acupuncture is one relatively modern innovation where large numbers of patients are treated regularly by a relatively unskilled nursing staff. Machines will inevitably substitute for some of these treatments. Evidence linking acupuncture treatment on the anterior forearm (*xinbao* 心包 6) with the symptomatic relief of nausea has spawned a range of arm bands that assist in travel sickness. But an accreditation of only those elements of acupuncture and moxibustion that are consistent with realities defined under the conditions and confinements of biomedical trial will certainly do permanent damage to the conduct of the profession.

To my mind the most intractable problem is in isolating the elements of therapy that link to a desired therapeutic outcome. Few seem to acknowledge the levels of diversity in practice – an artifice created on the one hand by a desire in the profession to represent a normative view of acupuncture and moxibustion, one amenable to standardised teaching and assessment – and on the other by the necessity to render the technique reproducible within controlled situations. Both, by necessity, impoverish 'the arts' of acupuncture and moxibustion. To my knowledge no studies directly compare different styles of individual complementary therapies, let alone the many different forms of acupuncture that exist internationally – and even within the confines of one clinic. There are a multitude of individual styles of practice as well as individual issues of competence, all of which introduce an untenable amount of variables and undermine any trial of 'acupuncture and moxibustion' as a unitary phenomenon.

One study of depression undertaken in an Arizona hospital does at least attempt a proper definition of its form of acupuncture. The model introduces the idea of limited flexibility in treatment through the identification of a number of syndromes commonly identified in 'Standardised Chinese Medicine' as most common in depression. They then randomly allocate patients to a group receiving specific treatment for their depression or, alternatively, another valid treatment directed towards another perceived pattern of disharmony in their health. This protocol, which allows for differential diagnosis within a limited, and well defined choice of treatment options, represents one step towards clarifying conditions of trial by describing the therapy that is being tested.[67]

Any holistic approach to therapy will describe the desired therapeutic effect on any individual symptom in its relation to the whole complex of a person's health. The essential defining elements of the therapy in a modern context, as much as in early imperial times, will not only include technical details of how and where to manipulate the needle, but also the mode of delivery, conditions of the room, state and intention of the practitioner etc. Consider for example the desired therapeutic conditions specified in *Huangdi neijing lingshu*. The Han dynasty practitioner is instructed to prepare the room and wait for the right moment:

67 Rosa Schnyer, *Bridging the Gap: Acupuncture in the Treatment of Depression. A Manual for Research and Clinical Practice*, (forthcoming).

> He (the practitioner) stays in an isolated and quiet place, firmly holding the coming and going of the spirit; he closes the doors and shut the lattices and the *hun* 魂 and the *po* 魄 'souls' do not scatter; he concentrates the intention and unifies the spirit and refines the division of *qi*; he does not hear human voices in order to gather their (the patient's) essence and unify their spirit; he commands the intent into the needle.[68]

In order that he should not damage the patient he must cultivate his attention

> . . . as if peering over a deep abyss and not daring to sink down; the hand, as if holding a tiger, desires its sturdiness; the spirit, without managing a crowd of other things, quietly and with intent observes the patient without looking to left or right; as for being righteous, without being deflected downwards, he must have principle through being upright; as for having to make the spirit upright, he must regard the patient's eye to govern their spirit, in order that the *qi* moves easily.[69]

The modern delivery of traditional Chinese medicine does not necessarily mimic these conditions, especially in the pressurised conditions of the PRC health-care system. But each culture will define the context of the therapeutic encounter differently. The culture of complementary medicine in Britain, for example may demand equivalent attention to issues of hygiene, design, quality and amount of attention, the simultaneous education in alternative forms of health-care, dietary and exercise advice, instruction in new perspectives on health and sickness as well as the personal bearing of the practitioner. All these factors may combine to create a new culture of health care that is an integral part of the delivery of that therapy.

Many will argue that anything other than the needle, the informed choice of points, and the techniques of stimulation, are incidental features of the therapeutic encounter, and that the effect of the incidental elements must needs be psychologically mediated. But the notion of psychological mediation is also culture specific. Outside of the field of psychology where do we set the boundaries of the mind in the realms of 'human interaction'? Can we not consider and evaluate the success of different forms of traditional medical practice on their own terms, whether those terms are framed with reference to historical experience or through a closer comparison of the intention of the practitioner with a patient centred examination of treatment satisfaction. Should we not marvel at the epistemological leaps performed by most modern practitioners of traditional medicine as they mediate classical wisdom, clinical experience and biomedical knowledge in their daily practice? Here we slip into the realms of medical anthropology and developments that I expect to shape the future of the evaluation of traditional medicines in the modern context.

68 *Lingshu juan* 2, *pian* 9. *Sibu beiyao* vol. 205, fasc. 1, 12a.
69 *Suwen juan* 14, *pian* 54. *Sibu beiyao* vol. 204, fasc. 3, 7.

What future is there for the history of Chinese medicine? There is a growing demand for new research arising in the colleges of traditional Chinese medicine, at academic centres for the history of medicine, Chinese studies, departments of medical anthropology as well as, to a certain extent, from those still involved in the justification of acupuncture from a biomedical point of view. Despite a certain flow of information between these different disciplines, each emphasises topics that are of immediate concern within its own field. Thus where Harper's *Early Chinese Medical Literature: The Mawangdui Medical Manuscripts* covers medicine and society in the late Warring States and Han period, and is written to the high standards of a sinological audience, histories addressing scientists or the Chinese medical profession in Europe and America are often written by those with little or no sinological training. They do, however, reveal different priorities, often driven by current disputes between the growing number of different acupuncture and moxibustion traditions available outside of Asia. Birch's *Understanding Acupuncture*, one of the best introductory works for contemporary patients and practitioners, begins with a diachronic history that summarises English-language histories available to him, and describes the acculturation and re-acculturation of acupuncture throughout Asia and in Europe. He then proceeds to highlight the danger of the hegemony of a single teaching tradition, often based on misconceptions arising from faulty translation.[70]

Better quality translations of a small number of the thousands of transmitted Chinese medical texts, and of the newly excavated texts, are slowly emerging. Textbooks such as Deadman and Al-Khafaji's Manual of Acupuncture are beginning to provide information about sources and give references for the facts they transmit.[71] But these are just chipping at the tip of the iceberg. Together with in-depth studies of critical times when the theory and practice of Chinese medicine was in transition the new scholarship will gradually seep into the quality of history available to students of Chinese medicine. It is clear that the success of any medicine owes as much to its cultural acceptance as to its perceived efficacy in biomedical terms. Increasing historical awareness is therefore a matter of critical importance to quality control and professional development in both the modern teaching and practice of traditional Chinese medicine. With increased investment in Chinese studies and history as a source of medical competence it will be interesting to see whether basic Chinese-language and medical history will become a requirement of those involved in teaching the profession.

Personally, I feel a deep sense of nostalgia for Lu and Needham's enterprise, whether we perceive that as founded on faith in a progression towards a Christian paradise, socialist utopia, or a universe of repeatable scientific truths. It gave us *Celestial Lancets*, still the most comprehensive introduction to the history of Chinese acupuncture and the starting point for successive generations of researchers. The modern research environment is no less a product of prevailing sociopolitical trends.

70 SJ Birch and R Felt, *Understanding Acupuncture* (Churchill Livingstone), Edinburgh, 1999.

71 Peter Deadman and Mazin Al-Khafaji with Kevin Baker, *A Manual of Acupuncture* (Hove: Journal of Chinese Medicine Publications, 1998).

Whatever the virtue in concentrating resources on localised realities there is a dark side to diversity and devolution, one that seems to stumble inexorably towards alienation and conflict. Nevertheless, the shift in the research agenda towards thickening our perception of medical cultures in their own time has undoubtedly ushered in an exciting new era in the field of history, and especially in the history of ideas about the body – which is, after all, the most fundamental reflection of our changing human condition.

ACUPUNCTURE AND MOXIBUSTION

(1) Introduction

Acupuncture and moxibustion (*chen chiu*[1]) are two of the most ancient and characteristic therapeutic techniques of Chinese medicine. The one may be defined broadly as the implantation of needles to different depths at a great variety of points on the surface of the human body, points gathered in connected arrays according to a highly systematised pattern with a complex and sophisticated, if still essentially medieval, physiological theory behind it; this technique was anciently called *chen shih*,[2] *pien shih*[3] or *chhan shih*[4].[a] The needles unquestionably stimulate deep-lying nerve-endings, hence their evocation of some far-reaching results; though the classical theory was based on conceptions, still of much interest, of a continuous circulation of *chhi*[5] and blood (*hsüeh*[6]) round the body.[b] The other technique consists in the burning of *Artemisia* (*ai*[7]) tinder (moxa), either in the form of incense-like cones (whether or not directly on the skin), or as cigar-shaped sticks held just above it, the points chosen for application being in general identical with those of the acupuncture system; this is called *ai jung chiu*[8][c] or *ai chiu*[9].[d] Depending on the degree of heat applied it may be either a mild thermal stimulus like a fomentation, or alternatively a powerful counter-irritant cautery. Very broadly speaking, the acupuncture technique was from ancient times onwards thought most valuable in acute diseases, while the moxa was considered more appropriate in chronic ones.[e]

It is interesting to take note of an ancient tradition that the main components of traditional Chinese medicine originated in different geographical parts of the homeland. At least two chapters of the *Nei Ching*[f] enlarge on the theme that varying

[a] Cf. *NCSW*, ch. 8, (p. 142).

[b] Contrary to a pneumatological emphasis often found in Western acupuncture literature, these two should never be thought of separately. Gk. *pneuma* is, by and large, the nearest equivalent to *chhi*. See on p. 16.

[c] Or, as *NCSW/PH*, ch. 12, (p. 72) says: 'cauterise with burning (tinder)', *chiu jo*[10] (ordinarily, *jui*).

[d] The second word in this phrase is sometimes written *chih*,[11] but incorrectly. *Chih* primarily means to broil, burn or toast in general, hence in medical texts it is more closely associated with the decoction of drug-plants, as in the book-title *Phao Chih Lun*[12] (cf. *SCC*, Sect. 44). *Phao*[13] of course also means a gunpowder weapon, especially a bomb thrown from a trebuchet (cf. Sect. 30), as well as to fry or roast, for which latter the form *phao*[14] is preferable however. Moreover, the *Phao* of such titles is sometimes written *phao*,[15] which has the more appropriate connotation of boiling and bubbling. There is another word for moxibustion, *chiao*,[16] but we have never encountered it in medical texts.

[e] Cf. Chhêng Tan-An (*1*), pp. 51–2.

[f] The *Huang Ti Nei Ching* (Yellow Emperor's Manual of Corporeal Medicine) is the oldest and most famous of the Chinese medical classics (cf. pp. 88, 101 below). We date the *Su Wên* part of it (Questions (and Answers) about Living Matter) in the −2nd century, and the *Ling Shu* (Vital Axis) in the −1st. At various times we have compared it with the Hippocratic Corpus, for it was, like that,

1 鍼灸 2 鍼石 3 砭石 4 鑱石 5 氣 6 血 7 艾
8 艾絨灸 9 艾灸 10 灸焫 11 炙 12 炮炙論 13 炮 14 炰
15 泡 16 爝

methods of treatment had been found appropriate for people living in the diverse conditions of the several provinces and the four quarters.[a] Different environments gave rise to different incidences of endemic disease, hence the invention of different therapeutic methods (*i fa fang i*[1]). Thus moxibustion (*chiu jo*[2]) came mainly from the North, materia medica and pharmacy (*tu yao*[3]) from the West, and gymnastics, remedial exercises and massage (*tao yin*,[4] *an chhiao*[5]) from the Centre. But acupuncture (*pien shih*[6]) originated in the East, where people suffered greatly from boils and carbuncles; while its elaborations (in the form of the nine needles, *chiu chen*[7])[b] came up from the South. As for apotropaics (exorcisms, magical spells, and sacrifices to the gods and ancestors, *chu yu*[8]), this, it was considered, had been fairly universal from the earliest times. In part, it may be, this ancient proto-historical presentation was following the system of symbolic correlations, five types of medical treatment being analogised with the fivefold classification and especially the five directions of space, but there may be rather more to it than that.[c] For we know that ancient Chinese society was built upon, or greatly influenced by, a number of 'local cultures', environing societies which brought various distinguishable traits into the eventual common Sinic stock.[d] In this case, acupuncture would have been associated with the south-eastern quasi-Indonesian aquatic element, while moxa would have come down to join it from the northern quasi-Tungusic nomadic element, and the pharmaceutical influence would have come from the western Szechuanese and quasi-Tibetan element. Further research will doubtless sift the plausibility of this interpretation.

In our main work the system of acupuncture, unique to Chinese medicine, has been mentioned from time to time, but not so far fully discussed. It is among the most ancient components of Chinese medical art, and constitutes perhaps its most complicated feature. It is a system of therapy—and the relief of pain—which has been in constant use throughout the Chinese culture-area for some two and a half thousand years; and the labours of a multitude of devoted men through the centuries have given it a highly developed doctrine and practice. Nevertheless its study presents great difficulties, partly because the books on acupuncture written in different dynasties have been elements in a long and gradual development, not always self-consistent and not free from loop-line elaborations now more or less abandoned; but even more because the physiology and pathology of the system are themselves so ancient that the clear-cut definitions and conceptions of modern science cannot be expected. As the centuries passed, different masters emphasised somewhat different aspects and

the first systematisation, not by a single hand, not too different in date, and embodying the clinica experience and theories of half a dozen previous centuries (Needham & Lu Gwei-Djen (8), repr. Needham (64), p. 270). When we first said this we did not know that Willem ten Rhijne, the first expositor of acupuncture to the Western world (cf. pp. 271 ff. below), had made essentially the same comparison in +1685; see Carrubba & Bowers tr. (1), p. 379.

[a] *NCSW*, ch. 4, (p. 69), *NCSW/PH*, ch. 12, (p. 71).
[b] See p. 103 below.
[c] On the fivefold correlations cf. *SCC*, Vol. 2, pp. 261 ff.
[d] Eberhard (1, 2, 3).

[1] 異法方宜 [2] 灸焫 [3] 毒藥 [4] 導引 [5] 按蹻 [6] 砭石
[7] 九鍼 [8] 祝由

procedures as a result of their own deep study and practical expertise (*hsin tê* [1]);[a] and they handed on their understanding as clearly as they could to their particular disciples or in the schools of medicine by means of personal instruction and demonstration. Some wrote down specific guidance in the form of mnemonic rhymes (*fu* [2] and *ko* [3]) which the student could learn by heart and recite.[b] Since the revolution of 1949, however, a new phase has appeared in that the instruction given in the schools of traditional Chinese medicine is now being systematically set forth in volumes of the *chiang i* [4] (or lecture-notes) type, and these are of great value to all who wish to occupy themselves with the subject.[c] Moreover, as is well known, China has developed a system in recent decades by which some physicians fully trained in modern-Western medicine continue their studies in colleges of traditional-Chinese medicine, while conversely others beginning with traditional medicine, including acupuncture, go on to qualify in modern medicine afterwards.

At the present time the traditional medical men in China are working side by side with the modern-Western-trained physicians in full cooperation. This is a very remarkable fact, which we ourselves have seen during four extended stays in China since the revolution. It has been brought about by the revaluation of all national traditions in the country's mid-century renaissance, the convictions of her political leaders, the social needs and conditions, especially rural, and the relative paucity of medical men trained in modern scientific medicine. The two types of physicians have joint consultations and joint clinical examinations, and there is the possibility for patients to choose whether they will have their treatment in the traditional way, including acupuncture, or the modern way; in other cases the physicians themselves decide which is best and proceed to apply it. There is, moreover, a steadily growing tendency to take all that is best from both traditions and combine them—elsewhere we shall discuss, for example, the treatment of fractures, where prolonged consideration has decided that in fact there were many valuable features in the traditional methods,[d] and what is now practised is a mixture of the two, the Chinese and the Western. Such fusion is destined, we believe, to occur more and more, giving rise to a medical science which will be truly modern and oecumenical, not qualifiedly modern-Western. And an example outstandingly relevant here is the successful application of acupuncture in recent years to induce analgesia in major surgery. This we shall discuss later on in its place (pp. 218 ff.), but it certainly constitutes a remarkable marriage between traditional-Chinese and modern-Western medicine.

Acupuncture then is a method of therapy (including sedation and analgesia), developed first during the Chou period (– 1st millennium), which involves the implanta-

[a] A brief but valuable summary of these different schools is given in Anon. (*98*).

[b] Many good examples will be found in *CCCY*, chs. 4A, B. The language is liable to be laconic and beautiful, though often archaic and unintelligible to the vulgar; but ten of them have been done into modern language and explained by Chhen Pi-Liu & Chêng Cho-Jen (*2*).

[c] A brief account of this type dealing with the history of Chinese medicine will be found in Anon. (*83*).

[d] Here the permissive use of very slightly flexible bamboo splints is contrasted with the invariable immobilisation of the limb in plaster. See the series of papers by Fang Hsien-Chih *et al.* (1).

[1] 心得 [2] 賦 [3] 歌 [4] 講義

tion of very thin needles (much thinner than the familiar hypodermic needles)[a] into the body in different places at precisely specified points according to a charted scheme based on ancient and medieval yet intelligible physiological ideas. Indeed the theory and the practice were, one finds, already well systematised in the –2nd century, though much development was to follow. We ourselves have many times seen the way in which the implantation of the needles is done, attending acupuncture and moxa clinics in several Chinese cities (and in Japan also); and one can say that the technique remains in universal use in China at the present day. It also permeated centuries ago all the neighbouring countries of the culture-area, and for three hundred years past has awakened interest, together with a certain amount of practice, throughout the Western world.[b] In what follows we shall describe first the *ching-lo*[1] circulation system and its classical theory, then delineating the historical growth and development of the specialist literature concerning it, and studying the effect which the technique had in other cultures. We shall go on to examine its role in Chinese medicine, and finally take up the possible physiological interpretations which look like giving it a rationale in terms of modern science.

That acupuncture is a system of cardinal importance in the history of Chinese medicine is not disputed by anyone, but its actual value in objective terms remained until recently, and to some extent still remains, the subject of great differences of opinion. It is possible to find in East Asia modern-trained physicians both Chinese and Occidental who are wholly sceptical about its value, but it is notable that in China they are very few, and that the vast majority of medical men there, both modern-trained and traditional, do believe in its capacity to cure, or at least to alleviate, many pathological conditions. Presumably no one will ever really know the effectiveness of acupuncture (or the other special Chinese treatments) until an adequate number of case-histories has been analysed according to the methods of modern medical statistics — but the accomplishment of this may well take half a century, so great are the difficulties of keeping medical records in a country of eight hundred million people, where the ratio of highly qualified physicians to the general population is relatively low, and the need for medical and surgical treatment of all kinds is so great and urgent. We cannot wait that long in our work, and are therefore obliged to embark upon our historiography with a mild preference in one direction or the other. What that is will be stated in a moment, but first there are two points to be made. On the matter of published statistics it would not be fair to say that the Chinese medical literature contains no quantitative figures, and we shall be quoting some of them from time to time. But secondly the whole subject has taken a rather dramatic turn during the past fifteen years on account of the remarkable successes which have been achieved in China by the application of acupuncture for analgesia in major surgery. Here there

[a] This is generally the case today, but as we shall see (p. 70 below), instruments of very varying material and different forms, often of course much less fine, were used in ancient times.

[b] We shall return later on to the question of transmission (p. 262). Korea, Vietnam and Japan received the inheritance rather fully, but it is a little puzzling that Arabic culture was so much more influenced by Chinese sphygmology than by acupuncture.

[1] 經絡

is no long and tortuous medical history to be followed up, no periods of remission or acute relapse, no chronic conditions with uncertain responses, no psycho-somatic guesswork. Either the patient feels intolerable pain from the surgical intervention, or he does not, and the effectiveness can be known within the hour, or even quicker. More than any other development, this acupuncture analgesia (or 'anaesthesia', as it is usually called, with undeniable but infelicitous logic)[a] has had the effect of obliging physicians and neuro-physiologists in other parts of the world to take Chinese medicine seriously, almost for the first time. In due course we shall describe it, and consider its possible explanations in terms of modern knowledge of the physiology of the nervous system.[b]

Now for our preference, it derives, one might say, from a kind of natural scepticism. But scepticism can work in more ways than one. What we find hard to believe is that a body of theory and practice such as acupuncture could have been the sheet-anchor of so many millions of sick people for so many centuries if it had not had some objective value; and it strains our credulity as physiologists and biochemists by training to believe that the effects were wholly subjective and psychological. One might almost think in terms of a calculus of credibility, pending that time which to us seems likely to be far ahead when all the mysteries of psycho-somatic causation will have been resolved.[c] It seems to us more difficult to suppose that a treatment practised among so great a number of human beings for so long a time had no basis in physiology and pathology, than that it has been of purely psychological value. Of course it is true that the practices of phlebotomy (blood-letting)[d] and urinoscopy in the West had exceedingly little physiological and pathological basis on which to sustain their extraordinary and long-enduring popularity, but none of these had anything like the subtlety of the acupuncture system. Possibly blood-letting had some value in hypertension and hyper-viscosity,[e] and extremely abnormal urines could tell their story, but neither contributed much to modern practice.[f]

A view commonly expressed (mostly by Westerners) is that acupuncture has acted primarily by suggestion, like many other things in what they often call 'fringe' medicine; and some do not hesitate to equate surgical acupuncture analgesia with

[a] See p. 221 below.

[b] It is fair to say that neuro-physiological interpretations were already adumbrated by Churchill (1, 2) as early as 1823.

[c] 'No testimony', wrote Hume, in a famous sentence, 'is sufficient to establish a miracle, unless the testimony be of such a kind, that its falsehood would be more miraculous, than the fact, which it endeavours to establish.'

[d] Contrary to certain impressions, this was never a part of classical traditional Chinese medicine. Only blood from the superficial capillaries was drawn in one variant of acupuncture procedure (*tzhu lo*[1]) now performed with a cluster of five or seven pins (*mei hua chen*[2]). We discuss the matter on p. 164 below.

[e] Cf. Taylor (1).

[f] On these see the books of Keele (1) and Brockbank (1). Keele rightly congratulates the ancient Chinese physicians on their freedom from 'magico-religious concepts of disease', though he calls their traditional medical philosophy 'metaphysical', as we should not; but he might have added that they were always free from that individual genethliacal astrology which played so painfully prominent a part in medieval European medicine, as he himself shows (cf. Mercier, 1). At the same time folk-medicine in China always contained a large element of exorcistic-magical apotropaics.

[1] 刺絡 [2] 梅花針

hypno-anaesthesia, in spite of many differences which we shall point out in due course.[a] To extend the term 'hypnosis' to cover a general belief entertained by hundreds of millions of rational people for two millennia, and hence by prospective surgical patients today, would surely be a gross misuse of a term. Of course we are far from wishing to deny the importance of a certain measure of suggestion and suggestibility, such as is known to be inevitable in all therapies which man has ever developed. But animal experiments, where the psychological factor is largely ruled out, support our view that physiological and physico-chemical things are happening in the nervous system under acupuncture, and animal experiments are increasingly being performed in laboratories investigating the technique—we shall mention several as occasion arises. And not only this, but acupuncture has been a constituent part of veterinary medicine in China at least since the great treatises of the Yuan period, and continues to this day in widespread use for animal diseases.[b] Theories of suggestion are here comparatively at a loss.

Our belief is, then, that the scientific rationale of acupuncture will in due course be established. Without anticipating what we shall have to say about the possibilities (pp. 213 ff. below) it is fair to hint that many are now lying open. Apart from the classical theories of the circulation of the *chhi* through the *ching-lo* system and its way-stations, shortly to be described, it is quite clear that in terms of neuro-physiology the needles stimulate various receptors at different depths which send their afferent impulses up the spinal cord and into the brain. Perhaps they trigger events in the hypothalamus which activate the pituitary gland and lead to an increase of cortisone production by the suprarenal cortex. Perhaps they stimulate the autonomic nervous system in such a way as to lead to an increased output of antibodies from the reticulo-endothelial system. Both these effects could be of great importance from the therapeutic point of view, and others also could easily be visualised. Perhaps in another situation they monopolise afferent input junctions in thalamus, medulla or cord, in such a way as to prevent all pain impulses getting through to the cortex regions of the brain, and so successfully inducing analgesia. But we must leave the working out of these suggestions until later; here it should only be added that there are many other neuro-physiological phenomena which deserve consideration in the context of acupuncture, e.g. the Head Zones of the skin in mammals which relate superficial regions to the viscera, and the multifarious effects of referred pain. So too some of the sensations experienced by patients undergoing acupuncture may have had no small effect on the formulations of the classical theory.

Still something more remains to be said about the theoretical setting of acupuncture —and indeed also other traditional Chinese methods, such as the medical gymnastics for example, which originated very early in that culture.[c] We have in mind the relative value placed in Chinese and Western medicine respectively on aid to the healing and protective power of the body, as against direct attacks on invading influences. A

[a] Pp. 238, 260 ff. below.
[b] See p. 239 below.
[c] See the relevant sub-section in *SCC*, Vol. 5, pt. 5, as also pp. 302 ff. here. And the old paper of Dudgeon (1) is always worth reading. One may mention also the book of Huard & Huang Kuang-Ming (7).

physiological mind might think of this as strengthening the response *vs.* diminishing the stimulus.[a] Now both in Western medicine and in Chinese medicine these conceptions are both to be found. On the one hand, in the West, besides the seemingly dominant idea of direct attack on the pathogen, we have also the idea of the *vis medicatrix naturae*,[b] a theme of resistance and the strengthening of resistance to disease which is strongly embedded in Western medicine from the time of Hippocrates and Galen onwards. On the other hand, one can equally affirm that in China, where the holistic approach might be thought to have dominated, there was also the idea of combating external disease agents, whether these were malign or sinister *pneumata*, the *hsieh chhi*[1] from outside, of unknown nature, or distinct venoms or toxins left behind for example when insects had been crawling over food (this is a very old conception in China);[c] so that the attack on external agents was certainly present in Chinese medical thought too. This may be called the *chhü hsieh*[2] aspect (or, in pharmacological parlance, *chieh tu*[3]); and the other one, the *vis medicatrix naturae*, was largely what the Taoists meant in China by *yang shêng*,[4] the nourishment of life and the strengthening of it against disease.[d] It should by now be clear that whatever the acupuncture procedure does, it must be along the lines of strengthening the patient's resistance (e.g. by increasing antibody or cortisone production); and not directly fighting the invading *pneumata* or organisms, venoms or toxins, i.e. not the characteristic 'antiseptic' attack which has naturally dominated in the West since the time of origin of modern bacteriology. This is shown by the significant fact that while Westerners are often prepared to grant value to acupuncture in affections such as sciatica or lumbago (for which modern-Western medicine can do very little anyway), Chinese physicians have never been prepared to limit either acupuncture or the related moxa (mild or severe cautery and heat-treatment) to such fields; on the contrary they have recommended it and practised it in many diseases for which we all now believe we know clearly the causative organisms, e.g. typhoid, cholera, or appendicitis, and they have claimed at least remissions if not radical cure.[e] The effect is thus in principle cortisone-like or immunological. It is assuredly very interesting that both these conceptions (i.e. the exhibition of hostile drugs, and the strengthening of the body's resistance) have developed in both civilisations, in the medicine of both cultures; and one of the things which any really adequate comparative history of world medicine would have to do would be to elucidate the extent which these two contrasting ideas dominated in the thought of East and West at different times.[f]

[a] One could liken this to the contrast between brushing off a mosquito and being immune to the effects of its bite.

[b] The father of one of us (J. N.), who was still in general practice when he was a small boy, constantly used to talk to him about this, and he has never forgotten it.

[c] Cf. the study on hygiene by Needham & Lu Gwei-Djen (1).

[d] A great deal on the *yang shêng* idea will be found in our account of physiological alchemy, *SCC*, Vol. 5, pt. 5.

[e] One of us (G. D. L.) has vivid recollections of the dramatic recovery of her mother in Nanking from cholera after acupuncture.

[f] Inglis (1), in his interesting and not at all uniquely condemnatory book on unorthodox medical systems, which he groups under the term 'fringe medicine', puts the point that however bizarre some

[1] 邪氣 [2] 去邪 [3] 解毒 [4] 養生

In addition there was of course always a third, that springing from the idea of balance or *krasis*, just as Chinese as it was Greek, in accordance with which, disease was essentially a malfunction or imbalance, one or other component entity in the body having unnaturally gained the lead over the others. Since the development of modern endocrinology this conception has indeed taken a new lease of life, but it was present from the beginning in both civilisations. European blood-letting and purging was a direct, if crude, result of it, since the thought was that 'peccant humours' had to be got rid of; but in China a defective balance between Yin and Yang or deviant relationships between the Five Elements were generally diagnosed and altered in a more subtle way, and it is very much to the point that acupuncture was the first court of appeal in this matter also. No one could miss in the following exposé the overwhelming importance of the Yin and Yang in the governance of the system which acupuncture undertook to affect, and we have little doubt that many interventions of this kind did return the living human body with its nerves and hormones to a more even keel, though exactly how the medieval physicians visualised the interplay of the two great forces remains, as always, hard for us to understand fully because of their philosophical nature. Neither they, nor the unitary *chhi* of which they formed part, nor the Five Elements either, were readily capable of giving rise to a quantified science.[a] Never mind, the results were what mattered, and once again acupuncture could accomplish something health-giving.

One would hardly expect to find a vivacious passage dealing with the power of suggestion and the *vis medicatrix naturae* in a seventeenth-century text, and that by a lay hand. Yet Cyrano de Bergerac, in his 'philosophical voyage' to the countries of the Moon and the Sun, written in +1659, accomplished just this. His guide was none other than the Daemon of Socrates, who turned out to be a very *libertin*, free-thinking Spirit. In the course of an argument about miracles Cyrano bursts out:

'But I have seen supernatural things happen—I have known more than twenty miraculous cures of men who were sick unto death!'

'Ah', he interrupted, 'you say that these people were cured miraculously, but you little know that the power of the Imagination is capable of combating all diseases, on account of a certain natural Balsam,[b] distributed throughout our bodies, which contains Qualities

of them may be (ranging from 'radiaesthesia' and 'naturopathy' to the long-established, if still in many ways unconvincing, homoeopathy), all are primarily directed towards assisting the *vis medicatrix naturae*, and none towards attacking invading pathogenic organisms. He includes acupuncture in his survey, treating it with the respect due to its venerable antiquity in China, and recognising that without the sphygmology and the psycho-somatic organicism it can be but a poor imitation of the original. But he goes no further into Chinese medicine, nor does he treat of the Ayurvedic and Unani systems of India. In all of these, of course, the direct attack on parasites of all kinds preceded the coming of bacteriology by many centuries.

[a] This does not mean that ancient Chinese medical science was unconscious of the value of measurement. Respiration rate is considered with relation to blood circulation in *NC* (pp. 2–3); heart-beat with relation to respiration rate in *NCSW/PH*, ch. 18, (pp. 99ff.); the exact length of the acu-tracts is given in *NCLS/PH*, ch. 17, (pp. 187ff.), cf. ch. 48, (p. 353); and a wealth of osteological measurements in *NCLS/PH*, ch. 14, (pp. 175ff.). Indeed, the measurement of weight and lengths of organs was a feature of ancient Chinese anatomy (cf. *SCC*, Sect. 43).

[f] Cf. *SCC*, Vol. 5, pt. 2, pp. 75–6, with the Paracelsian background. And in John Donne's 'Ecstasie': 'Our hands were firmly cemented, By a fast Balm which thence did spring...' Mazzeo (1) is excellent on this.

antagonistic to those of every illness that attacks us. Our Imagination, alerted by Pain, goes and searches in the right place for the specific Remedy, which it opposes to the poison, and so heals us. This is why the ablest physicians on your earth advise a Patient rather to take an Ignorant Doctor, whom he esteems to be very knowing, than a Skilful Physician, whom he imagines to be ignorant. For they consider that our Imagination, labouring to recover our Health, is capable of curing us, with hardly any aid from Remedies, while the most powerful Medicines will be too weak if the Imagination does not apply them. Are you surprised that the most ancient Men of your world lived to so many Ages without the least knowledge of Physick? Their Nature was yet in its force, their constitutions were resilient, and that universal Balsam had not yet been dissipated by the Drugs wherewith your Doctors consume you. It was enough then for the recovery of one's Health earnestly to wish for it, and to imagine oneself cured; so that all at once their clear, vigorous and taut Fancy plunged into that vital Oyl, extracting the Elixir of it, and bringing the active to bear upon the passive —when, lo and behold, almost in the twinkling of an eye, they were as full of health as they had been before...'[a]

Who could ask for a more insightful visualisation of the power of central nervous and endocrine mechanisms in immunological and corticoid protection and response?

This brief introduction may end with a few words on modern secondary sources which can be of great help to the enquirer, though never any substitute for the study of the original texts themselves, those in fact which we shall be describing in the survey of the historical literature. Pride of place must necessarily be given to books in the Chinese language, inaccessible though they are, alas, to so many Western medical scientists who could gain so much by reading them. Reference has already been made to books of the *chiang i* (lecture-notes) type, and here the best concerned with acupuncture are Anon. (*90*) and (*91*), prepared respectively by the Shanghai and Nanking Colleges of traditional medicine.[b] Among the more outstanding recent full-dress treatises are those of Chu Lien (*1*) and Anon. (*107*),[c] with which we would associate the two books of Chhêng Tan-An (*1*, *2*), the former of 1956, the latter of 1931 with its pioneer photographs of surface anatomy with the tracts drawn upon the living body.[d] It remains true, however, that no real understanding can be attained without the basis of the *Huang Ti Nei Ching*, *Su Wên* and *Ling Shu* (The Yellow Emperor's Manual of Corporeal (Medicine); Pt. I, the Questions (and Answers) about Living Matter; and Pt. II, the Vital Axis),[e] those Early Han texts of the −2nd and −1st centuries which correspond in large measure with the Hippocratic Corpus. Therefore it is good to have recourse to Anon. (*81*), the lecture-notes on its general

[a] White ed., pp. 68–9, Eng. auct., adjuv. Lovell, Aldington and Strachan trs.

[b] One version of the former has been translated into English by Ågren (1). Cf. H. C. Lu (1).

[c] Here Anon. (*124*) must also be mentioned, though containing more scientific interpretation than historical tradition.

[d] Cf. Fig. 1. Here, however, he had been to some extent anticipated by the work of Wang Yu-Chung & Chang Ping-Yüeh (*1*) in 1906, for in their discussion of the similarities and differences between Chinese-traditional and modern-Western medicine they gave many diagrams of modern anatomy, superimposing on it charts of the acu-tracts. But their book is now rare, and we know of only one copy, that which we had the pleasure of examining in the collection of Dr Kimura Koichi in Kyoto in 1964.

[e] Our reasons for translating the titles in this way are set forth elsewhere (Needham & Lu Gwei-Djen (8), p. 263, repr. Needham (64), p. 271). Cf. also p. 88 below.

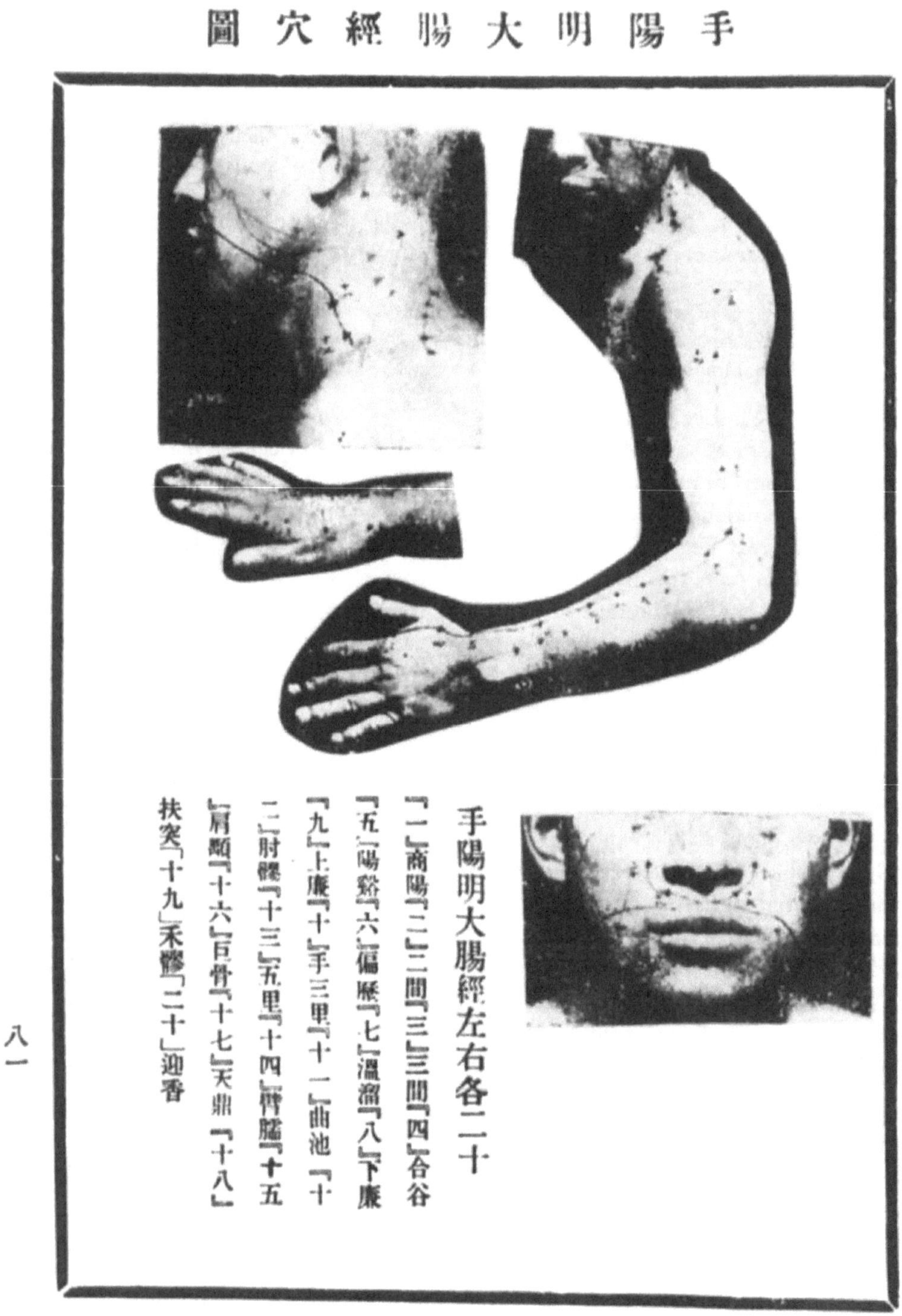

Fig. 1. Pioneer photographs of surface anatomy with acu-points and acu-tracts drawn upon the living body; from Chhêng Tan-An's book of 1931.

medical system. Indispensable also are the versions of the ancient text done into modern colloquial style (*pai hua*[1]), since these show exactly how the traditional physicians of the present day understand the meaning of the old statements; here we have the *Su Wên* by Chou Fêng-Wu, Wang Wan-Chieh & Hsü Kuo-Chhien (*1*), the *Ling Shu* by Chhen Pi-Liu & Chêng Cho-Jen (*1*), and the *Nan Ching* by Chhen Pi-Liu (*1*).[a] Smaller books by Phêng Ching-Shan (*1*) and Yeh Ching-Chhiu (*1*) may also be mentioned, while specialised techniques such as the multiple needle device are discussed by Wu I-Chhing (*1*). Lastly the contributions of Japanese medical scholars are not to be disregarded, since much of value can be found in Homma Shōhaku's book (*1*) on the *ching-lo* system, and that of Sugihara Noriyuki (*1*) on the general theory of traditional Chinese medicine.

Books on acupuncture in Western languages can only be regarded as a second-best. Though there are many more recent books in European languages, those of Soulié de Morant have not been superseded. From 1901 he studied directly under two eminent physicians named Yang and Chang respectively, at Peking and Shanghai; then thirty years later, on returning to France, he set forth at length the classical system of acupuncture (2, 3).[b] Among the writings derivative from this tradition are those of Baratoux (1); Baratoux & Khoubesserian (1) and Lavergne & Lavergne (1). Since then several different strains of transmission have led to Europe. From Formosa (Thaiwan) the influence of Wu Hui-Phing (1, 2) generated the books of Lavier (1, 2); Moss (1); and Lawson-Wood & Lawson-Wood (1). From Vietnam that of Nguyen Van Nha affected those of Mann (1–5). Other writers, such as Tan, Tan & Veith (1), Rubin (1) or Manaka & Urquhart (1), have sought to translate the instructions in contemporary Chinese practical manuals. Japanese studies, of varying worth, have also exerted influence in Europe, e.g. Nakayama (1) and Sakurazawa (1). Then in the years when the socialist countries of Eastern Europe were in close touch with China an authentic current flowed westwards through them, giving rise to works such as that of the Czech Heroldová (1) devoted to acupuncture in particular, and that of the Hungarian Pálos (1) which sought to set this art in the cadre of Chinese medicine as a whole, not unsuccessfully. Similar[c] attempts have been made, on a rather popular level, by Beau (1) and Huard & Huang Kuang-Ming (10).[d]

In approaching acupuncture through the works of representatives of the present-day practitioners in the Western world some reserve should be exercised, for the

[a] The significance of these lies partly in the fact that students of Chinese traditional medicine today have only two years in which to learn a system that customarily demanded diligent study for more than a dozen years. The amount of attention they can devote to the theories and the history is therefore necessarily restricted.

[b] The former embodied an atlas of acupuncture in which the loci and acu-tracts were superimposed upon a background of modern myology and osteology (Fig. 77). This development of Wang Yu-Chung's system was continued in several later atlases, notably those of Dufour (1) and Mann (3).

[c] At this time many Soviet students went to China to learn acupuncture.

[d] Besides these and other books in Western languages, such as Duke (1) in Italian and Børdahl (1) in Danish, there has grown up, especially in Europe, a large periodical literature, on which we may draw from time to time in what follows. This has aroused considerable interest in China, as can be seen from the book of Thao I-Hsin & Ma Li-Jen (*1*), which lists some 350 papers and translates into Chinese 50 articles. Cf. Chhêng Tan-An (*3*), p. 31.

[1] 白話

following reasons: (*a*) very few of them have had reliable linguistic access to the voluminous Chinese sources of many different periods, (*b*) it is often not quite clear how far their training has given them direct continuity with the living Chinese clinical traditions, (*c*) the history in their works is liable to be minimal or unscholarly, (*d*) their accounts of theory are generally very inadequate, (*e*) they tend to adopt a too simplistic assimilation of classical Chinese disease entities to those of modern-Western medicine, (*f*) the cardinal importance of sphygmology in Chinese differential diagnosis is almost ignored, and (*g*) their works are naturally so much influenced by modern-Western concepts of disease aetiology and semeiography that they seem not to practise the classical Chinese methods of holistic classification and diagnosis. Nevertheless this literature has its value. By comparison, a brief and anonymous but authoritative statement on acupuncture issued by the National Academy and Research Institute of Chinese Traditional Medicine a dozen years ago (Anon. 80) is an important document.[a] Now that acupuncture analgesia has awakened so much interest in the Western world,[b] and with the growing tendency to interpret acupuncture in terms of modern neuro-physiology and neuro-chemistry, submitting its techniques to experimental research of this kind, the quality of the Western literature may be expected to rise. But a truly happier state of affairs can hardly be hoped for until (*a*) some Western acupuncturists acquire linguistic fluency in Chinese, and (*b*) political conditions permit of a substantial number of them spending some years in China as direct disciples of the exponents of the central and autochthonous tradition.[c]

We confess indeed to a certain anxiety in the presence of the practitioners' manuals now appearing in the Western world, too greatly simplified, as it seems to us, even when directly derived from Chinese handbooks in current use. In China the situation is quite different because the rural paramedical personnel (*chhih chiao i shêng*[1]), who are taught to make good use of very simple acupuncture manuals,[d] have always at their back the profound expertise of the best acupuncture physicians in the major hospitals, to whom any difficult case can quickly be referred. Not everyone with a modern-Western medical qualification can immediately perform all the traditional-Chinese therapeutic feats. Pulse diagnosis, for example, as well as a very organicist psycho-somatic approach, is a fundamental feature of the traditional art, which after all depends on much subtle theorising, not of course in the modern style, but not non-sense either. We offer, therefore, a word to the wise in due season.

So did Hsü Ling-Thai (+1690 to +1771) in the latter half of the +18th century. In his *Chen Chiu Shih Chhuan Lun* [e] he wrote:

[a] Since then this has been expanded to a book (Anon. 135). There is also now the booklet of Fu Wei-Khang (1), more historical in treatment.

[b] Accounts of acupuncture and the analgesia it can produce keep appearing in the most unlikely places, e.g. *Whitaker's Almanack* for 1975, p. 1016—a remarkably well-informed article too.

[c] It is good to report that during the past few years several three-month foreign-language courses have been held in China for medical Westerners, and the expectation is that this programme will expand.

[d] For example, the one produced by the Hopei Health Department (Anon., *200*), and translated into English by Silverstein, Chang I-Lo & Macon (1).

[e] Part of *I Shu Chhüan Chi*, in ch. 1, (p. 96).

[1] 赤脚醫生

To seek for a good horse according to a map (i.e. at a given place where the animal is known to have been, but forgetting that it may no longer be there) is to know its traces only approximately, and not to know it as it really is. Thus when someone like this (who has only learnt by rote) attempts to cure the diseases of men (with acupuncture), his intervention can be effective, but just as often not.

Throughout the present century, from Soulié de Morant onwards, the accent was on spreading the medical practice of acupuncture in the Western world. More disinterested studies, which took an objective look at acupuncture as practised in traditional China, are far rarer, though naturally the classical histories of Chinese medicine, such as those of Hübotter (1) and Wang Chi-Min & Wu Lien-Tê (1), devote to acupuncture as much space as they see fit. Among the former the monograph of Morse (4) occupies a special position, and there is still much to be learnt from it. Morse was an anatomist who taught for many years at the West China Union University at Chhêngtu in Szechuan,[a] and in this work he tried to come to grips with the cosmological philosophy underlying Chinese medical techniques.[b] He made considerable study of the classical books on acupuncture which we shall describe later on, he explained the acu-tracts, he gave a complete list of the acu-points with translations of their names, and he caused Chinese workmen to carve blocks for four folding charts embodying the surface anatomy of the system in use.[c]

(2) THE *CHING-LO* SYSTEM AND ITS CLASSICAL THEORY

In the following pages it will be our object to describe the array of acupuncture points and channels on and in the human body in its more or less fully developed form, for only after acquiring a fairly clear idea of what the system is will it be possible to appreciate how it came to be. As is well enough known, then, there exist on the surface of the body a large number of well-defined points, *hsüeh*[1] (loci or acu-points),[d] at which hair-fine metal needles of varying length are inserted by the physician in different specified manners.[e] We can get further light on how these acu-points were thought of by taking a look at the other technical terms which were at different times applied to them.

Among such standard names in various historical periods were *shu*,[2] *chhi fu*,[3] *chhi hsüeh*[4] and *khung hsüeh*,[5] the first being particularly continuous from ancient till

[a] He gave a remarkable description of the practice of an itinerant acupuncturist at Suifu, who first awakened his astonishment and interest.

[b] He was not averse, however, to unsatisfactory attempts at modernising interpretations.

[c] On various points he went somewhat astray, as in his idea that the acupuncture needles were intended to allow 'morbid juices' to escape, and that the system could therefore be likened to the old Galenic humoral pathology, in which the 'peccant humours' had to be drawn away.

[d] The sense here is indeed something like 'cavities', and particularly 'transmission cavities'; but we cannot accept the Latin and English equivalents proposed by Porkert (1, 2, 3, 5), *foramina inductoria*, and still less 'sensitive points', for reasons given in Needham & Lu Gwei-Djen (9). See also p. 52.

[e] As already noted, in the past the needles were of very various materials, forms and thicknesses; and even now other types are sometimes used. On the ancient system of nine needles and their applications, see p. 102 and Table 16 below.

1 穴 2 俞 3 氣府 4 氣穴 5 孔穴

recent times. *Hsüeh* itself means a hole or a minute cavity or crevice. *Shu* is normally pronounced *yü*,[a] but as a technical medical term it took from the beginning the sound of *shu*[1],[b] 'to transport, to pay' or 'to hand over'.[c] *Shu* (*hsüeh*)[2] has thus the sense of transmission cavities, 'where the *shen chhi*[3] (*pneuma* of life)[d] goes in and out', as the *Ling Shu* says, adding that they are neither in the skin nor the flesh, neither in the muscles nor the bones.[e] This shows how abstract and invisible the *chhi* channels were thought to be. *Shen chhi* here is the equivalent of *ching chhi*[4],[f] and 'going in and out' meant following the channels and passing from depth to surface and *vice versa*. As for *chhi hsüeh*,[5] the *Su Wên* defines them as pores or interstices in the flesh conveying and harbouring the *ying chhi* and the *wei chhi*;[g] liable also to be invaded by malign *chhi* (*hsieh chhi*[6]) from outside, an invasion which acupuncture can repel.[h] The term *khung hsüeh*,[7] meaning tiny pores, was one of the earliest appellations, and occurs in titles of ancient lost books;[i] it has been adopted officially to denote acu-points (*kōketsu*) in Japan, corresponding to *shu* (*hsüeh*) in China, where *hsüeh tao*[8] and *tzhu chi tien*[9] are now also used.

The oldest extensive texts describing the acu-points occur in that part of the *Huang Ti Nei Ching*[10] (Yellow Emperor's Manual of Corporeal Medicine) which is now known as the *Ling Shu*[11] (Vital Axis). Though nothing permits an exact dating, the most satisfactory time to which to ascribe these is the −1st century, and as we shall mention later on, it is probable that the *Ling Shu* is the present name for that portion of the *Nei Ching* which appears in Han bibliographies under the title *Chen Ching*[12] (Manual of the Needles). Since the *Su Wên*[13] part of the Corpus (the Questions (and Answers) about Living Matter), which dates from the previous century, also contains a good deal about the acu-points, it is clear that the system must have been well advanced in development during the Warring States period—but we shall in due course return to the historical issues. The *Nei Ching* says in several places that there

[a] There are many trained acupuncture physicians today, especially in the West, who know no other usage.

[b] Since the absence of Rad. no. 159 (carriage) was liable to lead to confusion, it seemed good in some periods to add other radicals, e.g. no. 130 (flesh), making *shu*,[14] as especially in the Sung.

[c] *NCSW/PH*, ch. 3, (p. 17); cf. Hsieh Li-Hêng (*2*), vol. 2, p. 1748.

[d] We recognise the banality of this expression, yet we are unable to follow Porkert (*1*), pp. 173, 176, 181, in his confident alternative. He defines *shen* as actively organising and individuating configurative and transformative force, while *chhi* would be configurational energy substantiating or 'structing' certain qualities, i.e. the 'structive aspect of an energetic configuration'. As in many of his other contexts, the models here are (*a*) the inductor and the competent substrate in experimental morphology and embryology, and (*b*) modern knowledge of energy in physics, and the inter-convertibility of its many forms. We have set forth elsewhere (Needham & Lu Gwei-Djen, 9) the reasons for our reluctance to read back modern scientific ideas as sophisticated as these into the minds of the naturalists and physicians of the Chhin and Han.

[e] *NCLS/PH*, ch. 1, (p. 9); cf. Anon. (*90*), p. 101.

[f] Cf. *SCC*, Vol. 5, pt. 5. *Ching chhi* could be translated 'generative morphogenetic *pneuma*', one of the 'three primary vitalities'.

[g] Cf. p. 28 below for an explanation of these, and *NCSW/PH*, ch. 58, (p. 298).

[h] *NCSW/PH*, ch. 10, (p. 64).

[i] See p. 120 below.

1 輸　2 兪穴　3 神氣　4 精氣　5 氣穴　6 邪氣
7 孔穴　8 穴道　9 刺激點　10 黃帝內經　11 靈樞　12 鍼經
13 素問　14 腧

are 365 acu-points in all,[a] by symbolic correlation with the number of degrees (*tu*[1]) in the celestial circles, to which indeed it likens them, as also to the number of days in the year;[b] and in Han times this number was also supposed to comprehend the number of bones in the human body.

Here we see the importance of that macrocosm–microcosm philosophy which always lay at the basis of acupuncture theory. But actually the *Nei Ching* only mentions 160 by name, and not more than 295 in all can be deduced from its descriptions, so that the theoretical number may have been a counsel of perfection only.[c] Until the last half-dozen years the total number was stabilised at 670, but in the burst of further advance which has accompanied the development of acupuncture analgesia, as well as acupuncture treatment of deaf-mutism and paralysis, a considerable number of effective new acu-points has been added, especially in the region of the external ear.[d] At the same time it may be that some of the older acu-points have fallen out of use, and processes of this kind have doubtless been going on all through the history of the technique. It must be appreciated that each one of the acu-points has a distinctive technical name which has clung to it through the ages (cf. Table 4).[e] As in all the classical Chinese taxonomic sciences a certain amount of synonymy grew up, so we find some of the best authors carefully listing the overlaps and sorting out the confusions.[f] Till recently it was estimated that about 450 acu-points were in current use, but those most commonly used now do not exceed 40 to 50 in number.[g]

If this were the whole story, a recognition of hundreds of points on the body where it was safe to insert a needle, the system would have been indeed empirical, but it is far from that. One hesitates even to call it quasi-empirical, since the theories elaborated with regard to it were complex and subtle, though not of course theories in the sense of modern science. If, pursuing the ancient astronomical analogy, we think of the acu-points as microcosmic equivalents of the stars in the heavens, we find at once that they were not scattered at random but tied together in patterns like the asterisms and constellations. They were connected with each other in a complicated reticulate system, resembling at first sight to modern eyes a map of the underground railway system in a great city. But it was fundamentally circulatory in nature, a system of channels for transporting energy or vital force (*pneuma* or *chhi*,[2] Yang in nature) to

[a] See e.g. *NCSW/PH*, ch. 54, (p. 281), ch. 58, (p. 290), ch. 59, (pp. 299, 307). Also *NCSW/WMC*, ch. 58, (p. 482), ch. 59, (p. 500).

[b] See *SCC*, Vol. 3, p. 268.

[c] See Anon. (*91*), p. 12, and below, pp. 99 ff.

[d] Of course most of these are outside the twelve classical acu-tracts.

[e] Naturally most of the names apply to two points, one on each side of the body, since the twelve tracts are paired in mirror-image fashion.

[f] E.g. *CCTC*, ch. 7, (pp. 234.2 ff.).

[g] And often not more than 20 (F. Mann, priv. comm. 1973; Chang Chien-Ying, priv. comm. 1972). The standard set authorised in recent years by the Monpushō (Ministry of Education) in Japan comprised 70 (Yeh Ching-Chhiu (*1*), p. 57). At times there has been a tendency on the part of famous physicians to emphasise only very few of the acu-points; thus in the Sung Ma Tan-Yang[3] recommended no more than 12, and Tou Kuei-Fang[4] only 8. There was also a belief that many diseases could be cured by inserting needles at five points only (IG 4 and 10, V 36, VU 54 and P 7; see Table 4 below). These were called the 'four panacea points' (*ssu tsung hsüeh*[5]), four because San-li[6] occurred twice in them (IG 10 and V 36), one in the arm and one in the leg.

[1] 度 [2] 氣 [3] 馬丹陽 [4] 竇桂芳 [5] 四總穴 [6] 三里

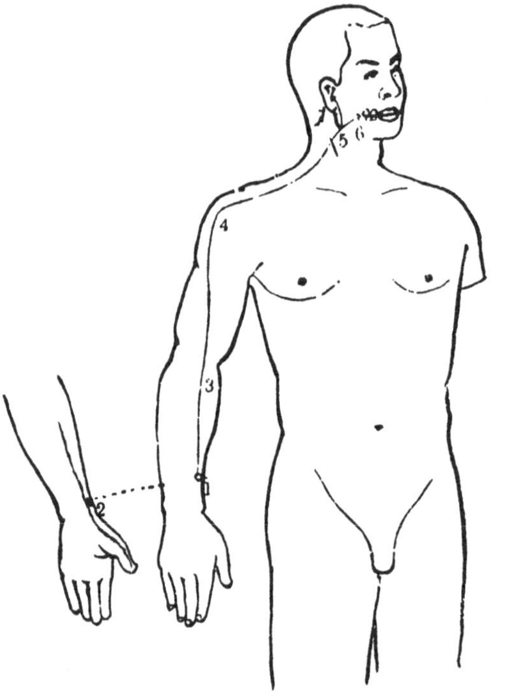

Fig. 2. Diagram to show an acu-junction; from Anon. (*90*).

all tissues round the body,[a] just as the vital juice (*haima* or *hsüeh*,[1] Yin in nature) passed round in the blood-vessels. Yang implies as usual the formless and insubstantial, Yin the palpable and material. But this should not be taken to mean any too radical separation of the Yang and the Yin, for one must always remember that neither is ever so pure as not to contain a trace of its opposite within itself.[b] The main channels are the *ching*[2] (tracts or acu-tracts, as we call them), twelve in number, known as regular tracts (*chêng ching*[3]).[c] Each has at least one *lo*[4] (junction or acu-

[a] From these hesitating equivalents it can be seen that we do not yet know how best to translate *chhi*, which is why (ever since *SCC*, Vol. 2, pp. 22–3, 41, 76, 369, 472) we have consistently left it untranslated. We even doubt whether there could ever be a justified one-word European translation. In Vol. 2 we said that *chhi* was something like *pneuma*, i.e. subtle spirits, tenuous matter, something resembling air, or a gas or a vapour, but also something which could have the character of radiant energy like radioactive emanation, or X-rays, or very highly penetrating particles. In later Chinese (Neo-Confucian) philosophy, 'matter-energy' may do well enough, but for these earlier periods we should not like to particularise too finely. We certainly cannot adopt the terminology proposed by Porkert: 'configurational energy' (1), p. 167, or 'patterned energy' (2, 3), to the exclusion of all other conceptions. For the *ching chhi*[5] with which we are here concerned he has, (1), p. 169: 'cardinal conduit energy' or 'circulating energy', but again this seems to us too narrowly non-material. Our criticisms of Porkert's integral and exclusive energetics theory have been set forth in Needham & Lu Gwei-Djen (9). But 'energy' shows signs of becoming established as the occidental translation of *chhi* in medical texts; cf. Schatz, Larre & de la Vallée (1), esp. p. 144; Mann (11), p. 39; Schuldt (1).

[b] Cf. *SCC*, Vol. 5, pt. 5, *passim*, as also Vol. 2, p. 276.

[c] It has become customary for Western writers to translate *ching* as 'meridians' but the analogy with astronomical hour-circles or terrestrial longitude is so far-fetched that we do not adopt the term.

[1] 血 [2] 經 [3] 正經 [4] 絡 [5] 經氣

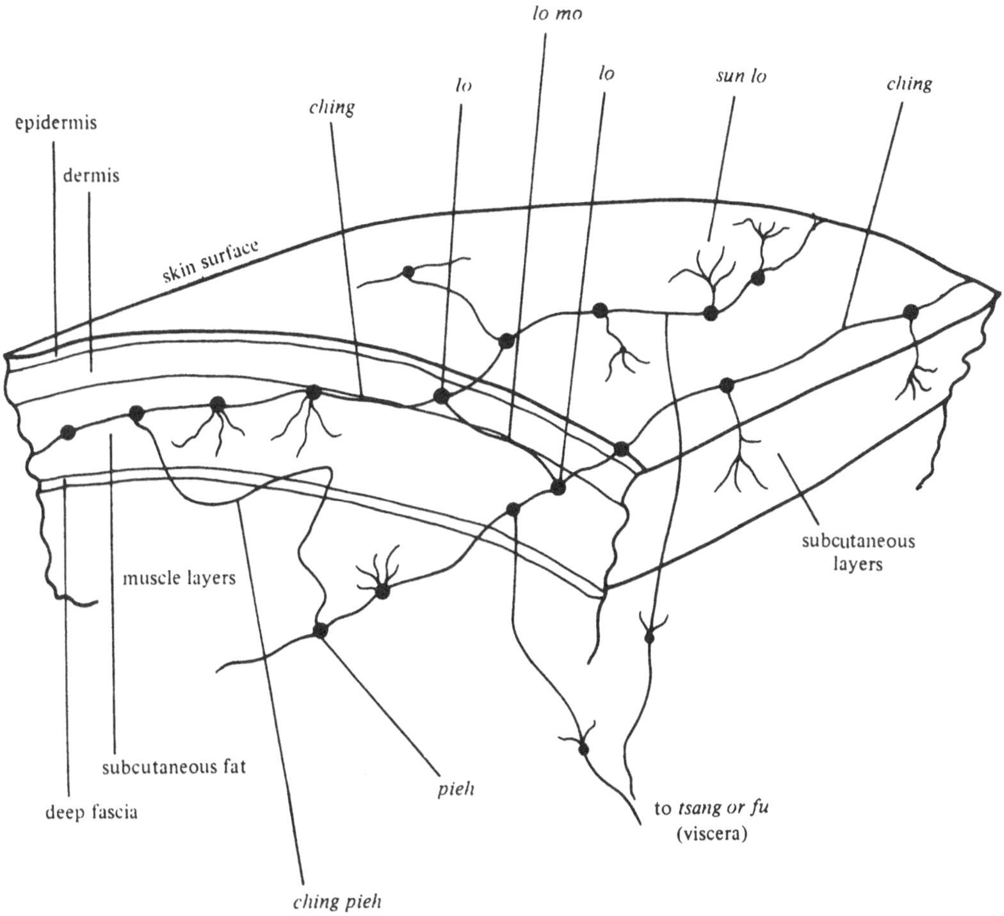

Fig. 3. Diagram to elucidate the *ching* (acu-tracts), *lo* (acu-junctions), tract-connecting branches (*lo mo*), dendritic 'capillary' micro-branches (*sun lo*), acu-junctions for long tract-connecting cross-channel branches (*pieh*), and these long connections themselves (*ching pieh*). Orig. drawing.

junction)[a] whereby it connects with one or more neighbouring tracts through short branches (*lo mo*[1]).[b] The *ching* and *lo* are indeed invisible, running along, like the principal blood-vessels and nerves, under the surface, as it were, of the city.[c] They

'Tract' is as nearly non-committal as possible for the supposed channel of the *chhi*, and perhaps the established use of the word for the bundles of neuron fibres in the spinal cord may be a recommendation for our usage rather than the reverse. We applaud the attack of Huard & Huang Kuang-Ming (1) on the translation 'meridians'. As for the 'sinarteries' and 'sinarteriology' of Porkert (1), we fear that this is going further and faring worse. To put a syllable indicating 'Chinese' in front of 'arteries', when (*a*) they were never really visualised as tubes, (*b*) they did not radiate from the heart, and (*c*) they also performed a quasi-venous function, seems to us more quixotic than helpful.

[a] Porkert (1), p. 203, has 'reticular conduit', not entirely unacceptable, though cloaking the importance of the actual points of branching as such.

[b] Cf. Fig. 2. These *lo mo* are confined to the forearms and the lower parts of the legs.

[c] Later on (p. 186) we shall consider what efforts have been made to assign a material and histological reality to the tracts.

[1] 絡脈

were always thought of (cf. Fig. 3) as lying in what we should now call the subcutaneous tissues rather than on the surface of the skin itself.[a] As for the *lo*, it is as if one had separate transport companies with exchange points for the public provided at places where they come near to each other; thus the *lo* may be called anastomotic loci or acu-points. Later we consider the question whether historically the *hsüeh*[1] as individual points antedated the tracts which strung them together, or whether it was the other way round (p. 85). In any case, the *lo* (acu-junctions) were not confined to those which made connections from one tract to another, for there were said to be

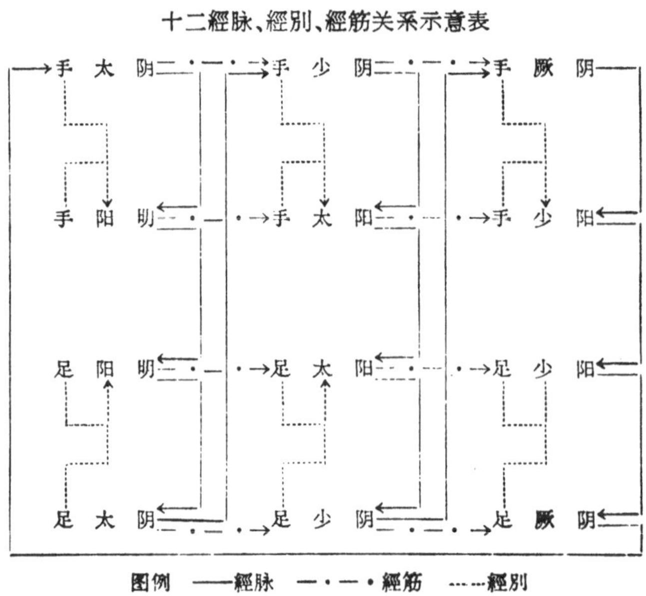

Fig. 4. Chart of the long cross-connections (*ching pieh*); from Anon. (*91*).

innumerable *sun lo*,[2] dendritic acu-junctions and short branches, which left the tract and lost themselves in the superficial tissues of the body.

This conception of radiating 'capillary vessels', as we should call them, was a real insight of ancient Chinese physiology, evidently based on observations of the arterioles, venules and nerve-branchings. In the +8th century, Wang Ping, commenting upon a chapter of the *Nei Ching Su Wên*, quoted a *Chen Ching*[3] as saying:[b]

The tracts and channels (*ching mo*[4]) are inside the body and the branches (*chih*[5]) which connect them horizontally are the *lo*.[6] And the *lo* again have further branches which are called *sun*.[7]

[a] Various depths are specified in ancient descriptions, as will be seen from the translations given on pp. 96 ff. below. An erroneous impression may have developed in the minds of those who look at standard charts without being able to read the very detailed accounts in the original texts.

[b] *NCSW* (ch. 17), ch. 62, (p. 306), tr. auct.

[1] 穴 [2] 孫絡 [3] 鍼經 [4] 經脉 [5] 支 [6] 絡 [7] 孫

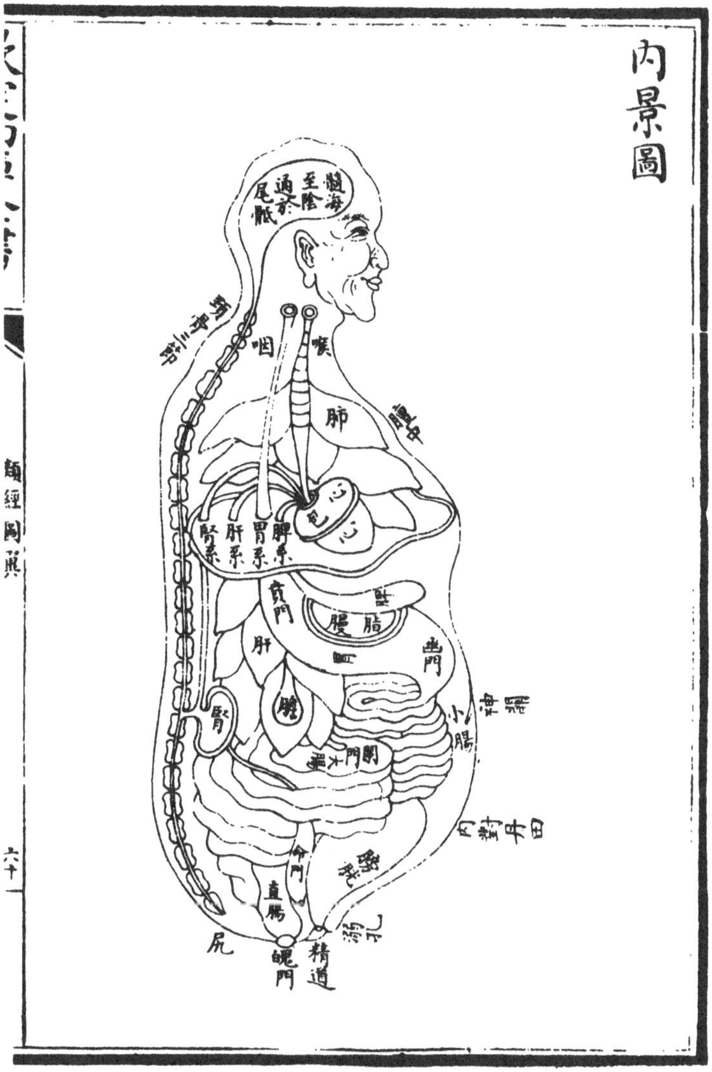

Fig. 5. Traditional drawing of the twelve viscera, from the *Lei Ching* of Chang Chieh-Pin, +1624 (Ssu Khu Chhüan Shu edition).

The *Chen Chiu Ta Chhêng* (+1601) also says that:

apart from the 12 regular tracts and the 15 acu-junctions (*lo mo*[1]) there are also horizontal branches (*hêng lo*[2]) and dendritic branches (*sun lo*[3]), the arrangement of which no one really knows, though there must be at least 300 of these *chih mo*[4] scattered through the body.[a]

The twelve main or regular tracts (*chêng ching*[5]) of the body run cephalo-caudally, to or from the extremities. They are linked by long cross-channels (*ching pieh*[6]) running between the *ching*, and joining them just as a contour canal joins two rivers,[b] even

[a] Ch. 2, (p. 40.2), tr. auct.
[b] Cf. *SCC*, Vol. 4, pt. 3, pp. 299ff.

[1] 絡脈 [2] 橫絡 [3] 孫絡 [4] 支脈 [5] 正經 [6] 經別

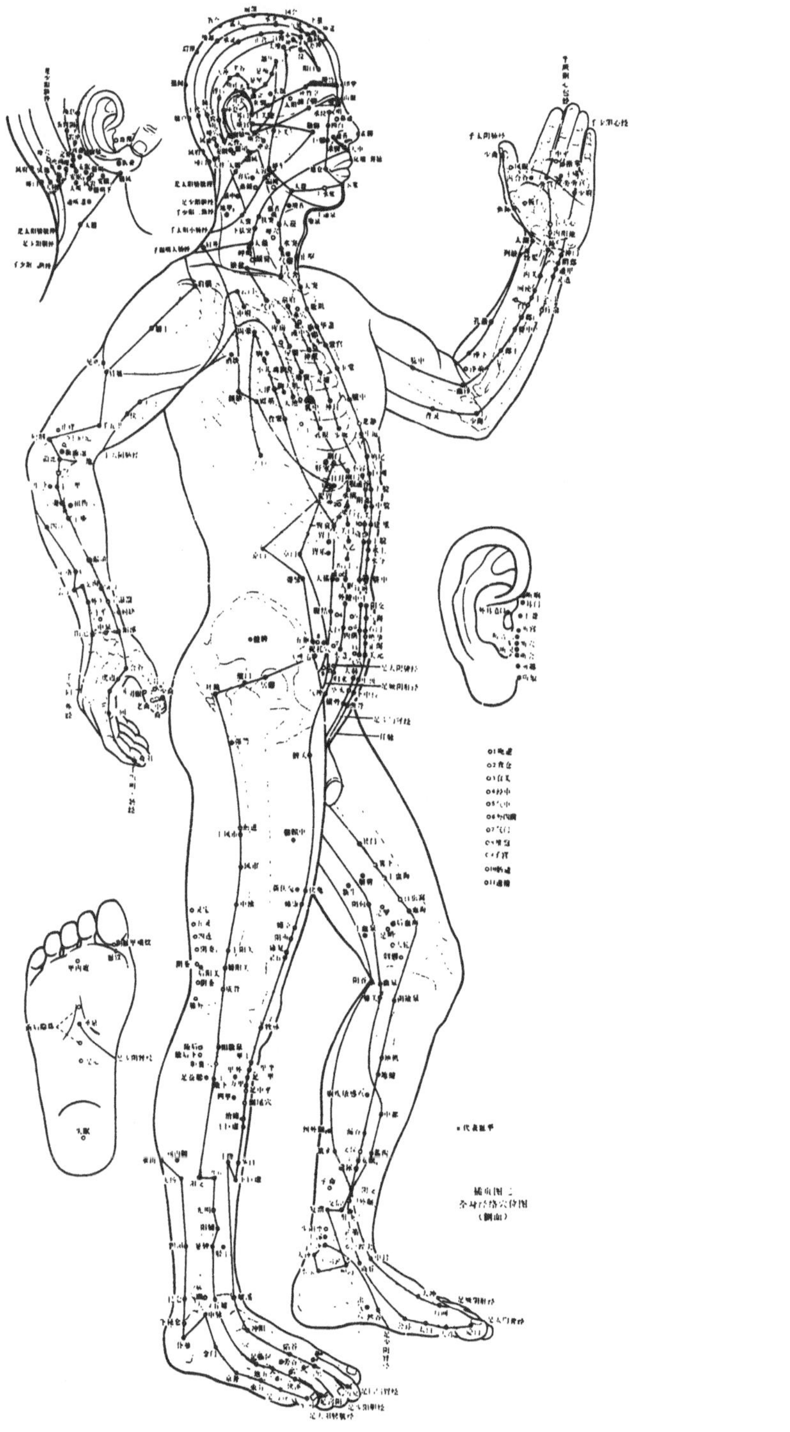

Fig. 6. Side view of the male human body with acu-points and acu-tracts shown against an osteological background. Anon. (*123*).

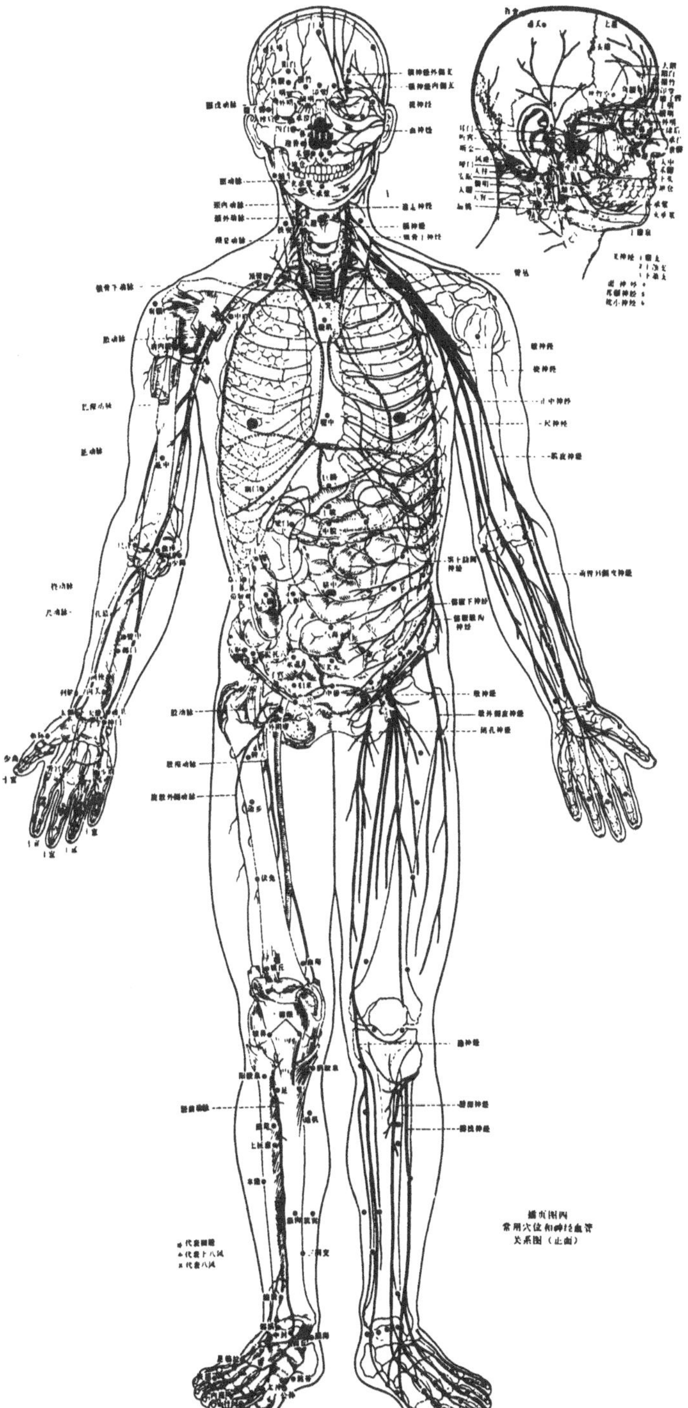

Fig. 7. Anterior view of the human body with the acu-points marked on an osteological, neurological and splanchnological background. Anon. (*123*).

though they may be flowing in opposite directions (Fig. 4).[a] The points where these cross-channels originate are called *pieh*.[1] Even more important, each one of the regular tracts is connected with one or other of the twelve viscera (Fig. 5)[b]—the six hollow organs (*fu*[2]) which are Yang, and therefore 'outer' (*wai*[3]);[c] and the six solid organs (*tsang*[4]) which are Yin, and therefore 'inner' (*nei*[5]).[d] It is fundamental to the system that each one of the twelve *chêng ching* not only pertains to (*shu*[6]), and so connects with, that internal organ which gives its name to the tract in question; but also has a direct association (*lo*[7]), and connection with, the internal organ belonging to the tract next in the series (cf. Table 2). Each Yin tract is connected primarily with a Yin viscus (*tsang*[4]), but also secondarily with a Yang one (*fu*[2]). Let us illustrate this by a concrete example taken from Table 2. The first of the tracts, the Shou Thai-Yin Fei Ching (cheirotelic pulmonic Thai-Yin tract), passes indeed to the lungs, but further connects with the large intestine, which gives its name to the succeeding tract in the series.[e] All this applies only to the regular tracts; the auxiliary ones (*chhi ching*[8]) were never associated directly with visceral organs.

What exactly, one asks, was the relation of the tract-channel system to anatomy as we understand it today? This is a question to which we shall have to return in several places, partly when we describe and translate the *Nei Ching* accounts of the courses of the tracts,[f] partly when we consider claims that specific structures underlie them,[g] and partly in connection with the growth of anatomical knowledge in China considered in Sect. 43. Modern books on acupuncture, both Chinese and Western, generally show the chart system of the tracts (as we ourselves do in Figs. 6 and 7) superimposed upon modern anatomical diagrams, whether superficial, myographic or osteographic. It is interesting that this practice began in China and not in the West, for in 1906 two physicians, Wang Yu-Chung[9] and Chang Ping-Yüeh,[10] published a work entitled *Chung Hsi Hui Tshan I Hsüeh Thu Shuo*;[11] as we have seen, this included much modern anatomy combined with charts of the principal acu-tracts and acu-points.[g] Nearly all later books have followed the same practice, e.g. Chhêng Tan-An (*2*) in 1933.

We have spoken of stars and railways but the really classical analogy was with earthly water-works. There is no doubt that in the *ching-lo* system we have to deal with a very ancient conception of a traffic nexus with a network of trunk and secondary channels and their smaller branches. From the beginning these were thought of in terms analogous to those of hydraulic engineering,[h] involving rivers, tributaries,

[a] Cf. *NCLS/MC*, ch. 11, (pp. 1043 ff.); Anon. (*90*), pp. 80 ff., 509 ff.

[b] From what we say about these elsewhere it emerges that originally there were only ten, two groups of five symbolically correlated with the Five Elements, but as time went by an ancient specifically medical sixfold classification asserted itself and two more were added. These were the 'three coctive regions' and the 'pericardium' (cf. p. 40).

[c] Therefore also patefact (*piao*[12]); see p. 43.

[d] Therefore also subdite (*li*[13]); see p. 43.

[e] In this way there arose the appellation *liu ho*,[14] the 'Six Pairs'.

[f] P. 93 below.

[g] Cf. Fig. 1 and p. 9 above.

[h] Readers of *SCC* will long have appreciated the outstanding importance of hydraulic engineering in the shaping of Chinese culture; cf. Vol. 4, pt. 3, pp. 211 ff.

1 別 2 腑 3 外 4 臟 5 內 6 屬 7 絡
8 奇經 9 王有忠 10 章秉鉞 11 中西滙參醫學圖說 12 表 13 裡
14 六合

derivate canals, reservoirs, lakes, etc.; and this analogy is quite explicit in the *Ling Shu*. For example, each one of the twelve regular tracts listed in Table 1 below was placed in symbolic correlation with one or other of the great rivers of the Chinese home-land. Thus the pulmonic tract was analogised with the Yellow River (Ho shui[1]), the crasso-intestinal tract with the Yangtze (Chiang shui[2]), the felleic tract with the Wei River (Wei shui[3]), etc.[a] As we go on we shall see many examples of names of acu-points and types of points which indicate traffic and transmission, e.g. *shu*.[4] Some of the acu-points bear names suggesting tanks or reservoirs (*hai*[5]),[b] others again have names which indicate pools or lesser reservoirs (*chhih*[6]).[c] We are thus clearly in the presence of an important doctrine arising from the idea of the microcosm, the body of man representing the macrocosm in little;[d] and the basic idea of a circulation, which was already unmistakably present in the Earlier Han period, may well have been associated with a recognition of the meteorological water-cycle—the exhalations of the earth rising into the clouds and falling again as rain, that rain which filled the great rivers to overflowing, nourished all reservoirs and made canal transport possible and easy.[e]

It is not at all difficult to support the foregoing paragraph with textual evidence. In the *Kuan Tzu*[7] book there is a chapter on water and the earth, probably written about the late −4th century during the Warring States period.[f] At the beginning of this we read:[g]

> (One can say that) water is the blood and the *chhi* of the earth, because it flows and penetrates everywhere (just in the same manner) as the circulation (of the *chhi* and the blood) in the *ching-chin*[8] (nerve, muscle and tendon) and the *ching-mo*[9] (tract and channel, including blood-vessel) systems.

The analogy therefore is quite clear, and the microcosmic parallel evident, but the text has a special interest because it may well be a century or two older than the

[a] This is often described, as by Sun Chin-Chhing (*1*). The essential references are *NCLS*, ch. 12, (p. 21), *NCLS/MC* (pp. 1047ff.), *NCLS/PH* (pp. 155ff., with a table of the correlations on p. 162). The text compares in parable form (*yü*[10]) the characteristics of the tracts with those of the rivers in terms of size, deepness, width and distance, relating thereto the proper depth of insertion of the needle and the time it ought to be left in place.

[b] These could be analogised with the *torculum Herophili* of anatomy, the large pool of blood at the base of the skull. Thus we have Chhi-hai[11] (JM 6) and Chhi-hai-shu[12] (VU 24), the torcular of the *chhi*. Then there is the torcular of the blood (Hsüeh-hai[13]) at LP 10, the lesser torcular (Shao-hai[14]) at C 3, and the small torcular (Hsiao-hai[15]) at IT 8. The meaning of these abbreviations will become clear immediately; see Table 4 on p. 53.

[c] These could be called lacunae or sinuses. For example, there is a 'celestial sinus' (Thien-chhih[16]) at HC 1, a sinous sinus (Chhü-chhih[17]) at IG 11, and a sinus of the Yang (Yang-chhih[18]) at SC 4.

[d] Cf. *SCC*, Vol. 2, pp. 294ff.

[e] Let it not be thought that these cosmic analogies were fruitlessly fanciful on the part of the Chinese. William Harvey himself, as Pagel (4, 6, 19, 20, 24, 25, 26) showed long ago, was powerfully influenced by similar thoughts, likening, for example, the sun to the heart, and the blood-circulation to the apparent diurnal motion of the stars.

[f] It may have been the product of the Chi-Hsia Academicians (*SCC*, Vol. 2, pp. 234–5).

[g] Ch. 39, p. 1*a*, tr. auct. The words are: *Shui chê ti chih hsüeh chhi, ju chin mo chih thung liu chê yeh.*[19] We gave a rough translation of the whole of this chapter at a previous stage (Vol. 2, pp. 42ff.), but here it is necessary to be more precise, to bring out the full meaning.

1 河水 2 江水 3 渭水 4 兪 5 海 6 池 7 管子
8 經筋 9 經脉 10 喩 11 氣海 12 氣海兪 13 血海 14 少海
15 小海 16 天池 17 曲池 18 陽池 19 水者地之血氣如筋脉之通流者也

Huang Ti Nei Ching itself. This means that the *ching-chin*[a] and *ching-mo*[b] systems were already well understood before that systematisation was put down in the writing that we have now, a fact which adds further weight to what we shall say later (pp. 111 ff.) about the long antecedent background of the *Nei Ching*. In another place, earlier on, we encountered a further example of the analogical use of the term *mo*, also worth recalling here. At the end of his life (−210), the general Mêng Thien,[1] accused of impiety and all sorts of imaginary crimes during his service to the Chhin emperor, remarked: 'How could I build the Great Wall without cutting through the veins of the earth?'[c] So *ti mo*[2] was a commonplace in those days, and indeed the expression *shan mo*[3] for a range of mountains has continued on in physiographical usage until the present time.

Thus it was entirely in accord with the ancient hydraulic engineering metaphor of this physiology that disease should have been visualised as arising often from the abnormal flow of the Yang and Yin in the tract-channel system, as we shall call it. The current could be excessive, or the volume too great (*yu yü*[4]), or conversely, perhaps by some blockage or other,[d] deficient (*pu tsu*[5]).[e] These were the kind of derangements which could be restored tc normality by acupuncture and moxibustion. But the concept of a circulatory flow was just as important as the hydrodynamic idea itself. The circulation of the Yang *chhi* in the *ching-lo* system was considered to go on side by side with the circulation of the blood (*hsüeh*[6]) and its Yin, travelling within the blood-vessels (*mo*[7]). The accepted speed of this circulation was comparatively fast, not indeed as rapid as that established in modern physiology since the time of William Harvey, but not so much slower as has often been supposed. Without trespassing too much on the content of the physiological Section 43, these facts must now be demonstrated by textual references and quotations.

(i) *The circulation of* chhi *and blood*

So far we have been speaking mostly of the *ching-lo*[8] system, that of the acupuncture tracts and their branches, only too commonly thought of in the West as the be-all and end-all of the medical theory lying behind acupuncture.[f] But in the ancient, medieval and traditional texts we meet frequently with another expression, much wider in significance, *ching mo*.[9] This may be translated as the tract-and-channel network

[a] See p. 51 below.

[b] See p. 92 below.

[c] *Shih Chi*, ch. 88, p. 5*b*; cf. *SCC*, Vol. 4, pt. 1, p. 240, and Bodde (15), pp. 61, 64, 65.

[d] This idea, more perhaps than anything else, may best account for the ultimate origin of needling. One could clear the channels of the *chhi* just as one would take a cane or stick to unblock a gutter or drain-pipe choked with autumn leaves. On the concept of *stasis*, widely present in ancient Chinese natural and medical philosophy, see *SCC*, Vol. 1, p. 219, Vol. 4, pt. 3, p. 268.

[e] These two terms have great general importance in Chinese medicine, as we shall see in *SCC*, Vol. 6. Its exponents were assuredly not wrong in recognising the manifold ills which can follow from impedances of the circulation in man—thromboses, embolisms, aneurisms, abnormalities of blood flow and volume, etc. etc.

[f] Huard & Huang Kuang-Ming (1) deserve credit for appreciating the vanity of this.

1 蒙恬 2 地脉 3 山脉 4 有餘 5 不足 6 血
7 脉 8 經絡 9 經脈

system. Here we write it just as it appears in all the texts of the classical tradition; but there is another way of writing *mo*,[1] and this it is which has been adopted in contemporary Chinese printing, always avid of simplifications, for *ching mo*.[2] Since we have two orthographic forms at our disposal we propose to adopt a different and more useful convention. The word *mo* was used in a variety of senses. The first meaning that comes to the mind of an ordinary translator is 'pulse', and this is right enough, but the word also meant blood-vessels in general, the vessels which carried the *hsüeh*, and could even by extension refer to the heart. The characters *mo*[3] and *mo*[1] are normally completely interchangeable, but it will be convenient to use the first form mainly for statements about the pulse, restricting the second form mainly to talk about the channels of blood (with their contained *hsüeh*); and we shall try consistently to do this. Thus we write the typical phrases for the pulse of the blood in the arteries as forms of *mo hsiang*,[4] but when we say that 'the blood moves in the vessels' we write *hsüeh hsing mo nei*[5].[a] Thus we shall write *ching mo*[6] to mean 'the tracts and the pulse', and *ching mo*[2] to mean 'the tracts and blood-channels' (more or less equivalent to the modern anatomically precise idea of blood-vessels and capillaries).[b] But the widest meaning of *ching mo* in general remains 'the tract-and-channel network system' and this we shall often call it. The moment is now ripe for developing both these two conceptions a little, but first there is something more to be said about the relation of *ching mo* and *ching lo*.

The expression *ching mo* was often used almost synonymously with *ching lo*,[7] partly because the ancient Chinese physicians had a great deal more at the back of their minds than the modern student of Chinese medical history, and partly because they did not always make the same kind of sharp distinctions that we find in modern science, even modern biology and physiology. It will be remembered that the word *mo* also occurred in inter-connections between the tracts (*ching*[8]) as *lo mo*,[9] though their dendritic capillary terminations resumed the name of *lo* as *sun lo*.[10] As we shall see in a moment, the Yang circulated through the *chhi* tracts, *ching*, while the Yin was carried round in the blood through the vessels. So just as a *mo* appeared on the Yang side, a *lo* appeared on the Yin one, for the blood-containing capillaries in the epidermis were termed *hsüeh lo*[11].[c] Thus there was a certain terminological overlap, and one can only say that on the whole, and broadly speaking, the *ching* and *lo* were channels for Yang and *chhi*, while the *mo* were channels for blood and Yin. Undoubtedly the typical abbreviation *ching lo*[12] can be confusing to those uninitiated in classical Chinese medical literature, since *mo* is left out of it and hence the basic theoretical parallelism is obscured. Of course practical acupuncture itself was done mainly at points along the tracts,[d] but it was based on a much wider body of theory which involved channels

[a] As we have just seen, *mo* in ancient times meant all kinds of channels, lines or ridges in the macrocosm as well as the microcosm.

[b] See *NCLS/PH*, ch. 10, (pp. 104 ff.).

[c] *NCLS/PH*, ch. 39, (p. 302).

[d] Mainly, because as time went on more and more points outside them were discovered and used, especially in modern times; and also because certain techniques do draw capillary blood from superficial vessels (cf. p. 5 above and p. 164 below).

[1] 脉 [2] 經脉 [3] 脈 [4] 脈象 [5] 血行脉內 [6] 經脈
[7] 經絡 [8] 經 [9] 絡脉 [10] 孫絡 [11] 血絡 [12] 經絡

other than the tracts. It also involved sphygmological diagnosis (*mo hsiang*[1]), and the study of the inter-relations between the internal organs (*tsang hsiang*[2])[a] in accordance with the principles of patefact and subdite (*piao li*[3]) phenomena.[b]

The expression *ching mo*[4] is an important one, too much overlooked in modern attempts to introduce therapeutic acupuncture into the Western world. 'Tracts and pulse' had a most intimate relation, because it was only the very delicate observation of the 28 different types of pulse which could give a clue as to which tracts were needing acupuncture. After all, these were the waves stemming from the heart beat, and that would be expected to be responsive to diseased conditions in various other parts of the body, especially the viscera. In a page or two we shall learn from original texts how intimately connected the Yang and Yin were thought to be—by scrutinising the latter in the blood, therefore, it ought to be possible to know what was going wrong with the former in the tracts. This was the link, then, which the physicians were arguing about in the Warring States and Early Han periods. Only the blood side could tell you what to do with the needles on the tract side (Fig. 8).

Let us turn now to the other expression, *ching mo*.[5] As we saw, this can be translated 'tracts and blood channels', certainly including what we think of as the gross vascular system today but also embodying the subtlest and finest pores through which blood can pass. It is quite interesting that the conception of capillary vessels never seems to have caused any difficulty for the Chinese physiological thinkers, because in the West the delay in recognising them was one of the greatest barriers in the +17th century to the acceptance of the Harveian circulation of the blood; perhaps the fact that in the Chinese system there was a parallel set of vessels and pores for the circulation of the almost infinitely vaporous *chhi* encouraged the idea that blood also would have no difficulty in seeping through the tissues on its way back to the heart. And indeed the idea of a pumped circulation of both *chhi* and blood was vital to the Chinese conceptions, a circulation quite unequivocally stated, as will in a moment appear.[c] First, then, one has to understand that the Yin was in the vessels with the blood, while the Yang was circulating in the tracts. Both Yin and Yang components had a double origin, partly inherited from the parents (the *hsien thien*[6] endowment), and partly derived from ingested nourishment (the *hou thien*[7] main-

[a] This is the expression europeanised by Porkert (1), pp. 3, 107ff., as 'orbis-iconography' or the 'imagery of functional orbs'. We think it unnecessary to adopt such phraseology. Porkert's point is that the names of *tsang* and *fu* in Chinese thought refer by no means only to the anatomical organs in question, but rather to the whole complex of what we should call their physical structure, physiological function, and range of pathological abnormalities. *Hsiang* implies the study of these, the visualisation of their condition, and the understanding of the inter-relations between one *tsang* or *fu* and the others at any given time. Once this is clearly appreciated there is surely no need for a term such as 'orb', with all its astronomical undertones of concentric motion, quite misleading in this context, and unsuitable for the microcosm.

[b] Cf. p. 43 below.

[c] This has been well recognised by Liang Po-Chhiang (1); Kapferer (1) and Huard & Huang Kuang-Ming (1). Yet many Western writers still go about to dismiss it as 'mystical' (e.g. Boenheim (1), a paper in any case full of sinological mistakes). The quotation from the *Nei Ching* given in translation in a brief paper by Benkov & Pei Lung-Tang (1) was the source of a well-known statement in the book of Hogben (3), p. 800. Its wording came, not surprisingly, from Wang & Wu (1), p. 35.

1 脈象 2 臟象 3 表裡 4 經脈 5 經脉 6 先天
7 後天

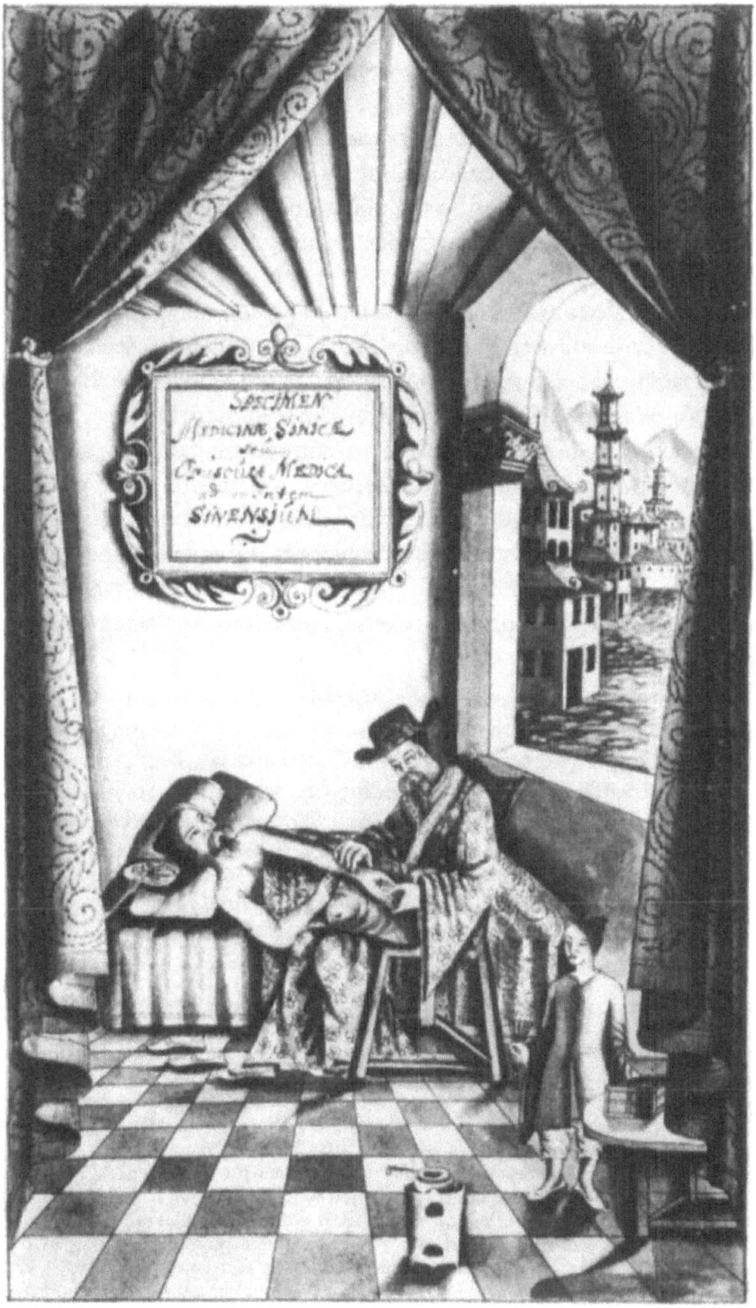

Fig. 8. Frontispiece of the manuscript copy of Andreas Cleyer's *Specimen Medicinae Sinicae* of +1682 (see p. 277 below) in the Berlin Staatsbibliothek (MS. Lat. fol. 92). The Chinese physician is taking the pulse of the patient while his boy stands ready with the box of acupuncture needles, moxa and drugs. A stove for their concoction is seen in the foreground. The picture illustrates well the close link between sphygmology and acupuncture.

tenance). Thus the Yin component was partly a permanent *hsüeh chhi*[1] (blood *chhi*), inherited from the maternal parent, and partly an ever-renewed *ying chhi*[2] (or *mo chhi*[3]), i.e. what we might call an intravascular nutritive Yin component.[a] Again it is rather remarkable that the ancient Chinese medical physiologists, destined never to know anything about amino-acids or monosaccharides, should nevertheless have thought out an internal nutritional concept quite resembling in principle that of the *Bausteine* of the German biochemists of the beginning of the twentieth century. On the other hand the Yang component was partly a permanent *ching chhi*[4] (seminal *chhi*),[b] inherited from the paternal parent,[c] and partly an ever-renewed *wei chhi*,[5] i.e. what we might call an extravascular protective Yang component.[d] This too was in no wise contradictory with modern knowledge, since the nutritive molecules certainly have to leave the blood-vessels at some point, and pass through the lymphatic and intercellular fluids to reach their destination in the cytoplasm of the living cells.[e] With all these ideas in mind we shall be able to appreciate fully the demonstrative quotations which follow. What the old Chinese physicians were essentially saying was, in our language, that under normal conditions of health, all parts of the body are supplied with the essential constituents to replace metabolic loss and effect bodily repair by means of a circulation of *chhi*; if anything interferes with the free flow of this, illness will result, but acupuncture and moxibustion can restore the normal situation.[f] As the *Ling Shu* says:[g]

Whether a man goes on living in health, or whether a disease arises; whether it is in human power to control it, and whether the patient can be cured; whether one is only at the beginning of the study of acupuncture (and moxibustion), or whether one has come to the fullness of it—all depends on (an understanding of the functions of) the twelve-tract network system of Yang and Yin channels (*ching mo*[6]). To the slap-dash practitioner or the tyro it all seems very easy; only the great physician knows how difficult it really is.

And in another place it speaks very clearly of the system:[h]

The function of the tract-channel network system (*ching mo*,[6] of the human body) is to

[a] The word *ying* here means not camp or barracks but rather constructional, supplying, furnishing. If a modern coined word should be convenient, one could call it 'endo-trophic' *chhi*. For Porkert (1), pp. 27, 170, 188–9, *ying chhi* is of course another form of energy, 'the structive aspect of indeterminate physiological energy'; essentially metabolic in character—as we would agree.

[b] We appreciate the unsatisfactory character of this rough and ready translation, but doubt whether Porkert's 'free usable unattached structive potential energy', (1), pp. 27, 169, 176, 178–9, (2), expresses the thought of the ancient medical philosophers any more justifiably.

[c] On the ancient doctrine, so widespread, that 'the father sows the white, and the mother sows the red' see Needham (2), pp. 24 ff., 60. Parts of the body were called 'spermatical' or 'sanguineous' according to their colour and their presumed origin. We discuss certain Chinese parallels in *SCC*, Vol. 5, pt. 5.

[d] The word *wei* here certainly means guarding or protective, 'exo-phylacteric' *chhi*, as one might say, and in the light of what we know about the susceptibility of ill-nourished tissues to infection and attack, the thought was by no means far-fetched. Porkert (1), p. 170, is content with 'defensive energy', but as usual we feel uneasy at confining the meaning wholly to energetics.

[e] Classical passages on the circulation of the endo-trophic and exo-phylacteric *chhi* are: *NCLS/PH*, ch. 18, (pp. 192 ff.), *NCLS/MC* (pp. 1077 ff.).

[f] Cf. the presentation of Wu I-Chhing (*2*), repr. in Chhêng Tan-An (*3*), p. 32.

[g] *NCLS/PH*, ch. 11, (p. 149), tr. auct.

[h] *NCLS/PH*, ch. 47, (p. 340), tr. auct.

[1] 血氣 [2] 營氣 [3] 脉氣 [4] 精氣 [5] 衛氣 [6] 經脉

promote a normal passage (*hsing*,[1] i.e. circulation) of the blood and the *chhi*, so that the vital essentials derived from man's food can nourish (*ying*[2]) the Yin and Yang (viscera), sustain the muscles, sinews and bones, and lubricate the joints.

The *Su Wên* defines the blood-vessels as 'the habitation of the blood' (*fu mo chê hsüeh chih fu yeh*[3]).[a] And from the time of the *Ling Shu* onwards it is always said that 'the (Yin) *ying*[2] *chhi* travels within the blood-vessels (*mo*[4]), while the (Yang) *wei*[5] *chhi* travels outside them'.[b] At the same time the two *chhi* were regarded as intimately connected. Blood *chhi* and tract *chhi* have different names, says Chhi Po at one place in the *Ling Shu*, but they belong to the same category (*i ming thung lei*[6]).[c] Both are derived from the liquid and solid ingesta (*shui ku chih ching chhi yeh*[7]).[d] And the Ting commentary on the *Nan Ching* says that 'the flow of the blood is maintained by the *chhi*, and the motion of the *chhi* depends on the blood, thus coursing in mutual reliance they move round (*hsüeh liu chü chhi, chhi tung i hsüeh, hsiang phing erh hsing*[8])'.[e]

Now for the statements of the circulation. The *Ling Shu* says: 'What we call the vascular system (*mo*[9]) is like dykes and retaining-walls (forming a circle of tunnels) which control the path that is traversed by the *ying*[10] *chhi*, so that it cannot escape or find anywhere to leak away (*yung o ying chhi ling wu so pi*[11]).'[f] A commentary on this written by Wu Mao-Hsien[12] of the Ming (but earlier than +1586) adds: 'it means that the *ying*[2] *chhi* travels within the blood vessels round and round, day and night, meeting nothing to stop or oppose it (*chou yeh huan chuan, wu so wei ni*[13]), and that is what the blood vessels are'.[g] This is only the first of a number of instances of affirmations which historically could not have been derived from William Harvey's famous publication of +1628. But there is no need to quote from Ming texts, because seventeen centuries earlier we can find statements such as this in the *Su Wên*, where Chhi Po says that 'the flow in the tract and channel (network system, of the body) runs on and on, and never stops; a ceaseless movement in an annular circuit (*ching mo liu hsing pu chih, huan chou pu hsiu*[14])'.[h] Clearly the circulation of the blood and *chhi* was standard doctrine in the −2nd century, a situation contrasting rather remarkably with the long uncertainty in the Western world, with its ideas of air in the arteries, or a tidal ebb and flow of the blood.[i]

[a] *NCSW/PH*, ch. 17, (p. 91), *NCSW/WMC* (p. 160). If the status of a material liquid such as one can study in a laboratory test-tube is denied to *hsüeh*, it is impossible to make sense of ancient Chinese thought on the circulation. Yet this is what Porkert (1), pp. 27, 185, does. For him, *hsüeh* is 'individually specific structive energy', i.e. that form of energy in the body which responds to active energies by morphogenetic activity and physiological function.

[b] *NCLS/PH*, ch. 18, (p. 193), *NCLS/MC* (p. 1077), parallel passages in *NCLS/PH*, ch. 10, (p. 139), ch. 52, (p. 375). Cf. also *Nan Ching Chi Chu*, Nan no. 30, pp. 27*b* ff., and *Lei Ching*, ch. 8, (p. 192.2).

[c] *NCLS/PH*, ch. 18, (p. 198), *NCLS/MC* (p. 1088). On the conception of categories, cf. *SCC*, Vol. 5, pt. 4, pp. 305 ff.

[d] *NCLS/PH*, ch. 32, (p. 237), *NCLS/MC* (p. 1152). Cf. *Lei Ching*, ch. 29, (p. 703.1).

[e] *NCCC*, Nan no. 30, p. 28*a*.

[f] *NCLS/PH*, ch. 30, (pp. 267–8).

[g] *NCLS/MC*, ch. 30, (p. 1153); cf. Wang Ping's commentary in *NCSW/WMC*, ch. 23, (p. 251).

[h] *NCSW/PH*, ch. 39, (p. 212), *NCSW/WMC* (p. 359).

[i] Cf. Singer (25).

1 行 2 營 3 夫脉者血之府也 4 脉 5 衛 6 異名仝類
7 水穀之精氣也 8 血流據氣氣動依血相憑而行 9 脉 10 營
11 壅遏營氣令無所避 12 吳懋先 13 晝夜環轉無所違逆 14 經脉流行不止環周不休

The more detailed theory of the circulation may be well seen in a passage in the *Nan Ching*, and the commentaries upon it. This text says:[a]

The *ying*[1] (or *jung*[2])[b] *chhi* runs within the blood vessels, while the *wei*[3] *chhi* travels outside them (in the tracts). The *ying chhi* circulates endlessly, never coming to a stop (save at death). After fifty revolutions the two *chhi* meet again, and this is called a 'great meeting' (*ta hui*[4]). The Yin and Yang *chhi* go along with each other in close relation (*hsiang kuan*[5]), travelling in circular paths which have no end (*ju huan wu tuan*[6]). So one can see how the *ying* and the *wei* mutually follow one another.[c]

Yü's commentary on this explains that the 50 revolutions take place during each day and night of 12 double-hours or 100 quarters.[d] This the *Ling Shu* had already stated,[e] pointing out that it corresponded both with the time taken by the sun to traverse the round of 28 lunar mansions,[f] and with 13,500 respiratory cycles of inspiration and expiration.[g] Rough measurements of the lengths of the tracts and principal blood-vessels gave a length of 162 ft. as the distance to be traversed on the complete cycle,[h] so that the circulation repeated fifty times gave a total distance of 8,100 ft. (810 *chang*[7]),[i] and the blood and *chhi* must move onward just 6 in. during each individual respiration.[j] As for the 'great meeting', it was considered to take place at the *tshun khou*[8] position, i.e. one of the three places where the pulse was felt at the wrist. How tenaciously these figures were adhered to between the −1st and the +16th centuries may be seen from a book such as the *Hsün Ching Khao Hsüeh Phien*[9] (An Investigation of the Acu-points along the Tracts) which reproduces all of them precisely.[k] Since this was composed in +1575 one sees again how impossible it was that the Harveian discoveries could have had any influence on this classical Chinese tradition.

What then was the position of the heart in that system? It was summed up in the pregnant phrase, *hsin chu mo*,[10] 'the heart controls the blood-vessels'. 'The heart presides', says the *Su Wên*, 'over the circulation of the blood and juices (*hsüeh i*[11]), and the paths on which they travel.'[l] Wang Ping, commenting, repeats: 'The heart controls the blood-vessels, confining the *ying chhi* (in its circular course), and the speed of its movement corresponds with the rate of breathing.'[m] Chang Chieh-Pin, commenting further, says: 'The heart rules over the circulation of the blood and the pulse which it exhibits. In accordance with the motive power of the element Fire, it

[a] *NCCC*, Nan no. 30, pp. 27*b* ff., tr. auct.

[b] The commentators explain that *ying* is called *jung* when actually in transit.

[c] This text is closely similar to that in *NCLS/PH*, ch. 18, (p. 193), with parallel passages in ch. 10, (p. 139), ch. 52, (p. 375). Cf. *NCLS/MC*, ch. 18, (p. 1077).

[d] On the Chinese horary system see *SCC*, Vol. 4, pt. 2, pp. 439–40; and Needham, Wang & Price (1), pp. 199 ff.

[e] See *NCLS/PH*, ch. 15, (pp. 182 ff.), with parallel passage in ch. 17, (p. 192). Cf. *NCLS/MC*, ch. 15, (pp. 1068 ff.).

[f] Cf. *SCC*, Vol. 3, pp. 233 ff.

[g] Cf. *SCC*, Vol. 5, pt. 5.

[h] *NC*, Nan no. 23, p. 27, *NC/PH*, p. 44.

[i] Just over a mile and a half.

[j] *CIC*, ch. 9, (p. 13).

[k] Ch. 1, (pp. 11–12).

[l] This occurs in a list of 'controllers', *NCSW/PH*, ch. 23, (p. 145), also ch. 44, (p. 239).

[m] *NCSW/WMC*, ch. 23, (p. 251).

1 營 2 榮 3 衛 4 大會 5 相貫 6 如環無端
7 丈 8 寸口 9 循經考穴編 10 心主脈 11 血液

sends the blood to all parts of the body.'[a] We also find it said in the *Su Wên*: 'Asthma (*chia*[1]) will occur if there is no drumming in the vessel of the heart',[b] on which Wang Ping comments that 'if there is no working of the bellows (lit. drumming, *ku*[2]) then the blood will not flow round'. It seems likely, in view of all that has so far been said, that the heart must have been thought of through the centuries as a pump of some kind, working in systole to propel the blood through its system of tubes, and we can find at least one clear analogy with a forge-bellows in pre-Harveian times. For in the *Lei Ching*, Chang Chieh-Pin wrote: 'The heart and pulse (*mo*[3]) is not itself either *chhi* or blood (*hsüeh*[4]), but rather it is the bellows of the *chhi* and the *hsüeh* (*chhi yu chhi hsüeh chih tho-yo yeh*[5]).'[c] Since Chang was born in +1563, and brought out his compendium of medical physiology four years before the *De Motu Cordis*, it is evidently implausible to assume any influence of European ideas upon him, especially as the Harveian discovery had a long and uphill way still to go before gaining general acceptance.[d] Besides, he repeated his statement several times in his writings, so that it may have been first made as early as +1593. One can take note, too, of another pre-Harveian statement of the same period, the interesting words which Juan Thai-Yuan[6] used in the preface to the fourth edition of Matteo Ricci's world-map (+1603). 'I had the dim perception', he said, 'that the earth is fixed and the air in motion, the water circulating with the air, somewhat as the blood and *chhi* ceaselessly circulate unresting in the human body.'[e] It is a little unusual to find Chinese scientific thinking in advance of European as late as this (in contrast with earlier periods such as the Thang and Sung), but here there seems to be a particularly good case of it. However, we are concerned now to sketch only so much of circulation-theory as is indispensable for the study of acupuncture.

One point remains, nevertheless. Since the ancient, medieval and traditional Chinese thought in terms of two circulations rather than one, what organ did they take as responsible for the pumping of the *chhi*? There is a straightforward answer, the lungs. Sometimes this appears implicitly, sometimes explicitly. For example, Chhi Po says in one place: 'The heart (in the body) is like the monarch (in the State), fount of all clarity and brightness; the lungs are like the prime minister, from whom all control proceeds.'[f] Or again: 'All the blood pertains (*shu*[7]) to the heart; all the *chhi* pertains to the lungs.'[g] But Chang Chieh-Pin wrote: 'The (Yin) *chhi* within the

[a] *Lei Ching*, ch. 15, (p. 314.2). Closely similar ideas can be found in European physiology of the +16th and +17th centuries. M. A. Severino wrote that 'the heart is therefore analogous with fire, and is nourished by the air...' (*Antiperipatias*, +1659), cit. Schmitt & Webster (1), p. 63.

[b] *NCSW/WMC*, ch. 48, (p. 430). 'To drum' (*ku*) or 'drum and blow' (*ku chhui*) were standard classical verb forms for the operation of bellows, whether for metallurgical or other purposes (cf. Needham (32), p. 3, and *SCC*, Vol. 4, pt. 2, p. 139), probably because the most ancient types of bellows were rather like drums (cf. Forbes (7), p. 578).

[c] Ch. 8 (p. 192.2), auth. comm. On this technical term for bellows and pumps see *SCC*, Vol. 4, pt. 2, pp. 137ff. *Tho-yo* means literally bellows-and-tuyère. See also *Ching-Yo Chhüan Shu*, ch. 2, (p. 45.2), i.e. *Chhuan Chung Lu*, ch. 18.

[d] Cf. Bayon (1).

[e] See d'Elia (15), p. 142. *Ju jen shen hsüeh chhi chou liu chih wu chih hsi.*[8]

[f] *NCSW/PH*, ch. 8, (p. 51). [g] *NCSW/PH*, ch. 10, (p. 64).

1 瘕 2 鼓 3 脈 4 血 5 其猶氣血之橐籥也 6 阮泰元
7 屬 8 如人身血氣周流之無止息

channels (the vessels) flows on into the tracts, and the (Yang) *chhi* within the tracts all returns to the lungs. Indeed the hundred (tracts and) channels pay court to the lungs.'[a] This was classical doctrine, for Chang Chih-Tshung in the Sung, commenting on the *Su Wên*, affirmed that all the *chhi*, after each circulation, returns and meets at the lungs.[b] In modern terms, this theory was not so very absurd, for the lungs are, like the heart, an innervated pump, and they do ensure the exchange of vital gases with the blood-stream, even though the *Nei Ching* writers knew nothing of oxygen and carbon dioxide. Where this ancient physiology diverged from the modern was in the conception of two parallel circulations, one anatomically demonstrable, the other not. Nevertheless, all the medical texts, both classical and medieval, clearly recognised that the lungs exhaled useless *chhi*, taking in the *chhi* of the atmosphere (*thien chhi*[1]);[c] and they also closely associated, as we have just seen (p. 30), the blood circulation cycle with the respiratory cycles.

Having said this much of the Chinese ideas of the circulation which underlay the practice of acupuncture, it is unavoidable to take a glance at how they compare with those modern conceptions of blood circulation which came to a head in the work of William Harvey and developed subsequently to him. We treat this subject more extensively in Sect. 43 on physiology,[d] but here in as many paragraphs we feel bound to deal with four aspects of it: (*a*) the quantitative approach and the speed of the circulation, (*b*) the concept of the heart as a pump, (*c*) the role of the macrocosmic analogy, and (*d*) possible mutual influences and transmissions.

It is easy to calculate that on the classical Chinese estimate of 50 complete circulations in our 24 hours, each revolution of the blood stream would take 28·8 mins. In the light of modern knowledge this was about 60 times too slow, for the actual circulation time is only 30 secs.[e] However, Harvey himself never succeeded in attaining that figure, a product of relatively recent research.[f] On the same page of the *De Motu Cordis* as he reached the acme of his argument about the quantitative impossibility of the heart ejecting so much blood in a given time unless the blood returned to it through invisible channels, he added:[g]

> But let it be said that this does not take place in half an hour, but in an hour, or even in a day; in any case it is still manifest that more blood passes through the heart in consequence of its action than can either be supplied by the whole of the ingesta, or than can be contained in the veins at the same moment.

As Peller (1) urged, one can to some extent draw a dividing line between Harvey's quantification and all that had gone before, but his emphasis was on quantitative

[a] *Lei Ching*, ch. 3, (p. 61.1), ch. 29, (p. 687.1). This was based on *NCSW/PH*, ch. 21, (p. 130).

[b] *NCSW/WMC*, ch. 21, (pp. 227ff.).

[c] This is evident in the sub-section on the Taoist respiratory exercises in *SCC*, Vol. 5, pt. 5.

[d] Considering, for example, the question whether the Han physiologists fully recognised the distinction between arterial and venous blood.

[e] Starling (1), p. 770; cf. Samson Wright (1), pp. 407–8.

[f] It would be too much to ask of the ancient and medieval Chinese physiologists that they should have made the rather difficult measurements required, when even Harvey himself was content with relatively few, and relied more on quantitative reasoning.

[g] Ch. 9 (facsim. ed., tr. p. 52).

1 天氣

reasoning backed only by some measurements, and he remained indelibly Aristotelian, giving much weight to analogies of the universal macrocosmic–microcosmic type.[a]

It is worth pausing here a moment to compare the data which would have been available to the *Nei Ching* writers on the one hand and to William Harvey on the other. In ancient China they could easily relate the heart-beat to time, by the aid of delicate water-clock measurements,[b] and by the same token they could also give the respiratory frequency of inspiration and expiration in terms of time.[c] Moreover, they made measurements at an early date of the approximate lengths of the great blood-vessels, so that they could form an estimate of the length of course to be run.[d] Lastly they must have been quite familiar with the rhythmic spurting of blood from a severed artery, and since they were predisposed on general philosophical and cosmological grounds to accept the idea of a circulation, they must have assumed that somehow or other in the intact body the blood seeped back to the veins and the heart. Of course they offered to posterity no experimental evidence in the Renaissance manner, they simply stated their estimated conclusions about circulation-time as part of a general medical doctrine. Harvey, for his part, was impressed basically by two things, first the anti-regurgitation valves in the veins, a piece of information which had probably escaped the Chinese anatomists in all ages; and secondly the quantitatively measured amounts of blood sent forth by the heart, which showed without question that in the living body it must get back to the heart somehow. What is so incredible about the European experience is how long it took before the circulation was understood and accepted.

Secondly we have to consider the heart as a pump or bellows, like a forge-bellows, as in Chang Chieh-Pin's words of +1624. References to this analogy in Harvey's writings are few, as Pagel (21) has pointed out. The earliest is the famous description: 'as by two clacks of a water-bellows to raise water'; but it is not contemporary with the MS of the Lumleian Lectures in which it appears (+1616), rather a later insertion probably made not before +1628.[e] The next is in the Epitome of Harvey's 'Anatomical Observations' written about +1640, where he wrote that 'the panting of the heart is but the pumping about of the blood, in the expansion receiving, and in the contraction sending it out'.[f] The third is in the 2nd Letter to Joh. Riolanus, dating from as late as +1649.[g] Basalla (1) and Webster (2) have taken some trouble to ascertain exactly what sort of water-pump Harvey probably had in mind,[h] and

a Cf. Pagel (20); Jevons (1).

b On the 'stop-watch clepsydra' see *SCC*, Vol. 3, pp. 318, 326–7.

c On the measurement of respiration-rate among Taoist adepts in physiological alchemy, see *SCC*, Vol. 5, pt. 5.

d This quantitative concern for weights and dimensions was very characteristic of ancient Chinese anatomy; cf. Sect. 43.

e *Praelectiones Anatomiae Universalis*, fol. 80v, tr. Whitteridge (1), p. 273; cf. also the translation by O'Malley, Poynter & Russell (1).

f This work, in 34 aphorisms, was reported to the Royal Society in +1687.

g *Exercitatio Anatomica de Circulatione Sanguinis*.

h Cuneate collapsible leather-sided bellows were rarely used for pumping water, either in China or the West, but Basalla found an illustration of one in a +1511 German translation of Vegetius, 'Vier Bucher der Rytterschaft'. See Ewbank (1), p. 207. Chang Chieh-Pin would probably have been thinking of the box-bellows or piston-bellows, cf. Needham (64), pp. 155ff.

it seems likely to have been a contractile cylinder with corrugated leather sides, used widely as a fire-engine in the +17th century.[a] Nevertheless it remains the case that pending further evidence the earliest reference to the heart as a pump is by a hairsbreadth Chinese.[b]

The pump conception was a mechanistic one, but it is generally agreed, following the sustained expositions of Walter Pagel, that Harvey is not explicable without his 'dark side', that complex of cosmological ideas which partook of the nature of the Neo-Platonism, Hermetism and natural magic typical of Renaissance proto-scientific thinkers.[c] Harvey was a faithful Aristotelian, therefore he inherited the idea of the peculiar excellence of the circle as such which had so much inspired Giordano Bruno,[d] and he took the macrocosm–microcosm analogy seriously. There were revolutions, i.e. circulations, of the sun, moon, planets and fixed stars in the heavens, round some centre (whether the earth or the sun), there was the meteorological water cycle in the sublunary world, and there was the prince around whom everyone revolved in earthly States. Harvey's passages are well known, for example:[e]

> This movement we may be allowed to call circular, in the same way as Aristotle says that the air and the rain emulate the circular movement of the superior bodies; for the moist earth, warmed by the sun, evaporates; the vapours drawn upwards are condensed, and descending in the form of rain, moisten the earth again...

And overleaf:[f]

> The heart, consequently, is the beginning of life, the sun of the microcosm, even as the sun in his turn might well be designated the heart of the world; for it is the heart by whose virtue and pulse the blood is moved, perfected and made nutrient, and is preserved from corruption and coagulation; it is the household divinity which, discharging its function, nourishes, cherishes, quickens the whole body, and is indeed the foundation of life, the source of all action.[g]

And again, towards the end of his book:[h]

> ...and as the prince in a kingdom, in whose hands lies the chief and highest authority, rules over all, the heart is the source and foundation from which all strength is derived, and on which all strength depends in the animal body.

If we compare these statements with those of the Chinese writers of the Ming and Chhing given in the preceding pages we are conscious of a considerable similarity. The chief difference is that the Chinese writers had behind them a steady tradition of

[a] An illustration is to be found in Bate (1), +1654 ed., p. 16.

[b] We mean, of course, in the context of a general circulation. Galen already had made a comparison between the heart and the forge bellows (*De Usu Partium*, VI, 15, Daremberg tr., vol. 1, p. 434), but only to cause the tides in the vascular system. Cf. Pagel (26), p. 212.

[c] See especially (1, 4, 6, 24, 25). Here Robert Fludd's quick support for Harvey is of special interest, cf. (1), pp. 277–8, (24), pp. 25 ff.

[d] Pagel (9).

[e] *De Motu Cordis*, ch. 8 (facsim. ed., tr. p. 49).

[f] *Ibid.*, p. 50.

[g] Reading between the lines of both these passages one can sense a feature characteristic of both Cesalpino and Harvey, but not well understood until Pagel (19) expounded it, namely that by *circulatio* they both had in mind not only the *destillatio* of the chemists, but even reflux distillation, as well as the purely hydrodynamic circulation. Hence the complexes of ideas about heating and cooling, blood regeneration, etc.

[h] *Ibid.* ch. 17 (tr. p. 88).

blood and *chhi* circulation going back at least to the −2nd century. Pagel (25) has studied the earliest European intimations of this, beginning with Plato himself, but the statements are never anything like so clear and explicit as those of the Chinese texts. Nevertheless, by the latter part of the Ming, towards the end of the +16th century, there were leading intellectual figures in Europe who were asserting the circulation, well prior to Harvey's proofs. Giordano Bruno, for instance, in +1590, said it in so many words;[a] and he took the blood to be a kind of material vector for 'air' and 'spirit'—strangely recalling the Yin *chhi* carried along with the blood, if we did not know of the dominance of the Galenic theory of 'spirits' in the West.[b] In the following year, Bruno again mentioned the *circumcursare et recursare* of the blood and humours, which he said paralleled the meteorological water cycle.[c] And in another writing of the same date he anticipated Harvey's parallel of the heart with the sun in the macrocosm.[d]

Lastly, Bruno is considered by Pagel as a link of much importance between Andrea Cesalpino and Harvey. Cesalpino in +1571 was the first of the anatomists to use the word *circulatio*, and as is well known, he described more or less correctly the pulmonary circulation.[e] But here he had been preceded by several others, notably Realdo Colombo in +1559 and Michael Servetus in +1546. Even more extraordinary, he had been preceded by the Damascus physician Ibn al-Qarashī al-Nafīs (d. +1288).[f] Ever since the first discovery of the relevant Arabic text by al-Tatawi (1) in 1924 there has been controversy as to whether or not this Arabic knowledge could have been transmitted to Harvey's +16th-century precursors,[g] but the weight of evidence that has now become available indicates that there was indeed a transmission, not only of the idea but of the arguments used to support it.[h] What is more, al-Nafīs may have had more than an inkling of the general circulation itself, for he spoke of the aorta as the great vessel that circulates the animal spirits to all the organs of the body. Both the statement itself and its expression in terms of what we should call *chhi* (animal spirit), invite the question (or is it but a wild surmise?) as to whether Ibn al-Nafīs and his contemporaries in the Arabic world could have been influenced by Chinese medical physiology.[i] We have found nothing to suggest this in any of the

[a] In the *De Rerum Principiis et Elementis et Causis*; for the references see Pagel (9), who fully examined the position of Bruno and his relation to other thinkers, anatomists and experimenters.

[b] The exact relationship of Galenic 'spirits', natural (or vital), and animal, to the *chhi* of traditional Chinese physiology, remains a subject for serious concern. Cf. Sect. 43.

[c] In *De Innumerabilibus, Immenso et Infigurabili, seu de Universo et Mundis*, pp. 524–5 (bk. 6, ch. 8); cf. D. Singer (1), p. 154.

[d] In *De Monade, Numero et Figure*, p. 22 (ch. 2). Cf. Pagel (9).

[e] For excellent accounts of the development of knowledge of the circulation before Harvey's decisive break-through, one may consult Foster (1), pp. 22ff., 27ff.; Cohn (1); Bayon (1, 2, 3) and Pagel (23, 24, 26).

[f] Cf. *SCC*, Vol. 4, pt. 1, p. xxvii.

[g] Temkin (2) was extremely sceptical, and Meyerhof (1, 2) with Haddad & Khairallah (1) uncertain, though very informative on the Arabic side, but in 1956 O'Malley (1) found a Latin translation of some of al-Nafīs' writings dating from +1547.

[h] See Bittar (1); Coppola (1) and especially Schacht (1). One of the intermediaries has now been identified as Andrea Alpago, a Venetian consul-general resident in the Levant for many years, and an accomplished oriental scholar.

[i] We are not, we find, the first to propose such an influence, for Li Thao (*14*), p. 111, impressed by the dominance of Avicenna's pulse-lore in European medical schools such as Montpellier down to

pages of translations of his writings so far accessible, but it is established that Ibn Sīnā in the previous century was so influenced, especially in the sphygmology of his *Qānūn fi' al-Ṭibb*; and in our studies of the spread of alchemical thought and practice we found abundant evidence of transmissions from China to the Arabic world.[a] Here we must leave the question, however, and return to the exposition of acupuncture and its theoretical background.

Before doing this, let us just spare a thought for the suspicion which grew up in Europe in the second half of the +17th century that indeed the circulation of the blood had been understood in China long before William Harvey. It was voiced by a number of writers responding to echoes from the *Nei Ching* transmitted through Jesuit and other channels, and a full account of it would be interesting reading if some specialist on European reactions to China in those times would collect all the literary materials. Here it may suffice to take two or three representative examples.

Perhaps one of the first was Isaac Vossius in his *De Artibus et Scientiis Sinarum* of +1685, often quoted elsewhere in our volumes.[b] That the blood circulated round the body had been known in China, he said, for more than 4000 years.[c] Rumours of this had come from Venetian merchants and Jesuit fathers, but now the most important texts had become available in translation.[d] As he recalled, Andrea Cesalpino had been the first to write of it in the West, and Paolo Sarpi had approved, then an Englishman devoted a book to it, but finding no support suppressed it; finally William Harvey brought it all to light. But none of them knew that the motion of the blood had been appreciated so long before in China.[e]

The passing of the last months of the century found Thomas Baker, non-juring Fellow of St John's in Cambridge,[f] writing there his 'Reflections upon Learning, wherein is shewn the Insufficiency thereof...' etc. This was a book designed to emphasise the inadequacy of rational science, and indeed human understanding itself, in the interests of revealed religion. In the chapter on medicine Baker sought to show how speculative and uncertain all biology and physiology were, and how everyone disagreed—the Galenists, the chymists, the Chinese.

Some have gone as far as China [he wrote] to find out (the Perfect Man); of which People's Skill such Wonders have been reported, as the Chymists themselves can hardly pretend to.

a late date, though not mentioning al-Nafīs, felt that on this account there was a strongly Chinees background to the discovery of William Harvey.

---

[a] *SCC*, Vol. 5, pt. 4, pp. 323 ff.

[b] Vos (1); *Variarum Observationum Liber*. Cf. e.g. *SCC*, Vol. 4, pt. 3, pp. 417–18, 666; and in Vols. 3 and 4, pt. 2, *passim*.

[c] Pp. 71–2. He was of course taking the legendary date of Huang Ti. But some two thousand years would have been right enough.

[d] That Vossius had access to a good translation is shown by the fact that he gave the exact figures which occur in the ancient Chinese numerical computations (p. 30 above).

[e] Naturally Vossius gave a long paragraph to the sphygmology of the Chinese, which he said surpassed by much that of the Greeks and Christians. Progress had been very slow until they came across the writings of Avicenna, and Vossius actually said that he in his turn had got his pulse-lore from the Chinese of Cathaya Nigra, i.e. Qarā-Kiṭāi or Western Liao, which neighboured upon Ibn Sina's own birthplace. How right Vossius was in this remarkable guess we shall see in *SCC*, Vol. 6. Cf. Vol. 4, pt. 1, p. 332.

[f] +1656 to +1740.

The Circulation of the Blood, which with us is a modern Discovery, has been known there, according to Vossius, four thousand years; they have such Skill in Pulses as is not to be imagin'd, but by those that are acquainted with them; and the Arabians are there said, to have borrow'd thence their knowledge in Physick. Even the missionaries, who have reason to know them best, grant, that there is somewhat surprising in their Skill of Pulses, (and) tell us that they have made Observation in Medicine 4000 Years, and that when all the Books in China were order'd to be burnt by the Emperor Chiohamti, those in Physick were preserv'd by a particular Exception.[a]

But then he goes on to disparage the practical uses which the Chinese made of their inventions, and concludes that 'the most considerable Improvements are probably to be found at Home', yet subject always to bewildering controversies among the various schools.

Finally, the Spanish Benedictine humanist Benito Geronimo Feyjoo y Montenegro[b] averred in his 'Teatro Critico Universal',[c] published a few years later, that the Chinese 'in the region of King Hoamti four centuries before the Flood' knew the circulation of the blood, and the diagnosis of diseases by careful observations of the pulse. Ever since then similar statements have been made, with varying degrees of verisimilitude. The preceding paragraphs will now have shown, we hope, that as so often the real answer is 'yes, but not exactly'.

All these asseverations were of course derivative, and it may be that we ought to have given pride of place here to Willem ten Rhijne, the Dutch East India physician who in the same year as Vossius' publication, +1685, first brought acupuncture to the knowledge of the Western world, though he had known it only in Japan.[d] In his *Mantissa Schematica de Acupunctura* he wrote:

Although the Chinese physicians (who are the forerunners from whom the physicians of the Japanese borrowed these systems of healing) are ignorant in anatomy, they have nevertheless perhaps devoted more effort over many centuries to learning and teaching with very great care the circulation of the blood, than have European physicians, individually or as a group. They base the foundation of their entire medicine upon the rules of this circulation, as if they were oracles of Apollo at Delphi.

They do not expound the rites of their art (to which they do not indiscriminately admit anyone) with honeyed words or ambiguous comparisons, nor do they obscure them with contrived and controversial nonsense, but use mechanical devices to clarify doctrinal analogy. Thus among the Chinese the masters employ hydraulic machines to demonstrate the circulation of the blood to their disciples who have earned the title of physician; and in the absence of such machines the masters assist understanding with clear figures—ever paying chief honour to the authority of antiquity. The various movements of the blood must be learned through precepts and rules as laid down by the Chinese (and I promise, God willing, to present examples of these elsewhere) if a cure is to be undertaken according to their regimen...[e]

[a] Ch. 15, pp. 217–18 (+1714 ed.).

[b] +1676 to +1764.

[c] First published in eight volumes between +1726 and +1739. The passage is also in the Madrid edition of +1773, p. 315. We are much indebted to the late Dr Dorothea Singer for telling us of this in Feb. 1943.

[d] We discuss his work more fully on pp. 271 ff. below.

[e] Carrubba & Bowers tr. (1), p. 375.

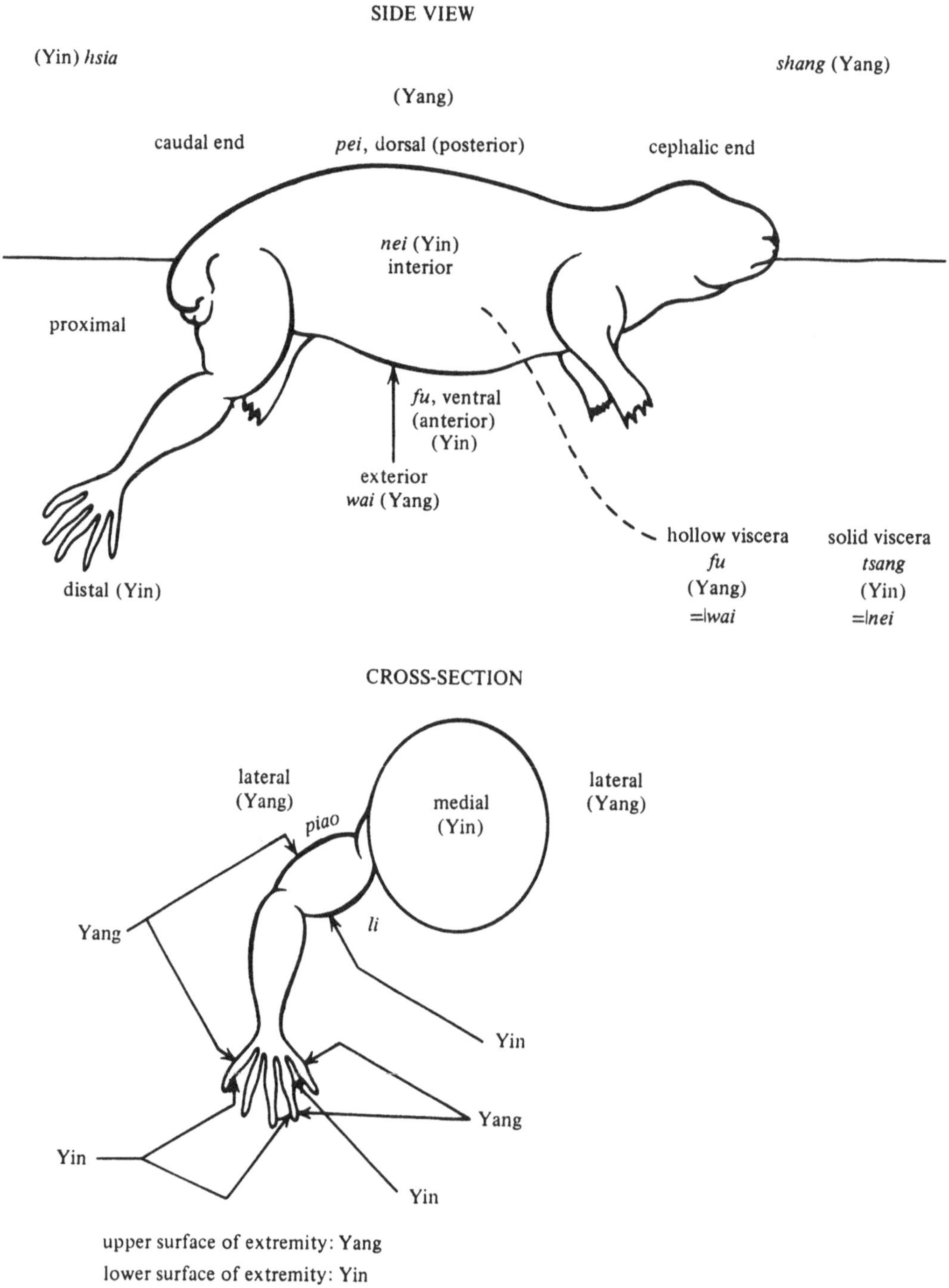

Fig. 9. Chinese usages of thought about Yin and Yang, inner and outer, above and below, etc., in relation to the mammalian body. Orig. drawing.

This is very intriguing. What visions does it not conjure up of Ming and Chhing medical teachers demonstrating the action of the heart with working models of double-acting piston bellows[a] or square-pallet chain-pumps,[b] with bamboo tubing cut to represent the lengths of the main vessels.[c] Of course ten Rhijne may have been thinking simply of the bronze acupuncture figures filled with water, and the wax covering which tested the accuracy of the student's choice of acu-point.[d] In any case the glimpse we get of demonstrations in Chinese medical teaching is a fascinating one.

(ii) *The tracts* (ching), *regular and auxiliary*

Since the tracts, like the viscera, were (and still are) sharply divided into Yang and Yin categories, we must pause here before going further to explain some of the standard usages of thought about the mammalian body, including that of man (Fig. 9). Cephalic, proximal and lateral directions were Yang; caudal, distal and medial directions were Yin. The dorsal or posterior regions (*pei*[1]) were Yang, the ventral or anterior regions (*fu*[2]) were Yin. Naturally the contents of the trunk was 'inner' (*nei*[3]) and Yin, while the exterior of the body was *wai*[4] and Yang; but as we know, the viscera were divided into five *fu*[5],[e] which were Yang,[f] and five *tsang*[6],[g] which were Yin.[h] These corresponded with the five elements, but from an early date a system of six *chhi*[7] became dominant in medical thought.[i] Hence in all medical literature there are two Fire elements, *chün huo*[8] (or simply *huo*), and *hsiang huo*[9].[j]

[a] See *SCC*, Vol. 4, pt. 2, pp. 135 ff. Chang Chieh-Pin's analogy is to be remembered.

[b] Vol. 4, pt. 2, pp. 339 ff. It may not be without significance that the Taoist anatomy and physiology embodied in the Nei Ching Thu diagrams always includes a square-pallet chain-pump. On this see Vol. 5, pt. 5.

[c] They had of course been measured with bamboo rods, as the texts say. If the force-pump for liquids had not been part of the indigenous Chinese engineering traditions (Vol. 4, pt. 2, pp. 142 ff.) generally speaking, certain forms of it were; and in any case European designs in this field were becoming available by +1600.

[d] See pp. 131, 135 below.

[e] The semantics of this term, deriving from 'palace' or 'official building', relate to the idea of transmission. Porkert (1), p. 26, reflecting the etymology has *orbes aulici*, from 'halls of audience', which we could only accept in the form of 'aulic organs' (cf. aulic counsellors), though we generally prefer not to give a translated equivalent.

[f] The large intestine (*ta chhang*[10]), stomach (*wei*[11]), small intestine (*hsiao chhang*[12]), bladder (*phang-kuang*[13]), and the gall-bladder (*tan*[14]). Mainly, therefore, hollow viscera, the function of which was the reception and absorption of food, with the transmission and excretion of waste. See *NCSW/PH*, ch. 11, (p. 69); *NCSW/WMC*, ch. 11, (p. 127).

[g] The semantics of this term, deriving from 'treasury', relate to the idea of storage. Porkert (1), pp. 26, 107, has *orbes horreales*, from 'granary', admissible as 'horreal organs', but again we prefer to leave the word untranslated.

[h] The lungs (*fei*[15]), spleen or lieno-pancreas (*phi*[16]), the heart (*hsin*[17]), the reins or reno-seminal system (*shen*[18]), and the liver (*kan*[19]). Mainly, therefore, seemingly solid viscera, the function of which was the storage of essential life-constituents (*ching chhi*[20]). See *NCSW*, *loc. cit.*

[i] Cf. Needham & Lu Gwei-Djen (8), repr. in Needham (64), pp. 265, 267.

[j] We came across both of these long ago, in *SCC*, Vol. 4, pt. 1, p. 65, but it was not opportune at that stage to examine them more closely. *Chün* connotes 'princely' and *hsiang* 'ministerial'. Cf. the ancient Chinese pharmacodynamic classification of drugs, where a third class, 'adjutant', was added (Sect. 38 in Vol. 6).

1 背	2 腹	3 內	4 外	5 腑	6 臟	7 氣
8 君火	9 相火	10 大腸	11 胃	12 小腸	13 膀胱	14 膽
15 肺	16 脾	17 心	18 腎	19 肝	20 精氣	

For this reason the heart was given a 'pericardium' (*hsin pao lo*[1]), making a sixth *tsang*;[2] and, by the same token, there was added to the five *fu*[3] a *san chiao*[4] ('three coctive regions') in addition to the small intestine.[a] For example, the *Su Wên* says:[b]

Speaking of the Yin and Yang of man, the external surface is Yang and the interior is Yin. (But when) speaking of his body then his back is Yang and his chest and abdomen is Yin. Furthermore, when speaking of viscera or internal organs, the *tsang* (i.e. liver, heart, spleen, lungs and reins) are Yin, while the *fu* (i.e. gall-bladder, stomach, small and large intestines, and bladder) are Yang. So also the pericardium is Yin and the three coctive regions Yang. For this reason it is desirable to understand what is meant by 'the Yin within the Yin (or Yang)' and 'the Yang within the Yang (or Yin)'. Why is this? (For example), disorders of the reins in winter are considered Yin within Yin, while heart disorders in summer are considered Yang within Yang. But (one also finds) liver disorders in spring, and that is a case of Yang within Yin; or again lung disorders in autumn, which represent Yin within Yang. When treating the diseases of the four seasons with acupuncture one should always base the selection of the points to be used with the relevant organ in mind.

This was only natural because a little earlier the *Su Wên* says that if the *chhi* of the four seasons does not follow its normal course, the five viscera are subjected to harmful influences.[c] As for the Yang within the Yin, and the Yin within the Yang, the great importance which these conceptions could play is abundantly seen in the descriptions of physiological alchemy.[d]

Much of the spatial terminology was familiar to all educated Chinese, if at times confusedly. In July, 1877, the first ambassador to the United Kingdom paid a visit to St Paul's Cathedral in London, and the talk turned to the traditional seclusion of women in China among the gentry.[e] Kuo Sung-Thao said that it was only natural for Yang things to come out and Yin things to stay in, and he instanced the head as Yang, which could decently be uncovered, while the lower Yin parts could not. But he erred in saying that the chest was Yang and the back Yin, so that the former could be bared and the latter not.[f] Their English guide was non-plussed by all this, and Kuo wrote: 'On account of the Westerners' temperament, when we can find reasons to debate with them, the clearer we are the more they respect us. Otherwise they think they are right, and their pride increases.'

A significance primarily anatomical also attaches to the six most fundamental terms relevant to acupuncture theory, i.e. the Three Yin and the Three Yang (*san Yin, san Yang*[5]). Thus we have Thai-Yin,[6] Thai-Yang,[7] Shao-Yin,[8] Shao-Yang,[9] Chüeh-Yin[10] and Yang-Ming.[11] Although the first four of these were regarded as the *chhi* of the four seasons,[g] and although the terms might give too great an impression of some

[a] We refrain from saying more about these matters here, since the subject is discussed fully in Section 43 on physiology.

[b] *NCSW/PH*, ch. 4, (p. 24); *NCSW/WMC*, ch. 4, (pp. 38–9). Tr. auct.

[c] *NCSW/PH*, ch. 2, (p. 20), *NCSW/WMC*, ch. 2, (p. 32).

[d] *SCC*, Vol. 5, pt. 5.

[e] Frodsham (2), entry for 23 July 1877.

[f] Of course the chest would be Yang relative to the abdomen, but the back could only be Yin if very caudal, and possibly it was something like this that Kuo had in mind.

[g] *NCSW/PH*, ch. 2, (pp. 8 ff.); *NCSW/WMC*, ch. 2, (pp. 11 ff., 17).

1 心包絡 2 臟 3 腑 4 三焦 5 三陰三陽 6 太陰
7 太陽 8 少陰 9 少陽 10 厥陰 11 陽明

scale of quantity or intensity,[a] their use here is essentially based upon the spatial positions of the internal organs.[b] And as we shall soon see, the six terms were and are used to denote each one of the six regular acu-tracts which have their beginnings or endings in the hand or foot respectively; and of course the visceral organs associated with them.

Continuing its definitions of parts and aspects of the body in Yin and Yang terms as just described, the *Su Wên* goes on[c] to imagine a man facing south so that the front of his body is sunlit, *kuang ming*,[1] i.e. Yang. Then the reins, at the lower part of the abdomen (Yin) will be associated with a tract called Shao-Yin (R),[d] while just above them (hence Yang to them) the bladder will be associated with a tract called Thai-Yang (VU), and this therefore is called a 'Yang within a Yin'. Similarly the upper part of the abdomen above the waist is also *kuang ming*,[1] i.e. Yang, and below it (hence Yin to it), the spleen will be associated with a tract called Thai-Yin (LP), while just in front of it (hence Yang to it) the stomach will be associated with a tract called Yang-Ming (V). This is again a 'Yang within a Yin' because the organs all occupy places in the interior and lower part of the body.[e] Each pair of tracts, moreover, is in a patefact-subdite (*piao li*[2]) relationship,[f] Thai-Yang and Yang-Ming being *piao* and Shao-Yin and Thai-Yin being *li*.[g] The system may seem arbitrary but its correlative linkages probably originated in the attempts of the ancient physicians to systematise their vast fund of clinical observations. Nor was there only a single scheme, for we shall find that the twelve regular tract names and the Three Yin and Three Yang terms were used in quite a different way in the *Shang Han Lun*[3] (Treatise on Febrile Diseases), and the literature which follows that tradition of treatment of pyrexia.

The oldest descriptions of regular tracts which we have are to be found in the *Ling Shu* of the *Huang Ti Nei Ching* (cf. the translations on pp. 93 ff. below). Anatomically oriented, they differentiate the acu-points and name many of them, grouping them out of the totality of points all over the surface of the body. One might see a parallel here with the identification of constellations from among the assembly of the stars. And just as the Chinese asterisms have almost nothing in common with the patterns which were seen by Westerners, so also nothing in any occidental physiological system, either ancient or modern, corresponds with the tracts of points on the body's surface. That of course does not deprive them of meaning, and we may well find that

[a] The Yin and Yang theory of ancient Chinese natural philosophy certainly always involved perpetual cyclic change. We saw this wave form long ago in Section 26 on physics (Fig. 277 on p. 9 of *SCC*, Vol. 4, pt. 1), and later we followed the thought of the alchemists on the subject in Section 33 on chemistry (Fig. 1515 in Vol. 5, pt. 4).

[b] It is interesting that in *NCSW/PH*, ch. 6, (pp. 41–2) Huang Ti asks why the medical use of the Yin–Yang concept in the *san Yin san Yang* theory differs from the ordinary cosmological usages of Yin and Yang. Chhi-Po goes on to explain, starting with the passage about the man facing south.

[c] *NCSW/PH*, ch. 6, (pp. 42 ff.).

[d] These standard letters will be explained immediately below, p. 44.

[e] For further details of this type of classification see *NCSW/PH*, ch. 4, (pp. 22 ff., esp. pp. 24–5).

[f] Cf. p. 46 below.

[g] *NCSW/PH*, ch. 5, (p. 32), ch. 6, (pp. 42 ff.).

[1] 光明 [2] 表裡 [3] 傷寒論

the tracts are in fact something like lines of equivalent physiological activity.[a] Thus we can see these physiological 'constellations' well established by the −1st century after what must have been a preparation several previous centuries long; and by the end of the +3rd the whole system was essentially complete.[b] The correlations with the viscera were established, and it was recognised that six of the regular tracts began or ended in the hands while six began or ended in the feet; three of each set being Yang and three Yin. Those which begin in the hand (Yang tracts) we designate as cheirogenic, and those which end there (Yin tracts) we call cheirotelic. Those which start from the foot (Yin tracts) we term podogenic, and those which end in the same extremity (Yang tracts) we refer to as podotelic. The other origins and terminations of all these are different also. The cheirogenic group terminates at the head, and the cheirotelic group originates in the chest region; while the podogenic group terminates at the abdominal region, and the podotelic group originates from the head.[c]

We are now in a position to look at the first table of the tracts (Table 1), where they are arranged in the Circulation Order.[d]

It needs a certain amount of explanation. The name of the tract and its translation is followed by the internationally accepted abbreviation,[e] with a note explaining the basis of this, and a letter differentiating the internal organs into the *fu*[1] group (Yang) and the *tsang*[2] group (Yin). At once it can be seen how this corresponds with the Yin or Yang character of the tracts themselves. The urino-genital system was not very clearly understood by the ancients, so we translate *shen*[3] in no. 8 as reno-seminal, and could well think of it as 'reins' as has been found convenient in translating texts of physiological alchemy in *SCC*, Vol. 5, pt. 5.[f] Then, as we have already seen, two out of the twelve internal organs are not among those recognised in modern physiology—the *hsin pao lo*[4] or 'pericardium' (but not exactly that structure as it is known in modern anatomy), and the *san chiao*[5] or 'three coctive regions'.[g] We shall not examine these more closely here, recalling only that they seem to have been necessitated by the very ancient sixfold medical classification as opposed to the philosophical system in which everything fitted into fives and groups of fives.[h] Now

[a] A somewhat similar thought is expressed by Mann (11), p. 38.

[b] This was the time when the *Chia I Ching* (cf. p. 119 below) set forth the corrleations between tracts and diseases; and in the *Shang Han Lun* the syndromes of different kinds of febrile diseases were referred to malfunctions of one or other of the regular tracts, six only however being used for this purpose (cf. p. 117 below).

[c] The Chinese titles themselves do not explicitly distinguish between the origins and terminations of the tracts, nor do the Latin equivalents used by Porkert (1), pp. 216 ff. He employs the term 'cardinal conduits' for the regular tracts. To this adjective we have no great objection, especially as we ourselves at one time thought of saying 'cardinal' and 'decumane' for *ching* and *lo* respectively. But though we have perforce used the word 'channel' in our explanations (e.g. p. 22), we fear that the term 'conduit' brings to mind too vividly the image of physical tubes, an idea of the *ching* which we cannot find in the classical literature, though of course the blood-vessels (*mo*) were certainly thought of in this way.

[d] Further information is also included there, but the explanation of that must be deferred for a few pages (cf. pp. 46, 48). The table is based upon that in Anon. (*107*), p. 10.

[e] Taken from Chhen Tshun-Jen (*3*), following Karow (3) and Bachmann (1).

[f] Perhaps one should also think of lienic as really lieno-pancreatic, since in ancient times the two organs were not clearly distinguished. Hence the symbol LP.

[g] Better, but rarely, written *chiao*.[6]

[h] Cf. *SCC*, Vol. 2, pp. 261 ff.; Needham & Lu Gwei-Djen (8), repr. Needham (64), pp. 266 ff.

[1] 腑 [2] 臟 [3] 腎 [4] 心包絡 [5] 三焦 [6] 膲

the order of circulation here given, starting with the pulmonic tract and ending with the hepatic one, after which everything begins all over again, is that which is found in the *Ling Shu* of the *Huang Ti Nei Ching*.[a] Thenceforward it continued as an invariably orthodox doctrine through the centuries, and holds good in traditional medical theory to this day.[b]

It can furthermore be seen from Table 1 that nos. 1, 4, 5, 8, 9 and 12 are Yin tracts; these are each related to a *tsang* organ, and each has a branch (*lo*[1]) which connects it with a *fu* organ. Most of their routes cover the medial sides (*nei tshê*[2]) of the four extremities, as well as the chest and the abdominal regions. Similarly, nos. 2, 3, 6, 7, 10 and 11 are Yang tracts; these are each related to a *fu* organ, and each has a branch (*lo*[1]) connecting it with a *tsang* organ or tract. These Yang tracts cover the lateral sides of the four extremities, the back, the head and the face.

Another way of demonstrating the circulation theory is seen in Table 2.[c] Here the acu-tracts and the thoraco-visceral organs corresponding with them are arranged on Yin and Yang sides, the former to the left and the latter to the right. Accordingly there is an implicit classification into the 'internal' and the 'external' categories,[d] for *li*[3] or 'subdite' phenomena[e] are those which are passing unseen within the body, while *piao*[4] or 'patefact' phenomena[f] are those which show themselves unfailingly as symptoms giving information to the physician. One can also see well the symmetrical relationship between the hand and foot beginnings and endings.

The tracts and the viscera were sometimes brought into correspondence with the series of twelve cyclical characters, *ti chih*[5],[g] as in the mnemonic rhymes on the circulation found in a number of books.[h] These cyclical characters also stood, of course, for many other things, such as months, double-hours of the day and night,[i] and compass-points.[j] The word used in the texts for this relationship is *na*,[6] meaning adoption or correlation.[k] Some Western writers, however,[l] have given the impression that the circulation was a single diurnal round which spent a whole double-hour in

[a] *NCLS/PH*, ch. 10, (pp. 104 ff.), ch. 11, (pp. 149 ff.), both in the third great chapter. This circulation is also the 'international order', quite rightly. It is found in the *Chen Chiu Ta Chhêng*[7] of Yang Chi-Chou[8] (+1601), who was following the *I Hsüeh Ju Mên*[9] of Li Yen[10] (+1575).

[b] The order also represents that of the twelve months of the year. A correlation is tabulated in Sugīhara Horiyukī (*1*), p. 15.

[c] Based on Anon. (*90*), p. 43. Cf. the explanatory figure given by Cleyer in +1682 (Fig. 10).

[d] These we discuss elsewhere in the context of the *pa kang*,[11] or 'eight principles of diagnosis'.

[e] The word is taken from *subditus*, the lining of a garment, a good parallelism both semantically and etymologically.

[f] The word comes easily from 'patent and obvious', something manifested and displayed externally. *Piao* is often now used in connection with indexes, charts, meters and gauges.

[g] Cf. *SCC*, Vol. 1, p. 79 and Vol. 3, pp. 396 ff.

[h] E.g. *CCCY*, ch. 3, (p. 248); *CCTC*, ch. 5, (p. 126). Cf. the diagram in Chhêng Tan-An, Chhen Pi-Liu & Hsü Hsi-Nien (*1*), p. 39.

[i] Cf. Needham, Wang & Price (1), pp. 199 ff.

[j] Cf. *SCC*, Vol. 4, pt. 1, pp. 297–8.

[k] In the same way, the twelve tracts were also correlated with the series of ten cyclical characters (*thien kan*[12]).

[l] E.g. Hübotter (1), pp. 89–90.

1 絡 2 內側 3 裡 4 表 5 地支 6 納
7 針灸大成 8 楊繼洲 9 醫學入門 10 李梴 11 八綱 12 天干

Table 1. *The twelve regular acu-tracts* (chêng ching) *and the eight auxiliaries* (chhi ching)

name of tract		internationally accepted abbreviation	internal organ with which the tract connects	*fu* (Yang) or *tsang* (Yin)
1 Shou Thai-Yin Fei Ching 手太陰肺經	Cheirotelic pulmonic Thai-Yin tract	P	lungs (*pulmones*)	T
2 Shou Yang-Ming Ta-Chhang Ching 手陽明大腸經	Cheirogenic crasso-intestinal Yang-Ming tract	IG	large intestine (*int. crassum* or *grandum*)	F
3 Tsu Yang-Ming Wei Ching 足陽明胃經	Podotelic gastric Yang-Ming tract	V	stomach (*ventriculus*)	F
4 Tsu Thai-Yin Phi Ching 足太陰脾經	Podogenic lieno-pancreatic Thai-Yin tract	LP	spleen (*lien*), (and pancreas)	T
5 Shou Shao-Yin Hsin Ching 足少陰心經	Cheirotelic cardiac Shao-Yin tract	C	heart (*cor*)	T
6 Shou Thai-Yang Hsiao-Chhang Ching 手太陽小腸經	Cheirogenic tenu-intestinal Thai-Yang tract	IT	small intestine (*int. tenue*)	F
7 Tsu Thai-Yang Phang-Kuang Ching 足太陽膀胱經	Podotelic vesical Thai-Yang tract	VU	bladder (*vesica urinaria*)	F
8 Tsu Shao-Yin Shen Ching 足少陰腎經	Podogenic reno-seminal Shao-Yin tract	R	kidneys (*renes*), 'reins'	T
9 Shou Chüeh-Yin Hsin-Pao-Lo Ching 手厥陰心包絡經	Cheirotelic pericardial Chüeh-Yin tract	HC	pericardial (*habitatio cordis*)	T

10 Shou Shao-Yang San-Chiao Ching 手少陽三焦經	Cheirogenic tricoctive Shao-Yang tract	SC	the three coctive regions	F
11 Tsu Shao-Yang Tan Ching 足少陽膽經	Podotelic felleic Shao-Yang tract	VF	gall-bladder (*vesica fellea*)	F
12 Tsu Chüeh-Yin Kan Ching 足厥陰肝經	Podogenic hepatic Chüeh-Yin tract	H	liver (*hepar*)	T
1 Tu Mo 督脉	Dorsal median tract (Regulative Yang auxiliary tract)	TM	no such connection	
2 Jen Mo 任脉	Ventral median tract (Regulative Yin auxiliary tract)	JM	no such connection	
3 Chhung Mo 衝脉	Tract-uniting quickening auxiliary tract	–	no such connection	
4 Tai Mo 帶脉	Tract-uniting cinctural auxiliary tract	–	no such connection	
5 Yang Chhiao Mo 陽蹻脉	Inter-connecting upstanding Yang auxiliary tract	–	no such connection	
6 Yin Chhiao Mo 陰蹻脉	Inter-connecting upstanding Yin auxiliary tract	–	no such connection	
7 Yang Wei Mo 陽維脉	Ligative Yang auxiliary tract	–	no such connection	
8 Yin Wei Mo 陰維脉	Ligative Yin auxiliary tract	–	no such connection	
Phi Ta Lo 脾大絡	the Great Acu-junction of the spleen	LP21	spleen (*lien*)	

Table 2. *The* chhi *circulation in the acu-tracts*

陰 YIN	裡 *li* (subdite)	cyclical characters	臟 *tsang*		腑 *fu*	cyclical characters	表 *piao* (patefact)	陽 YANG
Thai Yin	cheirotelic	寅	→pulmonic	→	crasso-intestinal ↓	卯	cheirogenic	Yang Ming
	podogenic	巳	lienic ↓	←	gastric	辰	podotelic	
Shao Yin	cheirotelic	午	cardiac	→	tenu-intestinal ↓	未	cheirogenic	Thai Yang
	podogenic	酉	reno-seminal ↓	←	vesical	申	podotelic	
Chüeh Yin	cheirotelic	戌	peri-cardial	→	tricoct-ive ↓	亥	cheirogenic	Shao Yang
	podogenic	丑	—hepatic (↑ to pulmonic)	←	felleic	子	podotelic	

passing through each tract. In the light of the classical doctrine that the blood and *chhi* circulate fifty times through the whole body in each day and night, this must be regarded as a misunderstanding of the texts. What would be consonant with them would be to say that the *chhi* of each tract occupies a dominant position at a certain regular double-hour during each day and night (cf. Fig. 10).

It has been customary to give the tracts in yet another order, keeping their groups of threes in accordance with their origins and terminations in one or other of the extremities, and at the same time demonstrating their *piao-li* (patefact-subdite) character.[a] Such tables demonstrate the remarkable symmetry of the system. But there is a different array which is even more interesting, because it illustrates the classical proto-quantitative thinking about the relative proportions of blood (*hsüeh*[1]) and *chhi*[2] normally present in each of the tracts.[b]

This system was called the 'standard proportions in the body of man' (*jen chih chhang shu*[3]), and it certainly shows that the amounts of blood and *chhi* in each tract were not rated at all the same. Perhaps this conclusion originated from anatomical observations that some tracts were more nearly running parallel to palpable blood-

[a] Cf. the tables and discussions in Anon. (*90*), p. 30 and Anon. (*91*), p. 12.

[b] This table is based upon *NCSW/PH*, ch. 24, (pp. 145–6); *NCSW/WMC*, ch. 24, (p. 252). We say 'proto-quantitative' because the estimates were not based upon any actual measurements, so far as one can see. The system is an interesting anticipation of that 'Science of the Balance', so important nearly a millennium later in the alchemy and proto-chemistry of the Arabic culture; cf. Vol. 5, pt. 4, pp. 393, 459 ff.

[1] 血 [2] 氣 [3] 人之常數

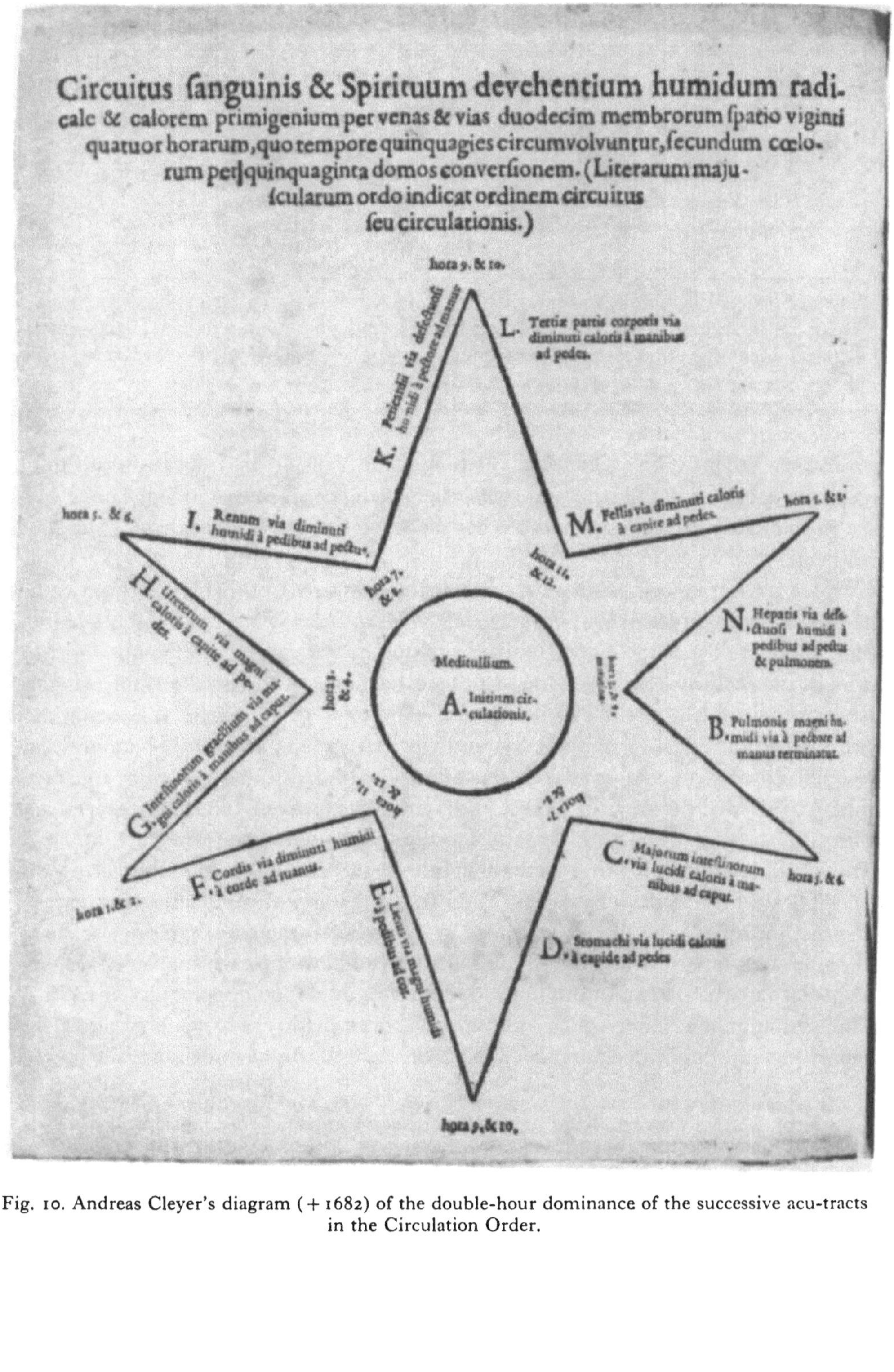

Fig. 10. Andreas Cleyer's diagram (+ 1682) of the double-hour dominance of the successive acu-tracts in the Circulation Order.

Table 3. *Relative proportions of blood and* chhi *in the acu-tracts*

									hsüeh	*chhi*
Piao	Thai-Yang	6	IT	cg	7	VU	pt		+++++	+
	Shao-Yang	10	SC	cg	11	VF	pt		+	+++++
	Yang-Ming	2	IG	cg	3	V	pt		+++++	+++++
Li	Thai-Yin	1	P	ct	4	LP	pg		+	+++++
	Chhüeh-Yin	9	HC	ct	12	H	pg		+++++	+
	Shao-Yin	5	C	ct	8	R	pg		+++++	+

The abbreviated name of each tract is here followed by its number in the circulation order, its international code-letter (cf. Table 1), and its course whether cheirogenic (cg), podotelic (pt), cheirotelic (ct) or podogenic (pg). 'Much' (*to*[1]) is represented by +++++, 'little' (*shao*[2]) is represented by +.

vessels than others. The exceptional position of the Yang-Ming tracts was said to be due to the fact that both blood and *chhi* 'originated' there. Illness brought imbalance to the standard proportions, and a knowledge of them was considered crucial in treatment.

We are now in a position to look again at the lower part of Table 1. Above come the twelve regular tracts (*shih-erh ching mo*,[3] *shih-erh chêng ching*[4]) just discussed, but below there are listed the eight auxiliary or supernumerary tracts,[a] famous for centuries as the *chhi ching pa mo*.[5] One of the most significant things about them is that although they are all lines of acu-points (*hsüeh*[6]) they were not regarded as connected with the main internal organs in the way that the regular tracts are. Therefore they were not grouped in the *piao-li* relationships. The Tu Mo[7] and Jen Mo[8] are tracts which run medially down the dorsal and ventral surfaces of the body respectively (Figs. 11, 12), so it was natural to associate the former with the Yang and the latter with the Yin, forces which they were thought to regulate or equalise in the *chêng ching* like spillways or overflow channels.[b] The two Tai Mo[9] run round the lower part of the waist just above the iliac crest, meeting the median tracts at right angles, hence the name 'belt-tracts'; while the Chhung Mo[10][c] run down on each side of the front of the body somewhat lateral to the Jen Mo. This affords a good opportunity of emphasising an important matter which has not so far been made clear, namely that all the regular tracts are duplicated as mirror-images on each side of the mid-line of the body,[d]

[a] See especially on these Anon. (*107*), pp. 208 ff., and Chhêng Tan-An (*2*), pp. 227 ff. Porkert (1), pp. 203, 273, employs the term 'odd conduits' (very odd, in English, better in German, p. 199, as 'unpaarigen'). But still this is unsatisfactory, since some of the auxiliary tracts are in fact duplicated as mirror-images while others are not.

[b] *NC*, Nan no. 28 (p. 33); *NC/PH* (p. 56).

[c] Now often abbreviated as *chhung mo*.[11]

[d] This can be seen, for example, in the way the *Chen Chiu Chhüan Shu* gives the note *erh hsüeh*[12] under particular acu-points, indicating their symmetrical doubling, left and right (cf. p. 131). See also *CCTC*, ch. 1, (p. 10, illustration).

1 多 2 少 3 十二經脉 4 十二正經 5 奇經八脉 6 穴
7 督脉 8 任脉 9 帶脉 10 衝脉 11 冲脉 12 二穴

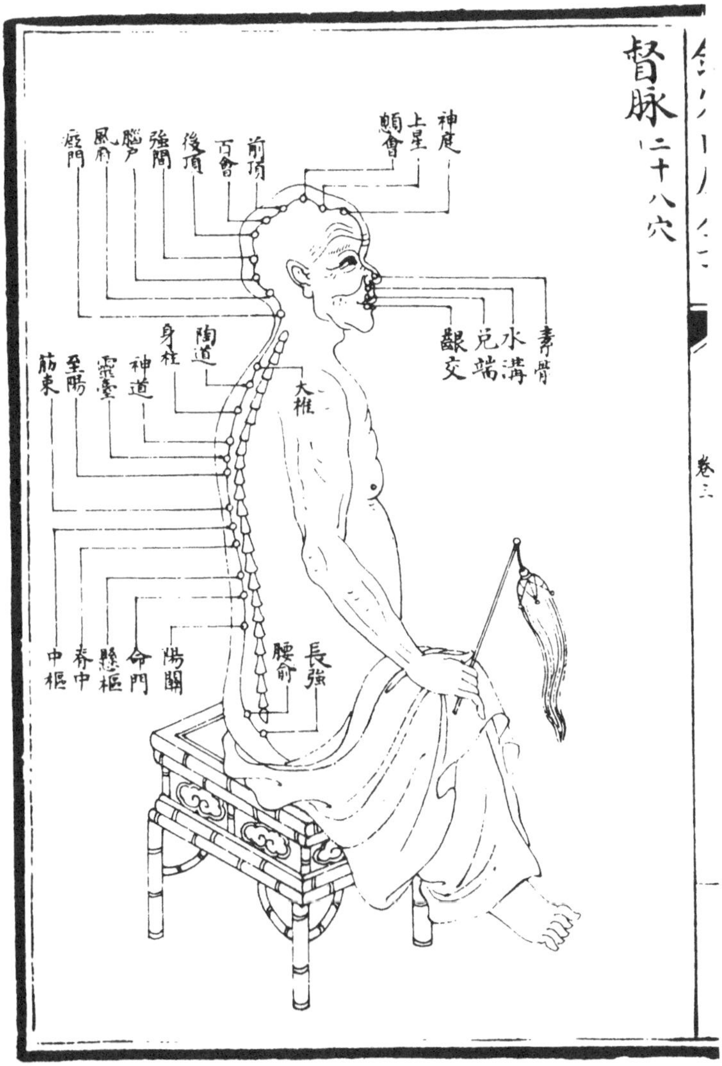

Fig. 11. The auxiliary tract Tu Mo (cf. Table 1), depicted in Chang Chieh-Pin's *Lei Ching* (+1624). *SKCS* edition.

while some of the auxiliary tracts are and some are not. Thus the Tu Mo and Jen Mo are necessarily single, but Tai Mo and Chhung Mo are double, and so are the other four (Yang Chhiao Mo,[1] Yin Chhiao Mo,[2] Yang Wei Mo[3] and Yin Wei Mo[4]). Thus, since only two tracts are unduplicated symmetrically, there are, in all, anatomically, 38 tracts ($12+6 = 18\times 2 = 36+2$).

Just as there were auxiliary tracts so also there were auxiliary internal organs, not among the familiar twelve. These were another kind of *fu*[5] (therefore Yang), the *chhi hêng chih fu*,[6] listed as follows: the brain (*nao*[7]), the bone-marrow (*sui*[8]), the bones

[1] 陽蹻脈 [2] 陰蹻脈 [3] 陽維脈 [4] 陰維脈 [5] 腑
[6] 奇恆之腑 [7] 腦 [8] 髓

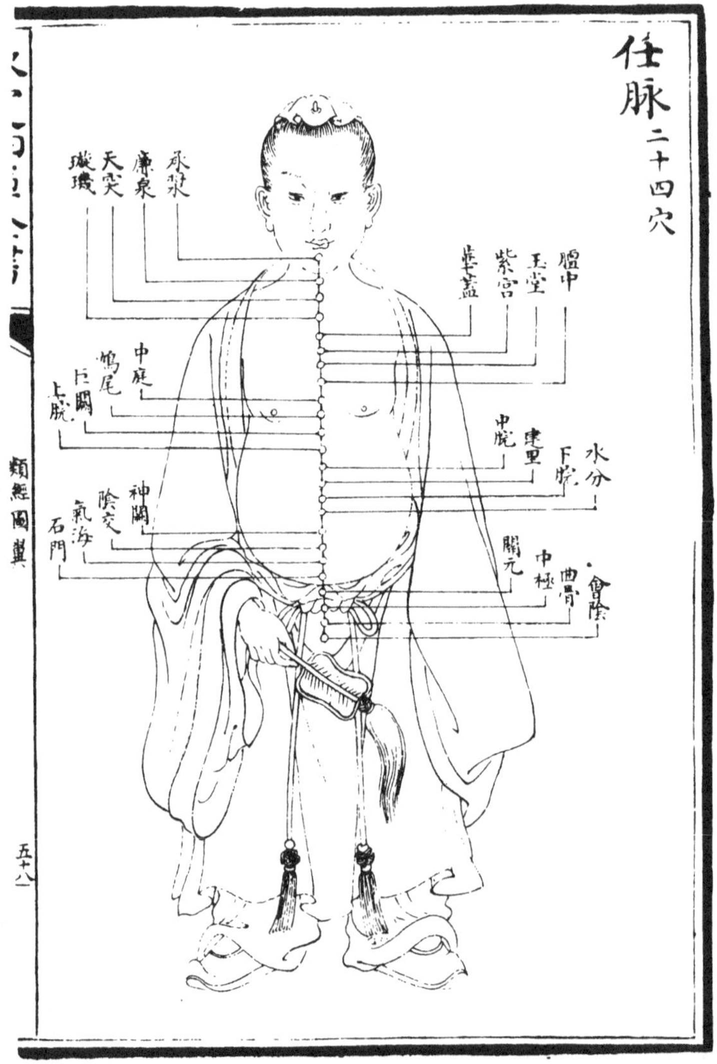

Fig. 12. The auxiliary tract Jen Mo (cf. Table 1), depicted in the same work. *SKCS* edition.

themselves (*ku*[1]), the blood-vessels (and lymphatics) themselves (*mo*[2]), the gall-bladder (*tan*[3])[a] and the uterus (*nü tzu pao*[4]).[b] The characteristic of all these was that they were thought to be concerned with *ching chhi*,[5] the vital *chhi* of vigour and health,[c]

[a] This was curious, for as we have seen, it also figured as a regular *fu*.

[b] See *NCSW/PH*, ch. 11, (p. 68), *NCSW/WMC* (p. 126), and *TSCC*, *I shu tien*, *tshê* 432, p. 14*b*.

[c] This expression is also met with in physiological alchemy (*SCC*, Vol. 5, pt. 5). There it refers primarily to seminal or reproductive *chhi*, *hsien thien chih chhi* or reno-seminal *chhi* (*shen chhi*[6]), but in the context of acupuncture the reference is rather to the *hou thien chih chhi*, the circulating life-constituents derived from the ingested nutriment (*ying chhi* and *wei chhi*, see p. 28 above). Acupuncture can only deal with the malfunctions of these. Cf. also pp. 14, 29 above.

1 骨 2 脉 3 膽 4 女子胞 5 精氣 6 腎氣

and they were supposed to hold it temporarily for the benefit of the body, passing it on to the tracts and the viscera; not voiding anything to the external world as the ordinary *fu* did. Probably this was the reason why the auxiliary tracts, especially Chhung Mo and Tai Mo besides the two median ones, were long extensively used in gynaecology.[a]

The eight auxiliary tracts differ considerably in importance, and also in frequency of use by acupuncture physicians. First, Tu Mo and Jen Mo are the only ones which have sets of named acu-points of their own;[b] all the others intersect with the regular tracts so frequently that their points are in fact identical with particular named *hsüeh* on those. For example, Tai Mo's three points, the only ones used in practice, are the same as three on the podotelic felleic Shao-Yang tract (i.e. VF 26, 27, 28), coinciding on its way down to the lower extremity. The special position of Tu Mo and Jen Mo is recognised by their being classed with the 12 regular tracts in the phrase 'the Fourteen Tracts (*shih-ssu Ching*[1])'. Another connection is that the Yang Chhiao Mo is regarded as a *pieh mo*[2] or branch[c] of the Tsu Thai-Yang Ching (the podotelic vesical tract), while Yin Chhiao Mo is a branch of the Tsu Shao-Yin Ching (the podogenic tract of the reins). Nevertheless the six minor auxiliary tracts were not regarded as on the main line of the *chhi* circulation.

Lastly, to complete the picture, one of the acu-junctions (*lo*[3]) was regarded as of special importance. It is known as the *phi chih ta lo*,[4] the Great Acu-Junction of the Spleen, and is in fact identical with the point Ta-pao[5] (LP 21).[d] It ranks indeed with the Fourteen Tracts themselves, and explains the phrase *shih-wu lo mo*,[6] the 'fifteen junctions and channels' (cf. Fig. 28).

Besides all the entities so far mentioned, ancient Chinese medical physiology recognised a further inter-connecting system of a distinctly neuro-muscular character, the 12 *ching chin*[7].[e] As in ancient Greek and Hellenistic anatomy, the distinctions between tendons, sinews, muscles and nerves were not particularly clear, and *chin* is a word which possessed all these meanings. The 12 *ching chin* bore the same names as the regular tracts (*chêng ching*[8]), but were thought of as passing more superficially through the tissues; all of them originated from the tips of the four extremities, and travelling upwards, ended on the head and face.[f] Unlike the *chêng ching* none of these tracts had any relationship with the twelve viscera; and acupuncture was done on them in a special way, i.e. with hot or cauterising needles (*fan chen*,[9] *huo chen*[10]), not at particular acu-points but at the site of the muscular or other pain.

In addition to all the tracts and acu-points discussed so far, there were classically

[a] Chu Hsiao-Nan (*1*).

[b] Hence they are also the only ones with international abbreviations, TM and JM.

[c] Cf. p. 22 above.

[d] Synonyms: Tsung-chhi[11] and Chhi-hai[12] (cf. p. 23 above). For an exposition of Phi-ta-lo see Anon. (*107*), p. 107. We may recall that the great repository of acu-point synonyms is *CCTC*, ch. 7, (pp. 234.2 ff.).

[e] The *loci classici* are *NCTS*, ch. 13, (p. 83), *NCLS/PH*, ch. 13, (pp. 163 ff.), *Chia I Ching*, ch. 2 (sect. 6), (p. 47).

[f] Drawings showing the paths of the *ching chin* will be found in Anon. (*90*), pp. 529 ff.

1 十四經 2 別脉 3 絡 4 脾之大絡 5 大包 6 十五絡脉
7 經筋 8 正經 9 燔針 10 火針 11 宗氣 12 氣海

a number of 'auxiliary points' situated away from any of the tracts, regular or auxiliary, and these were called *ching wai chhi hsüeh*.[1] For three of the 21 more important such loci listed by Chhêng Tan-An,[a] the drawing of capillary blood was specified, another two were also used for acupuncture, and the remainder were sites for moxibustion. Then there was the group of 'pain points' (*ah shih hsüeh*[2]), places where pressure could be particularly painful; these were known in the *Ling Shu* but first named thus by Sun Ssu-Mo in the +6th century.[b] And in addition to all these, modern practice, both in China and Europe, has in recent years used a considerable number more, especially on the hands and on the pinna of the external ear.

(iii) *The acu-points* (hsüeh), *ordinary and special*

We are now in a position to examine the list of acu-points on all the tracts drawn up in Table 4.[c] No one who undertakes to write them all out can fail to be impressed with the evocative, allusive, and sometimes quite poetical, character of the names which have grown up through long custom during the centuries.[d] A certain amount of synonymy favoured the facultative addition in some cases of words for limbs, trunk or head, to ensure certainty as to which acu-point was intended.[e] The order also differs slightly from one enumeration to another, but in Table 4 we follow the internationally-accepted order given by Chhen Tshun-Jen (*3*).[f]

A few of the synonyms have been indicated, but many more are likely to be en-

[a] (*2*), pp. 257ff. Some 938 are now recognised, as in the special treatise of Hao Chin-Khai (1).

[b] See Anon. (*90*), p. 104. Below, pp. 127, 175 also; the original reference is *CCCY*, ch. 3, (p. 203).

[c] Anon. (*121*) gives all acu-point names, and their anatomical positions, in both Chinese and English. Porkert (1), pp. 216ff., has now accomplished the remarkable feat of providing a Latin translation for each acu-point name; we cannot but think that this was a work of supererogation. At the same time he gives no translation of the synonyms, though they often do occur in the ancient and medieval literature.

[d] See, for example, the astronomical names occurring from JM 19 onwards, or TM 9 (details in Vol. 3, *passim*).

[e] Many anatomical terms are also naturally found in the list. Apart from some thirty commonplace names for the various parts of the body and its internal organs, we also find the skull (*lu*[3]) and its fontanelles or sutures (*hsing*[4]), the temporal region (*ping*[5] or *pin*[5]), the vertebral column (*lü*[6]), the pupil of the eye (*thung*[7]), the upper jaw (*chia*[8]) and the lower jaw or mandible (*han*[9]), also the gums (*yin*,[10] a word usually pronounced *khên*, to gnaw). Then there is the scapula (*nao*[11]), the rounded protuberance of the deltoid muscle (*yung*[12]), and muscles in general (*chin*[13]) though anciently these were not clearly distinguished from tendons and nerves. We also find the sternum (*han*[14]) and a less usual name for the breast (*ying*[15]); the diaphragm (*ko*[16]), and two curious words for the region between the heart and the diaphragm (*kao huang*[17]) often translated as 'the vitals', and losing their function as a more developed anatomy found nothing but the pericardial membrane between the heart and the central musculo-tendinous part of the diaphragm. Then comes the wrist (*wan*[18]), tubular visceral vessels, especially the urethra (*kuan*[19]), and the uterus (*pao*[20]). The disease radical (no. 104) provides two words, *chhi*,[21] and *ya*.[22] Finally, *liao*,[23] which occurs at least five times, properly denotes the pelvis; the Khang-Hsi Dictionary defines it as similar to *khuan*,[24] *kho*,[25] and *chia*,[26] but we may leave the elucidation of the exact meanings of these characters to Section 43 on anatomy. The acupuncturists, however, must have used the term for any place where bone is near the surface, for none of the acu-points so named is on or near the pelvis.

[f] It was set forth by Karow (3), cf. Bachmann (1), with German translations of most of the acu-point names. It was also adopted by the 7th International Congress of Acupuncture.

1 經外奇穴　2 阿是穴　3 顱　4 顖　5 鬢　6 膂
7 瞳　8 頰　9 頷　10 齦　11 臑　12 顒
13 筋　14 膻　15 膺　16 膈　17 膏肓　18 腕
19 脘　20 胞　21 瘈　22 瘂　23 髎　24 髖
25 髁　26 髂

Table 4. *The acu-points* (hsüeh) *on the tracts* (ching)

I Shou Thai-Yin Fei Ching (Cheirotelic Pulmonic Thai-Yin Tract)

P

1	Chung-fu	中府
2	Yün-mên	雲門
3	Thien-fu	天府
4	Hsia-pai	俠白
5	Chhih-tsê	尺澤
6	Khung-tsui	孔最
7	Lieh-chhüeh	列缺
8	Ching-chhü	經渠
9	Thai-yuan	太淵
10	Yü-chi	魚際
11	Shao-shang	少商

II Shou Yang-Ming Ta-Chhang Ching (Cheirogenic Crasso-intestinal Yang-Ming Tract)

IG

1	Shang-yang	商陽
2	Erh-chien	二間
3	San-chien	三間
4	Ho-ku	合谷
5	Yang-chhi	陽谿
6	Phien-li	偏歷
7	Wên-liu	溫溜
8	Hsia-lien	下廉
9	Shang-lien	上廉
10	San-li[a]	三里
11	Chhü-chhih	曲池
12	Chou-liao	肘髎
13	Wu-li[b]	五里
14	Pei-nao	臂臑
15	Chien-yung	肩髃
16	Chü-ku	巨骨
17	Thien-ting	天鼎
18	Fu-thu	扶突
19	Ho-liao	禾髎
20	Ying-hsiang	迎香

III Tsu Yang-Ming Wei Ching (Podotelic Gastric Yang-Ming Tract)

V

1	Thou-wei[c]	頭維
2	Hsia-kuan	下關
3	Chia-chhê[d]	頰車
4	Chhêng-chhi	承泣
5	Ssu-pai	四白
6	Chü-liao	巨髎
7	Ti-tshang	地倉
8	Ta-ying	大迋
9	Jen-ying	人迎
10	Shui-thu	水突
11	Chhi-shê	氣舍
12	Chhüeh-phên	缺盆
13	Chhi-hu	氣戶
14	Khu-fang	庫房
15	Wu-i	屋翳
16	Ying-chhuang	膺窗
17	Ju-chung	乳中
18	Ju-kên	乳根
19	Pu-jung	不容
20	Chhêng-man	承滿
21	Liang-mên	梁門
22	Kuan-mên	關門
23	Thai-i	太乙
24	Hua-jo-mên	滑肉門
25	Thien-shu	天樞
26	Wai-ling	外陵
27	Ta-chü	大巨
28	Shui-tao	水道
29	Kuei-lai	歸來
30	Chhi-chhung	氣衝
31	Phi-kuan	髀關
32	Fu-thu	伏突
33	Yin-shih	陰市
34	Liang-chhiu	梁邱
35	Tu-pi	犢鼻
36	San-li[e]	三里
37	Shang-chü-hsü	上巨虛
38	Thiao-khou	條口
39	Hsia-chü-hsü	下巨虛
40	Fêng-lung	豐隆
41	Chieh-chhi	解谿
42	Chhung-yang	衝陽
43	Hsien-ku	陷谷
44	Nei-thing	內庭
45	Li-tui	厲兌

IV Tsu Thai-Yin Phi Ching (Podogenic Lienic Thai-Yin Tract)

LP

1	Yin-pai	隱白
2	Ta-tu	大部
3	Thai-pai	太白
4	Kung-sun	公孫
5	Shang-chhiu	商邱
6	San-yin-chiao	三陰交
7	Lou-ku	漏谷
8	Ti-chi	地機
9	Yin-ling-chhüan	陰陵泉
10	Hsüeh-hai	血海
11	Chi-mên	箕門
12	Chhung-mên	衝門
13	Fu-shê	府舍
14	Fu-chieh	腹結
15	Ta-hêng	大橫
16	Fu-ai	腹哀
17	Shih-tou	食竇
18	Thien-chhi[f]	天谿
19	Hsiung-hsiang	胸鄉

[a] Alt. Shou-san-li 手三里 to distinguish from V 36.
[b] Alt. Shou-wu-li 手五里 to distinguish from H 10.
[c] In some enumerations, e.g. Anon. (*107*), V 4 is taken as V 1, and V 1, 2, 3 become V 8, 7, 6.
[d] On this name cf. *SCC*, Vol. 4, pt. 2, pp. 86, 347.
[e] Alt. Tsu-san-li 足三里 to distinguish from IG 10.
[f] Now often written with Rad. no. 85, so pronounceable *chhi* or *hsi*.

Table 4 (*cont.*)

20	Chou-jung	周榮
21	Ta-pao[a]	大包

V Shou Shao-Yin Hsin Ching (Cheirotelic Cardiac Shao-Yin Tract)

C

1	Chi-chhüan	極泉
2	Chhing-ling	青靈
3	Shao-hai	少海
4	Ling-tao	靈道
5	Thung-li	通里
6	Yin-chhi	陰郄
7	Shen-mên	神門
8	Shao-fu	少府
9	Shao-chhung	少衝

VI Shou Thai-Yang Hsiao-Chhang Ching (Cheirogenic Tenu-intestinal Thai-Yang Tract)

IT

1	Shao-tsê	少澤
2	Chhien-ku	前谷
3	Hou-chhi[b]	後谿
4	Wan-ku	腕骨
5	Yang-ku	陽谷
6	Yang-lao	養老
7	Chih-chêng	支正
8	Hsiao-hai	小海
9	Chien-chên	肩貞
10	Nao-shu	臑兪
11	Thien-tsung	天宗
12	Ping-fêng	秉風
13	Chhü-yuan	曲垣
14	Chien-wai-shu	肩外兪
15	Chien-chung-shu	肩中兪
16	Thien-chuang	天窗
17	Thien-jung	天容
18	Chhüan-liao	顴髎
19	Thing-kung	聽宮

VII Tsu Thai-Yang Phang-Kuang Ching (Podotelic Vesical Thai-Yang Tract)

VU

1	Ching-ming	睛明
2	Tshuan-chu	攢竹
3	Mei-chhung	眉衝
4	Chhü-chhai	曲差
5	Wu-chhu	五處
6	Chhêng-kuang	承光
7	Thung-thien	通天
8	Lo-chhio	絡却
9	Yü-chen	玉枕
10	Thien-chu	天柱
11	Ta-chu	大杼
12	Fêng-mên	風門
13	Fei-shu	肺兪
14	Chüeh-yin-shu	厥陰兪
15	Hsin-shu	心兪
16	Tu-shu	督兪
17	Ko-shu	膈兪
18	Kan-shu	肝兪
19	Tan-shu	膽兪
20	Phi-shu	脾兪
21	Wei-shu	胃兪
22	San-chiao-shu	三焦兪
23	Shen-shu	腎兪
24	Chhi-hai-shu	氣海兪
25	Ta-chhang-shu	大腸兪
26	Kuan-yuan-shu	關元兪
27	Hsiao-chhang-shu	小腸兪
28	Phang-kuang-shu	膀胱兪
29	Chung-lü-shu	中膂兪
30	Pai-huan-shu	白環兪
31	Shang-liao	上髎
32	Tzhu-liao	次髎
33	Chung-liao	中髎
34	Hsia-liao	下髎
35	Hui-yang	會陽
36	Fu-fên[c]	附分
37	Pho-hu	魄戶
38	Kao-huang[d]	膏肓
39	Shen-thang	神堂
40	I-hsi	譩譆
41	Ko-kuan	膈關
42	Hun-mên	魂門
43	Yang-kang	陽綱
44	I-shê	意舍
45	Wei-tshang	胃倉
46	Huang-mên	肓門
47	Chih-shih	志室
48	Pao-huang	胞肓
49	Chih-pien	秩邊
50	Chhêng-fu	承扶
51	Yin-mên	殷門
52	Fou-chhi	浮郄
53	Wei-yang	委陽
54	Wei-chung	委中
55	Chhêng-chin	承筋
56	Ho-yang	合陽
57	Chhêng-shan	承山
58	Fei-yang	飛陽
59	Fu-yang	付陽
60	Khun-lun	崑崙
61	Phu-shen	僕參
62	Shen-mo	申脉
63	Chin-mên[e]	金門
64	Ching-ku	京骨
65	Shu-ku	束骨

[a] Chhen Tshun-Jen (*3*) omits this acu-point, but it is a very important one, the unique Phi-ta-lo 脾大絡 (cf. Anon. (*107*), p. 107).

[b] Now often written with Rad. no. 85, so pronounceable *chhi* or *hsi*.

[c] Some enumerations, as in Anon. (*107*), have a different order between this point and VU 56. The chief difference is that VU 50–54 are brought upwards to precede the rest.

[d] Syn. Kao-huang shu 膏肓兪. Cf. p. 178 below. Dist. from R 16.

[e] Alt. Tsu-chin-mên 足金門, to distinguish from accidental confusion with VF 25.

Table 4 (*cont.*)

66	Thung-ku[a]	通谷
67	Chih-yin	至陰

VIII Tsu Shao-Yin Shen Ching (Podogenic Reno-seminal Shao-Yin Tract)

R

1	Yung-chhüan	湧泉
2	Jan-ku	然谷
3	Thai-chhi	太谿
4	Ta-chung	大鐘
5	Shui-chhüan	水泉
6	Chao-hai	照海
7	Fu-liu	復溜
8	Chiao-hsin	交信
9	Chu-pin	築賓
10	Yin-ku	陰谷
11	Hêng-ku	横骨
12	Ta-ho	大赫
13	Chhi-hsüeh	氣穴
14	Ssu-man	四滿
15	Chung-chu	中注
16	Huang-shu	肓兪
17	Shang-chhü	商曲
18	Shih-kuan	石關
19	Yin-tu	陰都
20	Thung-ku[b]	通谷
21	Yu-mên	幽門
22	Pu-lang	步廊
23	Shen-fêng	神封
24	Ling-hsü	靈墟
25	Shen-tsang	神藏
26	Yü-chung	彧中
27	Shu-fu	兪府

IX Shou Chüeh-Yin Hsin-Pao-Lo Ching (Cheirotelic Pericardial Chüeh-Yin Tract)

HC

1	Thien-chhih	天池
2	Thien-chhüan	天泉
3	Chhü-tsê	曲澤
4	Chhi-mên	郄門
5	Chien-shih	間使
6	Nei-kuan	内關
7	Ta-ling	大陵
8	Lao-kung	勞宮
9	Chung-chhung	中衝

X Shou Shao-Yang San-Chiao Ching (Cheirogenic Tricoctive Shao-Yang Tract)

SC

1	Kuan-chhung	關衝
2	I-mên	液門
3	Chung-chu	中渚
4	Yang-chhih	陽池
5	Wai-kuan	外關
6	Chih-kou	支溝
7	Hui-tsung	會宗
8	San-yang-lo	三陽絡
9	Ssu-tu	四瀆
10	Thien-ching	天井
11	Chhing-lêng-yuan	清冷淵
12	Hsiao-lo	消濼
13	Nao-hui	臑會
14	Chien-chiao[c]	肩髎
15	Thien-liao	天髎
16	Thien-yu	天牖
17	I-fêng	翳風
18	Chhi-mo	瘈脈
19	Lu-hsi	顱息
20	Chio-sun	角孫
21	Ssu-chu-khung[d]	絲竹空
22	Ho-liao	和髎
23	Erh-mên	耳門

XI Tsu Shao-Yang Tan Ching (Podotelic Felleic Shao-Yang Tract)

VF

1	Thung-tzu-liao	瞳子髎
2	Thing-hui	聽會
3	Kho-chu-jen[e]	客主人
4	Han-yen	頷厭
5	Hsüan-lu	懸顱
6	Hsüan-li	懸釐
7	Chhü-ping	曲鬢
8	Shuai-ku	率谷
9	Pên-shen[f]	本神
10	Yang-pai	陽白
11	Lin-chhi[g]	臨泣
12	Mu-chuang	目窗
13	Chhiao-yin[h]	竅陰
14	Chhêng-ling	承靈
15	Thien-chhung	天衝
16	Fou-pai	浮白
17	Wan-ku	完骨
18	Chêng-ying	正營
19	Nao-khung	腦空
20	Fêng-chhih	風池
21	Chien-ching	肩井
22	Yuan-i	淵液
23	Chê-chin	輒筋
24	Jih-yüeh	日月

[a] This is over the gastrocnemius muscle so it is not easily confused with the other of the same name, R 20, on the abdomen just below the sternum. But it is sometimes called Tsu Thung-ku 足通谷.

[b] See previous note, on VU 66.

[c] Or Chien-liao 肩髎

[d] Anon. (*107*) interchanges the numbering of SC 21 and 23.

[e] Syn. Shang-kuan 上關.

[f] The numbering between VF 9 and 18 differs in Anon. (*107*).

[g] Alt. Thou-lin-chhi 頭臨泣 to distinguish from VF 41.

[h] Alt. Thou-chhiao-yin 頭竅陰 to distinguish from VF 44.

Table 4 (*cont.*)

25	Ching-mên[a]	京門
26	Tai-mo	帶脉
27	Wu-shu	五樞
28	Wei-tao	維道
29	Chü-liao	居髎
30	Huan-thiao	環跳
31	Fêng-shih	風市
32	Chung-tu	中瀆
33	Yang-kuan	陽關
34	Yang-ling-chhüan	陽陵泉
35	Yang-chiao	陽交
36	Wai-chhiu	外邱
37	Kuang-ming	光明
38	Yang-fu	陽輔
39	Hsüan-chung	懸鍾
40	Chhiu-hsü	邱墟
41	Tsu-lin-chhi	足臨泣
42	Ti-wu-hui	地五會
43	Hsia-chhi	俠谿
44	Tsu-chhiao-yin	足竅陰

XII Tsu Chüeh-Yin Kan Ching (Podogenic Hepatic Chüeh-Yin Tract)

H

1	Ta-tun	大敦
2	Hsing-chien	行間
3	Thai-chhung	太衝
4	Chung-fêng	中封
5	Li-kou	蠡溝
6	Chung-tu[b]	中都
7	Hsi-kuan	膝關
8	Chhü-chhüan	曲泉
9	Yin-pao	陰包
10	Wu-li[c]	五里
11	Yin-lien	陰廉
12	Chi-mo	急脉
13	Chang-mên	章門
14	Chhi-mên	期門

XIII (= 1) Tu Mo (Dorsal Median Tract; Regulative Yang Auxiliary Tract)

TM

1	Chhang-chhiang	長強
2	Yao-shu	腰兪
3	Yang-kuan[d]	陽關
4	Ming-mên	命門
5	Hsüan-shu	懸樞
6	Chi-chung[e]	脊中
7	Chin-so	筋縮
8	Chih-yang	至陽
9	Ling-thai	靈臺
10	Shen-tao	神道
11	Shen-chu	身柱
12	Hsiung-tao	胸道
13	Ta-chhui	大椎
14	Ya-mên	瘂門
15	Fêng-fu	風府
16	Nao-hu	腦戶
17	Chhiang-chien	強間
18	Hou-ting	後頂
19	Pai-hui	百會
20	Chhien-ting	前頂
21	Hsing-hui	顖會
22	Shang-hsing	上星
23	Shen-thing	神庭
24	Su-liao	素髎
25	Shui-kou[f]	水溝
26	Tui-tuan	兌端
27	Yin-chiao	齦交

XIV (= 2) Jen Mo (Ventral Median Tract; Regulative Yin Auxiliary Tract)

JM

1	Hui-yin	會陰
2	Chhü-ku	曲骨
3	Chung-chi	中極
4	Kuan-yuan	關元
5	Shih-mên[g]	石門
6	Chhi-hai	氣海
7	Yin-chiao[h]	陰交
8	Shen-chhüeh	神闕
9	Shui-fên	水分
10	Hsiz-kuan	下脘
11	Chien-li	建里
12	Chung-kuan	中脘
13	Shang-kuan	上脘
14	Chü-chhüeh	巨闕
15	Chiu-wei	鳩尾
16	Chung-thing	中庭
17	Shan-chung	膻中
18	Yü-thang	玉堂
19	Tzu-kung[i]	紫宮
20	Hua-kai	華蓋
21	Hsüan-chi	璇璣
22	Thien-thu	天突
23	Lien-chhüan	廉泉
24	Chhêng-chiang	承漿

[a] Alt. Yao-ching-mên 腰京門 to distinguish from accidental confusion with VU 63.

[b] Alt. Tsu-chung-tu 足中都 to distinguish from inadvertent confusion with P 1, R 15 or SC 3.

[c] Alt. Ku-wu-li 股五里 to distinguish from IG 13.

[d] Alt. Yao-yang-kuan 腰陽關 to distinguish from VF 33.

[e] In some enumerations, e.g. Anon. (*107*); Chhêng Tan-An (*1*), this is followed by an acu-point named Chung-shu 中樞 as TM 7, after which the order continues until TM 28.

[f] Alt. Jen-chung 人中.

[g] Syn. Tan-thien 丹田.

[h] Alt. Fu-yin-chiao 腹陰交 to distinguish from the synonym of TM 27.

[i] Alt. Hsiung-tzu-kung 胸紫宮 to distinguish from other uses of this expression; the central polar region of the heavens (cf. *SCC*, Vol. 3, p. 259), the imperial palace at the capital (Vol. 4, pt. 3, p. 75), and Taoist heavens and temples (Vol. 5, pt. 2, p. 262).

ACU-POINT INDEX

Chang-mên	H 13
Chao-hai	R 6
Chê-chin	VF 23
Chêng-ying	VF 18
Chi-chhüan	C 1
Chi-chung	TM 6
Chi-mên	LP 11
Chi-mo	H 12
Chia-chhê	V 3
Chiao-hsin	R 8
Chieh-chhi	V 41
Chien-chên	IT 9
Chien-chiao	SC 14
Chien-ching	VF 21
Chien-chung-shu	IT 15
Chien-li	JM 11
Chien-liao	SC 14
Chien-shih	HC 5
Chien-wai-shu	IT 14
Chien-yung	IG 15
Chih-chêng	IT 7
Chih-kou	SC 6
Chih-pien	VU 49
Chih-shih	VU 47
Chih-yang	TM 8
Chih-yin	VU 67
Chin-mên	VU 63
Chin-so	TM 7
Ching-chhü	P 8
Ching-ku	VU 64
Ching-mên	VF 25
Ching-ming	VU 1
Chio-sun	SC 20
Chiu-wei	JM 15
Chou-jung	LP 20
Chou-liao	IG 12
Chü-chhüeh	JM 14
Chü-ku	IG 16
Chü-liao	V 6
	& VF 29
Chu-pin	R 9
Chüeh-yin-shu	VU 14
Chung-chhung	HC 9
Chung-chi	JM 3
Chung-chu	R 15
	& SC 3
Chung-fêng	H 4
Chung-fu	P 1
Chung-kuan	JM 12
Chung-liao	VU 33
Chung-lü-shu	VU 29
Chung-shu	TM 6·5
Chung-thing	JM 16
Chung-tu	VF 32
	& H 6
Chhang-chhiang	TM 1
Chhêng-chhi	V 4
Chhêng-chiang	JM 24
Chhêng-chin	VU 55
Chhêng-fu	VU 50
Chhêng-kuan	VU 6
Chhêng-ling	VF 14
Chhêng-man	V 20
Chhêng-shan	VU 57
Chhi-chung	V 30
Chhi-hai	JM 6
Chhi-hai-shu	VU 24
Chhi-hsüeh	R 13
Chhi-hu	V 13
Chhi-mên	HC 4
	& H 14
Chhi-mo	SC 18
Chhi-shê	V 11
Chhiang-chien	TM 17
Chhiao-yin	VF 13
Chhien-ku	IT 2
Chhien-ting	TM 20
Chhih-tsê	P 5
Chhing-lêng-yuan	SC 11
Chhing-ling	C 2
Chhiu-hsü	VF 40
Chhü-chhai	VU 4
Chhü-chhih	IG 11
Chhü-chhüan	H 8
Chhü-ku	JM 2
Chhü-ping	VF 7
Chhü-tsê	HC 3
Chhü-yuan	IT 13
Chhüan-liao	IT 18
Chhüeh-phên	V 12
Chhung-mên	LP 12
Chhung-yang	V 42
Erh-chien	IG 2
Erh-mên	SC 23
Fei-shu	VU 13
Fei-yang	VU 58
Fêng-chhih	VF 20
Fêng-fu	TM 15
Fêng-lung	V 40
Fêng-mên	VU 12
Fêng-shih	VF 31
Fou-chhi	VU 52
Fou-pai	VF 16
Fu-ai	LP 16
Fu-chieh	LP 14
Fu-fên	VU 36
Fu-liu	R 7
Fu-shê	LP 13
Fu-thu	IG 18
	& V 32
Fu-yang	VU 59
Fu-yin-chiao	JM 7
Han-yen	VF 4
Hêng-ku	R 11
Ho-ku	IG 4
Ho-liao	IG 19
	& SC 22
Ho-yang	VU 56
Hou-chhi	IT 3
Hou-hsi	IT 3
Hou-ting	TM 18
Hua-jo-mên	V 24
Hua-kai	JM 20
Huan-thiao	VF 30
Huang-mên	VU 46
Huang-shu	R 16
Hui-tsung	SC 7
Hui-yang	VU 35
Hui-yin	JM 1
Hun-mên	VU 42
Hsi-kuan	H 7
Hsia-chhi	VF 43
Hsia-chü-hsü	V 39
Hsia-kuan	V 2
	& JM 10
Hsia-liao	VU 34
Hsia-lien	IG 8
Hsia-pai	P 4
Hsiao-chhang-shu	VU 27
Hsiao-hai	IT 8
Hsiao-lo	SC 12
Hsien-ku	V 43
Hsin-shu	VU 15
Hsing-chien	H 2
Hsing-hui	TM 21
Hsiung-hsiang	LP 19
Hsiung-tao	TM 12
Hsiung-tzu-kung	JM 19
Hsüan-chi	JM 21
Hsüan-chung	VF 39
Hsüan-li	VF 6
Hsüan-lu	VF 5
Hsüan-shu	TM 5
Hsüeh-ha	LP 10
I-fêng	SC 17
I-hsi	VU 40
I-mên	SC 2
I-shê	VU 44
Jan-ku	R 2
Jen-chung	TM 25
Jen-ying	V 9
Jih-yüeh	VF 24
Ju-chung	V 17
Ju-kên	V 18
Kan-shu	VU 18
Kao-huang	VU 38
Kao-huang-shu	VU 38
Kho-chu-jen	VF 3
Khu-fang	V 14
Khun-lun	VU 60
Khung-tsui	P 6

ACU-POINT INDEX (*cont.*)

Ko-kuan	VU 41
Ko-shu	VU 17
Ku-wu-li	H 10
Kuan-chhung	SC 1
Kuan-mên	V 22
Kuan-yuan	JM 4
Kuan-yuan-shu	VU 26
Kuang-ming	VF 37
Kuei-lai	V 29
Kung-sun	LP 4
Lao-kung	HC 8
Li-kou	H 5
Li-tui	V 45
Liang-chhiu	V 34
Liang-mên	V 21
Lieh-chhüeh	P 7
Lien-chhüan	JM 23
Lin-chhi	VF 11
Ling-hsü	R 24
Ling-tao	C 4
Ling-thai	TM 9
Lo-chhio	VU 8
Lou-ku	LP 7
Lu-hsi	SC 19
Mei-chhung	VU 3
Ming-mên	TM 4
Mu-chuang	VF 12
Nao-hu	TM 16
Nao-hui	SC 13
Nao-khung	VF 19
Nao-shu	IT 10
Nei-kuan	HC 6
Nei-thing	V 44
Pai-huan-shu	VU 30
Pai-hui	TM 19
Pao-huang	VU 48
Pei-nao	IG 14
Pên-shen	VF 9
Phang-kuang-shu	VU 28
Phi-kuan	V 31
Phi-shu	VU 20
Phi-ta-lo	LP 21
Phien li	IG 6
Pho hu	VU 37
Phu-shan	VU 61
Ping-fêng	IT 12
Pu-jung	V 19
Pu-lang	R 22
San-chiao-shu	VU 22
San-chien	IG 3
San-li	IG 10
	& V 36
San-yang-lo	SC 8
San-yin-chiao	LP 6

Shan-chung	JM 17
Shang-chhiu	LP 5
Shang-chhü	R 17
Shang-chü-hsü	V 37
Shang-hsing	TM 22
Shang-kuan	VF 3
	& JM 13
Shang-liao	VU 31
Shang-lien	IG 9
Shang-yang	IG 1
Shao-chhung	C 9
Shao-fu	C 8
Shao-hai	C 3
Shao-shang	P 11
Shao-tsê	IT 1
Shen-chhüeh	JM 8
Shen-chu	TM 11
Shen-fêng	R 23
Shen-mên	C 7
Shen-mo	VU 62
Shen-shu	VU 23
Shen-tao	TM 10
Shen-thang	VU 39
Shen-thing	TM 23
Shen-tsang	R 25
Shih-kuan	R 18
Shih-mên	JM 5
Shih-tou	LP 17
Shou-san-li	IG 10
Shou-wu-li	IG 13
Shu-fu	R 27
Shu-ku	VU 65
Shuai-ku	VF 8
Shui-chhüan	R 5
Shui-fên	JM 9
Shui-kou	TM 25
Shui-tao	V 28
Shui-thu	V 10
Ssu-chu-khung	SC 21
Ssu-man	R 14
Ssu-pai	V 5
Ssu-tu	SC 9
Su-liao	TM 24
Ta-chhang-shu	VU 25
Ta-chhui	TM 13
Ta-chu	VU 11
Ta-chü	V 27
Ta-chung	R 4
Ta-hêng	LP 15
Ta-ho	R 12
Ta-ling	HC 7
Ta-pao	LP 21
Ta-tu	LP 2
Ta-tun	H 1
Ta-ying	V 8
Tai-mo	VF 26
Tan-shu	VU 19
Tan-thien	JM 5

Thai-chhi	R 3
Thai-chhung	H 3
Thai-hsi	R 3
Thai-i	V 23
Thai-pai	LP 3
Thai-yuan	P 9
Thiao-khou	V 38
Thien-chhi	LP 18
Thien-chhih	HC 1
Thien-chhüan	HC 2
Thien-chhuang	IT 16
Thien-chhung	VF 15
Thien-ching	SC 10
Thien-chu	VU 10
Thien-fu	P 3
Thien-hsi	LP 18
Thien-jung	IT 17
Thien-liao	SC 15
Thien-shu	V 25
Thien-thu	JM 22
Thien-ting	IG 17
Thien-tsung	IT 11
Thien-yu	SC 16
Thing-hui	VF 2
Thing-kung	IT 19
Thou-chhiao-yin	VF 13
Thou-lin-chhi	VF 11
Thou-wei	V 1
Thung-ku	VU 66
	& R 20
Thung-li	C 5
Thung-thien	VU 7
Thung-tzu-liao	VF 1
Ti-chi	LP 8
Ti-tshang	V 7
Ti-wu-hui	VF 42
Tshuan-chu	VU 2
Tsu-chhiao-yin	VF 44
Tsu-chin-mên	VU 63
Tsu-chung-tu	H 6
Tsu-lin-chhi	VF 41
Tsu-san-li	V 36
Tsu-thung-ku	VU 66
Tu-pi	V 35
Tu-shu	VU 16
Tui-tuan	TM 26
Tzhu-liao	VU 32
Tzu-kung	JM 19
Wai-chhiu	VF 36
Wai-kuan	SC 5
Wai-ling	V 26
Wan-ku	IT 4
	& VF 17
Wei-chung	VU 54
Wei-shu	VU 21
Wei-tao	VF 28
Wei-tshang	VU 45
Wei-yang	VU 53

ACU-POINT INDEX (*cont.*)

Wên-liu	IG 7	Yang-kuan	VF 33	Yin-mên	VU 51
Wu-chhu	VU 5		& TM 3	Yin-pai	LP 1
Wu-i	V 15	Yang-lao	IT 6	Yin-pao	H 9
Wu-li	IG 13	Yang-ling-chhüan	VF 34	Yin-shih	V 33
	& H 10	Yang-pai	VF 10	Yin-tu	R 19
Wu-shu	VF 27	Yao-ching-mên	VF 25	Ying-chhuang	V 16
		Yao-shu	TM 2	Ying-hsiang	IG 20
Ya-mên	TM 14	Yao-yang-kuan	TM 3	Yü-chen	VU 9
Yang-chhi	IG 5	Yin-chhi	C 6	Yü-chi	P 10
Yang-chhih	SC 4	Yin-chiao	TM 17	Yü-chung	R 26
Yang-chiao	VF 35		& JM 7	Yu-mên	R 21
Yang-fu	VF 38	Yin-hsi	C 6	Yü-thang	JM 18
Yang-kang	VU 43	Yin-ku	R 10	Yuan-i	VF 22
Yang-ku	IT 5	Yin-lien	H 11	Yün-mên	P 2
		Yin-ling-chhüan	LP 9	Yung-chhüan	R 1

countered, especially in ancient and medieval writings, hence the importance of the classical tables of synonyms mentioned already on p. 51. A little later on (p. 80) we shall see a good case of the difficulties of identifying an acu-point mentioned by an ancient writer—but they can usually be overcome.

If the number of acu-points in the table is added up, the total is 360.[a] But it is clear at a glance that the various tracts have very varying numbers of recognised acu-points, the largest being the bladder tract (VU) with 67, the smallest the heart tract (C) and the pericardium tract (HC) with 9 each. It then becomes evident, as the Yang and Yin sides are compared, that the Yang tracts tend to have a great many more acu-points than the Yin ones, in the proportion indeed of rather over two thirds to one third, for the former have 245 in all and the latter 115. Removing from these totals the 51 acu-points of the median unduplicated auxiliary tracts (27 in TM, and 24 in JM), and doubling the rest, we get 309 (i.e. $218+91) \times 2$, that is, 618. Adding the 51 unduplicated median points, the total is 669 (or one more). Presently we shall see this figure again in Table 15, which summarises the growth in number of the acu-points through the centuries.

We are now in a position to study a certain number of acu-points (*hsüeh*[1]) which were considered to have special qualities of one kind or another. First come the fifteen *lo mo hsüeh*,[2] junctions or acu-junctions (already mentioned on p. 17 above), between which *chhi*-bearing (pneumatophoric) channels (*lo*[3]) connected the main tracts together.[b] The classical source for this is the *Ling Shu*,[c] so the conception is very ancient. In Table 5, the *piao* (patefact) tracts are on the right, and the *li* (subdite)

[a] Or 361 if the extra TM 7 is included.

[b] Hence the term of Porkert (1), pp. 338–9, *foramina nexoria*, from nexus; which could give us 'nexic acu-points'.

[c] *NCLS/PH* (ch. 3), ch. 10, (pp. 142 ff.). An interesting account of these points with relation to synonymy, diagnosis and therapy, is given in *CCCY*, ch. 1, (pp. 135 ff.). Our table is constructed from the exposition in Anon. (*107*), pp. 55–6. Charts of the *lo mo* showing the connections will be found in Anon. (*90*), pp. 515 ff.

[1] 穴 [2] 絡脉穴 [3] 絡

Table 5. *The fifteen acu-junctions, or nexic acu-points* (lo mo hsüeh)

	Li tracts			*Piao* tracts		
SHOU (Cheiro-)	Shao-Yin	C 5	Thung-li	Thai-Yang	IT 7	Chih-chêng
	Chüeh-Yin	HC 6	Nei-kuan	Shao-Yang	SC 5	Wai-kuan
	Thai-Yin	P 7	Lieh-chhüeh	Yang-Ming	IG 6	Phien-li
TSU (Podo-)	Shao-Yin	R 4	Ta-chung	Thai-Yang	VU 58	Fei-yang
	Chüeh-Yin	H 5	Li-kou	Shao-Yang	VF 37	Kuang-ming
	Thai-Yin	LP 4	Kung-sun	Yang-Ming	V 40	Fêng-lung
Tu Mo TM 1 Chhang-chhiang (radiates in the cephalic region)						
Jen Mo JM 15 Chiu-wei (radiates in the abdominal region)						
Phi Ta Lo LP 21 Ta-pao[a] (radiates in the thoracic region)						

tracts on the left (as in Table 2), and the connection of each with each joins across the mid-line of the assembly.

These interconnections further ensured the integration of the whole body into a circulatory system, and the six *piao-li* pairs are known as the 'six unions' (*liu ho*[1]).[b] As for the *lo mo* of Tu, Jen and Phi, they are distributed over the front, back and sides of the body, increasing the efficiency of the *chhi* circulation. The 15 *lo mo* points are chiefly used for therapy in cases where *piao-li* symptoms are manifested at the same time, thus indicating that both Yang and Yin viscera have been affected by disease.

Next there are the eight *hui hsüeh*[2] and the many *chiao hui hsüeh*.[3] The *hui hsüeh* or 'assembly-points' were considered to be the points where the *chhi* of the viscera (both Yin and Yang), the *chhi* of the circulation, the *hsüeh*[4] (blood, more or less) and the blood-vessels, the *chhi* of the muscles, tendons, nerves and bones with their bone-marrow—in other words, as we should nowadays say, the diverse tissues of the body—each concentrated.[c] We enumerate them in Table 6.[d]

In so far as it was thought, then, that acupuncture at these particular points would affect all the tissues of the body the *chhi* of which congregated there, rather than anatomical regions as such where pain or discomfort might be felt, the idea was a rather sophisticated one. The *Nan Ching* directs that treatment should be given at these points in febrile diseases of the Yin type.[e]

[a] Syns. Tsung-chhi[5] and Chhi-hai.[6]

[b] A typical example of the habit common to physicians and philosophers of using common expressions with special highly technical meanings. Encountered in any ordinary text, *liu ho* would mean the four directions of space plus the zenith and the nadir, i.e. the universe.

[c] Hence Porkert's terms, (1), pp. 344–5, *foramina conventoria* for *hui hsüeh*, and *foramina copulo-conventoria* for *chiao hui hsüeh*. We dislike *foramina* (cf. Needham & Lu, 9), but the adjectives, if englished, might conceivably prove useful.

[d] Following Anon. (*107*), table 17.

[e] *CCCY*, ch. 1, (p. 139).

1 六合 2 會穴 3 交會穴 4 血 5 宗氣 6 氣海

Table 6. *The eight assembly-points* (hui hsüeh)

			hui hsüeh		
1	Tsang hui	臟 會	Yin viscera	H 13	Chang-mên
2	Fu hui	腑 會	Yang viscera	JM 12	Chung-kuan
3	Chhi hui	氣 會	*chhi*	JM 17	Shan-chung
4	Hsüeh hui	血 會	blood, etc.[a]	VU 17	Ko-shu
5	Chin hui	筋 會	muscles and tendons[b]	VF 34	Yang-ling-chhüan
6	Mo hui	脈 會	pulsating blood-vessels[c]	P 9	Thai-yuan
7	Ku hui	骨 會	bones	VU 11	Ta-shu
8	Sui hui	髓 會	bone-marrow	VF 39	Hsüan-chung[d]

The *chiao hui hsüeh* are, as their name implies, points of intersection where the tracts cross one another, i.e. 'communication, transfer and assembly points'.[e] Altogether there are 101 of them, some being junctions of more than two tracts simultaneously, and hence treatment at these acu-points could cure illnesses invovling several tracts. Although they occur all over the body, the intersections are particularly numerous on the head, face and trunk. The chief regular tract communication points are shown in Table 7.

Table 7. *Chief regular tract communication points* (chiao hui hsüeh)

1	Shou Thai-Yin	P	ct	P 1 Chung-fu	LP	pg	Tsu Thai-Yin	4
5	Shou Shao-Yin	C	ct	in the substance of the heart	R	pg	Tsu Shao-Yin	8
9	Shou Chhüeh-Yin	HC	ct	HC 1 Thien-chhih	H	pg	Tsu Chhüeh-Yin	12
6	Shou Thai-Yang	IT	cg	VU 1 Ching-ming	VU	pt	Tsu Thai-Yang	7
10	Shou Shao-Yang	SC	cg	VF 1 Thung-tzu-liao	VF	pt	Tsu Shao-Yang	11
2	Shou Yang-Ming	IG	cg	IG 20 Ying-hsiang	V	pt	Tsu Yang-Ming	3

The numbers at the extreme left and right indicate the positions of the tracts in the circulation order; their code-letters are given as well as the abbreviated names. The central column gives the *chiao hui hsüeh*. As before, ct, cheirotelic, cg, cheirogenic, pg, podogenic, pt, podotelic.

[a] *Hsüeh* was, and long remained, a word embracing meanings rather wider than 'blood', and sometimes probably ought to be taken as including the bodily juices in general, such as the *i*[1] so prominent in physiological alchemy (*SCC*, Vol. 5, pt. 5), lymph, chyle, interstitial fluids, and so on.

[b] The ancient physiology made little distinction between these and nerves.

[c] *Mo*[2] and *mo*[3] are orthographically interchangeable, but as already noted (p. 25) we use the former for pulse discussions only, keeping the latter for blood-vessels in general and acupuncture tracts.

[d] Formerly the synonym Chüeh-ku[4] was more common; see *CCCY*, ch. 1, (p. 139), ch. 4A, (p. 249), and *CCTC*, ch. 7, (p. 235).

[e] Cf. Anon. (*90*), p. 40.

1 液 2 脈 3 脉 4 絕骨

Table 8. *Auxiliary tract communication points* (chiao hui hsüeh)

chêng ching		*chhi ching*	communicating points *chiao hui hsüeh*	
Shou Chüeh-Yin	HC	Yin Wei Mo	HC 6	Nei-kuan
Tsu Thai-Yin	LP	Chhung Mo	LP 4	Kung-sun
Shou Thai-Yang	IT	Tu Mo	IT 3	Hou-chhi
Tsu-Thai Yang	VU	Yang Chhiao Mo	VU 62	Shen-mo
Shou Shao-Yang	SC	Yang Wei Mo	SC 5	Wai-kuan
Tsu Shao-Yang	VF	Tai Mo	VF 41	Tsu-lin-chhi
Shou Thai-Yin	P	Jen Mo	P 7	Lieh-chhüeh
Tsu Shao-Yin	R	Yin Chhiao Mo	R 6	Chao-hai

Besides this, all the three Yang tracts in the table on both sides have a common intersection with Tu Mo at Ta-chhui (TM 13); and the three Yin tracts in the table on the Tsu (foot) side have common intersections at Chung-chi (JM 3) and Kuan-yuan (JM 4). The three Yin tracts on the Shou (hand) side, however, depend on the intersection points of the three Tsu tracts with Jen Mo, connecting with that only through their *chiao hui hsüeh* such as Chung-fu (P 1). Thus in these ways the tracts of the body could exchange their *chhi* laterally, aiding further the general circulation by a kind of anastomosis.

The eight auxiliary tract *chiao hui hsüeh* are rather different. Their essential function was to link eight of the twelve regular (*chêng ching*) tracts with each one of the eight auxiliary tracts (*chhi ching pa mo*). This may be seen in Table 8.[a]

These *chiao hui hsüeh* were thus also a kind of *lo* or acu-junction, but it is interesting that four of the regular tracts were not involved; i.e. the crasso-intestinal, gastric, cardiac and hepatic (IG, V, C and H). Four of these *chiao hui hsüeh* are also *lo mo hsüeh* (as can be seen by a comparison of Table 8 with Table 5); and two of them are also *shu hsüeh*, yet another category, which we shall next explain. Before doing so, however, we may note that once again the *piao-li* relationship is present, because some malfunction of the auxiliary tracts would not be revealed except through their connections with the regular tracts. As for the function of these intersections, it will be remembered that the auxiliary tracts have no direct access to the viscera; therefore conditions indicating abnormalities of these tracts could be relieved by acupuncture at the eight communication points in Table 8.

The term *shu hsüeh*,[1] which may be translated as 'transmission points', has been and is, as we have seen (p. 13), applied to all the acu-points of the body. But as *wu shu hsüeh*[2,3] it is also a term for a special group of five acu-points in each tract distal to the knees and elbows, named to indicate increasing (or decreasing) strength of flow

[a] Constructed from Anon. (*107*), table 18 on p. 58.

1 兪穴 2 五輸穴 3 五兪穴

of the *chhi*.[a] It would almost be possible to use the analogy of speed, as if visualising an electric train gaining acceleration as it starts from the terminus of the line, and slowing down again as it reaches the other terminus—yet the thought here was of strength of flow rather than speed, amps, one might say, rather than volts. On the rising scale the successive stages were *ching*,[1] *yung*[2],[b] *shu*,[3] *ching*[4] and *ho*;[5] not really translatable, but at a pinch one might say: 'welling, fontane, flooding, fluent and confluent'. Each stage naturally had a symbolic correlation[c] with the Five Elements, and by the level of the main articulation (knee or elbow) the full power of the flow was attained.[d] Let us call them 'potency-level points'.

In the accompanying table (Table 9) several things are noteworthy. First it will be seen that the correlation between the *wu shu hsüeh* and the five elements differs for the two classes of tracts, Yin and Yang.[e] Secondly, it will be evident that the succession of the acu-points will be descending or ascending numerically in accordance with whether the tracts in question are cheiro- or podo-telic or -genic respectively, i.e. on whether they end at one or other of the extremities or whether they begin there. Third, all the twelve regular tracts are represented, but none of the auxiliary tracts or other linear arrays. It is furthermore interesting that none of the *wu shu* acu-points in the table have *shu* as part of their names; yet the word does occur in the lists (cf. Table 4), and quite frequently too—continuously from VU 13 to 30, and also elsewhere, e.g. R 16, and once in the leading position of the couplet (R 27). Twelve out of the eighteen along VU do in fact form the *pei shu hsüeh* of Table 11, as we shall see, but the origin of the others remains uncertain.

On the therapeutic side *ching*[1] points were (and are) used especially for anxiety states, *yung*[2] points for pyrexia, *shu*[3] for rheumatic, arthritic and muscular pains, *ching*[4] for coughs and bronchial affections, and *ho*[5] for illnesses of the digestive system and the Yang viscera. In using these points it has to be carefully borne in mind that since the correlations with the five elements differ as between Yin and Yang tracts, their relations with the viscera and also their symptoms will be quite different.

Another series of acu-points, the *yuan hsüeh*,[6] comprised those where the primordial *chhi* (*yuan chhi*[7]),[f] i.e. the pneumatic endowment inherited from the parents at birth, before the action of any external or environmental influences, in fact, the *hsien thien chih chhi*,[8] was supposed to collect in special amount or activity. It was thought of as

[a] One could perhaps think of them as transmission points *par excellence*. Porkert (1) speaks of the 'five inductories', presumably with the same idea in mind, but in view of the dangers inherent in the morphogenetic induction model (cf. p. 14 above) we think that such a term had better be avoided. He certainly means to invoke such induction here (his p. 336), for he says that 'all foramina are points of transmission of actual influences', i.e. 'inductive transmitters'.

[b] Sometimes written *jung*,[9] but wrongly. Meaning a small stream, it can also be pronounced *jung*, and it occurs in place-names as *ying* and *hsing*.

[c] Cf. *SCC*, Vol. 2, pp. 261 ff.

[d] See the account in Anon. (*107*), pp. 53–4. The *locus classicus* is *NCLS/PH*, ch. 2, (pp. 14 ff.).

[e] An early tabulation of these correspondences may be seen in *CCIF*, ch. 26, (p. 316.1), *c.* +660.

[f] Much has to be said about this in the discussion of physiological alchemy, *SCC*, Vol. 5, pt. 5.

1 井 2 滎 3 輸 4 經 5 合 6 原穴 7 元氣
8 先天之氣 9 榮

Table 9. *The five potency-level points in each acu-tract* (wu shu hsüeh)

Yin tracts		*ching* W		*yung* F		*shu* E		*ching* M		*ho* w	
Shou	P	11	Shao-shang	10	Yü-chi	9	Thai-yuan	8	Ching-chhü	5	Chhih-tsê
	HC	9	Chung-chhung	8	Lao-kung	7	Ta-ling	5	Chien-shih	3	Chhü-tsê
	C	9	Shao-chhung	8	Shao-fu	7	Shen-mên	4	Ling-tao	3	Shao-hai
Tsu	LP	1	Yin-pai	2	Ta-tu	3	Thai-pai	5	Shang-chhiu	9	Yin-ling-chhüan
	H	1	Ta-tun	2	Hsing-chien	3	Thai-chhung	4	Chung-fêng	8	Chhü-chhüan
	R	1	Yung-chhüan	2	Jan-ku	3	Thai-chhi	7	Fu-liu	10	Yin-ku
Yang tracts		*ching* M		*yung* w		*shu* W		*ching* F		*ho* E	
Shou	IG	1	Shang-yang	2	Erh-chien	3	San-chien	5	Yang-chhi	11	Chhü-chhih
	SC	1	Kuan-chhung	2	I-mên	3	Chung-chu	6	Chih-kou	10	Thien-ching
	IT	1	Shao-tsê	2	Chhien-ku	3	Hou-chhi	5	Yang-ku	8	Hsiao-hai
Tsu	V	45	Li-tui	44	Nei-thing	43	Hsien-ku	41	Chieh-chhi	36	San-li
	VF	44	Tsu-chhiao-yin	43	Hsia-chhi	41	Tsu-lin-chhi	38	Yang-fu	34	Yang-ling-chhüan
	VU	67	Chih-yin	66	Thung-ku	65	Shu-ku	60	Khun-lun	54	Wei-chung

The symbols for the elements here are as in *SCC*, Vol. 2, p. 253, W for Wood, F for Fire, E for Earth, M for Metal and w for Water.

Table 10. *Primordial* chhi *collector points* (yuan hsüeh)

Shou Yin	lung	P 9	Thai-yuan
Shou Yin	'pericardium'	HC 7	Ta-ling
Shou Yin	heart	C 7	Shen-mên
Tsu Yin	liver	H 3	Thai-chhung
Tsu Yang	gall-bladder	VF 40	Chhiu-hsü
Tsu Yin	spleen	LP 3	Thai-pai
Tsu Yang	stomach	V 42	Chhung-yang
Shou Yang	'three coctive regions'	SC 4	Yang-chhih
Tsu Yin	reins	R 3	Thai-chhi
Shou Yang	large intestine	IG 4	Ho-ku
Shou Yang	small intestine	IT 4	Wan-ku
Tsu Yang	bladder	VU 64	Ching-ku

radiating from the three regions of vital heat (*tan thien*[1]) but especially perhaps from the one in the abdomen.[a] Tentatively one could translate *yuan hsüeh* as 'primordial *chhi* collector points'. There is one in particular on each of the twelve regular tracts, as can be seen in Table 10.[b]

It will be noticed that six of these (all the Yin ones) coincide exactly with the Yin tract *shu hsüeh* points in Table 9, while the six Yang ones are displaced by one acu-point from those in that table. This occurs in the proximal direction both in the case of the three cheirogenic tracts, and (curiously also) in that of the three podotelic ones.

A further series of 'transmission points' is that comprising the *pei shu hsüeh*[2] or 'transmission points on the back'; they are situated along the bladder tract (VU), running cephalocaudally about 1½ in. from the centre line where Tu Mo (TM) is (Table 11). These acu-points were supposed to carry the *ching chhi*[3] of the various viscera, or to be particularly rich in it; twelve in number, they allowed for the two additional entities as well as the anatomically obvious thoracic and visceral organs.[c] In addition to this set there are six others with similar names (VU 16, 17, 24, 26, 29 and 30) including one for Tu Mo and one for the diaphragm. In recent times a new point for the pancreas (I-shu[4]) has been added between VU 17 and 18. Lastly, there is Yao-shu[5] (TM 2) for the kidneys, and that completes the muster of dorsal transmission points. When there is malfunction of any of the internal viscera it will be reflected at these points in the form of pain on pressure, swelling, unusual sensations of heat or cold, itching, etc., so that diagnosis can be made and acupuncture therapy applied.

A similar series of transmission points was recognised on the front of the thorax

[a] See also on this Vol. 5, pt. 5.

[b] The list is an ancient one, as we shall see on p. 85 below.

[c] A special study has been devoted to these acu-points by the Western acupuncture physician Baruch (2), who draws attention to their relation with the dorsal dermatomes (cf. p. 207 below).

[1] 丹田 [2] 背輸穴 [3] 經氣 [4] 胰輸 [5] 腰輸

Table 11. *Dorsal transmission points* (pei shu hsüeh)

	organ	acu-points		position in relation to vertebra number
P	lung	VU 13	Fei-shu	3rd thoracic
HC	'pericardium'	VU 14	Chüeh-yin-shu	4th thoracic
C	heart	VU 15	Hsin-shu	5th thoracic
H	liver	VU 18	Kan-shu	9th thoracic
VF	gall-bladder	VU 19	Tan-shu	10th thoracic
LP	spleen	VU 20	Phi-shu	11th thoracic
V	stomach	VU 21	Wei-shu	12th thoracic
SC	'three coctive regions'	VU 22	San-chiao-shu	1st lumbar
R	reins	VU 23	Shen-shu	2nd lumbar
IG	large intestine	VU 25	Ta-chhang-shu	4th lumbar
IT	small intestine	VU 27	Hsiao-chhang-shu	1st sacral
VU	bladder	VU 28	Phang-kuang-shu	2nd sacral

and abdomen, and these were called *mu hsüeh*[1].[a] Six of these were double because of the bilateral symmetry, but six were situated on the median line, and therefore single. The above scheme lists them (Table 11). In this case also visceral malfunctions would manifest themselves at the points, and acupuncture was applied to them.

Both these sets of points, dorsal and ventral, have a particular interest in the light of what we know today about the superficial manifestations of injury or malfunction in the thoracic and abdominal viscera and the pleural and peritoneal membranes which enclose them. One has only to open a treatise on applied physiology to see that the visceral afferent nerve-fibres have effects radiating much more widely than simple reports to the brain.[b] For example, while pressure on the parietal pleura gives a sharp pain located with considerable accuracy over the site of the irritation, any interference with the central diaphragmatic pleura leads to sharp referred pain in those parts of the neck supplied by the 3rd and 4th cervical posterior nerve roots. On the other hand the peripheral diaphragmatic pleura will cause referred pain in the body-wall either at front or back in the area innervated by the 6th to 12th thoracic nerves, i.e. the lower thorax, the lumbar region or even the abdomen. And in all cases pain may be accompanied by tenderness on pressure, and the reflex motor effects of

[a] In ancient Chinese anatomical terminology *mu yuan*[2] means any kind of membrane, such as the pleura, peritoneum, mesentery, etc. *Mu* is generally written with the *li* component (Rad. no. 19) in medical texts, but perhaps this was a convention for *mu*,[3] a curtain, with the *chin* component (Rad. no. 50), which would have been much more appropriate semantically. Here the reference may be, then, to the abdominal wall. Porkert, however, (1), p. 337, following a different line of thought, took *mu*[4,5] in its usual verbal sense, as meaning to summon, levy, collect or raise funds. Hence his translation *conquisitoria abdominalia*, emphasising the collection function (*conquisitor*, Lat., a recruiting officer).

These points have given rise to special studies by Western acupuncture physicians, notably Trubert (1); and Quaglia-Senta (1), who seeks to establish a relationship with the parasympathetic system.

[b] Samson Wright (1), pp. 207 ff.; cf. Moss (1), pp. 68 ff.

[1] 募穴 [2] 募原 [3] 幕 [4] 募 [5] 幕

Table 12. *Ventral transmission points* (mu hsüeh)

		dupl.	median	
P	lung	P 1		Chung-fu
HC	'pericardium'		JM 17	Shan-chung
C	heart		JM 14	Chü-chhüeh
H	liver	H 14		Chhi-mên
VF	gall-bladder	VF 24		Jih-yüeh
LP	spleen	H 13		Chang-mên
V	stomach		JM 12	Chung-kuan
SC	'three coctive regions'		JM 5	Shih-mên
R	reins	VF 25		Ching-mên
IG	large intestine	V 25		Thien-shu
IT	small intestine		JM 4	Kuan-yuan
VU	bladder		JM 3	Chung-chi

muscular rigidity. There may also be localised hyperalgesia, i.e. a condition in which a light pin-prick normally causing only slight discomfort brings about a strongly painful reaction; this would have been very clearly noticed by the acupuncture physicians. Similarly, the pain of cardiac ischaemia is felt in the sternum, not the heart, and renal colic manifests itself in the loin and scrotum, not the lumbar region. So also with the viscera in general, both solid and hollow. Although many pathological processes can occur in them without causing any pain at all, there are others which do, even if often referred to remote parts of the body, and therefore the ancient acupuncture tracts, and especially the sets of acu-points on the trunk, can be interpreted in the light of modern physiological knowledge. Indeed the general principle of the recognition of internal malfunction by means of external signs is fully reflected in the ancient *piao-li* diagnostic system.

The last series of which we have to speak here is that of the *chhi hsüeh*[1].[a] The word *chhi* is to be interpreted here as meaning a chink or small space, but the function of these acu-points is explained as collection centres for the *chhi*[2] of the tracts (*ching*[3]).[b] Here the relevant circulating *chhi* (*ching chhi*) especially collects, and these acu-points were important in practice especially for therapy in acute cases of disease diagnosed as associated with that particular tract. Each one of the regular tracts (*chêng ching*[4]) has one, as also 4 out of the 8 auxiliary tracts (*chhi ching*[5]), but not Chhung Mo or Tai Mo, nor the two median ones Tu Mo and Jen Mo (Table 13).[c]

These points were, and still are, used in acute conditions pertaining to the different

[a] *Chhi* here is equivalent to *chhi*[6] and *chhi*,[7] but it is always written as the first of these three forms in medical texts, and read as *hsi*. Cf. Anon. (*107*), p. 56.

[b] Porkert (1), p. 338, has *foramina rimica*, to translate the idea of tiny clefts, so one could conceivably speak of 'rimic acu-points'.

[c] As will be seen, the term *chhi* occurs twice in the list of acu-point names.

1 郄穴 2 氣 3 經 4 正經 5 奇經 6 郤 7 隙

Table 13. *Collection centres* (chhi hsüeh)

Shou Thai-Yin	P 6	Khung-tsui
Shou Chüeh-Yin	HC 4	Chhi-mên
Shou Shao-Yin	C 6	Yin-chhi
Shou Yang-Ming	IG 7	Wên-liu
Shou Shao-Yang	SC 7	Hui-tsung
Shou Thai-Yang	IT 6	Yang-lao
Tsu Yang-Ming	V 34	Liang-chhiu
Tsu Shao-Yang	VF 36	Wai-chhiu
Tsu Thai-Yang	VU 63	Tsu-chin-mên
Tsu Thai-Yin	LP 8	Ti-chi
Tsu Chüeh-Yin	H 6	Tsu-chung-tu
Tsu Shao-Yin	R 5	Shui-chhüan
Yang Chhiao Mo	VU 59	Fu-yang
Yang Wei Mo	VF 35	Yang-chiao
Yin Chhiao Mo	R 8	Chiao-hsin
Yin Wei Mo	R 9	Chu-pin

regular tracts. For example, Yang-lao (IT 6) can be acupunctured in cases of colic,[a] and Khung-tsui (P 6) in laryngitis, cough paroxysms, asthma, tonsillitis, etc.[b]

It remains now only to mention the existence of the so-called 'forbidden points' (*chin hsüeh*[1]).[c] The dangers of acupuncture were somewhat exaggerated by Old China Hands in the last century, but they saw it at its worst, often performed by ignorant medical pedlars;[d] nevertheless, apart from the obvious dangers of striking the greater nerves and blood-vessels, much care and skill was always necessary, especially when penetration exceeded half an inch or so.[e] By the +7th century standard lists of forbidden acu-points had been established.[f] Although modern technique has reduced the number, there are still a few where acupuncture is contra-indicated—for example, V 17 (Ju-chung), directly on the nipple.[g] In three other examples (TM 24, Shen-

[a] Chhêng Tan-An (*1*), p. 103; Anon. (*107*), p. 119.

[b] Chhêng Tan-An (*1*), pp. 61–2; Anon. (*107*), p. 65.

[c] Cf. Chhêng Tan-An (*1*), pp. 22–3.

[d] A typical paper from those days describing iatro-genic mishaps due to unskilled acupuncture is that of Yin (1). But all skilled acupuncture physicians would agree that there are very real dangers which it is necessary to avoid, and warnings therefore reasonably continue; cf. Carron, Epstein & Grand (1).

[e] There was also the question of pain caused to the patient. In certain cases we have encountered it was almost unbearable, but in the vast majority of insertions when the thin needles of today are used, they cannot be felt at all, and we have observed in clinics that the patient rarely winces. One of us (J. N.) could hardly feel insertions.

[f] Sun Ssu-Mo gives a good one in *Chhien Chin Yao Fang*, ch. 29, (p. 516). But there were substantial discussions already in *Chia I Ching*, ch. 5, (pp. 107ff.) and in *NCSW/PH*, ch. 52, (pp. 271ff.). There, for example, it was stated that acupuncture at Nao-hu (TM 16) could cause sudden death; and still today the use of this point is confined to moxibustion (Anon. *107*, p. 215). Cf. *NCLS*, ch. 73, p. 2*b*.

[g] See Anon. (*107*), p. 86.

[1] 禁穴

thing, high on the forehead; V 12, Chhüeh-phên, just above the clavicle, and SC 18, Chhi-mo, behind the lower part of the pinna of the ear)[a] it is laid down that only superficial penetration is permissible.[b] We shall return to this matter later on in connection with physiological interpretations, for the reason that the lore of danger-points in acupuncture has interesting connections with other fields of observation. Already in the late Sung period the *Hsi Yuan Lu*,[1] the father and mother of all books in all cultures on forensic medicine (+1247), recognises that blows on certain points of the body are particularly dangerous, and it specifies them by means of acu-points. Similar sensitive points are well known in forms of physical combat such as karate, and there was the characteristically Indian science of elephant control, where a sharp-ended stick is applied by the mahout to various points on the animal's body. When the time comes we shall look into this matter more fully.[c]

(3) Historical Growth of the System

With the completion of our account of the system of acupuncture physiology in its fully developed state the way is now open for the study of its history and the successive landmarks constituted by the series of great books which were written about it as the centuries passed.[d] Here our point of departure has already been indicated, namely the basic fact that the *Huang Ti Nei Ching, Su Wên* of the −2nd century, has a great deal to say about acupuncture, and the *Huang Ti Nei Ching, Ling Shu* of the −1st, has even more. Starting then from this Former Han dating we must investigate the centuries both earlier and later, first to see what can be said about the formative phases of the system, and then to follow the course of developments after this classical 'Hippocratic' period. But before doing anything else it will be advisable to examine certain ancient traditions about the materials of which acupuncture needles were made.

(i) *Origin and nature of the instruments*

There is fair proof, as we shall see, that the oldest extant mentions of acupuncture take us back to the middle of the Chou period, somewhere around −600, and this, it is interesting to note, antedates the flourishing of iron and steel technology in China by one or two centuries. But needles, of a sort, could have been made of bronze (Fig. 13*a*, *b*), and even conceivably copper or tin, to say nothing of finely beaten-out gold and silver, precious metals no doubt available, in limited amounts, to the people

[a] Op. cit., pp. 217, 85 and 175 respectively.

[b] On adverse reactions, contra-indications and complications in general see Peacher (1). It was always recognised that under certain circumstances, acupuncture at any point could cause fainting (*yün chen*[2]); cf. *CCCY*, ch. 4B, (p. 261).

[c] Cf. pp. 302 ff. below.

[d] Huard & Huang Kuang-Ming (8) have essayed a brief history of acupuncture, but so far there is no really adequate treatment of it in any Western language. The guidance has to be sought in Chinese books and papers, among which we may mention those of Anon. (*90*), pp. 14 ff.; Li Yuan-Chi (*1*); Sung Ta-Jen (*3*); Chang Chün-I (*1*) and Li Ching-Wei (*2*). But naturally no secondary sources can dispense one from the study of the original works themselves, including some of the ancient encyclopaedias. For example, there is a section on acupuncture in *TPYL*, ch. 830, pp. 10*b* ff.

1 冤　2 暈鍼

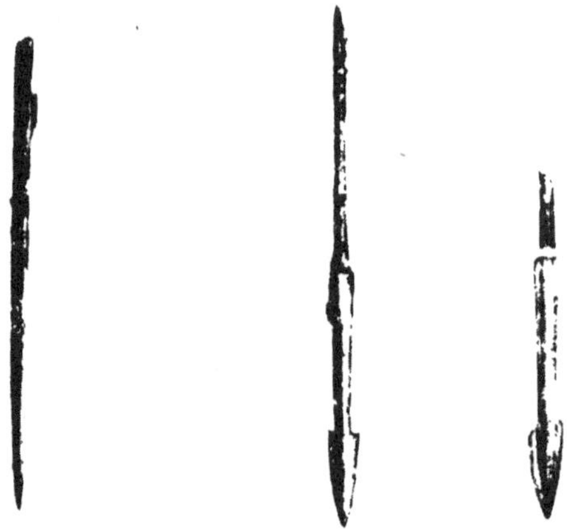

(*a*) (*b*)

Fig. 13. (*a*) A bronze needle from the Late Chou period (Anon. (*20*), pl. 74, fig. 6). (*b*) Bronze arrow-head needles from the Late Chou period (Anon. (*20*), pl. 67, figs. 3, 4).

of the Shang. We do not have certainty that the Shang practised acupuncture, but if they did they could also have used perishable substances available to all Asian men everywhere, i.e. thorns of various plants, slivers of bamboo (high in tensile strength), sharpened picks made of bone or horn. It might be imaginable that their Neolithic predecessors made use of stone, and so it comes as rather a shock to find that this was exactly the material which later Chinese tradition unanimously maintained had been used by the oldest of all the acupuncturists.

The word *pien*,[1] already used on the opening page of this monograph, and often translated curiously by lexicographers as 'stone probe', was familiar to Hsü Shen,[2] who in his *Shuo Wên*[3] of +121 defined it as 'a piece of (pointed) stone for pricking (to cure) illnesses (*i shih tzhu ping yeh*[4])'.[a] But probably the oldest mentions of stone needles occur in the *Shan Hai Ching*[5] (Classic of the Mountains and Rivers), that strange work composed perhaps largely around the −5th century, though containing materials ranging from the −11th to the +2nd, and while in many ways legendary or fabulous not without real geographical descriptions and interesting statements giving insight into ancient ideas and practices. Here we learn that on the mountain called Kao-shih chih Shan[6] 'there is much jade at the top, while at the bottom there are many needle-like stones (*chhi shang to yü, chhi hsia to chen shih*[7])'.[b] The same statement occurs again about Fu-li chih Shan,[8] with the added information that there is gold as well as jade at the top.[c] The commentators are all clear that these needle stones were for acupuncture; thus Kuo Pho[9] (+3rd cent.) says that they were given

[a] Ch. 9B, (p. 195.2).

[b] Ch. 4, p. 3*a*; cf. de Rosny (1), p. 158. *Chen shih* here is equivalent to *chen shih*,[10] as also *chhan shih*[11] cf. pp. 71, 105).

[c] Ch. 4, p. 7*a*; de Rosny (1), p. 169.

[1] 砭 [2] 許愼 [3] 說文 [4] 以石刺病也 [5] 山海經
[6] 高氏之山 [7] 其上多玉其下多箴石 [8] 鳧麗之山 [9] 郭璞
[10] 針石 [11] 鑱石

a sharp point and used for lancing swollen boils (*chih yung chung chê*[1]), while Wang Fu[2] of the Chhing remarks that the men of old made *pien*[3] out of them to cure diseases.

The tradition was then fixed by numerous mentions in the *Huang Ti Nei Ching*. For example, at one point Chhi Po says: 'In this present age it is necessary to bring forward powerful drugs to combat internal illnesses, and to use acupuncture with sharp stone needles (*chhan shih chen*[4])[a] and moxa (*ai*[5]) to control the external ones'.[b] Similar texts are found in other chapters, often mentioning the *pien shih*[6].[c] The general impression is that stone needles were not able to penetrate far into the tissues, and this is reasonable enough.[d]

By the Chin time, however, and outside professional medical circles, there was scepticism that needles could ever have been made of stone. Writing soon after +300 Ko Hung has an interlocutor saying to him:

> Even (Kungshu) Phan[e] and (Mo) Ti[f] could not make sharp needles out of shards and stones...The very gods and spirits cannot make possible what is really impossible; Heaven and Earth themselves cannot do what cannot be done...[g]

This is in the course of an argument about the possibility of Taoist material immortality, and though Pao Phu Tzu does not answer all his points directly, he goes on to a brilliant reply in which he shows that Nature contains many queer and paradoxical phenomena not covered by common-sense generalisations. 'There are more things in heaven and earth, Horatio...' etc.[h]

Yet it is rather difficult now to imagine what kind of mineral substance could have been used in ancient China for acupuncture 'needles'. The most obvious candidate might be obsidian or volcanic glass, but China was not a region of active volcanoes, and no material of this kind has been recognised in any of the descriptions in the pharmaceutical natural histories. China has flint,[i] knives of which can be sharp, but could it have been made sufficiently pointed? Possibly some hard sort of mica (*yün mu*[7])[j] might have been shaped to the purpose, or even some variety of asbestos (*shih*

[a] It may be said here that the characters *chen*[8,9,10] are all normally interchangeable, and we have not adopted any policy concerning them, except to use the simplest form (*chen*[10]) for all late writings and the bamboo form when appropriate (see immediately below).

[b] *NCSW*, ch. 14, p. 7*a*, *NCSW/C*, ch. 14p. 67*a*, *NCSW/PH*, ch. 14, (p. 79). Cf. on this Sung Ta-Jen (*3*). It does not of course necessarily mean that stone needles were still in use in the Han, for the text is an archaising one.

[c] E.g. *NCSW/PH*, ch. 12, (pp. 71–2), ch. 13, (p. 74). Other ancient references occur in some commentaries on the *Li Chi*, ch. 10.

[d] According to Sung Ta-Jen (*3*), p. 9, the *Shuo Yuan*[11] of Liu Hsiang[12] (−20) contains the saying (ch. 2) that 'if the disease is deep in the muscles (*chi fu*[13]), the stone needles will not be able to reach it'.

[e] The semi-legendary engineer of the State of Lu, *c.* −470 to −380, patron saint thereafter of all mechanicians.

[f] Founder of the philosophical artisan school of Mohism, living in the same period, later revered as an engineer and alchemist.

[g] *PPT/NP*, ch. 2, p. 2a.

[h] We gave a translation of much of this chapter in *SCC*, Vol. 2, pp. 437 ff.

[i] Torgashev (1), p. 414; di Villa (1), p. 47.

[j] RP 39, 93.

1 治癰腫者 2 汪紱 3 砭 4 鑱石鍼 5 艾 6 砭石
7 雲母 8 箴 9 鍼 10 針 11 說苑 12 劉向
13 肌膚

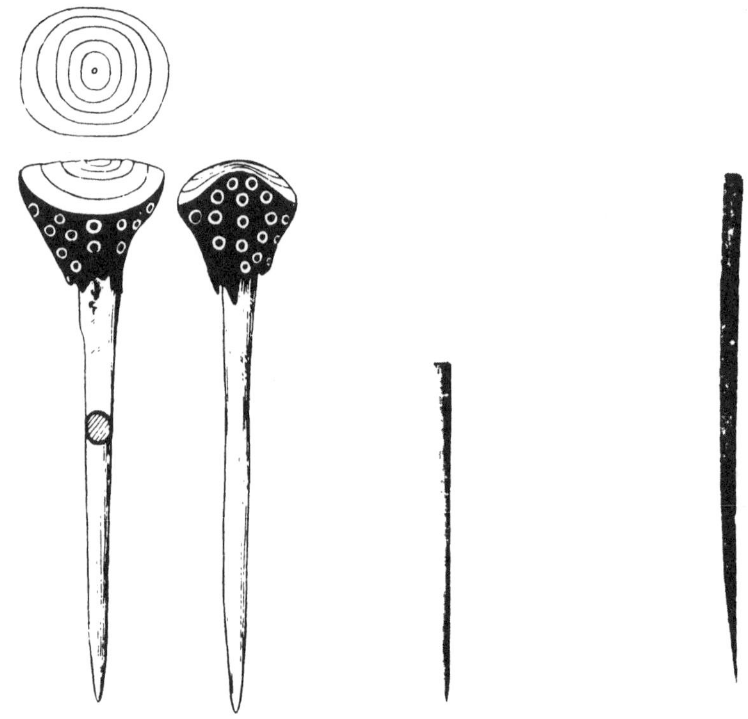

(*a*) (*b*) (*c*)

Fig. 14. (*a*) Bone needles of the neolithic period (Anon. (*194*), fig. 1). (*b*) A bone needle of the Late Chou period (Anon. (*20*), pl. 30, fig. 6). (*c*) Another from the same time (*Ibid.*, pl. 72, fig. 9).

ma[1]) like crocidolite,[a] with its fibres 3 in. long; but mica would have been difficult to work into spikes, and all asbestos fibres tend to be flexible. One could of course think of single needle-shaped crystals but these would surely have been too brittle. Perhaps jade, so tough, fibrous and hard to work, should not be excluded, especially in view of its unique position in the Chinese mind;[b] and artificial glass has been proposed, but apart from beads, plaques and tomb-ornaments it was not much known before the Han.[c] The subject remains open for speculation, and a probable solution has yet to be suggested.[d]

Two ideas mentioned in the preceding paragraphs deserve further remark. Kuo

[a] RP 35*f*, 56, 75.

[b] See *SCC*, Vol. 3, pp. 663 ff.

[c] See Vol. 4, pt. 1, pp. 101 ff. Whether glass needles could then have been drawn remains a moot point; they would have been disagreeably brittle.

[d] One striking find must however be recorded. Mrs Sarah Tomlin informs us that during the excavation at Shen Wan bay near Tung-ao Wan village on Lamma Island near Hongkong in 1973-4 directed by Dr Shih Hsüeh-Yen, they found half-a-dozen natural needles of quartz ranging around 1·5 in. long and roughly triangular in section; some had been broken off flat but several were quite sharp at the points. This raised beach site had been the haunt of late neolithic sea people, and inhabited as late as the Warring States period. Perhaps here is the clue to the puzzle.

[1] 石麻

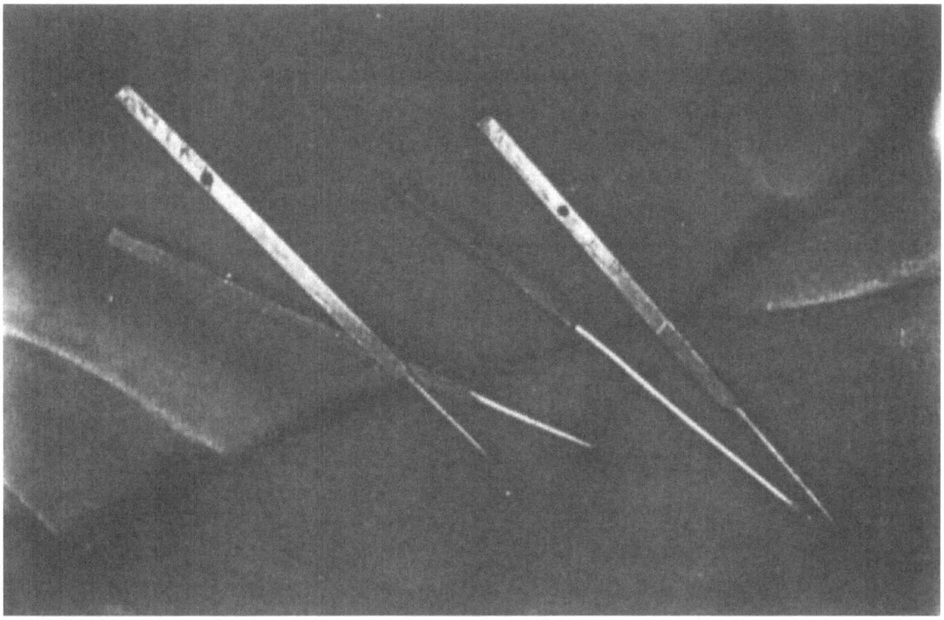

Fig. 15. Gold needles from the tomb of the Han prince Liu Shêng at Man-chhêng (−113). Orig. size, from Chung I-Yen (*1*).

Pho's statement about lancing boils reminds us that on one view at any rate the origin of all acupuncture needles lay in the ancient primitive instrument, whatever it was, used for opening abscesses to drain the pus from them.[a] Secondly it may be noted that the *Shan Hai Ching* uses the ancient form of the character for needle, *chen*,[1] with the bamboo radical (no. 118) at the top, reminding us that freshly whittled slivers of that material could have been very effective in medical use as well as for many other purposes.[b] Bone 'needles' too (*ku chen*[2]) have often been found in tombs and excavations, not only of neolithic age (Fig. 14*a*, *b*, *c*)[c] but also from Warring States burials, as at Erh-li Kang[3] near Chêng-chow.[d] They are often ground to sharp points at both ends, though never competing with wire for thinness. And the acupuncture technique could never reach the height of its effectiveness, administering its stimuli while causing the minimum of injury to the tissues, without wire-thin, and therefore metallic, needles.

The oldest traces of acupuncture which have come down to us, essentially from Middle Chou times, were all long preceded by the availability, and mastery, of copper, bronze, gold and silver; so that any of these metals could have been used in pin or

[a] This is expressed by many modern writers, for example, Anon. (*83*), p. 4.

[b] The point is often made, as by Chu Lien (*1*).

[c] Cf. Anon. (*194*) and *NCNA* Chinese bulletin, 29 June 1961, tombs near Shanghai. For bone needles of the Shang period, considered as hairpins, see Anon. (*195*), pl. 35, figs. 3–7, pl. 36, fig. 5.

[d] Anon. (*23*), pl. 15, figs. 15–17; pl. 27, figs. 4–7.

1 箴 2 骨箴 3 二里岡

needle form by the earliest acupuncturists. Probably the wire would have been forged and hammered out, for the use of the draw-plate[a] in any antique civilisation is not certainly established,[b] and we have no special evidence for it in ancient China. Recently four rather thick gold needles which may have been used in acupuncture[c] came to light in the tomb of the Han prince Liu Shêng[1] at Man-chhêng[2] (Fig. 15);[d] they are all about 3 in. long, round of cross-section though in one case triangular, while their square-sectioned 2-in. shanks have a small round hole at the far end.[e] They could hardly be considered very delicate instruments, but of course the precious metals had the advantage of not rusting or corroding.[f]

Nevertheless, steel (*kang*[3]), once known, was bound to replace all other materials for its strength and fineness. Any consideration, therefore, of the history of the physicians' needles is bound to involve us with the rather complicated question of the development of iron and steel technology in China.[g] Here the first thing that becomes apparent is (as already noted) that the oldest references to acupuncture seem to belong to the −6th or even −7th century while the first mentions of iron (*thieh*[4]) in China occur only from around −500 onwards. This surely indicates that materials other than iron were indeed used in ancient times. But before glancing at the most salient texts let us summarise what is known of China's iron and steel. At once we are surprised by the fact that although the age of iron came relatively late there (some seven centuries after the Hittites in Asia Minor), the Chinese could cast it almost as soon as they knew of it at all—an extraordinary achievement[h] when one recollects that blast-furnace cast iron (high-carbon iron) did not come in Europe until the +14th century. Furthermore China seems to have had no initial phase of bloomery furnaces yielding wrought iron (pure iron) only. The Chinese had however crucible

[a] A plate of a harder metal pierced with small holes through which are drawn by force lengths of slightly thicker wire. If the metal is malleable and ductile enough, the process will produce wire of almost any desired thinness.

[b] Wire in antiquity was generally beaten, but Maryon (2), pp. 481–2, studying a Persian rhyton of the −5th century, found that the gauge of its 136 ft. of gold wire was so uniform that it must, he thought, have been made with a draw-plate.

[c] Anon. (*106*), pl. 16B; Chung I-Yen (*1*), pl. 6.

[d] It may be relevant to remember here the eight pounds weight of gold wire which was used to sew together the jade scales of the body-cases of the Prince and his consort.

[e] The medical interpretation is somewhat strengthened by the fact that other objects found in the tomb are clearly inscribed as intended for the use of the Royal Physician; see Anon. (*111*), p. 13; Chung I-Yen (*1*). For example, there was a bronze bowl marked *I kung phan*.[5]

[f] This may be the place to refer to the continuing use of the precious metals for acupuncture needles down to the present time. How far they were used in medieval China we cannot readily say, but in modern times there has been a persistent idea that gold stimulates (reinforces, *pu*[6]) while silver sedates (reduces, *hsieh*[7]). The very inconclusive Western literature on this may be approached through the papers of Prinzing (1) and Prodescu, Stoicescu & Bratu (*1*); there were also Chinese and Japanese contributions, e.g. Sung Tê-Su (1); Fujita & Minami (1). All sorts of measurements have been made, as of 17-keto-steroid excretion, bile secretion and allergy relief. The question has aroused considerable interest in modern China too, and there are many references in the bibliography of Anon. (*149*); it remains in dispute. For a Chinese view of the Western experiments see Liu Yung-Shun (*2*).

[g] We faced a similar problem once before, when thinking about the availability of good steel needles for magnetic compasses; cf. *SCC*, Vol. 4, pt. 1, pp. 282ff. For further discussions of the history of iron and steel technology see Vol. 5, pt. 1 and in the meantime Needham (32, 72).

[h] Reasons for this can be adduced, but we must not recapitulate them here.

1 劉勝 2 滿城 3 鋼 4 鉄 5 醫工槃 6 補 7 瀉

methods using coal, which produced both cast iron (*shêng thieh*[1]) and wrought iron (*shu thieh*[2]) together, and if such techniques were known as early as the Warring States times their wrought iron could have been obtained that way; otherwise they must have made it from cast iron by some kind of puddling process in an oxidising hearth. Since they had so much more cast iron than wrought iron, they generally made steel not (as in Europe) by cementation (adding carbon to pure iron) but by finery (*pai lien*[3]) decarburisation methods (removing carbon from cast iron), i.e. a more controlled use of the same technique which if carried further would lead to wrought iron. Then somewhere about the +4th century a Chinese metallurgist of genius invented the sophisticated co-fusion method in which steel (*kuan kang*[4]) was produced by bathing wrought iron billets in molten cast iron, thus equalising the carbon content by diffusion; subsequent forging gives good eutectoid steel.

Now for some datings. A focal point is the casting of iron cauldrons (*ting*[5]), inscribed with Fan Hsüan-Tzu's[6] legal code, by Chao Yang[7] in the State of Chin in −512.[a] About the same time famous swords of iron were cast by Kan Chiang[8] for the prince of Wu (modern Chiangsu), Ho Lu[9] (r. −514 to −496).[b] That ancient calendar, the *Yüeh Ling*[10] (Monthly Ordinances of the Chou), speaks of 'metal and iron' as if the latter were something strange, and the best date for it is the −5th century.[c] Then in the −4th comes the famous passage in the *Kuan Tzu*[11] book on the iron tax, which says that every woman needs a needle and a knife, every farmer a hoe and a ploughshare, and every cartwright his axe, saw and chisel.[d] By this time we have ample material evidence of cast iron in the shape of actual tools, and moulds for making tools, in many Chinese museums. And this is supplemented in the Han not only by modern excavations of iron-works, but also by several striking textual descriptions of blast-furnace break-outs.

On general principles the knowledge of steel should not lag behind that of cast iron, so it may not be surprising that we can find the first reference to it also in the −5th century; this occurs in the Yü Kung[12] chapter of the *Shu Ching*[13] (Book of History). There the 'Tribute of Yü' says that Liangchow (approximately modern Szechuan, Shensi and Kansu) produces both iron and steel (*yu thieh yu lou*[14]).[e] The next important reference is that in the *Hsün Tzu*[15] book, *c.* −250, speaking of the spear-heads from Nanyang in Honan, made of 'great iron (*chü thieh*[16]), sharp as a bee's

[a] *Tso Chuan*, Duke Chao, 29th year; tr. Couvreur (1), vol. 3, p. 456.

[b] *Wu Yüeh Chhun Chhiu*, ch. 4, tr. Needham (32), p. 4. There is an aura of legend about these characters, and the source is late, but they are quite historical, and there is no reason to doubt the essentials of the tradition.

[c] It is incorporated in the *Li Chi*, ch. 6, p. 56*b*; tr. Legge (7), vol. 1, p. 265. Some of the astronomical data in the *Yüeh Ling* may be of the −7th century but it would be unsafe to put the text as a whole earlier than the −5th.

[d] Ch. 72, cf. Than Po-Fu *et al.* (1), p. 114. Parallel passage in ch. 81, tr. p. 182.

[e] Ch. 6, tr. Legge (1), p. 71; Karlgren (12), p. 15. The word *lou* later came to mean carved, engraved or inlaid, but all commentators agree that anciently it meant steel. Though some of the material in the Yü Kung seems to go back to the −9th or −8th century, scholars still do not dare to date it as a whole earlier than the −5th.

1 生鉄 2 熟鉄 3 百煉 4 灌鋼 5 鼎 6 范宣子
7 趙鞅 8 干將 9 闔廬 10 月令 11 管子 12 禹貢
13 書經 14 有鉄有鏤 15 荀子 16 巨鉄

sting'.[a] By this time, as we can deduce from certain texts written a little later, great advances were being made in steel manufacture, quenching, tempering, and 'the harmony of the hard and the soft (*kang juan chih ho*[1])', which probably means the pattern-welding of hard and soft (high and low carbon) steels.[b] Besides, from Chhin and Han times there remain many swords of iron and steel in Chinese museums, generally of course corroded but testifying by their length, so much greater than that of the older bronze ones, the characteristics and quality of the new metal.[c] And a number of other pieces of evidence demonstrate that by the −2nd century there was a well-developed steel industry in China.[d] Thus we may feel much confidence in the conclusion that by the time of the older part of the *Huang Ti Nei Ching* needles of wrought iron and mild steel were readily available to the physicians for their acupuncture.[e] This would have set the style for all later times.

But these thin pointed rods or wires must have been forged and hammered out, not drawn through a draw-plate. There is a special classical verb, *na*,[2] meaning to sharpen iron to a point by hammering; and in the West, at any rate, wire-drawing was a late medieval invention. The oldest description of it occurs about +1130, in the *De Diversis Artibus* of Theophilus Presbyter (Roger of Helmarshausen),[f] but it must have started a little before that. By the middle of the +14th century water-power was applied to the drawing of iron wire, and by the +15th it was a widespread industry.[g] Hence it is natural to find a picture of iron wire-drawing in the *Thien Kung Khai Wu*[3] (Exploitation of the Works of Nature) of +1637,[h] but so far no earlier illustration has come to light. Sung Ying-Hsing[4] says that the drawn and cut-off needles, after having been filed and ground to a sharp point, are packed in a cementation pot over a slow fire and then heated, quenched or tempered so as to give various grades of steel. This is significant because it is much easier to draw soft wrought iron than hard high-carbon steel.

Probably it is the carbon content which accounts for the great reputation that horse bits (*ma hsien thieh*[5]) had as the starting-point for acupuncture needles;[i] they would

[a] Ch. 15, pp. 16*a*ff.; tr. Dubs (8), p. 216 but transferred by him to ch. 19 for textual reasons. The passage appears also in *Shih Chi*, ch. 23, p. 6*b*. Again, all the commentators have recognised this special expression as referring to steel. The name afterwards standard, *kang*[6] or *kang thieh*,[7] came only later.

[b] E.g. Wang Chia's[8] *Shih I Chi*[9] (Memoirs on Neglected Matters), ch. 5, p. 1*a*, tr. Needham (32), p. 24; *San Fu Huang Thu*[10] (Illustrated Description of the Three Cities of the Metropolitan Area), ch. 30, tr. Dubs (2) vol., 1, p. 34; also *TPYL*, ch. 8345, p. *a* on a famous smith, Juan Shih.[11] There is more about him in Yang Chhüan's[12] *Wu Li Lun*[13] (Discourse on the Principles of Things). The first of these works dates from about +370, the two others from the end of the +3rd century if not before the end of the Later Han.

[c] On this and its consequences see Bodde (15).

[d] See Needham (32), p. 7.

[e] A few pages below (p. 79) we shall meet with a piece of textual evidence which bears this out particularly well.

[f] III, 8, 62 and 76; Hawthorne & Smith (1) tr. pp. 87–8, 138, 155; Dodwell (1) tr., pp. 68, 119–20, 137. Theophilus mentions mostly wire of gold, silver, copper, tin and lead, but one passage (III, 81, tr. Hawthorne & Smith, p. 159, Dodwell, p. 143) shows that he drew iron wire also.

[g] See Feldhaus (1), cols. 199ff.; Gille (14), p. 655; Forbes (8), pp. 74–5; F. C. Thompson (1).

[h] Ch. 10, p. 7*b*, reproduced in *SCC*, Vol. 4, pt. 1, p. 283, Fig. 332, and Needham (32), pl. 27, fig. 46; see also Sun & Sun (1), pp. 188, 193, 196.

[i] Cf. Anon. (*90*), p. 16. *CCTC*, ch. 4, p. 9*a* (p. 88.1).

1 剛軟之和 2 鈉 3 天工開物 4 宋應星 5 馬銜鉄 6 鋼
7 鋼鉄 8 王嘉 9 拾遺記 10 三輔皇圖 11 阮師 12 楊泉
13 物理論

have been made of mild low-carbon steel, still fairly fibrous, tough and malleable, not of brittle cast iron or soft wrought iron. The theorists developed appropriate explanations in the antique style, as one can see from passages like that in the *Chen Chiu Chü Ying*[1] of +1537, where we read as follows:[a]

Iron needles

According to the pharmaceutical natural histories (*pen tshao*[2]), the iron of horse bits and bridles (*ma han hsien thieh*[3]) is free from poison. Jih Hua Tzu[4] says that old bars of this (*thing*[5]) are good for making needles, and some believe that the needles used by the acupuncture practitioners always come from these sources.[b]

[Comm. by the author, Kao Wu[6]] When the pharmaceutical natural histories talk about soft iron they mean wrought iron (*shu thieh*[7]), and that has some poison in it. But the toxic effects are avoided by using iron from horse bits and bridles. Now the horse (according to the 'Book of Changes') belongs to the cyclical character (and double-hour) *wu*,[8] and that corresponds to the element Fire. Since Fire subdues Metal, this influence disperses the poison, and thus the iron of bits has been recognised as good for (acupuncture) needles. The ancients named these needles *chin chen*[9] (not because they were golden but) to indicate their preciousness. *Chin* was of course also the collective name for all metals, copper and iron, gold and silver.[c]

We cannot be sure that the needles in Kao Wu's time were wire-drawn rather than hammered out, though it would seem quite possible. They also had to go through many other processes, as we learn from him and similar writers, being boiled and heated with various chemicals, cementated, quenched and so on, all to the end of attaining optimum hardness and sharpness.

The subject of needle-making in China would repay much further research. We get a glimpse of it in the +10th century from Thao Ku's[10] *Chhing I Lu*,[11] where he says that

seamstresses or medical men will tell you the merits and disadvantages of different kinds of needles in just as much detail as Confucian scholars talking about brush pens.[d]

The most prized ones were those made of yellow steel and capped with gold heads (*chin thou huang kang hsiao phin*[12]). Later on we shall see (p. 105) what the *Huang Ti Nei Ching* has to say about the nine kinds of needles and pointed instruments used by the physicians of the −2nd century.

(ii) *The oldest references*

These preliminaries done, we can now have a look at the oldest references to acupuncture in Chinese literature. One of the first is to be found in the *Tso Chuan* commentary on the *Chhun Chhiu*, that record of the affairs of the feudal States between

[a] Ch. 3, (p. 189), tr. auct.

[b] This is the *Jih Hua Chu Chia Pên Tshao*[13] of +972, by Ta Ming.[14]

[c] An important statement because of the belief widely held in later times, and by Europeans especially, that gold and silver needles had a special virtue.

[d] Ch. 2, p. 23*b*, tr. auct.

1 針灸聚英 2 本草 3 馬啣銜鉄 4 日華子 5 鋌 6 高武
7 熟鉄 8 午 9 金鍼 10 陶穀 11 清異錄
12 金頭黃鋼小品 13 日華諸家本草 14 大明

the −8th century and the −5th. Under the date of −580 one finds the following passage.[a]

The Prince of Chin, being gravely ill, sent word to Chhin to ask for a physician. The Prince of Chhin accordingly sent his Doctor Huan (I Huan[1]) to attend him. Before he arrived, the sick prince suddenly saw in a dream as it were two young serving-men (within his own body) and he heard them talking together about his disease. One was saying to the other: 'Huan is a clever physician; I fear he will do us great harm. How can we escape from him?' To which the other replied: 'Let us take up our station between the heart and the diaphragm (*huang chih shang, kao chih hsia*[2])[b] — then what can he do to us?'

Having arrived (and made his examination) the physician (Huan) said: 'This disease is incurable. It has settled in the region between the heart and the diaphragm, and therefore cannot be attacked by us.[c] No (needle) can penetrate to it, no drug can reach it. There is nothing to be done.' The prince exclaimed: 'What an excellent physician!' Then he caused him to be treated with great honour, and sent him back to Chhin.

Perhaps not every patient nowadays would applaud so selflessly the honesty of his doctor, though some might appreciate more candour than they actually get; in any case the story is still another indication of the very rational and scientific spirit which animated the early centuries of Chinese medicine. Although the word for needle is not in the text, the idea of the penetration of some instrument, and the characteristic coupling of that with the ingestion of drugs, has justified all commentators in regarding the reference as one to acupuncture.

We are not much given to etymological arguments, but the word *i* for 'physician' and 'medicine',[d] as in I Huan's title, cannot do without a note in the present context. The upper half of the character consists of a quiver-full of arrows on the left and a spear or lance on the right. The common explanation has been that these pointed weapons represented the pangs of the patient or the shafts shot by disease demons, or else the arrows directed by shamans in ceremonies against the evil forces; but there is no real authority for any of these interpretations. May it not be suggested instead that these sharp stilettos denoted from the outset the needles used in acupuncture?[e] Arrows (or needles?) appear also in the bone or bronze forms of other characters, denoting illnesses.[f] Originally the lower half of the character *i* was *wu* (a shaman or wizard)[g] but by the Han time already it had been permanently changed to *yu*,[h] meaning 'ripe' or 'fuller fermented', the phonetic of *chiu* (wine); and the

[a] Duke Chhêng, 10th year; tr. Couvreur (1), vol. 2, pp. 84–5, eng. et mod. auct.

[b] On this expression cf. *NCSW/PH*, ch. 54, (p. 272) and pp. 52, 54 above.

[c] Perhaps the second half of this sentence should read 'Moxibustion will do it no good'. Some regard *kung*[3] here as a technical term for this procedure. Similarly, *ta*,[4] 'to penetrate', is regarded by some commentators as a technical term for acupuncture. The third great therapeutic division, materia medica, is already explicit in the text.

[d] K/958; Chang Hsüan (*1*), p. 789.

[e] This has been hinted also by others, e.g. Schatz, Larre & de la Vallée (1), pp. 30–1.

[f] Lu Gwei-Djen & Needham (4), figs. 2, 5, 6.

[g] See *SCC*, Vol. 2, pp. 132ff.

[h] Rad. no. 164.

[1] 醫緩 [2] 肓之上膏之下 [3] 攻 [4] 達

ancient lexicographers were agreed that this was because of the importance of alcoholic extracts of materia medica in therapeutics.

There is another story in the *Tso Chuan* from a few decades later with an even clearer reference to acupuncture, though its context remains a little puzzling. It concerns the relationships between the families of three high officials of the State of Lu, Chi Sun,[1] Mêng Sun[2] and Tsang Sun,[3] and the background is one of disagreements and intrigues relating to the choices of succession of elder and younger sons of various wives and concubines. We can dispense with these details, noting only that Chi Sun was fond of Tsang Sun, who had helped him with an inheritance problem, while Mêng Sun hated him. In −549 Mêng Sun died, but Tsang Sun came and lamented at his lying-in-state. On leaving, his charioteer asked him why he had done this, since everyone knew of the enmity. Tsang Sun replied:[a]

> Chi Sun was attracted to me because my slight recurrent fever (*chi chhen*[4]) gave me a handsome hectic flush. Mêng Sun disliked me because I took drugs and acupuncture (*shih*[5]) to cure it. But the most becoming fever is not as good as the worst stone needle, for that could keep me alive instead of spreading poison through me as the fever did. Now Mêng Sun is gone I shan't last long.

And indeed that same winter he had to flee to Chu.[b]

The story has an interesting pendant because it was referred to again in the late +6th century, about the beginning of the Sui, when people were discussing the origins of acupuncture, and in so doing preserved a Han commentary on the passage. In the biography of Wang Sêng-Ju[6] in the *Nan Shih*[c] it is related that Chhüan Yuan-Chhi[7] consulted him on medical history before embarking on his commentary on the *Nei Ching Su Wên* and *Ling Shu*, the first that was attempted. Chhüan asked Wang about the stone acupuncture needles (*pien shih*[8]), and he replied that all the ancient texts spoke of stone—*Shan Hai Ching*, *Shuo Wên*, *Erh Ya*, etc.—instancing also this passage in the *Tso Chuan*. Then he went on to quote a commentary by Fu Chhien:[9] '"Stone" here means stone acupuncture needles. By the end of the previous dynasty good stone was no more available, so people used iron as a substitute.' Since Fu Chhien's *floruit* was +165 to +185, in the Later Han, this statement would agree well enough with other evidence as to the first introduction of iron needles (p. 75), whether he meant to refer to the Earlier Han or to the Chhin.

Another very old reference, which has the advantage of being seemingly precise about the acu-point used, occurs in the biography of Pien Chhio,[10] the famous Chou physician of rather uncertain date, in the *Shih Chi*.[d] Passing through the State of

[a] Duke Hsiang, 23rd year; tr. auct.

[b] The meaning of the story is not quite clear. Couvreur (1), vol. 2, p. 400, interpreted it in his translation purely figuratively and ethically, widely diverging from the rendering adopted here, which is based on Yü Yün-Hsiu (*1*), pp. 350–1. It hardly makes sense to take the fever as metaphorical, yet a hectic flush would hardly seem the kind of thing that would attract one patrician to another.

[c] Ch. 59, p. 15*a*. The biography in the *Liang Shu* omits the incident. The *Nan Shih* text writes Chin[11] instead of Chhüan, but there can be no doubt as to who is meant.

[d] Ch. 105, p. 6*a*, tr. auct., adjuv. Bridgman (2), p. 22, and others named in what follows.

1 季孫 2 孟孫 3 臧孫 4 疾疢 5 石 6 王僧孺
7 全元起 8 砭石 9 服虔 10 扁鵲 11 金

Kuo[1] on one occasion, he was called to attend the crown prince, who was lying in a coma (*shih chüeh*[2]). After examination:

> Pien Chhio ordered his disciple Tzu-Yang[3] to sharpen the needles on the grindstone (*li chen chih shih*[4]) so that acupuncture might be performed at the San-yang Wu-hui[5] point (or points). After a moment the Prince came to, and presently sat up...

Two things here call for remark, first the dating, and then the identification of the acu-point or points.[a] The dates of Pien Chhio have always been difficult to determine; traditionally his life fell in the −6th century, contemporary with Confucius perhaps, but various indications point rather to the −4th. The text dates of course from about −100, but whatever the time of the curing of the crown prince of Kuo it must have been much earlier than that. On the other hand some of the Kuo States seem too early; the most renowned of them was extinguished by Chin in −654, but not until it had left for us the tomb with the great park of chariots at Shang-tshun Ling near the San-mên gorge of the Yellow River excavated in 1958.[b] Eastern Kuo was earlier still, but Western Kuo, centred near Paochi in the Wei Valley, was rather later, and if that was the crown prince's State it would bring Pien Chhio to his traditional time, the −6th century.[c] The association of the physician with Kuo State may have been a later fable, but it would be hard to make that later than the −4th century, and such a date is already remarkable for the naming of one or more particular acu-points. Let us turn now to the problem of their identification.

Here the great difficulty is that we do not know much about the dates of origin of the individual acu-point names, not enough, in fact, to give us certainty in the interpretation of so ancient a text as this. However, something can be said (see Table 4). The bald-headed approach would naturally be to take San-yang[6] as 'the three Yang' something, and Wu-hui[7] as 'the five Hui' — presumably either tracts or acu-points. The former was what modern translators have done, thinking of tracts Yin and Yang; as we shall see in a moment. The latter was just what the commentator Chang Shou-Chieh did in the +8th century when he collected a list of *hui* from some version of the *Nei Ching* then available to him. But if one is familiar with the array of acu-point names, and accustomed to the synonym register in the *Chen Chiu Ta Chhêng*, one is wary of such simple solutions and conscious that the two doublets might be acu-point names themselves. Since triplets and quadruplets are also possible in such names we can state at once the first alternative, namely that Pien Chhio and his student meant one single point only, TM 19, on the top of the head, for San-yang-wu-hui is in fact one of the accepted synonyms of what is most commonly called

[a] There are several other references to Pien Chhio's skill in acupuncture, but mostly later than this text, or much later. For example there is the passage about preventive medicine in the *Ho Kuan Tzu* book, which we quote in the sub-section on hygiene—meanwhile see Needham & Lu Gwei-Djen (1), pp. 434–5, repr. in Needham (64), p. 345.

[b] See Anon. (27), and mentions already in *SCC*, Vol. 1, p. 94, Vol. 4, pt. 2, pp. 77, 246.

[c] Cf. here Bridgman (2), p. 55.

[1] 虢 [2] 尸厥 [3] 子陽 [4] 厲鍼砥石 [5] 三陽五會 [6] 三陽
[7] 五會

Pai-hui.[a] But one has to reckon with the possibility that this quadruplet came to be applied to TM 19 only in later centuries, derivatively from the *Shih Chi* passage and not antecedent to it. Still, both of the doublets themselves, San-yang and Wu-hui, are also classically synonyms of this point.[b] A second alternative would be to assume that two separate points were meant. In this case one could take San-yang as equivalent to Pai-hui but have recourse also to Jen-ying, V 9, one of the synonyms of which is Wu-hui. This would mean Pien Chhio doing acupuncture both on top of the head and beside the sternomastoid muscle. Then there is a third alternative, namely that his San-yang meant SC 8, now called San-yang-lo, a point on the outer surface of the forearm over the extensor muscles beside the ulna. For some reason or other this was always regarded as a dangerous spot (a *chin hsüeh*[1]), and even contemporary treatises say that moxa only should be used there,[c] but nevertheless — and this is what makes it interesting — it has been traditionally used for arousal from coma.[d] Then the accompanying Wu-hui point could have been either TM 19 (20) or V 9. Lastly, a fourth possibility is that San-yang could have been either of the two points already mentioned (TM 19 (20) or SC 8), while Wu-hui could really have been five in number, i.e. the five of the commentary, identified as far as possible in Table 14 (V 9, JM 8, SC 13, VF 2 and JM 17). Thus there are four main interpretations of Pien Chhio's treatment.

The translation of this passage is such an object-lesson of the difficulties which beset historians of ancient Chinese medicine that it is worth giving some of the versions which have so far been offered. Thus we may quote as follows:

Bridgman (2): '(prepared the needles) to attract to the exterior the three Yang (pulses) and the five "reunions" '.[e]

Hübotter (4): '(prepared the needles) and punctured the meeting-places of the three Yang (tracts)'.[f]

Barde (5): '(prepared the needles) so as to extract (the air?) from the five *hui* points of the three Yang (tracts)'.[g]

Nguyen Tran-Huan (3): '(prepared the needles) and inserted them at the San-yang and Wu-hui points'.[h]

Thus the tendency has been to interpret San-yang as the three Yang tracts as a whole.

[a] TM 20 in Chhêng Tan-An (*1*), p. 182, who accepts the quadruplet synonym, however. Sung Ta-Jen (*3*) was sure that this single point was meant, pointing out that it is also Wei Hui,[2] i.e. the meeting-point of the two auxiliary tracts (*wei mo*[3]) which bear this name (cf. Table 1), on the upper surface of the cranium.

[b] *CCTC*, ch. 7, (p. 236.1).

[c] Anon. (*107*), p. 172.

[d] Hsieh Li-Hêng (*2*), s.v. Under quite other conditions, in a seeming paradox, it is now sometimes used for acupuncture analgesia.

[e] Bridgman (p. 60) was well aware of the commentary giving the five names from *NCSW*, and quoted it, but did not take the further step of trying to identify them with traditional acu-points.

[f] There are, of course, six, or ten if the auxiliary tracts are counted.

[g] Unfortunately the five *hui* points of the commentary are not all on Yang tracts (cf. Table 14).

[h] He interpreted San-yang here, however, as meaning many points along three of the Yang tracts (not further specified), and the Wu-hui as being the five of the commentator's list, though he found difficulty in identifying Chhi-hui and Hsiung-hui.

[1] 禁穴 [2] 維會 [3] 維脉

Table 14. *Synonyms of acu-points possibly used by Pien Chhio*

Yang or Yin	acu-point	synonyms from *CCTC*[a]	synonyms from *NCSW*[b]	anatomical position
Yg	Jen-ying 人迎 V 9	= Wu-hui 五會 = Pai-hui	Pai-hui 百會	edge of sterno-mastoid muscle in neck, close to the great vessels
Yn	Thien-chhih 天池 HC 1	= Thien-hui 天會		over mammary gland, lateral to nipple
Yn	Shen-chhüeh 神闕 JM 8	= Chhi-hui 氣會	Chhi-hui 氣會	on the abdominal wall at or very near umbilicus
Yn	Ti-chi 地機 LP 8	= Phi-hui 脾會		medial to tibia, over soleus muscle
Yg	Nao-hui 臑會 SC 13	= Nao-liao 臑髎	Nao-hui 臑會	back of upper arm, above but near lower edge of deltoid muscle
Yg	Pai-hui 百會 TM 19 (or 20)	= Wu-hui 五會 = San-yang 三陽 = San-yang-wu-hui 三陽五會	Pai-hui 百會 (alt.)	top of head over sagittal suture in parietal region
Yg	Thing-hui 聽會 VF 2	= Thing-ho 聽河 = Hou-kuan 後關	Thing-hui 聽會	in front of the anterior edge of the ear pinna at the level of the intertragic notch
Yn	Shan-chung 膻中 JM 17	= Hsiung-chung 胸中	Hsiung-hui 胸會	over sternum at the level of the fused insertion of the 8th, 9th and 10th ribs
Yg	San-yang-lo 三陽絡 SC 8			a point on the outer surface of the forearm over the extensor muscles beside ulna above extensor retinaculum band

[a] Ch. 7, (pp. 234.2 ff.).

[b] The names of these five *hui*, not the same in any particular as the later *hui hsüeh* and *chiao hui hsüeh* listed in Tables 6, 7, 8 and above, are not to be found in the *Su Wên* part of the *Huang Ti Nei Ching* now, but were supplied by one of the *Shih Chi* commentators, Chang Shou-Chieh,[1] in his remarks on the passage in question about Pien Chhio, written in +737, presumably from some version of the *Nei Ching* available to him then. Hence Hsieh Li-Hêng (*2*), in his medical encyclopaedia, vol. 1, p. 401, could quote them only from the *Shih Chi* commentary.

[1] 張守節

We should not like to deny that the doublet may often have been used in this sense, adding also that it seems sometimes to have been applied to the two Yang Ming tracts alone, but then we can have no idea which acu-points in particular Pien Chhio used.

We have gone into this much detail because it is of such great interest that Ssuma Chhien should have preserved from his documentary sources or oral tradition what may have been the actual names of one or two of the acu-points used by the physicians of the late Chou, Warring States and Chhin periods, i.e. the time preceding the compilation of the *Nei Ching*. One would hesitate to adopt any of the above interpretations, however, before enquiring whether there was any tradition among medieval Chinese medical writers concerning the procedure of Pien Chhio. And in fact there was such a tradition, as may be seen from the *Tou Thai-Shih hsien-sêng Liu Chu Chih Yao Fu*[1] (The Encomium of Mr Regius Professor Tou on the Essentials of the (Circulation of the Chhi according to the) Time Cycle Theory),[a] written in +1315. There Tou Chieh[2] (the younger) says clearly that Pien Chhio used Wei-hui as the acu-point. Chhêng Tan-An (*2*)[b] and Sung Ta-Jen (*3*) continued this tradition. Unfortunately Wei-hui is a name not found in the existing lists of synonyms, but a parallel opinion, also old, and expressed for example in the *Hsün Ching Khao Hsüeh Phien*[3] (An Investigation of the Acu-Points along the (Fourteen) Tracts), a work written about +1580, probably by Yen Chen-Shih,[4] supported San-yang-wu-hui as the single place. Wei-hui may have been therefore a former name for Pai-hui (TM 19), the point 'of the hundred meetings' on the upper surface of the cranium where the Tu Mo tract collects or 'ties together' all the 'three Yang' (*san Yang*) *chhi* of the body.[c] Thus the conclusion is that the point generally known at the present day as Pai-hui was probably the only one used by Pien Chhio,[d] and this is supported by several recent writers.[e] On the whole, therefore, Nguyen Tran-Huan understood the matter best, though even he was apparently unaware of the traditional interpretation in the Chinese medical literature, which indicates a single point alone.

Finally, after all these historical excursions, it is pertinent for the physiologist to ask how acupuncture needles could possibly arouse a patient from coma anyway. That they can effect this is in all the Chinese books, but recent experiments throw new light on the mechanism. Chhen & Erdmann (1), using an electrical method of measuring the partial pressure of oxygen in the rat brain, found that needling at Jen-chung (TM 25 or 26) will cause an immediate rise in tissue oxygen in the frontal cortex, due to sudden vaso-dilation and an intensification of the capillary perfusion rate. Further research will certainly enlarge our knowledge of the neurological connections which lead to this effect.

[a] In Tu Ssu-Ching's *Chi Shêng Pa Sui* (*Fang*), ch. 2, p. 7*a*.
[b] P. 34.
[c] Anon. (*107*), pp. 11, 216. An alternative view, however, is expressed by Chhen Pi-Liu & Chêng Cho-Jen (*2*), p. 51, who identify Wei-hui with JM 3, Chung-chi,[5] a point located medially four inches below the umbilicus.
[d] It is still in use for arousal from coma, and also classically for migraine; see Chhêng Tan-An (*1*), p. 348.
[e] Jen Ying-Chhiu (*1*), p. 8; Thao I-Hsün & Ma Li-Jen (*1*), p. 313.

[1] 竇太師先生流注指要賦 [2] 竇傑 [3] 循經考穴編 [4] 嚴振識 [5] 中極

There is still more to say about Pien Chhio and the coma of the Crown Prince of Kuo, and it concerns a very curious passage which Ssuma Chhien wrote in the form of a dialogue between the great physician and a Royal Tutor (Chung Shu Tzu[1]), a lover of the technical arts (*hsi fang chê*[2]), when he first appeared at the palace gate. Enquiring how long the prince had been 'dead', he was told that he had been unconscious for half a day, and had not yet been encoffined.

So Pien Chhio said: 'Pray announce that I am Chhin Yüeh Jen[3a] from Po-hai in Chhi, of a family from Chêng. Say that I have not hitherto had the pleasure of viewing the splendour of this Court, nor of paying my respects to the royal presence. Now I hear that the Crown Prince is dead — yet I believe I can revive him.'

The Royal Tutor exclaimed: 'Are you, Sir, not boasting of your powers? Is it possible you claim that you can bring back the Prince to life? I have heard that in very ancient times there was a physician named Yü Fu[4].[b] In curing diseases he did not use decoctions of drugs (*thang i*[5]), nor alcoholic extracts (lit. sprinklings of sweet wine, *li sa*[6]), nor needles of stone (*chhan shih*[7]), nor yet remedial exercises for stiff joints (*chiao yin*[8]), nor massage of different kinds (*an wan*[9]), nor even warmed plasters placed on poisoned lesions (*tu yün*[10]). By a single examination[c] he knew the cause of the illness, and its reflection in the acu-points (*shu*[11]) of the five viscera. Then he would set about cutting open the skin and dissecting the flesh, taking hold of the vessels and rejoining the muscles, handling the brain and the nerves, examining the diaphragm and scraping the membranes; or else he would wash out the intestines and the stomach, or rinse the five viscera themselves—in short, his techniques were so subtle that he could change the patient's form entirely (and make it like new). If, Sir, your methods are as good as his were, then perhaps the Prince can be revived. But if they are not, then whatever your wishes may be, even a child would not keep faith in you for a single day!'[d]

Pien Chhio replies with an important speech embodying the holistic, organicist and psycho-somatic principles so characteristic of Chinese medicine, but it does not concern us here.[e] In due course he has audience with the sovereign of the State, and achieves his seemingly miraculous cure. But what is so interesting about this passage? Of course it is semi-legendary, for Ssuma Chhien died a couple of thousand years ago, and not even he could know the course of a conversation which took place between people who had lived perhaps half a millennium earlier still—it is, if you like, history

[a] This name has given rise to much discussion. It has been thought to mean 'the man of Yüeh practising in Chhin', but Pien Chhio was not prominently connected with either of those States. Recent Chinese medical historians prefer to regard it as a family name and a given name — Chhin Yüeh-Jen. Cf. Chao Yü-Chhing & Khung Shu-Chên (*1*) and Ma Khan-Wên (*1*).

[b] One of the legendary ministers or technicians of Huang Ti (cf. *SCC*, Vol. 1, p. 51).

[c] Here the wording strongly suggests the pulse, for *po mo*[12] is to this day a colloquial expression for the more classical *chhieh mo*.[13] Alternatively—or additionally — it may mean that he felt for tenderness or pain at the acu-points in question.

[d] *Shih Chi*, ch. 105, pp. 3*b*, 4*a*, tr. auct. adjuv. Bridgman (2), pp. 19ff., 56–7; Barde (5), pp. 15–16, 45–6; Nguyen Tran-Huan (3), pp. 62–3, 73. We diverge widely from all these translators, however, on a number of points, especially the interpretation of the pregnant words: *i po chien ping chih ying, yin wu tsang chih shu*.[14]

[e] We deal with it in another place, *SCC*, Vol. 6.

1 中庶子 2 喜方者 3 秦越人 4 兪附 5 湯液 6 醴灑
7 鑱石 8 蹻引 9 案玩 10 毒熨 11 輸 12 撥脈
13 切脈 14 一撥見病之應因五臟之輸

in romance form. But it remains quite valid for the ideas of the historian's own time, and it may enshrine a valuable hint concerning the earliest history of acupuncture. At first sight it seems to have strayed in here from a paragraph on the earliest history or pre-history of surgery in China, and indeed we may look at it again from that point of view, for both the surgery and the anatomy of the ancient Chinese have been greatly undervalued by medical historians in general. Furthermore the opening sentences on the techniques that Yü Fu did not use include acupuncture needles (though, curiously, not moxibustion). But then when the Imperial Tutor comes to the great secret of Yü Fu's diagnostic genius he reveals that the *shu*,[1] acu-points (cf. Tables 4, 9, 11 above), were what he chiefly depended upon. Hence the prospect opens in front of us that individual 'acu-points' may indeed have been recognised long before their assembly into 'constellations', i.e. the patterns of the tracts. And there can be little doubt that visceral malfunction of many kinds can be reflected in all sorts of ways in phenomena ascertainable on palpation. Thus the course of the most ancient developments grows a little clearer.

Can we form any idea of what acu-points were so important for Yü Fu? Commenting on this text in +737, Chang Shou-Chieh gave a list of the *yuan*[2] acu-points by name[a] drawn, he said, from the *Nan Ching*. They correspond exactly with those given in Table 10 above, except that Tui-ku[3] (C 7) is now known as Shen-mên.[4] Chang was doubtless thinking of the statement in the *Ling Shu*: 'If you clearly understand the *yuan* acu-points and attentively observe their reflections (by the pulse or palpation), you will know the site of the disease among the five viscera.'[b]

It is time that we took leave of Pien Chhio, but we still cannot do so because he is connected with some singular stone reliefs which have recently come to light among the inscribed Han sculptures preserved at the Confucian Temple at Chhü-fou in Shantung. Of these we illustrate three (Fig. 16 *a*, *b*, *c*).[c] In each case a human-headed bird with arms is holding an elongated object in one hand, and the wrist of a kneeling person with the other. There may be one or more similar persons behind, seemingly waiting their turn. Liu Tun-Yuan (*1*), the discoverer of these reliefs, regards them as scenes of acupuncture, moxibustion and pulse diagnosis, with the human-headed bird representing Pien Chhio by a kind of pun on his given name.[d] The taking of the pulse by the bird-man seems clear enough, and the position of the uplifted arm does certainly suggest the action of acupuncture.

It is hard to know just what to make of these reliefs. There is indeed the echo of the name; and the stones almost certainly came from Liang-chhêng Shan[5] in Wei-shan

[a] We have assumed that *shu* in the above passage refers to any acu-points connected with the five *tsang* viscera, but it will be remembered that there are a number of points on the back specifically combining that term with the several *tsang* and *fu* viscera in their names (Table 11), and furthermore that the Yin set of *yuan hsüeh* is identical with the set of *shu hsüeh* in its most restricted sense (cf. Tables 9 and 10). So it may be that in this old text some more specific meaning was intended.

[b] *NCLS/PH*, ch. 1, (p. 11).

[c] The last was reproduced by Capon & McQuitty (1), pp. 174 (text), 186 (fig.). We are indebted to Prof. H. Karplus for bringing this to our attention. Cf. Li Tsung-Ying (1).

[d] *Chhio*,[6] also written *chhio*,[7] means primarily the magpie, *Pica sericea* (R 303).

[1] 輸 [2] 原 [3] 兌骨 [4] 神門 [5] 两城山 [6] 鵲 [7] 䧿

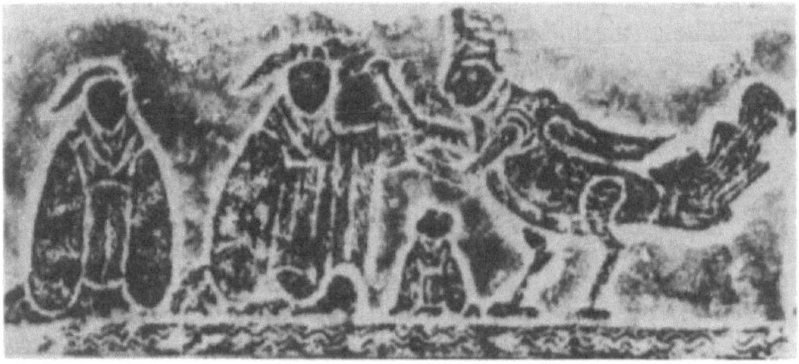

(a)

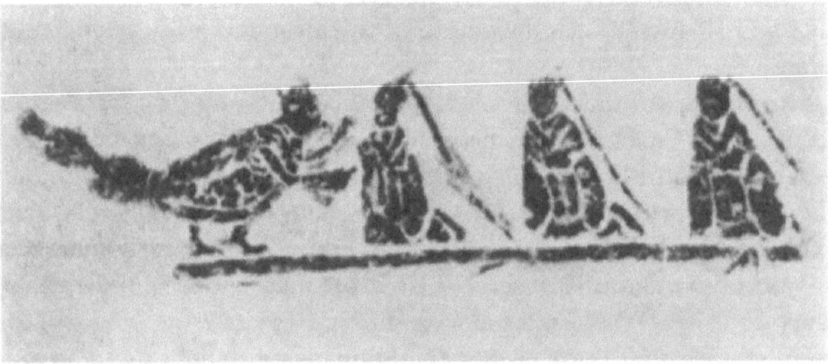

(b)

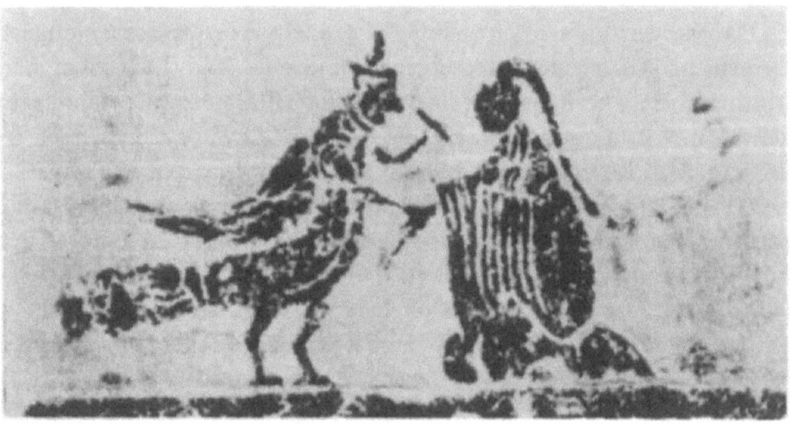

(c)

Fig. 16. The case of Pien Chhio and the human-headed bird. Three of the Later Han stone reliefs preserved at Chhü-fou in Shantung, and almost certainly from Wei-shan Hsien, his birthplace in the same province; from Liu Tun-Yuan (*1*). (*a*) Ornitho-android figure taking the pulse of a kneeling patient, and about to perform acupuncture. A child looks on and another patient waits behind (fig. 1). (*b*) Another scene with patients queuing up (fig. 2). (*c*) The human-headed bird as doctor, a scene illustrating again the close connection of acupuncture with sphygmology (fig. 4).

Hsien,[1] Shantung, the land of Pien Chhio's birth.[a] The literature contains occasional links between stone needles and birds' beaks; for example the *Kuang Ya* (+230)[b] says: 'Stone needles are called *tsui*[2].' On this Kuo Pho (*c.* +310) comments: '*Tsui*[2] is the name for the sharp point; so also a bird's beak or bill is called *tsui*[3]—the meaning is more or less the same.' But it is hard to find any textual passages explaining a myth of human-headed birds, or their relation with medicine. Human-headed birds are not rare in Han reliefs, for some fifteen examples are recorded in the motif-register of Finsterbusch (1).[c] They occur in two forms, first as one type among those weird beings that flit through tomb-wall scenery or round the sides of coffins, engaging in dream hunts with feathered immortals, or passant regardant in friezes.[d] Secondly they bear the sun and moon as their bodies, winging them on their scheduled flights through the skies.[e] It looks then as if there were three sorts of these ornitho-androids. Was one of them really a personification of Pien Chhio?

Casting the net wider, one recalls the *ba* birds of Ancient Egypt, the souls of the human dead.[f] The sirens of Greek mythology were also human-headed birds. But India yields something more relevant, the *gandharvas*, human-headed avian inhabitants of the skies since Vedic times, later prominent as a class of heavenly music-makers but originally, and traditionally, supposed to be good physicians.[g] Their iconography, however, starts rather late, hardly before the +1st century,[h] i.e. about the time of the Shantung medical bird-men, or very little after it. We are left then with the possibility that Liu Tun-Yuan's interpretation is right, and that in Eastern China during the Han some interplay occurred between the *gandharva* idea and the records or legends of the great physician whose given name meant 'magpie'. Although the relations between China and India at this early time have often been over-rated,[i] it might just be that Pien Chhio was given, or more probably took, his avian name on account of the *gandharva* myth. On all these questions the ledger remains open.

Before turning to the −2nd century, the Chhien Han period and the *Nei Ching*, we may pause for a moment to note another of the earliest references to moxibustion. It occurs in the *Chuang Tzu* book, in that brilliant chapter on the Robber Chih (*tao Chih*[4]) which we have had occasion to refer to, and quote, more than once already.[j] There Confucius, after having been worsted in his debate with the philo-

[a] They were found or excavated before the coming of modern scientific archaeology.

[b] By the lexicographer Chang I. Ch. 8A, p. 24*a*.

[c] See figs. 24, 91, 92, 288, 305, 326, 335 and 508 in her own album, and more in Fu Hsi-Hua (1), vol. 1, fig. 17, vol. 2, figs. 20, 25, 120, 146, 149.

[d] We can find one of the latter as late as the +5th century, in the Northern Wei tomb at Têng-hsien described by Hsü Hsün-Chan & Chhen Ta-Chang (*1*), colour pl. 2, p. 10.

[e] See Chêng Tê-Khun (7), figs. 12, 13; Rudolph & Wên Yu (1), figs. 94, 95; Wên Yu (*1*), pls. 86, 87; Nagahiro Toshio (*3*), p. 43, fig. 64 These seem rather characteristic of Szechuan.

[f] Bonnet (1), pp. 74ff.

[g] We are much indebted to Dr F. R. Allchin for information in this paragraph.

[h] See e.g. Rice & Rowland (1), pls. 76–7, 82 illustrating Begram finds; Smith (3); Joshi (1), p. 238, fig. 176. It will not be forgotten that Begram was one of the Afghanistan way-stations on the Old Silk Road (cf. *SCC*, Vol. 1, p. 182).

[i] Cf. Vol. 1, p. 206, Vol. 4, pt. 3, pp. 442–4.

[j] Cf. *SCC*, Vol. 2, pp. 101–2 and Vol. 5, pt. 2, p. 55.

1 微山縣 2 桀 3 觜 4 盜跖

sophical bandit on the origins of kingship, private property and the State, is made to say: 'I am like a man who has cauterised (i.e. applied moxa to) himself, without being ill at all.'[a] I never ought to have gone to talk with that fellow. There is some doubt whether this chapter was written by Chuang Chou himself in the −4th century, but it cannot be later than the −2nd because Ssuma Chhien refers to it, and the −3rd, the time of the ascendancy of Chhin, might be an acceptable date for it. There is not much doubt that the thermal treatments at a variety of strengths using *Artemisia* tinder go back to the Middle Chou at least.

(iii) *China's Hippocratic Corpus*

The mountainous landmark of acupuncture literature is indeed the *Nei Ching*, a Fujiyama visible from all times and angles. The *Huang Ti Nei Ching*, in our interpretative translation 'The Yellow Emperor's Manual of Corporeal (Medicine)', seems always to have consisted of two parts (though not necessarily under the same names as now), first the *Su Wên* (Questions (and Answers) about Living Matter), secondly the *Ling Shu* (the Vital Axis). There is also a third important recension, which mixes and redistributes material from both parts in an arrangement thought at one time to have been the original order; this is the *Thai Su*[1] (the Great Innocence),[b] due to a famous Sui editor Yang Shang-Shan[2] about +610. We must trace briefly the history of the parts of the book because it happens to be of particular significance for acupuncture.[c]

In his preface to the *Chen Chiu Chia I Ching*,[3] which we shall discuss presently (p. 119), Huangfu Mi[4] in +282 remarked that the *Chhi Lüeh*[5] (Bibliography in Seven Sections)[d] which Liu Hsin[6] had finished about +15 listed a *Huang Ti Nei Ching* in 18 chapters—now, he said, we have the *Su Wên* in 9 chapters and the *Chen Ching*[7] (Needle Manual) also in 9, hence these must have been the two parts which together constituted the *Nei Ching*. Later tradition reported that of old the *Nei Ching* had always come in two portfolios (*chih*[8]).[e] But the name of *Chen Ching* did not last into the Thang, for the bibliographies of both the official histories of that dynasty give a *Chiu Ling Ching*[9] (Manual of the Nine Mysteriously Effective (Instruments)[f]) as the second part of the *Nei Ching*; and it was now given a commentary, which did not survive, by a physician named Ling Pao[10].[g] Then in the neighbourhood of +762 the title attained its present form *Ling Shu*, changed again, it would appear, by the

[a] Ch. 29, tr. Legge (5), vol. 2, p. 176; *Pu Chu* ed., ch. 9B, p. 23*a*, writes *chiu* correctly.

[b] Our reasons for forming and retaining all these translations are given in Needham & Lu Gwei-Djen (8), repr. Needham (64), pp. 271–2.

[c] One of the best discussions of this subject is that of Chang Hsin-Chhêng (*1*), vol. 2, pp. 978 ff. Others will be mentioned immediately below.

[d] This was the basis of the *Chhien Han Shu* bibliography; cf. *SCC*, Vol. 3, p. 24.

[e] So Yang Hsüan-Tsao,[11] for example, of the early Thang.

[f] The justification for adding the word in brackets is that the number of types of needle described in both parts of the *Nei Ching* was precisely nine (the *chiu chen*,[12] on which see p. 102 below).

[g] This very extraordinary name, which looks like a Taoist pseudonym or pun, is nevertheless quite correct; cf. *SIC*, p. 244.

1 太素 2 楊上善 3 針灸甲乙經 4 皇甫謐 5 七略
6 劉歆 7 鍼經 8 帙 9 九靈經 10 靈寶
11 楊玄操 12 九鍼

great editor Wang Ping[1].[a] Knowing this background it would be tempting to replace the traditional translation of 'The Vital Axis' by 'The Mysteriously Effective Controllers (i.e. Instruments)'. *Shu* is well susceptible of this meaning of controlling, and it is clear now that at a certain stage *ling* was nine of something, while to begin with, the book had been all about needles.

The old title of *Chen Ching* (Needle Manual) persisted some time longer, however, as we know from a story of the late Northern Sung. Chiang Shao-Yü[2] tells us that under the emperor Chê Tsung some classical books were presented at court by a Korean embassy, and one of these was the *Huang Ti Chen Ching*. Wars and fires had destroyed so many copies in China that this recovery was greatly appreciated, and in +1093 it was imperially decreed that the book should be reprinted and circulated for the benefit of all physicians.[b] In spite of this, however, Shih Sung,[3] writing a preface for the *Ling Shu* about +1155, said:

> Unfortunately this work has been almost lost and very rare for a long time past, so that hardly anyone has studied it. Medical practitioners who study medical books can be effective in their therapeutics, but never was there seen one who could accomplish this without such reading. As for those who try to practise without it, and without having served their apprenticeship in good medical families, they harm and kill (their patients) more severely than if they took a knife and stuck it into them. That is why there is an old saying that scholars who do not study medical books (to help their parents) may be considered unfilial...[c] As for me, my family long conserved an old copy of the *Ling Shu* in 9 chapters and 81 sections, and now I have edited it in 24 chapters, adding excursuses at the end of each on the sounds and meanings of certain characters, so that all can be readily understood by those who are devoted to the preservation of life.

By the time of Wang Ying-Lin[4] in +1267, writing the *Yü Hai*[5] compendium, the *Ling Shu* was no longer in danger of disappearing, and he accepted the later majority view that the *Chen Ching* had been indeed its ancient title.[d] Of course none of the sceptical scholars of the Sung and Yuan believed that the two parts of the *Nei Ching* went back to the time of the Yellow Emperor himself, pre-Shang as that would have to have been.[e]

With regard to the dating, the consensus of scholarly opinion is that the *Su Wên* belongs to the −2nd century and the *Ling Shu* to the −1st;[f] only a few writers invert the sequence.[g] A few have preferred to make the *Ling Shu* Later Han (+1st or +2nd

[a] We suspect this from a later note inserted in the bibliography of the *Sui Shu*, according to Chang Hsin-Chhêng, op. cit., p. 979.

[b] See *Sung Chhao Lei Yuan*,[6] and *Yü Hai*, ch. 63, pp. 9*b*, 10*a*, 23*b*. Cf. *SIC*, pp. 228–9.

[c] *Wei jen tzu erh pu tu i shu yu wei pu hsiao yeh.*[7] We often find this rather powerful motivation for medical study in action; cf. pp. 119, 127 and 129. It was, for example, how Wang Thao[8] came to write his *Wai Thai Pi Yao*.[9]

[d] Cf. *ICK*, p. 50.

[e] Lü Fu[10] of the Yuan well expressed this. One could wish that their philological example had been followed by many writers in Western languages, both Chinese and Western, in our own century.

[f] Lung Po-Chien (*2*); Ho Ai-Hua (*1*); Anon. (*90*), p. 17.

[g] About +1586 Ma Shih[11] believed, from various pieces of internal evidence, that the *Ling Shu* was older as well as more important than the *Su Wên* (cf. *TSCC*, *I shu tien*, ch. 67, *I pu*, ch. 47, *NCLS/MC*, vol. 2, p. 903), but this was rebutted by Taki Mototane (*1*) in *ICK*, pp. 55–6. Yü Yün-Hsiu (*1*), p. 226, still favours such a view, however.

1 王冰 2 江少虞 3 史崧 4 王應麟 5 玉海 6 宋朝類苑
7 爲人子而不讀醫書由爲不孝也 8 王燾 9 外臺秘要 10 呂復 11 馬蒔

century).[a] Evidence has also been brought forward showing that whatever the exact dates may be, the *Su Wên* is earlier than the first of the pharmaceutical natural histories, the *Shen Nung Pên Tshao Ching*[1].[b] Liang Chhi-Chhao long ago maintained that the *Nei Ching* was unquestionably a Han work;[c] he pointed out that some expressions recall typical phrases of the Chhin period, with ways of thinking very like those of the *Lü Shih Chhun Chhiu* (−239). Then the fictional dialogue form, with Huang Ti[2] and his interlocutors, Chhi Po,[3] Lei Kung,[4] Shao Yü,[5] and Po Kao,[6] is very reminiscent of the conversations in the *Chuang Tzu* book, with Huang Ti and Kuang Chhêng Tzu,[7] for example;[d] and many another imaginary debate in the literature of the −4th and −3rd centuries. So suggestive are the parallels that doubt sometimes arises whether the *Nei Ching* were not better ascribed to the −3rd century, yet we may be content with the view that some passages in it may well be of that date, and that in any case it indubitably summarises the clinical experience of all the Chou and the Chhin. On the other hand the philosophical content, the dominant part played by the Yang and Yin and the Five Elements in the physiology and pathology, means that these theories at any rate could not be older than the time of Tsou Yen,[8] i.e. about −320.[e] But they may well have been worked in later than some of the cliinical material, and later also than the first more or less empirical usages of acupuncture.[f]

The Thang commentary of Ling Pao on the *Ling Shu* was not the first that the *Nei Ching* had had, for Chhüan Yuan-Chhi[9] had made one for the *Su Wên* either in the Sui period or not long before, but this also failed to survive. The oldest that we now have, for both parts, was due to Wang Ping[10] in +762. There is no doubt that he rearranged the order of some of the chapters, and it is widely believed that he supplied new text for some seven which by his time were missing.[g]

No one can read through the chapters of the *Su Wên* and more especially of the *Ling Shu* without realising that acupuncture, commonly referred to as 'pricking' (*tzhu*[11]), was prescribed in the majority of pathological conditions considered. It is much more prominent there than drugs, which in spite of the *Pên Ching* did not really come into their own as an equal and parallel armamentarium until the Later Han with Chang Chung-Ching.[12] Let us look at one of the key passages of the *Nei Ching* about acupuncture.[h]

Huang Ti said: 'I should like to know the Tao of acupuncture.' Chhi Po replied: 'The first thing in this art and mystery is that you must concentrate the mind (on the patient as

[a] E.g. Li Thao (*13*), Fan Hsing-Chun (*1*). Arguments based on place-names and astronomical references are always rather weak because such things were so easily updated.

[b] Chhen Chih (*1*).

[c] (*6*), pp. 154–5. Cf. Chang Hsin-Chhêng (*1*), vol. 2, pp. 969, 978.

[d] On Kuang Chhêng Tzu see *SCC*, Vol. 2, pp. 98–9.

[e] See Vol. 2, pp. 232 ff.

[f] After all, I Huan and Pien Chhio lived long before Tsou Yen.

[g] *NCTS*, Introd. by Hsiao Yen-Phing, *c.* 1899.

[h] *NCSW/PH*, ch. 25, (p. 151), tr. auct., adjuv. Chamfrault & Ung Kang-Sam (1), vol. 2, p. 107. Cf. Huang Wên (1), p. 10 and Veith (1), pp. 215–16. The classical commentaries are assembled in Anon. (*76*), pp. 261–2. Cf. Nguyen Van Nghi (3).

1 神農本草經 2 黃帝 3 岐伯 4 雷公 5 少兪 6 伯高
7 廣成子 8 騶衍 9 全元起 10 王冰 11 刺 12 張仲景

a whole), then, once you have decided on the state of his five viscera (whether *hsü*,[1] asthenic, or *shih*,[2] plerotic), as indicated by the nine pulse observations (*chiu hou*[3]), you can take the needle in hand. If you have felt no deathlike pulse, and heard no inauspicious sound, then the inner and outer signs are in correspondence. You must not rely on the external appearances (symptoms) only, and you must understand fully the coming and going (of the *chhi* in the tracts); then alone can you perform acupuncture on the patient.

(The conditions of) patients are either *hsü*[1] (asthenic) or *shih*[2] (plerotic); in the five former do not lightly apply the needles, in the five latter do not delay to do so.[a] When the *chhi* has arrived,[b] the needle must be withdrawn as quickly as possible. The twisting of the needles must be done in an even and regular way, quietly and attentively watching the patient to observe any minute changes that occur when the *chhi* arrives; such changes are so obscure that they can hardly be seen. When the *chhi* arrives[c] it is like a flock of birds, or the breeze in the waving millet—only too easily can one miss the fleeting moment.[d] The physician must be like a crossbowman pressing his trigger at the exact time, not an instant too soon, not an instant too late.'

Huang Ti went on: 'What does one do in the asthenic (*hsü*) condition, and what does one do in the plerotic (*shih*) condition?' Chhi Po answered: 'In a case of asthenia you should give acupuncture tending to plerosis; in a case of plerosis apply it so that it tends to asthenia. When the tract (Yang or Yin) *chhi* arrives, take great care that you do not lose it.[e] Whether the needle is inserted superficially or deeply depends on the acu-point chosen;[f] and whether the *chhi* arrives immediately or later (the needle must be pulled out as soon as it comes). Applying acupuncture is like treading the edge of a precipice; the hands should be firm and strong — as if grasping a tiger — and the mind oblivious of all other things.'[g]

A great many of the chapters in both the *Su Wên* and the *Ling Shu* are concerned mainly with acupuncture.[h] Some give anatomical descriptions, still very intelligible today, of where the twelve regular tracts begin and end, and what structures they pass through or over,[i] others describe the nine types of needles used by the Han

[a] Because sedation (*hsieh*[4]) is easy, but tonification (*pu*[5]) is more difficult. We return elsewhere to the practical significance of these terms, e.g. inserting the needle in accordance with, or against, the believed flow of the *chhi* in the tract (pp. 115, 119). Five because of the five Yin viscera (*tsang*[6]), on which see p. 39.

[b] I.e. when the patient has reported one or more of the characteristic subjective responses (cf. p. 192), or when the physician has experienced one or other of the typical sensations.

[c] Later technical terms for this, still used today, are *chen kan*[7] and *tê chhi*.[8] The former phrase evokes the whole Chinese natural philosophy of resonance (*kan ying*[9]), on which see *SCC*, Vol. 2, pp. 281–2, 304, Vol. 4, pt. 1, pp. 29ff., 233 and *passim*. In biological terms, this means stimulus and response. Today we should think of it as evidence of the stimulation of the deep receptor nerve-endings.

[d] These metaphors were intended to describe a kind of fluttering feeling experienced by the acupuncturist. Inexpert practitioners could easily miss it, and their practice would be ineffective.

[e] This again refers to the response reported by the patient. Apart from other effects, in *hsü* (asthenic) patients the arrival of the Yang *chhi* was experienced as a slight feeling of local warmth; in *shih* (plerotic) patients the opposite effect was a slight coolness at the place. This was called *chhi chih*.[10]

[f] Two whole chapters in the *Su Wên*, the Tzhu Yao Lun[11] and the Tzhu Chhi Lun,[12] are devoted to the specific depths of penetration appropriate for many acu-points; cf. *NCSW/PH*, chs. 50, 51, (pp. 268–9, 269–70). The points were regarded as lying at different depths below the surface of the skin, not all at one level, as might be mistakenly assumed from the usual diagrams.

[g] Cf. an enlarged parallel passage in *NCSW/PH*, ch. 54, (p. 279).

[h] For example, not attempting an exhaustive list, *NCSW*, chs. 12–14, 16, 20–1, 25–6, 32, 36, 41, 43, 50–5, 57–64, then *NCLS*, chs. 1–3, 5, 7, 10, 39, 55, 60–1, 67, 75, 78.

[i] *NCSW*, chs. 16, 20, 21, *NCLS*, chs. 2, 10.

1 虛 2 實 3 九候 4 瀉 5 補 6 臟 7 針感
8 得氣 9 感應 10 氣至 11 刺要論 12 刺齊論

acupuncturists,[a] and others again relate the physiology of the tracts to the diagnosis of disease by observations on the pulse.[b] One has only to look at some of the chapter titles in the *Su Wên* to appreciate its preoccupation with acupuncture—for example: Chen Chieh[1] (Study of Needles, ch. 54), Chhi Hsüeh[2] (the Acu-points, ch. 58), Tzhu Jê[3] (Acupuncture in Fevers, ch. 32), or Tzhu Nio[4] (Acupuncture in Malaria-like Diseases, ch. 36). Including moxibustion with acupuncture one could say without exaggeration that 70 to 80% of the total text is concerned with therapy by these treatments.[c] Circulation-theory, as we have already seen (p. 25), is closely correlated with the palpation of the 'pulse-image' (*mo hsiang*[5]), the types of pulse being divided into the three Yang and three Yin named just in the same way as the tracts.[d] Here the regular tracts are spoken of as *ching mo*,[6] because the circulation of blood (*hsüeh*,[7] a Yin thing) was thought of as occurring in the blood-vessels (*mo*[8]) just as that of the *chhi*[9] (a Yang thing) was conceived to occur through the invisible tracts. It was natural that tracts should be connected with pulses, for the viscera were the common aetiological origin; when these were affected by disease it would show itself in the pulses, and could be put right after diagnosis by acupuncture along the tracts. It is a striking fact that the anatomical courses of all of these have remained without any serious modification since the Early Han, for although the names of the acu-points show some differences from later enumerations, the places where the twelve tracts begin and end have never changed through two millennia. Sometimes the classifications are rather curious, such as that which divided the body of man into upper, middle and lower regions (*shang, chung, hsia*[10]) corresponding to the age-old cosmological division into heaven, earth and man (*thien, ti, jen*[11]).[e]

Always the text of the *Nei Ching* is truly difficult, not only for the laborious Western student but for any well-educated Chinese also, hence the inestimable value of the 'translations' into the modern language, done by scholars deeply versed in the centuries-old commentaries after many years of study. It cannot too much be emphasised that one of the greatest difficulties in following and translating ancient and medieval Chinese medical writings is that ordinary words are used in them with at least two meanings, the normal significance being called 'broad acceptance' (*kuang i*[12]), and the other 'restricted technical usage' (*hsia i*[13]). Thus to the unwary reader an expression such as *tu yao*[14] suggests that the medicament is poisonous, and that is how Western translators have usually taken it; but what it really means is that the drug contains one or more powerful active principles valuable in therapy. The converse (*wu tu*[15]) indicates that the drug simply has a mild beneficial effect on general health. So also the expression *jê ping*[16] may in broad acceptance mean all the group of *shang han*[17] fevers, but in the proper technical terminology *jê ping* designates only one of five divisions of the group of *shang han* fevers. In acupuncture similar ambiguities

[a] *NCSW*, ch. 54, *NCLS*, chs. 1, 7.
[b] *NCSW*, ch. 21.
[c] Cf. Anon. (90), pp. 17–18.
[d] *NCSW/PH*, ch. 21, (pp. 131–2).
[e] *NCSW/PH*, ch. 20, (p. 121).

[1] 鍼解 [2] 氣穴 [3] 刺熱 [4] 刺瘧 [5] 脈象 [6] 經脈
[7] 血 [8] 脉 [9] 氣 [10] 上中下 [11] 天地人 [12] 廣義
[13] 狹義 [14] 毒藥 [15] 無毒 [16] 熱病 [17] 傷寒

are encountered; for example, *shu*[1,2,3] denotes all the acu-points, but there is a smaller class of *shu*, the *wu shu hsüeh*, with special therapeutic properties (see Table 9), and within them again a smaller class of dorsal *shu* points (Table 11). Moreover, the usage of terms such as Thai-Yang, Thai-Yin, etc. in the Shang Han school following Chang Chung-Ching relates to the course of febrile diseases and is quite different from what is meant by them in the six tracts (*liu ching*[4]) of acupuncture.

It will now be well worth while to take a close look at some of the passages in the *Nei Ching* which describe anatomically the course of the tracts. In these passages one meets with a number of special technical terms which need preliminary attention, if only for the reason that (as so often) they are ordinary words employed in technical senses. Thus *chhi*[5] naturally refers to the point of origin of a tract. *Lo*[6] here is a term indicating that a tract makes a cross-connection linking it with another tract with which it has the *piao-li* relationship. Another term, *shu*,[7] denotes connection between a tract and the particular internal organ after which it is named. *Chih*[8] is any branch. When tracts or their branches unite it is called *ho*.[9] *Huan*[10] means that a tract doubles back on itself, *huan*[11] implies encircling, and *chhio*[12] signifies reversal of a tract followed by turning off in another direction. When a tract follows the natural course which would be expected of it from its Yang or Yin character, that is called *hsün*.[13] Ascent, along the cephalo-caudal and proximo-distal axes, is *shang*,[14] its opposite is *hsia*,[15] and level running is *hêng*.[16] The depth of acu-point reactivities under the surface of the body varies much, so that when a tract rises to a shallower position in or under the skin, this is called *chhu*,[17] and when it dives down deeper again, that is *ju*.[18] Anyone wishing to translate relevant passages in the ancient medical literature has to be aware of these usages.

Let us look, then, at some examples of *Nei Ching* texts giving anatomical descriptions of the tracts. Three of these *chêng ching*[19] appear in the following translations, and we shall note particularly the mentions of acu-points by their names. They come up in the usual circulation order, and first, the pulmonic tract (P), see Fig. 17:[a]

The Pulmonic Cheirotelic Thai-Yin Tract takes its origin in the central coctive region[b] and passes downwards, sending out (*lo*[20]) a connection with the large intestine (*ta chhang*[21]);[c] then it turns upwards towards the cardiac orifice of the stomach, penetrates the diaphragm (*ko*[22]), connects with (*shu*[23]) the lungs,[d] and goes through both trachea and bronchi (*fei hsi*[24]).

[a] *NCLS/PH*, ch. 10, (p. 105), tr. auct. Cf. *Chia I Ching*, ch. 2, (p. 29). See also Anon. (*90*), p. 45; Anon. (*107*), pp. 62 ff., 68. There are abridged précis in Chamfrault & Ung Kang-Sam (1), vol. 2, p. 358; and Huang Wên (1), p. 21, who thought it was all a description of arteries.

[b] The doctrine of the *san chiao*[25,26] we discuss elsewhere (*SCC*, Vol. 6). The upper one was in the thorax, and the other two in the abdomen, primarily disgestive and urino-genital respectively. See the comm. in *Shih Chi*, ch. 105, p. 5*b*.

[c] This is the viscus with which the pulmonic tract is particularly connected in the *piao li*[27] relationship; see Table 2 above. Tract IG is of course implied.

[d] *Shu* (or *chu*) is, as we have seen, an important technical term here indicating the special connection of the tract with the viscus from which it takes its name, and in relation to which it is *li*, not *piao*.

1 兪	2 輸	3 腧	4 六經	5 起	6 絡	7 屬
8 支	9 合	10 還	11 環	12 却	13 循	14 上
15 下	16 橫	17 出	18 入	19 正經	20 絡	21 大腸
22 膈	23 屬	24 肺系	25 三膲	26 三焦	27 表裡	

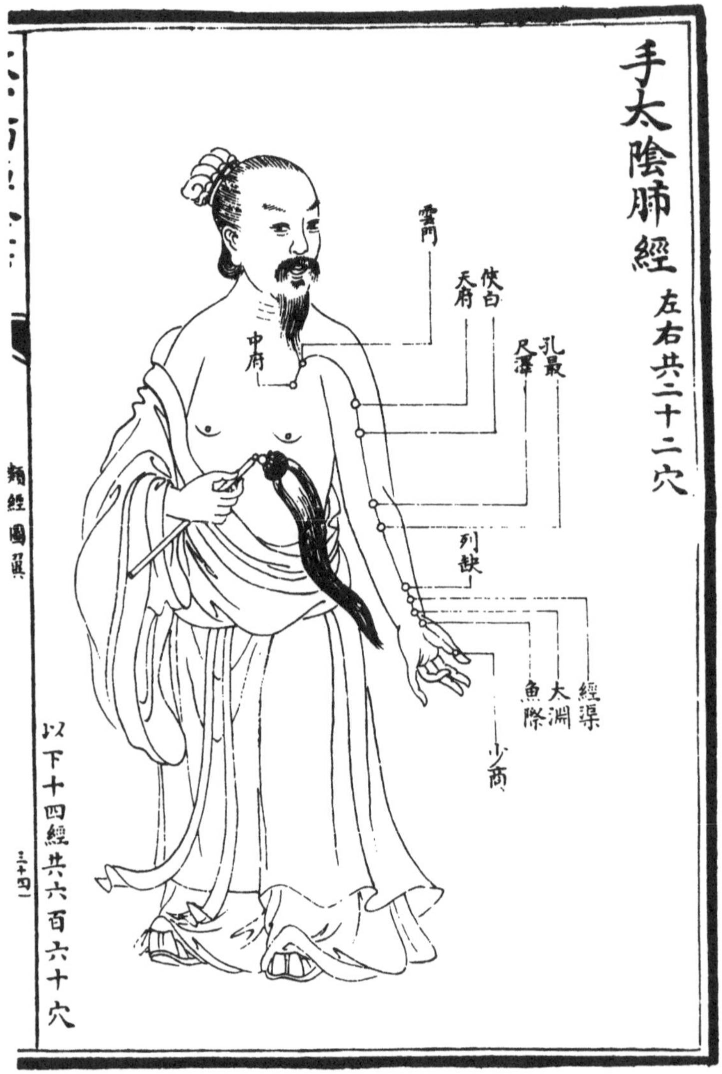

Fig. 17. The Cheirotelic pulmonic Thai-Yin acu-tract depicted in Chang Chieh-Pin's *Lei Ching* (+1624). The caption adds that there are 22 acu-points counting both left and right sides of the body. *SKCS* edition.

After that it turns sideways[a] and descends through the axilla (*i*[1]) running more superficially (*chhu*[2]) down the inner side of the arm, in front of the Cardiac Cheirotelic Shao-Yin Tract, to the cubital fossa (*chou chung*[3]). Then it continues down the inner side of the forearm to reach the edge of the lower end (*hsia lien*[4])[b] of the radius (bone, the 'oar-bone', *jao ku*[5])

[a] Here, where it surfaces, the line of acu-points begins.

[b] This expression is presumably anatomical here, meaning edge or corner; but Hsia-lien is also an acu-point name, IG 8, higher up towards the elbow. Perhaps it was derived precisely from the study of this ancient text through the ages, and several others may have originated in the same way.

[1] 腋 [2] 出 [3] 肘中 [4] 下廉 [5] 橈骨

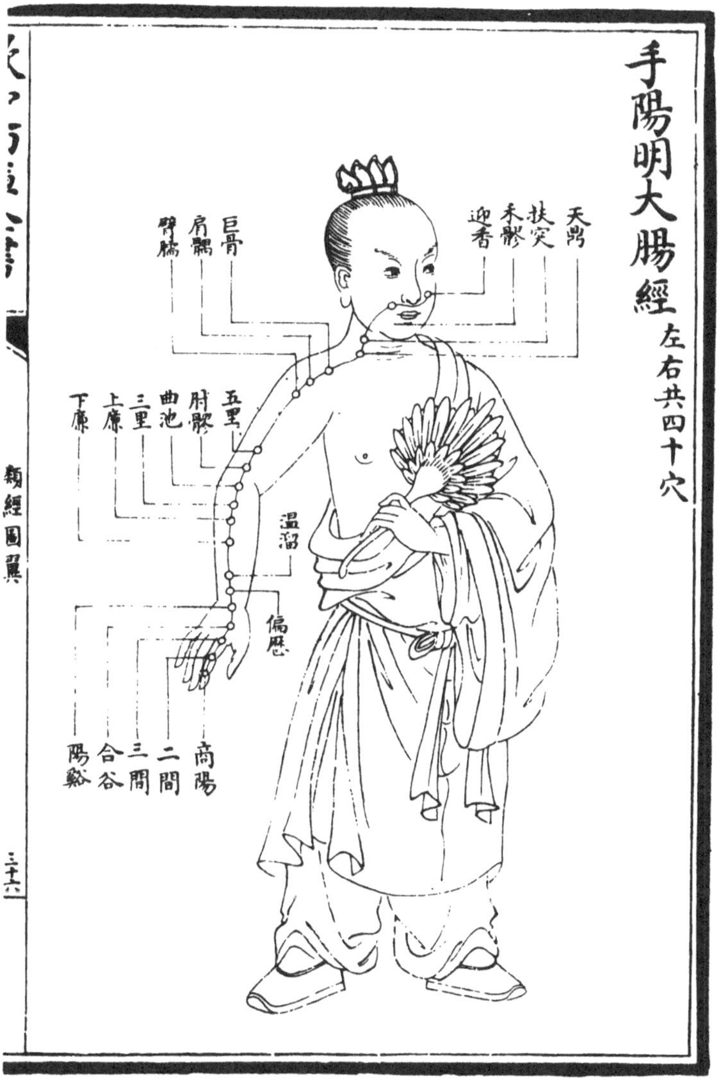

Fig. 18. The Cheirogenic crasso-intestinal Yang-Ming acu-tract depicted in the *Lei Ching*. The caption adds that counting both sides there are 40 acu-points. *SKCS* edition.

deeper in (*ju*[1]) by the radial artery (*tshun khou*[2]); passing afterwards across the thenar eminence at the Yü-chi[3] acu-point (P 10), and ending superficially at the tip of the thumb. It sends also a branch (*chih*[4]) across the dorsal surface of the wrist (*wan*[5]) to the tip of the index finger along its inner side.[a]...

And the text goes on to talk about the diseases that affect this tract. From the description one sees that like all the other regular tracts this one has an invisible line connect-

[a] It joins there the Crasso-intestinal Cheirogenic Yang-Ming Tract, which takes its origin at that point, handing on the circulation of the *chhi*.

[1] 入 [2] 寸口 [3] 魚際 [4] 支 [5] 腕

ing the visceral regions proper to it, almost reminiscent of an underground railway line coming to or near the surface for part of its length; and only after it has emerged can the series of acu-points (P 1 etc.) begin. Here one of them is prominently mentioned in the text by the same name that it continues to bear today.

Now for the second of the regular tracts (IG), that connected with the large intestine (Fig. 18).[a]

The Crasso-intestinal Cheirogenic Yang-Ming Tract originates from the thumb side of the tip of the index finger, and follows its edge (*shang lien*[1])[b] to cross the intermetacarpal fossa past the point Ho-ku[2] (IG4); then it runs up the hand at a deeper level between the two (extensor) muscles (*chin*[3]), rising (*shang lien*[1])[c] along the forearm still deeper to the outer side of the elbow (*chou*,[4] i.e. the lateral epicondyle of the humerus). Then it continues along the upper arm to the shoulder more superficially and goes through the joint between the clavicle and the scapula (*yü ku*[5])[d] out to an upper meeting-point at the cephalic end of the vertebral column (*chu ku*,[6] behind the neck).[e] Thence it descends (slightly deeper) to the supraclavicular fossa (*chhüeh phên*[7]).[f] Here there is a junction (*lo*[8]) going to the lungs (*fei*[9])[g] and further connecting (*shu*[10]) through the diaphragm (*ko*[11]) with the large intestine (*ta chhang*[12]). The branch (*chih*[13]) starting here runs upwards to the lower cheek and passes through the lower jaw and teeth; then doubling back at the sides of the mouth they[h] cross, going deeply at the Jen-chung[14] point,[i] the left passing up to the right and the right passing up to the left[j] on each side of the openings of the nostrils.[k] ...

And again the writer launches into an account of the relevant diseases. In this case, then, we have two acu-points mentioned by name, and possibly others disguised under the anatomical nomenclature. All these tracts, which have remained unchanged till now, can readily be followed on the diagrams in Figs. 6 and 7.

[a] *NCLS/PH*, ch. 10, (p. 108), tr. auct. Cf. *Chia I Ching*, ch. 2, (p. 29). See also Anon. (*90*), p. 48; Anon. (*107*), pp. 69ff., 78. Abridged précis in Chamfrault & Ung Kang-Sam (1), vol. 2, pp. 359–60, who recognised the acu-point names, and Huang Wên (1), p. 22.

[b] Now an acu-point name, Shang-lien, IG 9, but near the elbow, so here clearly anatomical.

[c] We take this phrase as purely directional, but doubtfully, because IG 9 is just in this place.

[d] The commentaries say that this includes *chia ku*,[15] the scapula, and *so ku*,[16] the collar-bone.

[e] This is the present Ta-chhui[17] acu-point (TM 13 or 14). The six Yang regular tracts meet here.

[f] Here presumably anatomical, but also the name of an acu-point, Chhüeh-phên, V 12, just above the centre of the clavicle.

[g] Tract P is of course implied.

[h] I.e. the symmetrical tracts from the right and left sides of the body.

[i] This lies at the centre of the infra-nasal groove or philtrum. The commoner name for the acu-point now is Shui-kou[18] (TM 25 or 26).

[j] The statement of the mid-line cross-over here is quite unmistakable. It is clearly shown in the drawing in *NCLS/PH*, p. 109; as also in Chhêng Tan-An's photograph of a living subject with the tract lines drawn on the skin, (*2*), p. 81. The diagrams in Anon. (*107*) are rather confusing, however, for while that on p. 69 shows it, that on p. 78 has the tract coming back and ascending on the same side. Possibly the cross-over is here intended to be 'taken as read', and all the acu-points on one side of the body shown, irrespective of which symmetrical tract they belong to. Derivative presentations also do this, either by a misunderstanding or with the aim of simplification (e.g. Mann, 3); but the manikin models made in China at the present day adhere to the ancient tradition.

[k] It is considered to end on each side of the lateral nasal processes, at Ying-hsiang[19] (IG 20).

1 上廉	2 合谷	3 筋	4 肘	5 髃骨	6 柱骨
7 缺盆	8 絡	9 肺	10 屬	11 膈	12 大腸
13 支	14 人中	15 胛骨	16 鎖骨	17 大椎	18 水溝
19 迎香					

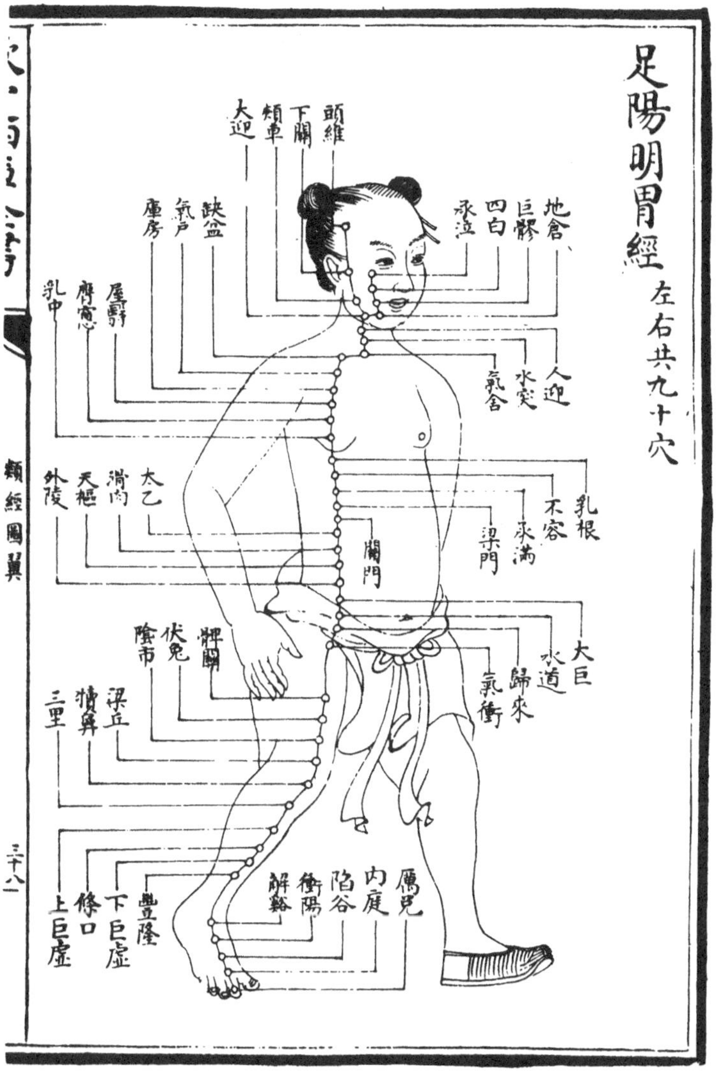

Fig. 19. The Podotelic gastric Yang-Ming acu-tract depicted in the *Lei Ching*. Reckoning bilaterally this tract has 90 points. *SKCS* edition.

And so we come to the third, the gastric regular tract (V), in a description very similar to that of the others (Fig. 19).[a]

The Gastric Podotelic Yang-Ming Tract originates at the sides of the bridge of the nose (*o*[1]), near the beginning of the Vesical Podotelic Thai-Yang tract, and it runs downwards along the sides of the nostrils entering deep into the upper jaw and teeth. It returns more

[a] *NCLS/PH*, ch. 10, (p. 110), tr. auct. Cf. *Chia I Ching*, ch. 2, (p. 30). See also Anon. (*90*), p. 50; Anon. (*107*), pp. 80, 97–8. Abridged précis in Chamfrault & Ung Kang-Sam (1), vol. 2, pp. 360–1, who recognised the acu-point names; and Huang Wên (1), p. 22.

[1] 頞

superficially, circling round the corners of the lips, and crosses (*chiao*[1])[a] at the Chhêng-chiang[2] acu-point,[b] proceeding backwards (laterally) along the lower edge[c] of the mandible (*i*[3]) and coming out at the acu-point Ta-ying[4] (V 5 or 8). Then it goes upwards over the ramus of the mandible (*chia chhê*[5])[d] in front of the ear past the acu-point Kho-chu-jen[6],[e] and follows the hair-line up to the forehead (*ê lu*[7]). But also from Ta-ying[4] (on the edge of the mandible) it sends a branch (*chih*[8]) downwards, passing first the acu-point Jen-ying[9] (V 9) along the throat (*hou lung*[10])[f] and then deeply into Chhüeh-phên[11] (V 12) in the supra-clavicular fossa.[g] Thenceforward it penetrates the diaphragm (*ko*[12]) to connect with (*shu*[13]) the stomach (*wei*[14]), sending off at a junction (*lo*[15]) a connection with the spleen (*phi*[16]).[h] From Chhüeh-phên[11] the main tract (*chih ching*[17]) descends on the inner edge of the breasts (*ju*[18]),[i] passing beside the umbilicus and going deeper to reach the Chhi-chhung[19] acu-point (V 30).[j] And there is another branch which starts from the cardiac orifice of the stomach (*wei khou*[20]) and descends within the abdomen (*fu*[21]) until it joins (*ho*[22]) the main tract at the Chhi-chhung[19] acu-point.[k] The tract then continues to the Phi-kuan[23] acu-point (V 31)[l] and further through the Fu-thu[24] acu-point,[m] past the patella (*hsi-pin*[25]),[n] and follows the lateral side of the tibia (*ching*[26])[o] to the upper surface of the foot (*tsu fu*[27]). Finally the tract runs more deeply along the medial side of the middle toe.[p] And it has a branch (*chih*[28]) which starts three inches below (the patella)[q] and runs down to the lateral side of the third toe.[r]

[a] I.e. the corresponding tract from the other side of the body. Here again the authorities are confusing, probably for the same reasons as those just given for tract IG. Some show an osculation at Chhêng-chiang, the centre point under the mouth (e.g. drawings in *NCLS/PH*, p. 112; Anon. (*107*), p. 80), followed by a return to the same side; others fail to show any such meeting at the mid-line at all (e.g. Chhêng Tan-An (*2*), p. 101; Mann (3); Anon. (*107*), p. 97). But the manikin models made in China at the present day adhere to the ancient description very faithfully.

[b] Now JM 24.

[c] *Hsia lien*[29] here must be part of the anatomical description, though Hsia-lien is also the name of an acu-point, IG 8, on the forearm, as we have just seen.

[d] This is also an acu-point, Chia-chhê, V 6, or 3, depending on the numbering system adopted for these branches.

[e] Now often called Shang-kuan,[30] VF 3, one of the felleic tract acu-points.

[f] About level with the laryngeal prominence (the thyroid cartilage) and hence on the sternohyoid and omohyoid muscles.

[g] From this point onwards two lines of tract are running in parallel, one deep in the body, one nearer the surface.

[h] Tract LP is of course implied here.

[i] Thus the text, but later illustrations and modern charts show the line descending centrally and passing through the nipple. See Chhêng Tan-An (*1*), p. 76; Anon. (*107*), pp. 80, 97; or Mann (3), fig. 1. This may be an example of development through the ages of practice, yet as we have seen (p. 68), V 17, at the nipple, is a 'forbidden acu-point' to this day.

[j] In the hypogastric region near the inguinal aponeurotic falx.

[k] Cf. Anon. (*90*), p. 51.

[l] Over the upper end of the sartorius muscle. The special medical pronunciation is Pei-kuan (*NCLS/MC*, vol. 2, p. 993).

[m] Over the quadriceps femoris muscle.

[n] The text actually says 'over the patella', but traditional descriptions (e.g. Anon. (*107*), p. 98) and modern charts (Mann (3), fig. 1) show the tract passing laterally.

[o] Along the tibialis anterior muscle.

[p] Lit. 'the space on the outer side of the middle toe'.

[q] I.e. at the Tsu-san-li[31] acu-point, V 36.

[r] Lit. 'the space on the outer side of the middle toe'.

1 交	2 承漿	3 頤	4 大迎	5 頰車	6 客主人
7 額顱	8 支	9 人迎	10 喉嚨	11 缺盆	
12 膈	13 屬	14 胃	15 絡	16 脾	17 直經
18 乳	19 氣衝	20 胃口	21 腹	22 合	23 髀關
24 伏兔	25 膝臏	26 脛	27 足跗	28 支	29 下廉
30 上關	31 足三里				

And yet another branch starts on the upper surface of the foot and passes down to the superficial tissues at the end of the big toe.[a]

Here then, in this ancient text, we find mention of no less than eight acu-points by the names which they still bear today.[b] In general, anyone reading over these luminous descriptions must allow a considerable degree of anatomical knowledge on the part of these founding fathers of Chinese human biology. It is much more than they have usually been credited with, and in another place (Sect. 43 on anatomy) we show that this was generally true through all the Chinese centuries, Western impressions having been derived mainly from the illustrations, which fell far behind the knowledge set forth in the texts. Lastly, the significance of these descriptions also lies in the fact that they clearly bring out the beginnings and ends of the tracts, and hence the continuity of the circulation of the *chhi*.

Having now had a close look at some of the Han anatomical descriptions we can clearly see that there was nothing vague or imprecise about the conception which the ancient physicians had of the courses of their acu-tracts, coming and going, shallow or deep, branching and re-joining, penetrating which organs and connecting with what areas of body surface. More than a dozen technical terms with exact meanings have already been discussed (p. 17), and a good many more could be added, but most notably missing is a comprehensive directional vocabulary. Terms like antero-posterior, dorso-ventral, proximo-distal, cephalo-caudal, would have been extremely useful to the writers of the *Ling Shu*, yet so far as one can see they were never developed in those early times. Nevertheless, the names of quite a number of the acu-points were imaginative, descriptive and definite, and most of them are still in use today. Since the gastric tract (V), our third example, had 45 such point names, and 90 in all because of bilateral symmetry, one can get an idea of the complexity of the array of points on the surface of the body available to the ancient physicians at least as early as the −1st century. The marvel is that the tracts were (and still are) anatomically invisible, thought of always as crevices or impalpable channels for vital *chhi*, not obvious tubes like the blood-vessels and lymphatics; and perhaps in the end it may turn out that what they really signify is a system of lines of equivalent physiological action.

There is no question that all the regular tracts (*chêng ching*) are minutely described in the *Nei Ching, Ling Shu*. However, in particular diseases acupuncture is often directed by means of approximate anatomical localisation rather than by the prescription of individual acu-point names, and directions are often given that it should be applied to specific tracts (*ching*) in general rather than to named acu-points themselves. One is then curious to look closer at the historical growth of the numbers of acu-points and names, and it is possible to draw up a table showing the course of the development.[c] In order to understand this it is necessary, without too much anticipat-

[a] Commentators say that this starts from the acu-point Chhung-yang,[1] V 42.
[b] And three more at least are present also by implication.
[c] We base this upon that given in Anon. (*91*), p. 12. See also Yeh Ching-Chhiu (*1*), pp. 24–5.

[1] 衝陽

Table 15. *Growth of the number of recognised acu-points*

	The 12 Regular Tracts (*chêng ching*)	The 2 Median Tracts (Tu Mo, Jen Mo)	Total no. acu-points named	Total no. acu-points including bilateral duplicates	Theoret. no.
Chhien Han					
Nei Ching, −2nd, −1st	135	25	160	295[a]	365
Hou Han, San Kuo & Chin					
Ming Thang Chih Yao, prob. +2nd *Chia I Ching*, +282	300	49	349	649	—
Thang					
Chhien Chin I Fang, c. +670	—	—	—	649	—
Sung & Yuan					
Thung Jen Ching, +1026 *Shih-ssu Ching Fa Hui*, +1341	303	51	354	657	—
Sung & Ming					
Tzu Shêng Ching, +1220 *Chen Chiu Ta Chhêng*, +1601	308	51	359	667	—
Now accepted (Anon. *91*)	309	52	361	670[b]	—

ing explanations which must follow later, to say a few words about the literary works which have to serve as our *points de répère*.

In Table 15 we begin with the *Nei Ching*, about which no more need be said, and go on to Huangfu Mi's[1] *Chen Chiu Chia I Ching*[2] (Treatise on Acupuncture and Moxibustion) of +282. As we know, he had at his disposal the *Su Wên* and the *Ling Shu* (originally the *Chen Ching*), but he also mentions in his preface a book now long lost, the *Ming Thang Khung Hsüeh Chen Chiu Chih Yao*[3] (Essentials of Therapy of the Human Body by the Application of Acupuncture and Moxa at the Acu-points),[c]

[a] Li Yuan-Chi (*1*) counts 313.

[b] This figure is the total for the acu-points classically recognised. Many more are now distinguished and in use, e.g. a group of 73 on the auricula or external ear (cf. Anon. (135), pp. 269 ff.; (*120*), pp. 297 ff.; (*123*), pp. 237 ff.). English definitions of anatomical positions are listed in Anon. (*121*).

[c] In the volumes of *SCC* there have been many references to the ancient imperial cosmic temple or ritual palace called Ming Thang (Vols. 2, 3, 4, pts. 1 and 3 *s.v.*). But from the Han time onwards the

1 皇甫謐　　2 針灸甲乙經　　3 明堂孔穴鍼灸治要

so this is included to indicate the continuity. In the Sung period human figures of bronze with little holes to indicate the acu-points became popular,[a] so we find a group of books with Thung Jen[1] in their titles — of these the most celebrated is that of the physician Wang Wei-I,[2] his *Thung Jen Shu Hsüeh Chen Chiu Thu Ching*[3] (Illustrated Manual of the Practice of Acupuncture and Moxibustion at (the Transmission) (and other) Acu-points, for use with the Bronze Figure). Side by side with this is placed the *Shih-ssu Ching Fa Hui*[4] (An Elucidation of the Fourteen Acu-tracts) by Hua Shou,[5] one of the greatest medical writers of Yuan times. The number of acu-points had now reached a nearly stable level, so in the next category are placed together a +13th-century work, Wang Chih-Chung's[6] *Chen Chiu Tzu Shêng Ching*[7] (Manual of Acupuncture and Moxibustion Profitable for the Restoration of Health), and a +16th-century one, Yang Chi-Chou's[8] *Chen Chiu Ta Chhêng*[9] (Principles of Acupuncture and Moxa). Finally the number of acu-points generally accepted at the present time is entered.

From this it can be seen that some 44% of the acu-point names still current are to be found in the *Nei Ching*, *Su Wên* and *Ling Shu*, while if those implicit in the texts are also taken into consideration, the figure rises to 70 or 80%.[b] But if we look at the number of names recorded by Huangfu Mi and his predecessors of Later Han and San Kuo times, the result is 96%. In general, then, one could say that the development of the whole system was approximately complete by +300, in the age of Ko Hung[10].[c] One must think too of the ancient idea of the theoretical total, for the *Nei Ching* says that there were 365 acu-points in all, to correspond with the number of days in the year and the number of degrees in the celestial circle.[d] Counting the bilateral duplicates, however, it mentions only 295. But after the Han there was little emphasis on any theoretical total, and the idea lived on mainly as a venerable statement.

Lastly there is the matter of synonymy, that characteristic noise or redundance which always accompanies the growth of systematic classifications in all cultures.

name was also applied, in accord with macrocosm–microcosm philosophy, to the human body, hence it became characteristic of anatomical and physiological-medical writings. We come across it in this sense in Vol. 5, pt. 5, where we quote one or two books which included it in their titles. Now we have it in connection with acupuncture. The volume in Huangfu Mi's library was not at all the only one of the kind, for we know also of a *Ming Thang Khung Hsüeh Thu*[11] which was current in the Liang and still extant in Thang (cf. *SIC*, p. 253), and a *Ming Thang Chen Chiu Thu*[12] (cf. *SIC*, pp. 265–6) of very uncertain date, attributed to Huang Ti, but perhaps not produced until the Sung. As Hsieh Li-Hêng says (*1*), p. 32*a*, the phrase Ming Thang always had a physiological rather than a purely anatomical nuance. Literary scholars often failed to get the point. For example, the *Shih Wu Chi Yuan* says (ch. 7, p. 38*a*) that books on acupuncture have this name because Huang Ti gave the first one to Lei Kung when sitting enthroned in the Ming Thang.

[a] See further, p. 131 below.
[b] Cf. Anon. (*90*), pp. 17–18.
[c] The great alchemical physician so often spoken of in *SCC*, Vol. 5, pts. 2 and 3.
[d] *NCSW/PH*, ch. 54, (p. 281) actually gives the number of *lo*[13] as 365 and says that the *sun lo*[14] (p. 19 above) are innumerable. Ch. 58, (p. 290) has 365 *chhi hsüeh*.[15]

1 銅人 2 王惟一 3 銅人腧穴針灸圖經 4 十四經發揮 5 滑壽
王執中 7 針灸資生經 8 楊繼州 9 針灸大成 10 葛洪
明堂孔穴圖 12 明堂鍼灸圖 13 絡 14 孫絡 15 氣穴

And just as Li Shih-Chen in the early nineties of the +16th century was making his tables of botanical and zoological superfluities in nomenclature for publication in the *Pên Tshao Kang Mu*,[a] so also a very few years later Yang Chi-Chou was drawing up his lists of synonyms in the names of acu-points.[b] The results were as follows:

	No. in lists	No. of extra names
Cases of one acu-point with two names	88	88
Cases of one acu-point with three names	26	52
Cases of one acu-point with four names	8	24
Cases of one acu-point with five names	2	8
Cases of one acu-point with six names	2	10
		182

Adding this total to the 359 names accepted at the beginning of the +17th century, one would get a grand total of 541, but that would be erroneously large because not all the synonymic names were completely different from any of those in the main list; there would be a number of confused overlappings which it is not worth while to analyse further.[c] But one could certainly take about 500 as the rough total of names applied through the centuries.

This conclusion is of course subject to one important proviso, namely that the figure for the number of names 'accepted today' in Table 15 no longer represents the state of the case. During the past dozen years, many new acu-points of importance have been recognised, partly in connection with the rapid development of acupuncture analgesia, and partly by the exploration of the properties of the auricula or pinna, the external ear. All these amount to at least 100, 73 being on the ear, and 33 on the hands.

We can turn now to another subject, the types of needles described in the *Nei Ching*. They are discussed several times in all the relevant texts, the *Su Wên*, the *Ling Shu* and the *Thai Su*,[d] as well as in many of the later treatises.[e] We have summarised the information in Table 16 for comparison with Fig. 20 drawn from the *Chen Chiu Ta Chhêng*[f] of +1601. It is of interest that only approximately three types survived into late times, and until now, and indeed the majority do look somewhat

[a] See *SCC*, Vol. 6, pt. 1.

[b] *CCTC*, ch. 7, (pp. 234.2 ff.).

[c] On the other hand, Yang Chi-Chou may have under-estimated the worst cases. For example Homma Shohaku (*1*) says that Chhang-chhiang[1] (TM 1) has 17 other names, and Kuan-yuan[2] (JM 4) has 26. But possibly this includes Japanese traditions, which for the most part, for lack of space, we have to pass over.

[d] *NCSW/PH*, ch. 54, (p. 280); *NCLS/PH*, ch. 1, (p. 6), ch. 7, (pp. 72 ff.), ch. 78, (pp. 545 ff.); *NCTS*, ch. 22, (p. 134).

[e] E.g. *Chia I Ching*, ch. 5, (p. 112). Among modern accounts we may mention Chu Lien (*1*), p. 41, and Anon. (*90*), pp. 16–17.

[f] Ch. 4, (p. 87.2), but we reproduce from an old edition, ch. 4, pp. 8*a*, *b*.

[1] 長强 [2] 關元

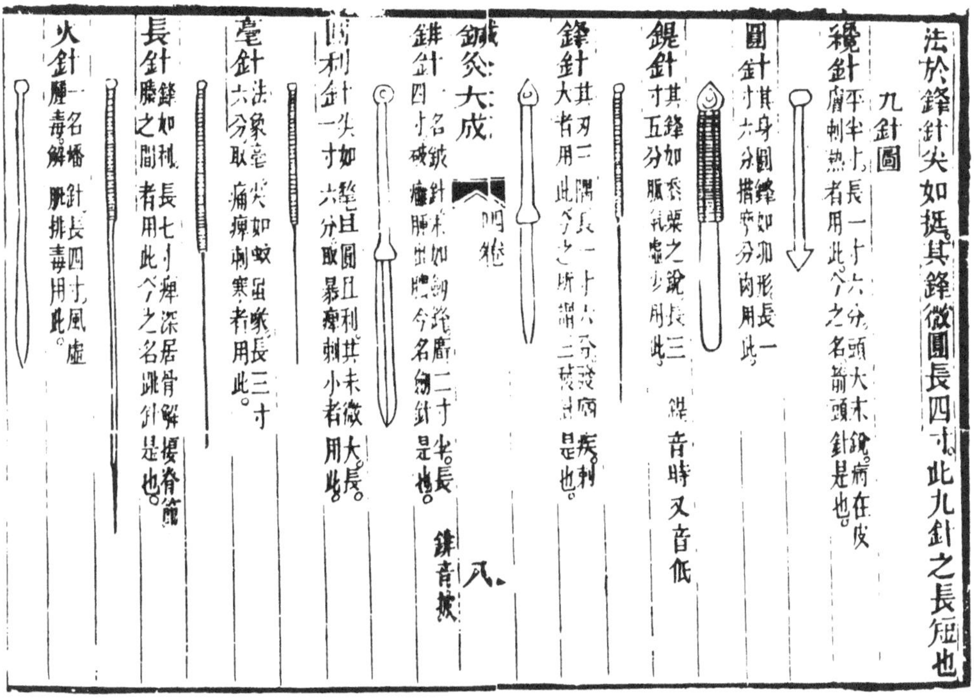

Fig. 20. The nine needles, an illustration from the *Chen Chiu Ta Chhêng* of +1601 by Yang Chi-Chou. Ch. 4, p. 8*a*, *b*.

crude, many as thick, no doubt, as present-day hypodermic injection needles or even thicker. The illustration may be compared also with Fig. 15 showing the needles of gold recovered from the tomb of Liu Shêng (d. −113). As we have noticed already, the number nine may have accounted for the name which the *Ling Shu* bore during Sui and Thang (p. 88 above), and it was of course one of the 'magic' ones in ancient Chinese cosmology and natural philosophy—Mayers (1) lists no less than 31 groups of nines in his list of the classifications. Various symbolic correlations were naturally attached to the nine needles but we need say no more of them here.[a] The ancient accounts may advantageously be compared with Fig. 21A which shows a typical acupuncturist's armamentarium of needles at the present day.

This may be the place to allude to a matter which we may have to raise again later but which cannot be excluded now, namely the possibility of iatrogenic infections brought about by the technique itself in the early days of acupuncture.[b] There are certain indications in the ancient texts of such unwitting inoculations due to unsterilised needles, but they are always attributed to the wrong use of the wrong needles, at improper places and unsuitable times, or for wrongly diagnosed conditions.[c] In

[a] See especially *NCSW/PH*, ch. 54, (p. 280) and *NCLS/PH*, ch. 78, (p. 545). The nature of the symbolic correlations and their role in ancient Chinese natural philosophy has been described in *SCC*, Vol. 2, pp. 261 ff.

[b] This was a typical gravamen of prejudice, doubtless not entirely unjustified, widespread among the early proponents of modern-Western medicine in China. Cf. p. 68 above.

[c] Cf. *NCLS/PH*, ch. 7, (pp. 72 ff.); *NCTS*, ch. 22, (p. 134.1); *Chia I Ching*, ch. 5, (p. 114).

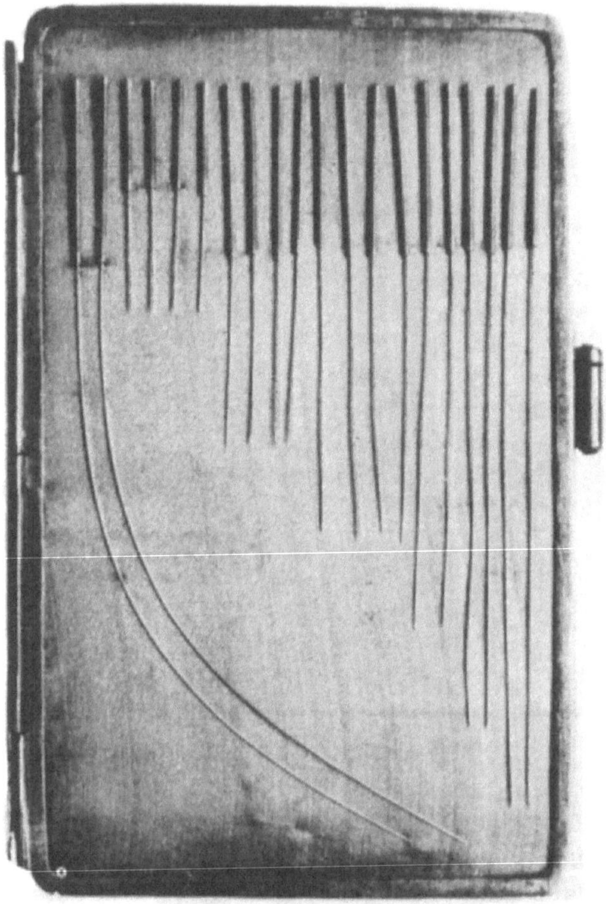

Fig. 21A. A contemporary Chinese physician's case of acupuncture needles.

later writings there is much to be read on 'boiling the needles' (*chu chen*[1]), but this was during their preparation, when they were heated with various drugs and chemicals, sometimes in water, sometimes dry, as part of the process whereby fine steel points were obtained (cf. p. 77 above).[a] But there were other techniques, used just before the moment of the acupuncture itself, which would have had a sterilising effect — for example *huo chen*,[2] in which the needle was raised to red heat in the flame of a sesame-oil lamp and then used hot to give a cauterising effect as well as the puncture.[b] Another form of sterilisation was called *wên chen*,[3] putting in the needle with a piece of dried *pai chih*[4] (*Angelica anomala*)[c] burning at the other end of it; this would surely have been effective but for some reason or other it was not thought very well of.[d]

[a] See *CCCY*, ch. 3, (p. 189) and *CCTC*, ch. 4, p. 9*a*.

[b] *CCCY*, ch. 3, (p. 189) and *CCTC*, ch. 4, p. 10*a*. Chang Chung-Ching was not at all in favour of this, and warned against it for some cases in his *Shang Han Lun*, Phang An-Shih comm. ed. ch. 2, pp. 23*a* ff.; an important point, proving that the practice must have been as old as the Later Han.

[c] Cf. Khung *et al.* (*1*), p. 304.2; Anon. (*109*), vol. 2, p. 1088.1.

[d] *CCTC*, ch. 4, p. 11*a* (p. 89.1).

1 煮鍼 2 火鍼 3 溫鍼 4 白芷

Table 16. *The nine types of needles described in the* Nei Ching

	name			length, ins.	employment
1	*chhan chen*[a]	鑱針	arrow-head needle	1·6	skin diseases and oedematous conditions
2	*yuan chen*	圓針	round-headed probe	1·6	massage
3	*tui*[b] *chen*[c]	鍉針	fine-pointed needle, 'with a sharpness like that of millet-grains'	3·5	used more for *shih* (plerotic) conditions than for *hsü* (asthenic) ones
4	*fêng chen*	鋒針	triangular-section lancet	1·6	sharp on all three edges, used for chronic diseases
5	*fei chen* or *phi*[a]	鈹針 鈹	sword lancet, or spear stylus	2·5	for lancing boils and imposthumes to rid the pus
6	*yuan li chen*[c]	圓利針	sharp round needle	1·6	of slightly larger diameter at the end, used in rheumatic conditions when there is much pain
7	*hao chen*[c]	毫針	capillary, or hair-thin, needle	3·6	'like a mosquito's sting', used often in rheumatic and painful arthritic conditions
8	*chhang chen*	長針	bodkin needle	7·0	for deep penetration of muscular and interstitial tissues
9	*huo chen*[d] or *ta chen*	火針 大針	cautery lancet great lancet	4·0	used in oedematous tissues near joints

[a] As already noted (p. 71) needles shaded into lancets for draining pus from swellings and wounds. Ancient literature has many references to the use of stone implements for this, e.g. *Chan Kuo Tshê* (*c.* −300), ch. 3, p. 20*a*, *b*; ch. 8, p. 38*a*, *b*, tr. Crump (1), pp. 74–5, 499 (both with reference to Pien Chhio); *Huai Nan Tzu* (*c.* −120), ch. 16, p. 4*b*. The *Kuang Ya* (+230) says that *chhan* needles are large like stiletto lancets (*phi*), as sharp as swords, yet made of stone (ch. 8A, p. 12*b*). We shall return to this subject when dealing with external medicine (*wai kho*).

[b] Here a special pronunciation; the character is normally considered interchangeable with *shih* or *chhih*,[1] meaning spoon or key.

[c] Only the types of needle so designated survived into recent centuries and are still in use. But there are also a number of new forms, such as the multiple needles (*mei hua chen*[2]).

[d] Also called *fan chen*, cf. p. 220.

1 匙　　2 梅花針

Finally there was *nuan chen*,[1] where the needles were carried on the person of the physician (or in his mouth) to keep them warm, and sometimes dipped in boiling or very hot water before use.[a] All these methods occur in books of relatively late date, so it will be interesting to see how far in history they can be taken back.[b]

(iv) *Developments in the Han and San Kuo periods*

This is as much as we need to write here concerning acupuncture in the *Huang Ti Nei Ching*. But, you may say, we have no irrefragable proofs that the *Nei Ching*, approximately as we know it, dates from the −2nd century. Up to a point this is true, and that is why it becomes of particular interest to see what confirmatory evidence can be got from historical sources unimpeachably of that time.[c] Fortunately we have at our disposal a text, already mentioned several times elsewhere, which meets this requirement very well, the extremely detailed biography of the physician Shunyü I[2] in the *Shih Chi*.[d] In the course of this Ssuma Chhien was inspired to copy out carefully from the archives no less than twenty-five clinical histories related by Shunyü I, as well as his replies to eight specific questions, all in response to an imperial decree of about −154 commanding him to explain the principles of his medical practice. Shunyü I, who stands out still as the most concrete, least shadowy figure of ancient Chinese medicine, was born in −216 in a part of the country which had formerly belonged to the State of Chhi;[e] and after receiving his professional education from Yang Chhing[3][f] and others built up a wide practice not only among commoners and officials but also the imperial princely families. Hence perhaps, on account of their influence at court, arose the accusation of malpractice which took him before judges in −167, but it failed and he was acquitted of all such charges. However, a similar incident occurred some thirteen years later, the interrogation so fortunate for historians of medicine living in long distant centuries, and relayed to us in Ssuma Chhien's text. Shunyü I lived on, doubtless still practising, afterwards, and died between −150 and −145. Most of the case descriptions thus recorded can be interpreted fairly readily in modern medical terms, if not always perhaps with certainty as between alternatives. Thus we have the precious gift of a deep insight into the

[a] *CCTC*, ch. 4, p. 10*a* (p. 88.2). It was thought that needles at body temperature facilitated the movement of the *chhi*.

[b] At the present day (1975) acupuncture needles in China are generally sterilised in 75% alcohol (cf. Kaada *et al.* (1), p. 421). Boiling for 15–20 minutes would however be safer in order to prevent the dissemination of hepatitis virus. The consensus of Western observers, such as Smithers *et al.* (1) and McLeod *et al.* (1), agrees with Kaada and his Norwegian colleagues here. Japanese practitioners use autoclaves.

[c] The *Chou Li* could be thought of, but its exact date is uncertain, and among its many medical officials (cf. Needham & Lu Gwei-Djen (1), repr. in Needham (64), pp. 346ff.) there is none whose job specification has anything of note to say on acupuncture.

[d] Ch. 105, pp. 7*b*ff., tr. Bridgman (2); Hübotter (3); Barde (5). On the general position of Shunyü I in the history of Chinese medicine see Needham & Lu Gwei-Djen (8), repr. in Needham (64), p. 273 etc.

[e] The point is significant, for the States of Chhi and Yen were just those which from the −4th century onwards had produced the majority of the Taoist thaumaturgical technicians whose importance for the early history of science and medicine in China can hardly be overrated (cf. *SCC*, Vol. 2, pp. 122, 232 and 240–1, as also Vol. 5, pt. 3, pp. 13ff.).

[f] Or Kungchhêng Yang-Chhing.[4]

[1] 煖鍼 [2] 淳于意 [3] 陽慶 [4] 公乘陽慶

thoughts, the knowledge and the practice of a Chinese physician of the −2nd century, just exactly at the time when we believe the *Huang Ti Nei Ching* was being written down.

Indeed there is reason for believing that Shunyü I possessed among his books, the titles of which have come down to us because he spoke of them to his interviewers, something which may have been an early version or portion of the *Nei Ching* under another name. This was the *Mo Shu Shang Hsia Ching*[1] (Treatise on the Pulse and Vessels, in Two Manuals);[a] and what is more, he seems to have received it from his teacher, for on the previous page he says that Yang Chhing told him to throw away his 'recipe books' (*fang shu*[2])[b] and follow instead the *Huang Ti Pien Chhio Mo Shu*[3] (Treatise on the Pulse and Vessels by the Yellow Emperor and Pien Chhio) a manuscript of which he would (and did) transmit to him.[c] Here the association with the name of Huang Ti would seem to be something more than a coincidence, and since Shunyü I would have been studying under Yang Chhing in the early years of the −2nd century (by −180), we have another rather strong indication that the *Nei Ching* (or at any rate parts of it) may belong rather to the −3rd. Even more, another of the titles given by Shunyü I seems to have been that of a text (whether a separate book or part of some corpus we do not know) specifically concerned with acupuncture, namely the *Chi Kai Shu*[4].[d] One hardly dares to translate this title, which has puzzled many through the centuries, but about +737 the commentator Chang Shou-Chieh[5] was clear that it referred to the Eight Auxiliary Tracts (*chhi ching pa mo*,[6] cf. p. 48 above), and he quoted a passage on them from the *Nan Ching* or 'Manual of Explanations of Eighty-one Difficult Points in the *Nei Ching*', a +1st-century text.[e] Thus if this be accepted, one of Shunyü I's books or tractates was especially connected with a branch of acupuncture, the use of the acu-points along the auxiliary tracts.

Enough for the moment on his books;[f] let us turn to some of his cases, and some of

[a] P. 9*b*, cf. Bridgman (2), pp. 26, 65. All earlier translators have taken this as referring to the pulse only (and so did we ourselves) but it is clear from p. 25 above that *mo* must have a much wider meaning here, including the channels of circulation of the *chhi* as well as the blood.

[b] Again significant, since Chhi was the land of *fang shih*[7] and *fang shu* par excellence. Shunyü I's first teacher, Kungsun Kuang,[8] had been a great master of recipes in relation to all kinds of natural phenomena, cf. p. 25*b*, tr. Bridgman (2), p. 48.

[c] P. 9*a*, cf. Bridgman (2), pp. 26, 65.

[d] P. 9*b*, cf. Bridgman (2), loc. cit.; Barde (5), pp. 21, 50. Earlier we englished it as 'The Art of Determining the Acu-points of the Eight Auxiliary Tracts' (Needham & Lu Gwei-Djen, 8); and this is still our interpretation. It is accepted too by modern authorities, e.g. Hsieh Li-Hêng (2), vol. 2, p. 1503.2. But Hsü Kuang,[9] who commented on the passage soon after +400, said that the first word should be pronounced *chi*, and that the second (normally pronounced *kho*) stood for *kai*.[10] Ku Yeh-Wang, about +560, remarked that this word meant skin and hair, but that does not fit in very well with the Shunyü I tradition. However, *chi kai* was a phrase used in Han times for any extraordinary and secret technique (cf. Morohashi dict., vol. 3, p. 572.3); so possibly the title disclosed no more of the contents than this. But even so, it could have been precisely on the auxiliary tracts, with a pun in its name. The importance of the interpretation we prefer is that it takes the *chhi ching* (p. 51) back into the centuries before the *Nan Ching*.

[e] P. 9*b*; he quoted it as *Pa-shih-i Nan*.[11]

[f] We discuss them in further detail elsewhere (Needham (64), *loc. cit.*).

1 脈書上下經　2 方書　3 黃帝扁鵲脈書　4 奇咳術　5 張守節
6 奇經八脉　7 方士　8 公孫光　9 徐廣　10 胲
11 八十一難

the questions of his interlocutors to which he gave precise answers. Case no. 3 was that of Hsün,[1] a palace superintendent in Chhi.[a] All the other physicians thought that he was suffering from *chüeh*[2],[b] and prescribed acupuncture at Jen-chung (TM 25 or 26),[c] but when Shunyü I examined him he said that this was wrongly done, for he was suffering from *yung hsien*[3],[d] and proceeded to cure him by a decoction of drugs. The modern interpretation of his trouble would be that he had vesical lithiasis with anuria and severe constipation, perhaps partly due to bilharzia infection. In this case therefore Shunyü stuck to pharmaceutical recipes and regarded acupuncture as inapplicable, but it shows that his colleagues were ready to use it. Erroneous use of acupuncture recurs several times. In Case no. 6 Tshao Shan-Fu,[4] a man of Chhi, and seemingly an epileptic, was suffering from a hepatic abscess of parasitic amoebic origin; Shunyü I predicted that he would die in eight days, and he did.[e] Previously however he had been attended by the Director of Medical Services in Chhi (Chhi Thai I[5]), who had ordered moxibustion[f] along the podotelic Shao-Yang tract (VF),[g] followed by a powerful purgative and then by more moxa[f] along the podogenic Shao-Yin tract (R). This, said Shunyü, ruined the liver, destroying deeply its firmness, so that the *chhi* of the patient was gravely affected and the fever was bound to intensify. The felleic (VF) tract was wrongly treated again in another instance (Case no. 10), that of a woman, Chhu-Yü,[6] the wife or concubine of a Minister of Works in Chhi, who had an acute cystitis due to lithiasis and probably bilharziosis.[h] All the other physicians thought that her disease lay in the lungs,[i] so they performed acupuncture along the podotelic Shao-Yang tract (VF), but Shunyü knew that the bladder was the chief site of the illness, so he applied moxas on the podogenic Chüeh-Yin tract (H) and gave a decoction of drugs, with the result that the girl was cured. Once again, both acupuncture and moxibustion were ready in the –2nd century at a moment's notice; the only problem for the doctors was whether or not, and where. It is noteworthy that Shunyü's decisions were in general based largely on his readings of the patient's pulse, which he always took.

Sometimes he himself proceeded immediately to give acupuncture after making his diagnosis. The old foster-mother nurse of a former Prince of Chi-Pei complained

[a] P. 11*b*, cf. Bridgman (2), pp. 28, 70 ff.

[b] On this term see Yü Yün-Hsiu (*1*), pp. 234, 322. It could mean locomotory difficulties with stumbling or falling, paralysis, catalepsy, prostration etc. and cold extremities.

[c] Cf. p. 56 above. The acu-point is now more often called Shui-kou, but also Kuei-kung.[7] Of the three translators noted above only Hübotter (3), p. 9, recognised the presence of an acu-point name, and located it correctly. Cf. Chhêng Tan-An (*1*), p. 184.

[d] I.e. swelling and retention; cf. also p. 135.

[e] P. 13*b* ff., cf. Bridgman (2), pp. 31–2, 74 ff., 169.

[f] And perhaps acupuncture also, as Hübotter (3), p. 12, assumed.

[g] The text suggests that this was done on the upper surface of the feet.

[h] P. 15*b* and 16*a*, cf. Bridgman (2), pp. 34–5, 82 ff. The tract which was wrongly treated was unfortunately omitted in his translation; and Hübotter (3), pp. 14–15, caught one or two points which were missed by the others.

[i] Some ancient MSS had liver here, according to Hsü Kuang's commentary.

[1] 循 [2] 蹶 [3] 涌疝 [4] 曹山跗 [5] 齊太醫 [6] 出於
[7] 鬼宮

that her feet felt hot, swollen and uncomfortable (Case no. 11).[a] Shunyü I therefore inserted needles at three acu-points in the sole of each foot[b] and applied compression so that there was no bleeding; soon the patient was greatly relieved. He considered that the attack had been brought on by a spell of drunkenness. The case is interpreted as one of gout following chronic alcoholism, but it has a special interest in several ways. First, it is as good as certain that Yung-chhüan (R 1) was the principal locus he used. Nowadays three other loci are recognised near it, one anterior and two posterior, all over the central part of the plantar aponeurosis and the flexor digitorum brevis; and one of them, Tsu-hsin,[1] 'sole of the foot', is named in the same words as those of our present text. Since Yung-chhüan has always been the only regular tract point on the sole of the foot Shunyü I must have been using acu-points off the tracts (*ching wai chhi hsüeh*[2]) — as was certainly done in later times and still is. Secondly his method of preventing bleeding was one of the adjuvant or tonic (*pu*[3]) techniques, keeping up a pressure with the finger immediately the needle is withdrawn. Thirdly the context indicates that his treatment was really for the relief of pain and accompanying symptoms rather than for what we should regard as a radical cure; and this indeed was one of the two great functions of acupuncture through the ages.

Shunyü I used acupuncture and moxa in many other cases. No. 13 was that of a Grand Prefect of Chhi who had bad carious teeth,[c] so he cauterised at acu-points along two regular tracts on the left side and gave him a mouth-wash based on *khu shen*[4] (*Sophora flavescens*),[d] after which the trouble cleared up. The difficulty here is to identify the tracts, for the text says *thai yang ming*[5],[e] but we think that this refers to the Shou Yang-Ming (IG) and the Tsu Yang-Ming (V) together since both include acu-points famous for their use in toothaches and extractions, Ho-ku (IG 4) in the former, and Chia-chhê (V 3) in the latter.[f] A somewhat similar case (No. 16) was that of a Prince of Tzu-chhuan[g] suffering from neuralgia in the head and shoulders;[h] here the text states very clearly that Shunyü I gave him acupuncture at three places along the same Tsu Yang-Ming (V) tract on both sides, and he was completely cured.

A few words more are needed on the questions and answers which Shunyü I exchanged with his interviewers in −154. In Question no. 2 he was asked why the course of an illness did not always correspond to the prognosis given.[i] He naturally

[a] P. 16*b*, cf. Bridgman (2), pp. 35, 83–4, but Barde (5), p. 29, gives perhaps the best translation of the three, though he mistook 'three acu-points' for 'thrice'.

[b] Cf. Anon. (135), p. 157; (*123*), p. 265.

[c] P. 17*a*, cf. Bridgman (2), pp. 36, 85–6.

[d] CC 1043–4; Khung *et al.* (*1*), pp. 689, 711; Anon. (*109*), vol. 2, p. 357.2.

[e] Bridgman, following some of the Chinese commentators in later books, thought that one should understand either Shou Yang-Ming or Shou Thai-Yang (IT) since the word *ming* tends to get left out in later quotations. Hübotter, op. cit., pp. 15–16, took the expression to mean both of these, while Barde, op. cit., pp. 30, 55, preferred Tsu Yang-Ming alone.

[f] Our interpretation is supported by Chamfrault & Ung Kang-Sam (1), vol. 1, p. 837; vol. 2, p. 427, from *NCLS*, ch. 26, recommending both V and IG for dental pain.

[g] Very probably Liu Hsien,[6] who was enfeoffed in −164.

[h] P. 18*b*, cf. Bridgman (2), pp. 38, 89. The pain may equally well have been rheumatic in origin. Shunyü traced its origin to the prince having 'caught a chill' after washing his hair.

[i] P. 24*a*, cf. Bridgman (2), pp. 46, 98.

1 足心 2 經外奇穴 3 補 4 苦參 5 太陽明 6 劉賢

replied that in different cases there were different conditions, whether of food and drink or of psychological factors, and also that some people take, or are given, inappropriate medicines, while others receive acupuncture or moxa at the wrong places and times; thus no prognosis can be absolutely reliable, and patients die when they should not. In Question no. 4 he was catechised about the long illness of a Prince Wên[1] who from the description had clearly suffered from myxoedema or a pituitary tumour with ensuing adiposity and genital infantility.[a] Shunyü I himself had not been called in, but said (very frankly in a pre-endocrine age) that the prince ought never to have been treated medically at all, and indeed in those days there was nothing that anyone could do. Later, he heard that the physicians had applied moxa at a number of acu-points, but that only made everything worse. They never ought to have given either acupuncture or moxibustion, Shunyü I concluded, for it could only have the effect of driving away the patient's *chhi*, i.e. his *chen chhi*,[2] or inborn vitality. Finally the inquisitors asked him about the principal pupils whom he had had (Question no. 7),[b] in reply to which he mentioned five. For example, the Prince of Chi-Pei had sent his Royal Physician, Wang Yü,[3] to sit at the feet of Shunyü I and study under him.

I taught him [he said] the course of the regular tracts and circulation vessels from head to toe, with the pulses corresponding to them (*ching mo kao hsia*[4]), together with the (principles of) action of the (eight) auxiliary tracts, and all the branches, under abnormal conditions (*chhi lo chieh*[5]),[c] and of course I had to explain the positions of the acu-points (*shu*[6]), (in each tract). I also told him how the *chhi* must now mount and now descend, how (at one moment) it issues forth and (at another) enters in, how there are malign and favourable kinds of *chhi*, and (what can be done to hinder them or help them by) the right management of the arrow-headed needles of stone (*chhi tang shang hsia, chhu ju, hsieh* (*chêng*) *shun ni, i i chhan shih*[7]). (Furthermore I also expounded) the proper way of determining how and where to apply acupuncture and moxibustion (*ting pien chih chhu*[8]). It all took more than one year...[d]

Nothing could illustrate more strikingly than does this passage the dominance of acupuncture and moxa treatments just in the century when the *Huang Ti Nei Ching* was taking shape. Since the *Shih Chi* text must have been completed by −90 there can be no further room for scepticism concerning the virtual consummation of the system's general outlines by the end of the −2nd century, and this must surely mean, as already suggested, that the beginnings of it must be older than that by several centuries.

That this is indeed the case has recently been demonstrated by the exciting and unexpected discovery of actual manuscripts of medical texts, written on silk, in the

[a] Pp. 24*b*, 25*a*, cf. Bridgman (2), pp. 47, 99 ff.

[b] Pp. 26*b*, 27*a*.

[c] The +8th-century commentator, Chang Shou-Chieh, notes that *chieh* is a technical term in sphygmology for intermittent pulse.

[d] Tr. auct., adjuv. Bridgman (2), pp. 49, 101; Hübotter (3), p. 28; Barde (5), pp. 42, 56.

1 文王 2 眞氣 3 王禹 4 經脉高下 5 奇絡結 6 兪
7 氣當上下出入邪(正)順逆以宜鑱石 8 定砭灸處

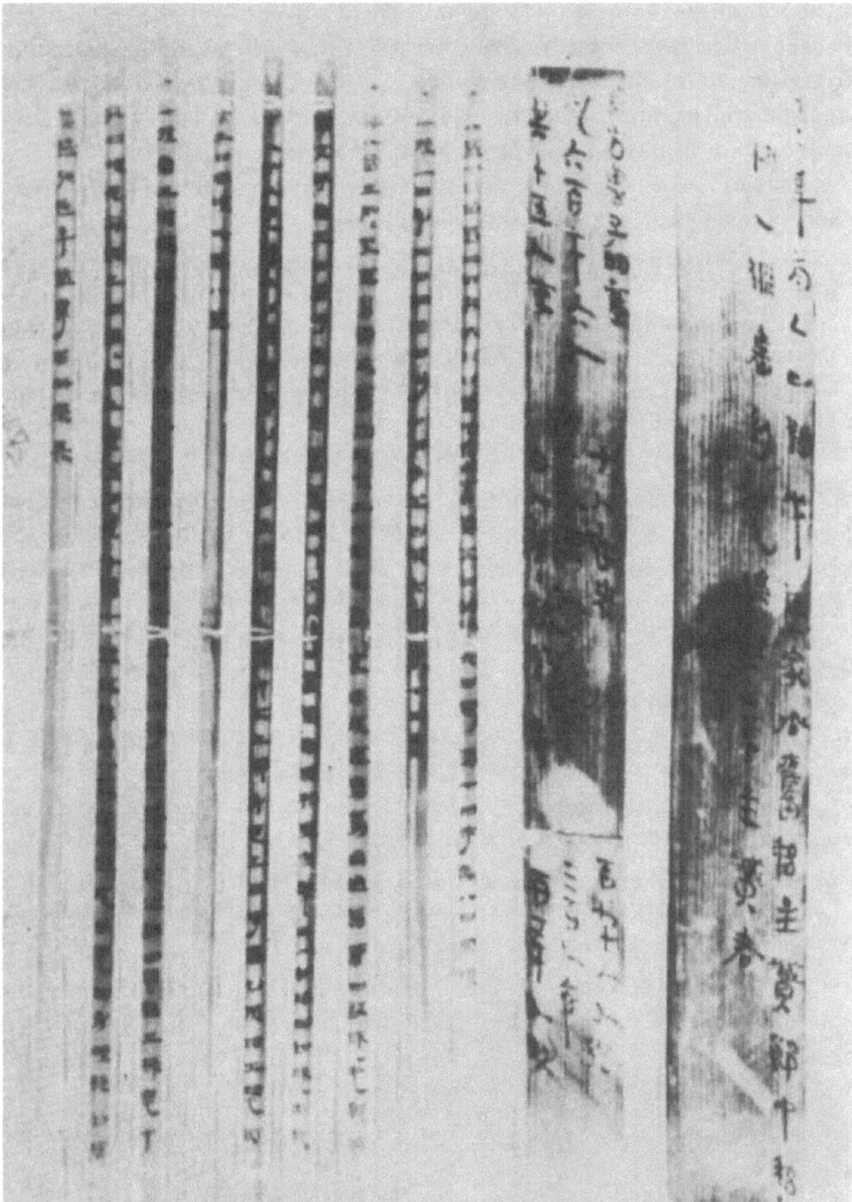

Fig. 21B. Some of the medical manuscripts from the tomb of the son of the Lord of Tai (Ma-wang-tui no. 3, near Chhangsha), who was buried in −168. This date is attested by the wooden slips on the right. The young lord's mother, whose body was preserved from corruption for two millennia by Taoist chemical art (cf. Vol. 5, pt. 2, p. 303), survived him only by about a couple of years, till −166 (corr. p. 304). Although most of the medical manuscripts are on sheets of silk, some on bamboo slips were found, and a few of these are illustrated here on the left. The style and content of the texts is similar to that of the *Nei Ching* but more archaic, so that they present a picture of Chinese medical thought during the two or three centuries preceding the formation of that great classic.

tomb of the son of the Lord of Tai,[a] a young man who died in −168 at the age of thirty or so.[b] The script resembles in some cases Chhin bronze inscriptions rather than those of the Han, so the manuscripts may well be of the −3rd century at least, and some linguistic considerations suggest an even earlier date, perhaps in the Warring States period (−4th century), perhaps even before the time of Pien Chhio.[c]

The manuscript texts (Fig. 21B) have themselves no titles but the transcribing palaeographers have given them the following names:

(1) *Tsu Pei Shih-i Mo Chiu Ching* (Moxa Manual of the Eleven Tracts on the Upper and Lower Limbs),
(2) *Yin Yang Shih-i Mo Chiu Ching* (Moxa Manual of the Eleven Tracts according to the Yin and Yang). This includes two sphygmological sections, one called *Mo Fa* (Method of Taking the Pulse) and the second *Yin Yang Mo Ssu Hou* (Fatal Prognoses determined by the Yin and Yang Pulses).
(3) *Wu-shih-erh Ping Fang* (Book of Fifty-two Illnesses and their Therapy).[d]

Other writings include short works on dietetics[e] and callisthenics (with illustrations),[f] both Taoist in character. Naturally none of these titles occur in the *Chhien Han Shu* bibliography, but the medical historians are inclined to identify the first two with a couple of lost books which it does contain, the *Chhêng Thien-Tsu Chiu Ching* and the *Tshao Shih Chiu Ching*, moxa manuals of Chhêng Thien-Tsu and Mr Tshao respectively.[g]

The picture of medical thought as a whole revealed by the manuscripts is clearly one a good deal older than that of the *Nei Ching*. The tracts number only eleven, not twelve,[h] and though all of them start from the heart, there is no concept of a continuous circulation through the whole system. There is no aetiological theory of disease, and very little about the Five Elements. The strong emphasis on moxibustion indicates once again that it may be even more ancient than acupuncture, but it is not correct to say that the latter is nowhere mentioned. True, metal needles (*chen*) do not appear, but the 'Book of Fifty-two Illnesses', though overwhelmingly pharmaceutical in character, has two clear mentions of 'stone needles' (*pien shih*)[i] and no more than that of moxa. All in all, the manuscripts now discovered reveal a whole phase of Chinese medical thinking previously unknown and characteristic of the two or three centuries before the compilation of the *Nei Ching*. The records

[a] On this family see *SCC*, Vol. 5, pt. 2, pp. 303–4, where we described the uncorrupt body of the Lady of Tai.

[b] The texts have been transcribed in Anon. (*197*, *199*) and discussed by Chinese historians of medicine in Anon. (*196*) by Ma Chi-Hsing (5) and by Harper (1). Some idea of the many other important texts which accompanied them may be gained from Hsiao Han (*1*).

[c] There are many archaic usages, such as the substitution of *wên* (warm) for *chiu*, and a different orthography of *Thai* when it comes in tract names.

[d] See Chung I-Yen & Ling Hsiang (*1*). The book contains 459 prescriptions and refers to 243 items of materia medica.

[e] See Thang Lan (*3*).

[f] See Anon. (*198*).

[g] Anon. (*196*).

[h] HC (the Shou Chüeh Yin Hsin-pao-lo Ching) is the only one left out, and curiously enough this is the only one not described in detail in the *Nei Ching*.

[i] Chung & Ling (*1*), p. 55.

concerning Shunyü I are therefore not only substantiated but much extended, and an important new chapter is added to the history of medicine in China.

Here another text, only slightly younger, deserves mention, the *Yen Thieh Lun*[1] (Discourses on Salt and Iron). As will be remembered,[a] this was an account of the great debate on the Han government's nationalisation policies which had been held in −81, written by Huan Khuan[2] in the style of a verbatim report soon afterwards, or at any rate some time during the following dozen years. The government ministers and high officials were opposed by a group of Confucian literati who looked back to quasi-feudal antiquity and objected to the growing bureaucratisation of imperial rule, both sides being strongly opposed to mercantile power.[b] In the course of the debate, and during a discussion of the balance between production and distribution, the literati introduced a medical analogy, only to have it turned against themselves by the bureaucrats, and the phrasing of this is what is of interest to us now. The passage runs as follows.[c]

The Spokesman of the Literati said: 'Only by feeling the pulse Pien Chhio could tell the origin of the patient's disease. If the (calid) Yang *chhi* was too abundant he would lessen it so as to bring it into harmony with the Yin. If the algid *chhi* (of Yin) predominated he would reduce it so as to harmonise it with the Yang. Consequently the *chhi* and the vessels were balanced and integrated so that there was no opportunity for malign *chhi* to remain (in the body). But ignorant and unskilled physicians (*chuo i*[3]) do not know the pores and patterns of the tracts and vessels (*mo li chih tshou*[4]) nor the differences between the blood and the *chhi*; they stab in their needles at random, without the least beneficial influence on the illness, and only succeed in injuring the flesh and the muscles. Now (the government) desires to subtract from the superabundant to assist the needy—and yet the rich grow richer and the poor grow poorer. With severe laws and arbitrary punishments it is intended to curb the tyrannical and suppress malefactors — yet wickedness continues as before. Possibly these measures differ from the way in which Pien Chhio used his (acupuncture needles of) iron and stone, so that the multitudes have not yet felt their salutary effects?'.

But the Imperial Secretary who was speaking had an answer to all this. First he recalled the great benefits which the unification of the empire after the Warring States had brought, and the vast resources now available to China. If all the staff of the Ministry of Finance were to disappear into the countryside and set up as farmers in the good old style nostalgically admired by the literati, the armies on the four frontiers would not get their rations. For a great country great and effective organisation was essential, and the old village ideologies would not do.[d]

It is not [he went on] that Nature provides us with only meagre wealth; (the problem is how to distribute it). This is not just a matter of using (acupuncture needles of) iron and stone to harmonise and equalise surplus and want, or to assist the needy. No, when His Excellency the Minister, in his capacity of Grain Intendant, took over the administration of

[a] From *SCC*, Vol. 2, pp. 251–2, Vol. 4, pt. 3, pp. 264, 518.

[b] We shall of course set the work in its full context in Sect. 48 in Vol. 7 on the social and economic background of Chinese science and technology.

[c] Ch. 14, p. 4*a*, tr. auct., adjuv. Gale (1), pp. 88–9.

[d] Cf. Gale (1), p. 87.

[1] 鹽鐵論 [2] 桓寬 [3] 拙醫 [4] 脉理之腠

the Imperial Treasury, he stimulated with his moxa and acupuncture the stagnant flow (of wealth), and opened up the hundred tracts and vessels for the general profit. As a result all commodities circulated, and the government obtained substantial revenue...This was certainly something like the skill and strength of Pien Chhio, and a great blessing derived from the nationalisation of the salt and iron industries.

To understand the full background of this one has to realise that the Confucian scholars believed in rural self-sufficiency, opposing both the improvement of communications[a] and the territorial expansion gained in frontier wars.[b] But here this does not matter; what concerns us is the use the two sides made of the medical analogy. It shows not only how universal acupuncture and moxa were by the −1st century, but also that the idea of the removal of obstacles and blockages in the circulation paths was one of the basic roots of the practical techniques.

The *Yen Thieh Lun* has another passage in which acupuncture is mentioned. Here the scholars are arguing that the ideal function of the magistrate is to prevent misdemeanours arising rather than to castigate them after they have arisen.[c]

The Spokesman of the Literati said: 'The law can punish a man but it cannot make him honest; it can execute a man but it cannot make him good. What is admired in a good doctor (*liang i*[1]) is his examining of the respiration (*shen hsiao hsi*[2]) so as to (advise how to) ward off malign *chhi* (*thui hsieh chhi*[3]); what is not admirable is his applying the needles of metal and stone (*chen shih*[4]) so as to bore into the skin and flesh. What is valued in a good (judicial) functionary (*li*[5]) is his excising of evil before it sprouts, thus preventing people from doing wrong; what is not valuable is his shutting them up in dungeons, and punishing or executing them.'

Thus once more we see how commonplace a thing acupuncture was in medical treatment at this time.[d]

Leaving now the formative period of the Early Han, we must say something about the two centuries of the Later Han, the century that saw the Three Kingdoms division, and then the main century of the Chin. This was the time that saw the appearance of the first books specifically and wholly devoted to acupuncture. The *Nan Ching*[6] was not one of these, but we must start with it.[e] As a title, the 'Difficulties Manual' is one of the most succinct in all Chinese literature, and it has to be expanded so as to say 'Manual of Explanations of Eighty-one Difficult Passages in the *Huang Ti Nei Ching*'. It is classically attributed to a Chhin Yüeh Jen,[7] but for reasons that will be

[a] Cf. ch. 10 (Gale (1), p. 65).

[b] Cf. ch. 16 (Gale (1), pp. 99ff.).

[c] Ch. 56, pp. 6*b*, 7*a*, tr. Derk Bodde.

[d] There are mentions in the *Lieh Tzu* book which may belong here, e.g. the consultation of Chi Liang with three physicians, one of whom refers to *yao shih*, i.e. 'drugs and stone (needles)'. Ch. 6, p. 10*b*, tr. Graham (6), pp. 128–9; Schatz *et al.* (1), pp. 163ff. This book contains some Warring States material, but its text was not completed till about +380. The same phrase occurs in the story of the exchange of hearts between Kung Hu and Chhi Ying effected by Pien Chhio's surgery; ch. 5, p. 16*b*, Graham tr. pp. 106–7.

[e] Apart from many separate editions of various dates, the almost complete text can be found in *TSCC*, *I shu tien*, chs. 89 and 90; repr. in *NCLS/MC*, vol. 2, pp. 1387ff. The important commentary of Hua Shou[8] (+1361), the *Nan Ching Pên I*, is in *ITCM*, pên 19–20. The writer, 'Chhin Yüeh Jen', whoever he was, took more from the *Ling Shu* than from the *Su Wên*, but he also used many textual quotations from other ancient sources not now identifiable.

1 良醫 2 審消息 3 退邪氣 4 鍼石 5 吏 6 難經
7 秦越人 8 滑壽

obvious this cannot mean Pien Chhio, whose sobriquet it had originally been; perhaps by this time the phrase had come to be a generic name for any great physician, something like 'the Hippocrates of our times'.[a] It must be later than the *Ling Shu* (or *Chen Ching*) and internal evidence shows that it must be earlier than the *Shang Han Lun*, which dates from the end of the Hou Han, i.e. about +200, so the +1st or +2nd century is a very probable time for it, and the former rather than the latter.[b] It was edited and explained by Lü Kuang,[1] who was a Director-General of Medical Services (Thai I Ling[2]) in the Wu State during the +3rd century; as he says, it 'discusses the structure and relations of the viscera, the observation of the pulse, and their relations with acupuncture and moxibustion'. These techniques are assumed throughout the book, indeed chs. 69 to 81 are concerned primarily with *chen fa*,[3] with much on methods of tonification and sedation (*pu hsieh*[4]), while the *ching lo*[5] circulation system of tracts figures prominently in chs. 23 to 29, and the transmission acu-points (*shu hsüeh*[6]) in chs. 62 to 68.[c] Covering no really new ground, it brings out many subtleties of theory and practice.[d]

Already the +1st century gives us the names of a number of eminent acupuncture doctors. There was, for example, Kuo Yü,[7] who became Royal Physician[e] to Han Ho Ti soon after +89; he was the expert who detected a male pulse when examining a patient seated behind a curtain in the interior apartments. He left no book, but certain famous phrases of technical terminology came down from him, and he can be heard discoursing on acupuncture in his biography in the dynastic history.[f] From this we know that his teacher had been a physician named Chhêng Kao,[8] and he in turn had been the disciple of a shadowy but intriguing figure, Fou Ong,[9] the old fisherman of the Fou River in Szechuan, who never put himself forward but did acupuncture like an angel if called upon.[g] There was a *Fou Ong Chen Ching*[10] needle manual current in the Later Han, but it was afterwards lost,[h] and a *Fou Ong Chen Mo Fa*,[11] or treatise on sphygmology, was also attributed to him, and also lost.[i] Working backwards, therefore, Fou Ong would have been active about +50, the likely age of the composition of the *Nan Ching*.

Here may be mentioned that important Taoist work, not primarily medical at all,

[a] The attribution seems not to antedate the editor Yang Hsüan-Tshao[12] of the early Thang, whose biography is preserved in *TPYL*, ch. 724.

[b] For discussions of the best dating see Hsieh Li-Hêng (*1*), p. 4*b*; Chang Hsin-Chhêng (*1*), vol. 2, pp. 984ff.

[c] The exposition narrows even to the *ching hsüeh*[13] (cf. p. 63 above) in chs. 63 to 65.

[d] Among modern studies cf. Anon. (*90*), p. 23; Li Thao (*13*).

[e] Thai I Chhêng.[14]

[f] *HHS*, ch. 112B, pp. 5*b*, 6*b*. Another biography is in *Li Tai Ming I Mêng Chhiu*,[15] ch. 2, p. 26*b*.

[g] At this time some of the knowledge of acu-points seems to have been still kept as a professional secret, for the lineage mentioned above was considered to record how it had been handed down, through a succession of favoured disciples.

[h] It was mentioned in bibliographies as late as the *Yü Hai* (+13th cent.), however, ch. 63, pp. 12*b* ff. See *SIC*, p. 230.

[i] *SIC*, p. 162.

1 呂廣 2 太醫令 3 針法 4 補瀉 5 經絡 6 俞穴
7 郭玉 8 程高 9 涪翁 10 涪翁鍼經 11 涪翁診脈法 12 楊玄操
13 井穴 14 太醫承 15 歷代名醫蒙求

the *Thai Phing Ching*[1] (Canon of Great Peace and Equality).[a] The first text belonged to the genre of apocryphal classics (*wei shu*[2])[b] and was most probably written about −25 by Kan Chung-Kho,[3] supposedly as a revelation from the immortal Chhih Ching Tzu.[4] But a second text, the *Thai Phing Chhing Ling Shu*,[5] appeared about +140, and this contains, among much material on fertility and magic, recipes for longevity in which acupuncture and sphygmology figure quite prominently.[c] There is a third text too, the *Thai Phing Tung Chi Ching*,[6] written at some date between the +1st and the +6th centuries, which though emphasising the idea that sickness was due to sin, gives many apotropaic talismans of a medical nature.[d] It also describes an arrangement of letter-boxes in the countryside for collecting extraordinary writings and special recipes, with the conscious idea, based on the circulation of blood and *chhi* in the body (cf. p. 26 above) that these contributions would be like vivifying fluids arriving at the capital and being redistributed around the body politic. We find further a remarkable description of medical experiments, the sages assembling and making observations on acupuncture and pulse. Nothing could exemplify better the universal prevalence of the technique of acupuncture at this early time. These texts, and others related to them, were directly connected with the development of the Taoist Church and the local or regional theocratic communities which flourished during the century preceding the establishment of the Chin dynasty.[e]

Another reference to acupuncture about this time (*c.* +150) occurs in the *Chhien Fu Lun*[7] (Comments of a Hermit Scholar) of Wang Fu,[8] a political writer who castigated the governments of his time for not seeking out and employing the best and most selfless men as their officials, and for doing nothing about urbanisation, wealth-accumulation, unemployment and injustice, trends which were indeed to bring about some decades later the collapse of the Han. In an eloquent passage, notable for his use of a medical microcosm doctrine,[f] he wrote:[g]

Superior physicians treat the body as a whole (lit. the State); inferior physicians simply treat the disease. Now anyone managing a State is certainly like someone treating an individual body. Disease is the sickness of the body; social chaos is the sickness of the State. In the body's illnesses we rely on medicine for a cure; in the chaos of the States we rely on men of ability and moral worth to regain order. For restoring order to the body, we have the arts of the Yellow Emperor; for restoring order to the world, we have the classics of Confucius. When an illness cannot be cured or when chaos in a State cannot be rectified, it is not that the method of acupuncture (*chen shih*[9])[h] is wrong, nor the teachings of the Five Classics perverted — the trouble is that those who use them are not the right men. 'If he is not the

[a] *TT* 1087. What follows is drawn from the interesting exposition of Kaltenmark (7).
[b] Cf. *SCC*, Vol. 2, p. 380 *et passim*.
[c] Cf. Vol. 5, pt. 2, pp. 103, 109, 126
[d] Cf. Vol. 5, pt. 3, pp. 6, 75.
[e] See Vol. 2, pp. 155ff. There has been much debate in China on whether the *Thai Phing Ching* group of texts emanated from milieux primarily 'peasant-progressive' or 'reactionary-religious' in nature; further study is needed.
[f] Cf. *SCC*, Vol. 2, pp. 294ff.
[g] Ch. 8, p. 6*a*, tr. auct., adjuv. Pearson (1).
[h] Lit. 'needles of metal and stone'.

1 太平經 2 緯書 3 甘忠可 4 赤精子 5 太平清領書
6 太平洞極經 7 潛夫論 8 王符 9 鍼石

right man',[a] then the compass will not (mark the) circle, nor the T-square right angles; the (inked) string will not lie straight, nor the balance be level; fire-drill and burning-mirror make no flame, nor can ores be smelted into metal; a whipped-up horse cannot be driven fast, nor a boat get way on her across water. All these eight processes are manifestations of the eternal Tao of Heaven, taking shape and appearing as things.

Next comes the *Shang Han Lun*[1] (Treatise on Febrile Diseases) of Chang Chung-Ching[2] (+142 to +210), one of the most cardinally important books in the history of Chinese medicine.[b] It needs no more than a mention here because Chang belonged to a different tradition, and laid more emphasis on drugs and other treatments; he was the first to set forth prescriptions in detail, and the first to classify febrile diseases into six main groups in accordance with the development of their syndromes, using the same terms as those which designate the twelve regular acupuncture tracts but with entirely different significances. Nevertheless he did not despise acupuncture, saying for example: 'In Thai-Yang Disease, when the fever will not abate, give acupuncture at Fêng-chhih (VF 20) and Fêng-fu (TM 15)...then one must do it at Chhi-mên (H 14).'[c] And he also mentioned different kinds of heated needles.[d]

Contemporary with Chang Chung-Ching there lived an equally great physician, Hua Tho,[3] a man whom we have occasion to mention in many other connections. He is often thought of as later in date, because although born near Hsüchow on the borders of Chiangsu and Anhui, his later life and practice were so much bound up with the places, people and leaders of a part of the country far away in the north-west, that part which soon afterwards became the northern kingdom of the San Kuo three, the State of Wei.[e] Here he acquired enduring fame for his skill in surgery and related disciplines,[f] his early use of some kind of anaesthesia,[g] and his discoveries and inventions in medical gymnastics.[h] Hua Tho was a very judicious acupuncturist. In his biography we read that

when moxibustion was called for, he cauterised only at one or two acu-point positions (*chhu*[4]), and after seven or eight applications (*chuang*[5])[i] the patients were cured. In cases

[a] A quotation from the *I Ching*, Hsi Tzhu appendix, pt. 2, ch. 8, p. 25*b*, cf. Wilhelm (2), Baynes tr., vol. 1, p. 374.

[b] Cf. Anon. (*90*), p. 18.

[c] *Chu Chieh Shang Han Lun*, ch. 2, (p. 66). But he also gave a decoction based on cinnamon (*Cinnamomum Cassia*), *kuei chih thang*[6] (p. 62). Cf. Anon. (*110*), p. 189, pl. 111.

[d] *Wên chen*,[7] *shao chen*,[8] *huo chen*;[9] cf. p. 104 above and pp. 135, 220 below.

[e] There has been much disagreement on the right dates for Hua Tho's life. Hübotter (1), pp. 14–15 placed him mainly in the San Kuo period (+190 to +265), while at the other extreme Chhen Tshun-Jen (*2*) made him earlier than Chang Chung-Ching, i.e. +110 to +207. Whether or not the story about his execution by Tshao Tshao is true, the general view is that he predeceased him, and as Hua's alleged age of 97 at the time of his death is also doubtful, the best estimate is perhaps that of Kung Shun (*1*), *c.* +145 to *c.* +208. But see also Chu Yen (*1*); Li Wei-Ching (*1*); and Anon. (*90*).

[f] Cf. *SCC*, Vol. 6.

[g] Cf. Sect. 45 in Vol. 6.

[h] See Vol. 5, pt. 5, and meanwhile, Needham (64), pp. 356–7.

[i] This was the standard term for the burning down of one moxa cone. It does not necessarily imply cauterisation leaving a permanent mark, for thin slices of ginger or garlic were often interposed between the cone and the epidermis. We shall say more of such things in the sub-section on moxa (pp. 171 ff. below).

1 傷寒論 2 張仲景 3 華佗 4 處 5 壯 6 桂枝湯
7 溫針 8 燒針 9 火針

where acupuncture was the most suitable treatment he also used only one or two acu-points. At the time of implantation of the needles he used to tell his patients what kind of sensations to expect, and asked them to say at once when they felt them. That would be the moment to withdraw the needle, and afterwards the patients were cured.[a]

Here was an excellent statement of the subjective responses known as 'getting the *chhi*' (*tê chhi*[1]), which have been so important in this technique from the beginning down to the present day, and which are now often interpreted as signals of the satisfactory stimulation of deep receptor nerve-endings.[b] The passage also suggests that Hua Tho had personal experience of these sensations, induced on himself, as do modern acupuncturists; and thirdly the restraint to few but effective points is an evidence of skill and experience closely paralleled by present-day tendencies (cf. p. 227).

In another place the dynastic history says:[c]

Tshao Tshao[2] (Wei Thai Tsu,[3] the posthumously consecrated emperor of the Wei)[d] heard of Hua Tho, and invited him to join his entourage. Now Thai Tsu suffered from migraine headaches (*thou fêng*[4])[e] accompanied by mental disturbance (*hsin luan*[5]) and dizziness (*mu hsüan*[6]). But Hua Tho gave acupuncture at a point in the sole of the foot[f] and the general was immediately cured.

There can be little doubt that this acu-point was Yung-chhüan (R 1),[g] and little reason for doubting its effectiveness. But in other cases, just as Shunyü I had criticised the wrong application of acupuncture, so also did Hua Tho; for example, another physician, Liu Tsu,[7] had tried to save a patient named Hsü I[8] by inserting needles in the stomach tract (V), but he got the liver tract (H) instead, which only made the sick man much worse, so that Hua Tho's prognosis of death in five days was borne out by the event.[h] Thus there can be no question that in the +2nd century acupuncture and moxa were in universal use, and the successes of acupuncture analgesia in our own time invite the speculation that just conceivably Hua Tho himself discovered this phenomenon, quite apart from the stupefying potions for which he became so

[a] *San Kuo Chih* (*Wei Shu*), ch. 29, p. 1*a*, tr. auct., adjuv. Hübotter (3), p. 32, who followed the shorter version in *HHS*, ch. 112B, pp. 6*b*, 7*a*, as reprinted in *TSCC*, *I shu tien*, ch. 525, p. 9*a* (or *tshê* 464, p. 54*a*).

[b] Cf. p. 192. But withdrawal as soon as the sensations were reported was quite the opposite of modern practice. Perhaps the historian slipped this in to enhance Hua Tho's clinical skill.

[c] *San Kuo Chih* (*Wei Shu*), ch. 29, pp. 3*b*, 4*a*, tr. auct., adjuv. Hübotter (3), p. 34, from the other sources just quoted.

[d] Because he lived (+155 to +220), eventually in a state of quasi-independence, under the Later Han.

[e] On the meaning of this expression see Yü Yün-Hsiu (*1*), p. 200.

[f] The text has the word *li*,[9] which can sometimes stand in old texts for *ko*,[10] the diaphragm, i.e. without Rad. no. 130; cf. Yü Yün-Hsiu (*1*), pp. 345–6. But anciently *li* was the name of pottery and bronze vessels with hollow feet (cf. *SCC*, Vol. 1, pp. 81–2), so it was natural for it to mean also the hollow of the foot. Since the diaphragm is not attainable by acupuncture, the word must mean something else here, and indeed R 1 is considered particular good for headache, dizziness and deranged vision. We have spoken of it in another context on p. 109 above.

[g] Cf. *CCTC*, ch. 8, (pp. 243–4); Chhêng Tan-An (*1*), p. 133; Anon. (*107*), p. 150.

[h] Cf. Hübotter (3), p. 38. The two tracts do in fact run more or less alongside each other on the front and sides of the abdomen and thighs.

1 得氣 2 曹操 3 魏太祖 4 頭風 5 心亂 6 目眩
7 劉租 8 徐毅 9 鬲 10 膈

famous—if so he kept it to himself and his immediate disciples so that the secret did not survive.[a]

(v) *Specialist writings and treatises, from Chin to Sung*

After the re-unification of the empire in +265 conditions permitted the production of what is now the oldest extant book entirely devoted to acupuncture and moxibustion—the *Chen Chiu Chia I Ching*,[1] finished by Huangfu Mi[2] some time between +256 and his death in +282. The title as it stands is untranslatable, for *chia* and *i* are the first two of the cyclical characters traditionally known as the ten *kan*[3] or 'celestial stems';[b] here they may have been intended to adumbrate the Yang and the Yin, or perhaps the work was originally in ten chapters numbered stemwise.[c] Huangfu Mi was a man of great parts, a scholar-official and historian from Kansu, who gave himself to the study of medicine partly in filial piety because of the paralysis of his mother and partly because of *fêng pi*,[4] rheumatism or neuralgia, from which he suffered himself. Huangfu Mi's 'Treatise on Acupuncture and Moxibustion'[d] deals systematically with physiology, pathology, diagnosis and therapy, plus an emphasis, rather original in the development of this literature, on prophylaxis.[e] What was also new in his writing was the grouping of the numerous acu-points (*hsüeh wei*[5]) under the heads of the various tracts (*ching*[6]) to which they belonged.[f] He gives their numbers and names all over the body, describes their positions and how to locate each of them,[g] names specific acu-points useful in the treatments of specific syndromes, and shows how the tracts relate to general classical medical theory.[h] He also adds much that had not been known or written down before concerning the practical side of the art, the *shou fa*,[7] giving details as to how deeply the needle should penetrate and the time during which it should be held in position, and how to manage tonification and sedation, or syndromic and enantiodromic effects (*pu*[8] and *hsieh*,[9] or *ying*[10] and *sui*[11]). For moxa, the number of cones or tinder sticks desirable at each acu-point is recorded. The book of Huangfu Mi was destined to exercise great influence abroad, especially in Japan, where it became one of the foundations of therapy from the +7th century onwards.[i] To this day the number and positions of the Japanese acu-points correspond exactly with those in the *Chia I Ching*. There was also at least one translation into Korean, as well as editions in classical Chinese printed in Korea.

[a] The fact that Hua Tho had such a reputation for curing headaches and other intractable pain conditions may be relevant here, since it was precisely from this background that surgical analgesia by acupuncture emerged.

[b] Cf. *SCC*, Vol. 1, p. 79 and other Vols., s.v.

[c] *ICK*, p. 311.

[d] Tr. Hübotter (5).

[e] Detailed studies of the contents will be found in Hsieh Li-Hêng (*1*), p. 11*a*; Anon. (*90*), p. 23.

[f] He discussed the tracts in a different order from that of the *Nei Ching*, grouping the acu-points of head, face, chest and back separately, and conserving the three Yin and three Yang tract classification only for the four limbs. See Li Yuan-Chi (*1*), pp. 266–7; Jen An (*1*), p. 33.

[g] He was the first to go over the human body in a systematic anatomical way, enumerating, for example, the 26 acu-points in the region of the shoulders.

[h] In their relation, for example, to the visceral organs.

[i] Jen An (*1*), p. 35.

1 針灸甲乙經 2 皇甫謐 3 干 4 風痺 5 穴位 6 經
7 手法 8 補 9 瀉 10 迎 11 隨

Huangfu Mi was by no means the only eminent practitioner and theorist of acupuncture in his time. For example, in +239, when Huangfu was already about 40, Lü Po[1] was appointed Director of Medical Services or Archiater-Royal in Wu State.[a] Lü was the writer of a *Yü Kuei Chen Ching*[2] (Needle Manual of the Box of Jade), long lost now, but influential in its time, and doubtless known to Huangfu Mi, though not actually mentioned by him.[b] Acupuncture writings, also lost, have even been attributed to Hua Tho, such as the *Chen Chung Chiu Tzhu Ching*[3] (Confidential Pillow Book of Moxa and Needling), but this may well have been a later compilation not available to Huangfu Mi.[c]

There can be no doubt that Huangfu Mi knew the *Su Wên* and the *Ling Shu* (or *Chen Ching*) by heart, as it were, but he also had the *Nan Ching* at his disposal, together with that shadowy specialist treatise, probably of the +2nd century, which we have had occasion to refer to already in connection with the growth in the number of acupoints (p. 100 and Table 15), namely the *Ming Thang Khung Hsüeh Chen Chiu Chih Yao*.[d] As we saw, the prefix *Huang Ti* was applied to at least one of these *Ming Thang* books, as it was to the *Nei Ching* itself; and it is quite probable that there were other Later Han books which Huangfu Mi took into account in his work though not mentioning them in his preface.[e] For example in the Liang, and perhaps much earlier, there was a *Ming Thang Hsia-Ma Thu*[4] (Toad Manual for the Human Body),[f] the strange title of which is explained by the longer one of another, also from those times, the *Huang Ti Chen Chiu Hsia-Ma Chi* (or *Thu*, or *Ching*)[5]—in other words, 'The Yellow Emperor's (Illustrated Manual of the) Preferential and Forbidden Days for Acupuncture and Moxibustion according to the Lunar Cycle', or, for short, 'The Yellow Emperor's Toad Manual'.[g] This bizarre appellation referred to the toad in the inconstant moon. We shall presently see (p. 138) that there was a great lore of favourable and unfavourable times and days for applying acupuncture and moxa in different ways at various loci, depending on the hour, the day in the lunation and the season of the year. We shall also suggest that modern knowledge of circadian rhythms, endocrine cycles and seasonal incidences of disease goes some way to justify these

[a] *TPYL*, ch. 724, pp. 6*a*, *b*.

[b] *SIC*, pp. 230–1. Lü Po has frequently been confused with Lü Kuang,[6] also a royal physician, whose *floruit* was much later, in the +6th century, towards the end of the Liang and the beginning of the Sui. Lü Kuang it was who wrote the first commentary on the *Nan Ching*. Cf. Fan Hsing-Chun (*12*).

[c] *SIC*, p. 232.

[d] Cf. *SIC*, p. 245.

[e] It would be interesting to know whether he was aware of the work of his contemporary Wang Shu-Ho,[7] whose *Mo Ching*[8] (Manual of Sphygmology), the fundamental treatise on the subject, appeared less than twenty years later, *c.* +300. The *Mo Ching* takes acupuncture as a matter of course, and has a good deal to say about it.

[f] Cf. *ICK*, p. 313; *SIC*, p. 248.

[g] Hsieh Li-Hêng (*1*), p. 11*b*, thinks *Chi* a mistake for *Ching*. Cf. *ICK*, p. 305; *SIC*, p. 246. The references in the *I Hsin Fang* (+982) to a *Hsia-Ma Ching* (ch. 2, (pp. 66.1, 68.1, 69.1, 71.1) etc.) may well be to this work. We know the name of at least one author of this type of book — Hsü Yüeh,[9] who produced in the Liang a *Lung Hsien Su Chen Ping Khung Hsüeh Hsia-Ma Thu*.[10] A text with the abbreviated title, almost impossible to date, is still allegedly extant in Japan.

[1] 呂博 [2] 玉匱鍼經 [3] 枕中灸刺經 [4] 明堂蝦蟆圖
[5] 黃帝鍼灸蝦蟆忌(圖, 經) [6] 呂廣 [7] 王叔和 [8] 脈經
[9] 徐悅 [10] 龍銜素鍼并孔穴蝦蟆圖

ancient scruples. That Huangfu Mi also had access to anatomical charts is indicated by some ancient titles which have come down to us, such as the *Huang Ti Shih-erh Ching Mo Ming Thang Wu Tsang Jen Thu*[1] (The Yellow Emperor's Charts of the Twelve Tracts (of Acupuncture) and the Five Viscera of the Microcosm, i.e. the Human Body).[a]

The *Chia I Ching* is a book full of interest for the history of Chinese medicine. For example, the preface says that 'the really excellent physician controls disease before any illness has declared itself, the man of middling art practices acupuncture before the disease has come to its crisis, and the inferior practitioner does it when the illness is dying away anyhow (or: when the patient is declining and dying)'.[b] Much of Huangfu Mi's teaching is comprised in this epigram.[c]

Here is where we find the acupuncture and moxa tradition touching for a moment the alchemical and the political. The wife of the great proto-chemical and thaumaturgical writer Ko Hung[2] was named Pao Ku.[3] She must have lived approximately between +288 and +343, and her father was also a Taoist, Pao Thai-Hsüan,[4] presumably the same as Pao Ching[5] the alchemist,[d] and none other than Pao Ching-Yen[6] the radical social thinker.[e] Pao Ku had a career of her own, for she became renowned as a specialist in moxibustion and cauterisation, especially against affections of the skin, perhaps benign neoplasms such as epitheliomas, perhaps eczemas and other dermatological malfunctions. Moreover, she transmitted her skills to pupils, especially Tshui Wei.[7] It is of much interest to find a woman expert in Chin times, especially one so close to the growing-points of unorthodox naturalistic thought.[f]

The next focal point in the acupuncture story is the life and work of Sun Ssu-Mo[8] (+581 to +673), in the Sui and early Thang dynasties, a great alchemist as well as an eminent physician and medical writer.[g] The best route to him, perhaps, lies in the thread of filiation of anatomical acupuncture diagrams and charts. As we have just seen (p. 120) there is a possibility that something of this kind already existed before the end of the Han, though there is no evidence that any were ever incorporated in the *Chia I Ching* of Huangfu Mi. Unfortunately neither of Sun Ssu-Mo's great works now has his charts,[h] but he does tell us clearly where he got them from, and how he improved them. It seems that about +460, in the Liu Sung time, a physician named Chhin Chhêng-Tsu[9] produced a *Yen Tshê Tsa Chen Chiu Ching*[10] (Manual of Acupuncture and Moxibustion Loci seen on the Recumbent Figure Laterally);[i] but

[a] Cf. *ICK*, p. 306; *SIC*, p. 254; Hsieh Li-Hêng (*1*), p. 32*b*.
[b] *Shang kung chih wei ping, chung kung tzhu wei chhêng, hsia kung tzhu i shuai.*[11]
[c] It derives from rather longer forms of the same saying in *NCLS*, ch. 4, p. 21*b* (*PH*, p. 42), and ch. 55, p. 17*b* (*PH*, p. 388). We consider these in other contexts elsewhere (*SCC*, Vol. 6).
[d] Cf. Vol. 5, pt. 3, p. 76.
[e] Cf. Vol. 2, pp. 434ff.
[f] The best study of her life is that of Sung Ta-Jen (*5*).
[g] Cf. *SCC*, Vol. 5, pt. 3, pp. 132ff. On his medical work see Li Yuan-Chi (*1*), pp. 263, 266, 269.
[h] They were lost even before the Yuan edition of +1307.
[i] Cf. *SIC*, p. 229, and Vol. 5, pt. 3, p. 45.

1 黃帝十二經脉明堂五藏人圖 2 葛洪 3 鮑姑 4 鮑太玄
5 鮑靚 6 鮑敬言 7 崔煒 8 孫思邈 9 秦承祖
10 偃側雜鍼灸經 11 上工治未病中工刺未成下工刺已衰

Sun Ssu-Mo found many deficiencies between these charts of Chhin and the detailed traditions of Huangfu Mi. However, there were later diagrams which were better, notably those contained in the *Ming Thang Jen Hsing Thu*[1] prepared by Chen Chhüan[2] about +610, probably as part of an acupuncture manual (*Chen Ching*) now long lost also.[a] It will be remembered that Chen Chhüan and his brother Chen Li-Yen[3] were also deeply interested in drugs, producing two of the pharmaceutical natural histories.[b] Sun's diagrams were in colour, five different inks being used for the regular tracts, with green for the auxiliary ones (*chhi ching pa mo*).[c] He still recognised 649 loci, combining Huangfu Mi's definitions with Chen Chhüan's charts in improved form, and he entitled his chapter Ming Thang San Jen Thu,[4] because he made three charts of the body, anterior, posterior and lateral.[d] Although Sun seems not to mention it, there was another work of about +610 which he may well have utilised, the *Huang Ti Nei Ching Ming Thang* (*Chu*),[5] (A Description of the Microcosm, i.e. the Human Body, to accompany the Yellow Emperor's Manual of Corporeal Medicine), certainly commented on by Yang Shang-Shan[6] and quite probably wholly written by him too.[e] This work, one chapter of which is still preserved in Japan, began with charts of the viscera of the human body, followed by a description of the *ching-lo* system, with details of acu-points and specific treatments for various syndromes. And there were many other relevant books produced in the Sui period, but all were lost, and now we have hardly more than their titles.

Sun Ssu-Mo is generally considered the first systematiser of the *thung shen tshun fa*[7] or 'module system', and if he had done nothing else than this it would suffice to keep his memory undimmed among acupuncturists. Throughout the preceding pages many readers must have wondered how the exact position of acu-points could be determined on the bodies of small men and women, or of children. The Chinese were well aware of this problem from early times, and the system was to chart out a 'standard body' with many measurements in inches (*tshun*[8]) (cf. Figs. 22, 23), then to apply these to bodies unusually small or unusually large so as to generate a set of measurements in relative inches accordingly.[f] For example if the height of a man was defined as 75″ (7½ Chinese feet), the actual height of a boy would be found to be much less, but it would still be counted as 75 relative inches each a good deal smaller in length,

[a] *SIC*, p. 255; Chang Tsan-Chhen (5).

[b] See Vol. 6, pt. 1.

[c] The use of coloured inks was one of those simple techniques which helped Chinese scholars so much in keeping texts and papers in order. Thao Hung-Ching had used it in his pharmaceutical work about +500, and the Sung Bureau of Historiography adopted it on a large scale (cf. Vol. 7, and meanwhile Needham (56), p. 13).

[d] Acupuncture and moxibustion appears in *Chhien Chin Yao Fang*, chs. 29, 30, (pp. 508.1 ff.) and in *Chhien Chin I Fang*, chs. 26, 27, 28, (pp. 308.1 ff.). The two accounts, the former *c.* +652, the latter *c.* +670, are by no means exactly the same.

[e] He was, of course, the editor, and probably the compiler or re-arranger, of the *Huang Ti Nei Ching*, *Thai Su*, on which see p. 88. On his *Ming Thang* book see *ICK*, pp. 306, 314; *SIC*, pp. 257–8; Anon. (90), p. 4.

[f] One rarely finds any mention of this module system in Western-language expositions, so the account of Karoff (1) is to be commended.

[1] 明堂人形圖 [2] 甄權 [3] 甄立言 [4] 明堂三人圖
[5] 黃帝內經明堂(注) [6] 楊上善 [7] 同身寸法 [8] 寸

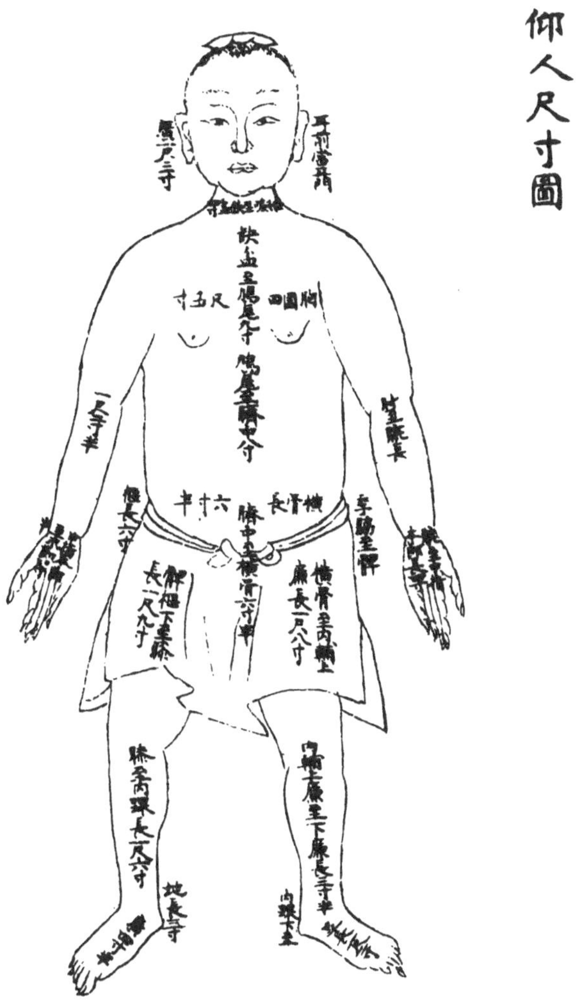

Fig. 22. The module system for determining the exact position of acu-points and moxa points on human bodies of very varying sizes, a standard set of measurements being reduced to 'relative inches' in accordance with the deviation of size from the normal human body taken as standard. For example, in this diagram an inscription just above the nipples says: 'the circumference of the chest (just under the armpits) is 4 ft. 5 ins. (i.e. 45 Chinese inches)'. This anterior view is from the *Hsün Ching Khao Hsüeh Pien* of +1575 or a little later (vol. 2, p. 374).

and all the positions of acu-points would be found by measurement in terms of these smaller units.[a] In other words, to every man his own inch. But how was it found? In the *thung shen tshun fa*, still widely used today, the variable, relative or modular inch is defined as the distance between the upper ends of the distal and middle interphalangeal folds formed by flexing the patient's middle finger (Fig. 24).[b] Each of

[a] See for example the discussions in Mêng Ching-Pi (*1*) and Chhêng Tan-An (*1*), pp. 57–8.
[b] Anon. (*121*), p. 3; (*172*), p. 74, Engl. tr. pp. 98ff. A figure is in *CCTC*, ch. 4, (p. 86.1).

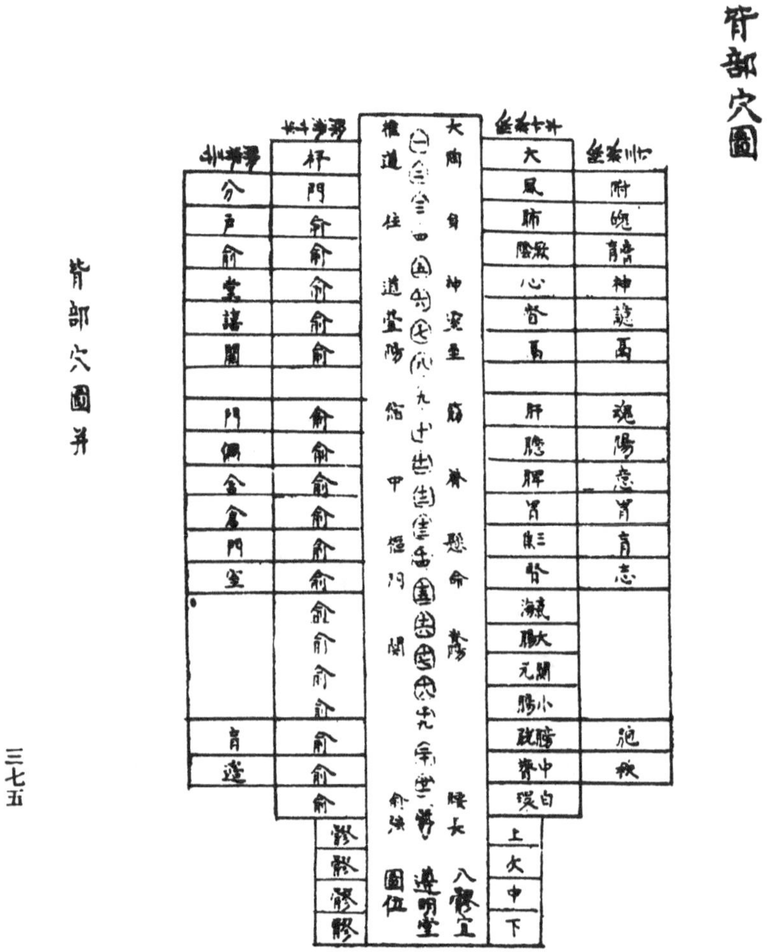

Fig. 23. Sometimes the acu-points were shown in a tabular array, as here in a diagram taken from the same work (vol. 2, p. 375), depicting the back of the body. The central column gives the points on or very near the spinal column, the vertebral processes being numbered, though not exactly in accord with modern practice. The two nearest columns on each side list the points 1·5 ins. away from the centre line to left and right, the two outer ones listing the points 3 ins. away to left and right. These are of course the standard measurements, to be converted to relative inches in accordance with the size and height of the patient.

these 'inches' was divided, from antiquity onwards, into ten *fên*,[1] a precision which could be important since the relative inch was used not only for locating acu-points but for measuring the depth of needle insertion. For the measurements people took strips of bamboo skin (*mieh*[2])[a] or rice-stalk pith (*tao kan hsin*[3]), or even paper or straw.[b]

[a] The importance of this in the technique of deep borehole drilling will appear in *SCC*, Vol. 5, pt. 1.

[b] The texts advise against the use of tape or string, which are liable to stretch.

[1] 分　　[2] 篾　　[3] 稻桿心

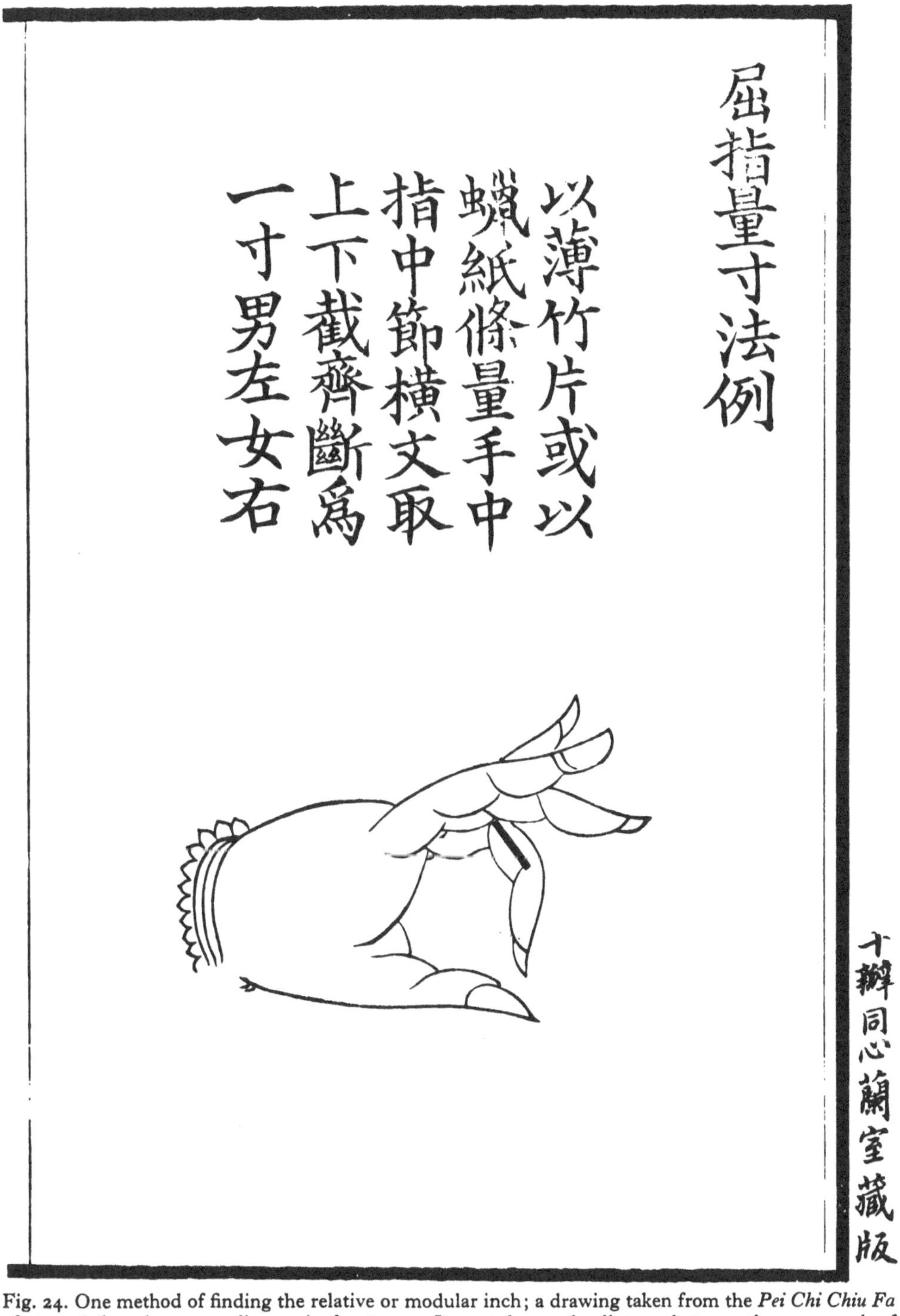

Fig. 24. One method of finding the relative or modular inch; a drawing taken from the *Pei Chi Chiu Fa* of +1226, based on an earlier work of *c.* +1112. It was taken as the distance between the upper ends of the distal and middle inter-phalangeal folds formed by flexing the patient's middle finger. The caption calls it the 'bent-finger technique for determining the inch' proper to the patient, and the text recommends using a little bamboo rule or a length of waxed paper for the measurement.

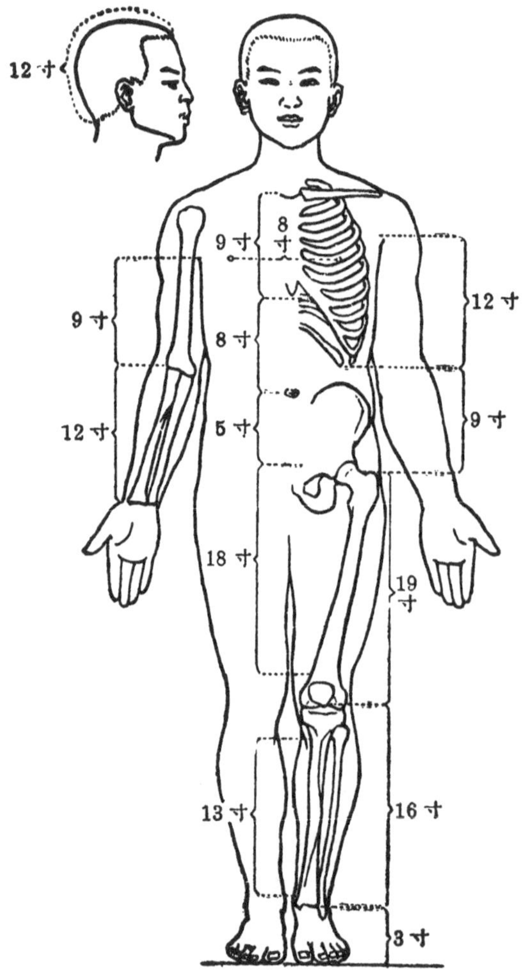

Fig. 25. Another module system depending on osteology (from Anon. (*91*), p. 27), perhaps older than the use of the knuckles. For example, the distance between the lowest point of the tenth rib and the upper surface of the greater trochanter of the femur is taken as 9 standard ins., these to be converted to relative ins. in accordance with the patient's height. The inset shows yet another way, the measurement of the distance between the anterior and posterior hair lines over the crown of the scalp—here 12 standard inches.

A determination of relative inches using bone markers in surface anatomy may be much older than the use of the knuckles; it was, and is, called *ku tu chê liang tshun fa*.[1] For example, the distance from the lower edge of the patella to the lateral malleolus at the ankle was defined as 16 modular inches, while the distance between the olecranon at the elbow and the head of the ulna at the wrist was counted as 12·5 modular inches (Fig. 25). Yet another way, less osteological, was to measure the distance

[1] 骨度折量寸法

between the anterior and posterior hair lines over the crown of the scalp (*chhien fa chi chih hou fa chi*[1]). The *ku tu*[2] idea is rather ancient, for the texts say: *chhi ku chieh chih ta hsiao chhang tuan ko chi ho*[3],[a] 'by taking the size and length of bones and joints we can know the average standard proportions'. And in the *Ling Shu*, Huang Ti says:[b] 'I should like to know the standard measurements of ordinary human beings (*yuan wên chung jen chih tu*[4]). (If we take) an average person's height as 75 inches what will be the sizes and lengths of all the bones?' And measurements of many parts of the body follow.

There is of course a considerable change in the proportions of the parts of the body between birth and old age,[c] but the traditional Chinese methods do not seem to have taken account of this. If they had, they would have been even more directly ancestral to d'Arcy Thompson's famous theory of morphological transformations,[d] and the classical work of Julian Huxley on unequal growth rates in animals.[e] For what they envisaged was the regular expansion of a co-ordinate system with increasing age, female bodies reaching their maxima at a lower stature than male ones; and this was surely the first step on the way to visualisation of co-ordinate distortions as relating different species of animals, and different ages of the same animal species.

In his two great books, the *Chhien Chin Yao Fang*[5] of +652 and the *Chhien Chin I Fang*[6] of about +670, Sun Ssu-Mo gave much attention to acupuncture and moxibustion. He described many disease syndromes and the treatments of this kind which they needed, he listed the transmission points (*shu hsüeh*,[7] in the narrow sense, cf. p. 62), he developed the use of the *ah shih hsüeh*[8] (cf. p. 52) especially on the back, inserting where the muscular pain was felt to be;[f] and he collected the special loci which had been discovered outside the 12 regular tracts (*ching wai chhi hsüeh*[9]). But it is also interesting that Sun gave serious warning of certain dangerous points (*chin hsüeh*,[10] 'prohibited loci'). The fact is that by his time it had become common knowledge that acupuncture could be quite perilous, especially in the hands of the ignorant or the careless, and at first he was not at all favourable to it though he changed his mind eventually and devoted five chapters to the subject. In the following century the aversion from acupuncture went further, and Wang Thao's[11] celebrated book, the *Wai Thai Pi Yao*[12] (Important (Medical) Techniques revealed by the Governor of a Distant Province), mentioned it only to record its dangerous or deleterious effects, which indeed he was the first to describe in detail.[g] Wang Thao was of course primarily a pharmacological therapist (*fang chi chia*[13]), but he was willing to devote a

[a] *Chia I Ching*, ch. 2, (pp. 50–1), and the same words are in *NCTS*, ch. 13, (p. 86.2).
[b] *NCLS/PH*, ch. 14, (p. 176); *NCLS/MC*, ch. 14, (p. 1062); *CIC*, ch. 2, (pp. 50ff.).
[c] Among many studies, see conveniently that of Medawar (1) in Clark & Medawar (1).
[d] d'Arcy Thompson (2), pp. 719ff.
[e] Heterogonic or heterauxetic growth; see Huxley (1); and on chemical heterauxesis Needham (12), p. 531.
[f] *CCCY*, ch. 3, (p. 203).
[g] Cf. *ICK*, p. 321; Anon. (90), p. 24.

1 前髮際至後髮際 2 骨度 3 其骨節之大小長短各幾何
4 願聞衆人之度 5 千金要方 6 千金翼方 7 腧穴 8 阿是穴
9 經外奇穴 10 禁穴 11 王燾 12 外臺秘要 13 方劑家

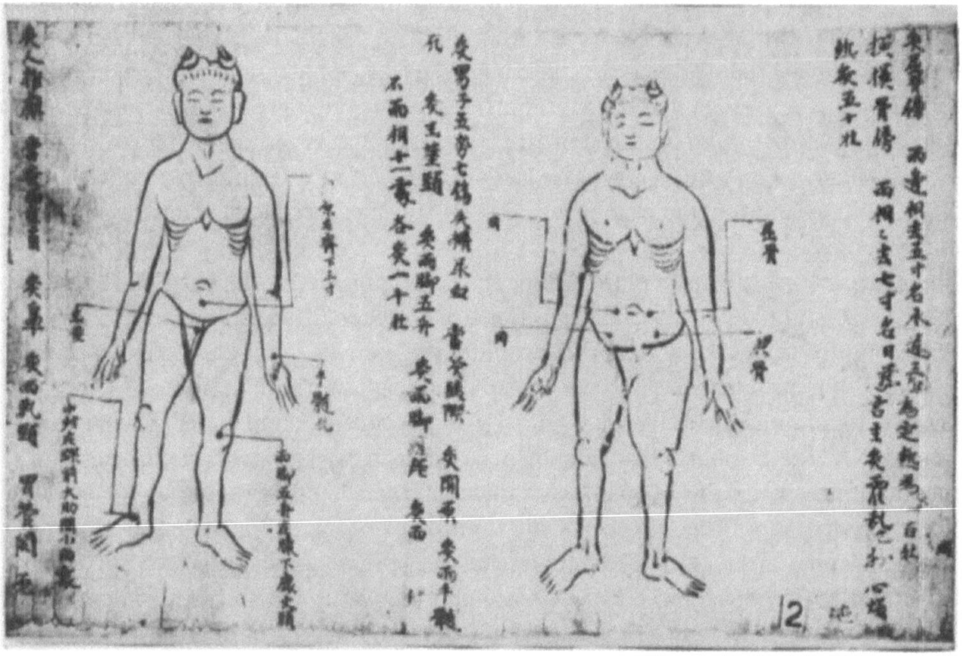

Fig. 26. A section of one of the paper scroll manuscripts in the Stein Collection at the British Museum (S/6168). It contains fragments of an untitled work, perhaps a notebook, by an anonymous physician of Thang date, on moxibustion for various diseases; the text is interspersed with rough sketches of surface anatomy with the moxa points marked on them. A full description has been given by Ma Chi-Hsing (*4*).

whole chapter (Ming Thang Chiu Fa[1]) to moxa,[a] for which a knowledge of the acu-points was essential.

From this time, and showing the same tendency, dates the interesting manuscript hand-scroll two fragments of which are preserved in the Stein Collection in the British Museum.[b] According to the description of Ma Chi-Hsing (*4*), its title is lost, but it contains eight diagrams of the human body, with accompanying captions and commentary (Fig. 26). It is not at all a systematic text but seems rather to record the personal experiences and practice of a plebeian physician (*ling i*[2]).[c] It mentions some twenty-seven diseases, and the names of about fifty acu-points, many of which are exactly the same as those used today.[d] Others, however, seem to have been popular synonyms used in the Thang period; and the writer has a habit of referring simply to the names of tracts (such as Shou Yang-Ming),[e] which may have been a way of directing moxibustion to be used all along them. Moxa, indeed, is the only treatment prescribed, and there are no references to needles, though possibly there may have been in the parts of the scroll now missing.

[a] Ch. 39, (pp. 1077.1 ff.).

[b] S 6168 and S 6262.

[c] Cf. Needham (64), p. 265.

[d] For example VU 11, 13, 15, 18, 23 and 28; VF 3, 17, 20; TM 15, 19; IT 16 and R 11. San-li, both IG 10 and V 36, is prominent.

[e] It is known that this was a customary thing in and before the Thang, but not in the Sung and later.

1 明堂灸法 2 鈴醫

The Sui and Thang periods were marked by great medical activity stimulated by changes of national importance.[a] It started with a rich basis, because the *Sui Shu* bibliography lists no less than 256 books, ten times as many as could be enumerated under the Han, even though some had been lost after the Liang. The invasions of the barbaric northern tribes had sent many scholars south to the Yangtze valley and beyond, where they came into contact for the first time with the characteristic illnesses of sub-tropical and tropical regions. Ko Hung's[1] *Chou Hou Pei Chi Fang*,[2] for instance, had been written in the Lo-fou Shan mountains just north of Canton. Improvements in papermaking, and, as the age wore on, the introduction of block printing, necessarily affected medical writings, and even more perhaps, medical illustration. The continual competition of Taoists and Buddhists for political influence aided the development of psycho-physiological therapies and the introduction of fragments of Indian medical thought. Another important factor was the fuller establishment of an Imperial Medical Service (Thai I Shu[3]), and the regularisation of the Imperial Medical College (Thai I Hsüeh[4]), assuredly by a long way the oldest teaching medical institution in the world. Acupuncture always figured in it, with a departmental Professor (Chen Po Shih[5]), Lecturers (Chen Chu Chiao[6]) and Demonstrators (Chen Shih[7]); later this Department was divided into three Sections. Since a similar College of Medicine was established in every province, though on a smaller scale, as early as +629, it seems certain that the College at the capital must have been functioning from the beginning of the dynasty, i.e. in +618, all the more so as there had been an analogous institution under the Sui, and the origins of the system can even be traced back to a Northern Wei reorganisation in +493.[b] Acupuncture figured prominently enough at the Thang imperial court, for we read of the cure of the emperor Thang Kao Tsung, who in +683 was suffering from an eye affection with migraine and dizziness, by a Royal Physician named Chhin Ming-Hao[8].[c] So also a Vice-President of the Imperial Secretariat, Tshui Chih-Thi,[9] was sufficiently involved, probably for personal or family reasons, to produce a book entitled *Ku Chêng Ping Chiu Fang*[10] (Moxibustion for Conditions like Tubercolosis),[d] or *Chiu Lao Fa*,[11] about +670.

The incident of the emperor's cure by Chhin Ming-Hao was one of those occasions when there is mention of a little blood produced by the pricking (*tzhu*[12]). A modern term often used for this is *fang hsüeh*,[13] or 'liberation of blood'.[e] This term might give rise to a misconception, for the procedure is not, and never was, a variant of phlebotomy or venesection in the Western sense. Sir William Temple, writing about +1695, was perfectly right when he said: 'The Chinese never let blood'.[f] Their

[a] A good survey of these is to be found in Li Thao (*4*), and Li Yuan-Chi (*2*) has written specifically on the development of acupuncture and moxa during the Thang period.

[b] Full details will be given in *SCC*, Vol. 6, pt. 3; meanwhile see Lu Gwei-Djen & Needham (2), and Chhen Pang-Hsien (*1*), 2nd ed., p. 188.

[c] *TCTC*, ch. 203, (p. 6415); *CCTC*, ch. 7, (p. 221.2). The main acu-point used was Pai-hui, on which cf. p. 82 above.

[d] *SIC*, p. 250.

[e] See Anon. (*173*), p. 72, Eng. tr., p. 96.

[f] In his essay 'Upon Health and Long Life', in 'Miscellanea', pt. 3, 1701 ed., p. 168.

1 葛洪 2 肘後備急方 3 太醫署 4 太醫學 5 鍼博士
6 鍼助教 7 鍼師 8 秦鳴鶴 9 崔知悌 10 骨蒸病灸方
11 灸勞法 12 刺 13 放血

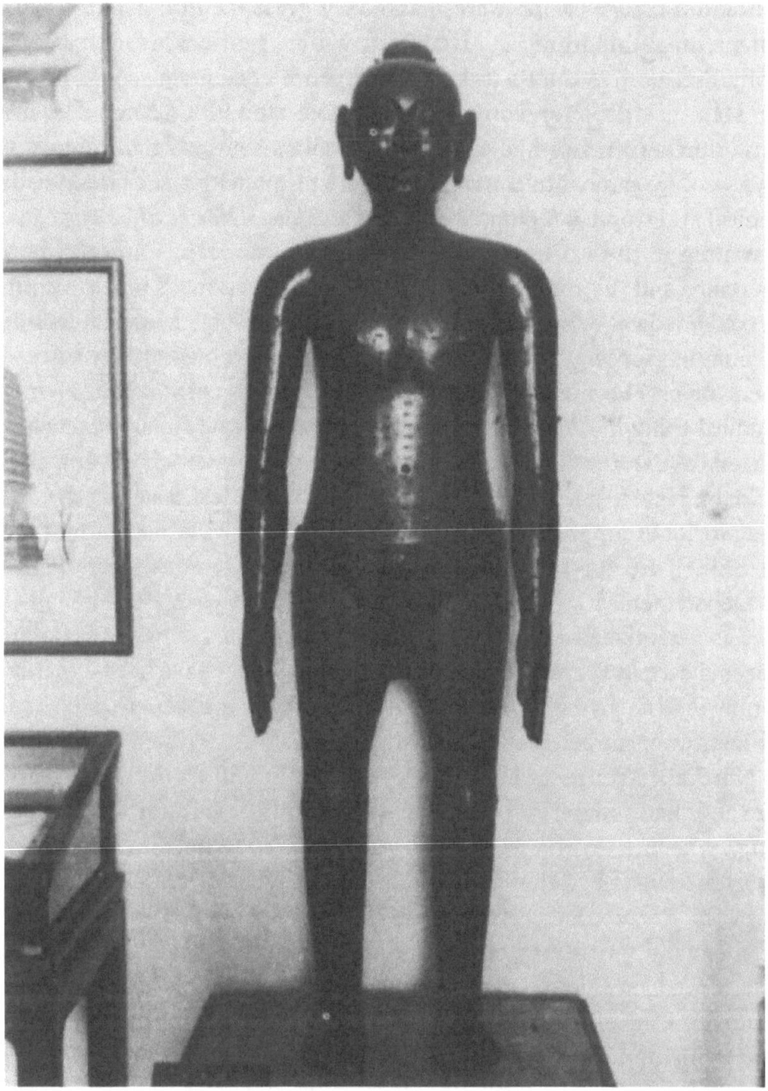

Fig. 27. Life-size human figure in bronze with the acu-points indicated by small holes and marked with their names. The first of these was cast by Wang Wei-I in +1027, but this one dates from the Ming, either between +1436 and +1449 or +1457 and +1464, most probably in +1443, and its maker was Hsü Ao. Photo: National Historical Museum, Peking.

practice included only the drawing of blood in very small amounts from the capillary vessels, and in recent times this has generally been done with the aid of groups of needles at one end of a handle, such as the *mei hua chen*[1] which has five,[a] or the *chhi hsing chen*[2] which has seven.[b]

[a] On the 'plum-blossom needles' see Anon. (*173*).
[b] On the 'seven stars needles' see Wu I-Chhing (*1*).

[1] 梅花針 [2] 七星針

During the late Thang and Wu Tai periods there was little new development, but less than a century after the country had been re-united by the Sung, a landmark was reached in the first casting of life-size human acupuncture figures in bronze (Fig. 27).[a] This was the work of Wang Wei-I[1],[b] commissioned in +1026 and finished in the following year.[c] The metal walls of the figures were pierced with small holes corresponding to the principal loci for acupuncture and moxibustion, then covered with wax, filled with water, and used for the examination of medical candidates from the central and provincial colleges.[d] If they located correctly the acu-points which they suggested needling (as the result of their diagnoses), drops of water would appear, otherwise they would fail their test.[e] It appears that Wang Wei-I made two of these *thung jen*,[2] one being placed in the I Kuan Yuan[3] or Central Medical Institute, and the other in the Hall of Benign Assistance (Jen Chi Tien[4]) in the Ta Hsiang Kuo Ssu[5] temple at the capital, Khaifêng.[f] Moreover, Wang Wei-I prepared an illustrated manual to accompany the figures, with the title *Thung Jen Shu Hsüeh Chen Chiu Thu Ching*;[6] it was afterwards several times reprinted in different dynasties (Fig. 28). After long examination of the literature, Wang recognised and listed 354 loci, as against the 313 and 349 that had previously been counted (cf. Table 15).[g]

Probably the best original description which we have of the bronze figures is that contained in Chou Mi's[7] *Chhi Tung Yeh Yü*[8] (Rustic Talks in Eastern Chhi) of +1290. Chou Mi wrote:[h]

> Once I heard my maternal uncle Chang Shu-Kung[9] say that formerly, when he was a Sub-Prefect in Hsiangchow, he protected and investigated one of the bronze acupuncture figures. The statue was made of fine bronze (*ching thung*[10]), and both the *tsang* and *fu* viscera were all complete.[i] The names of the acu-points were marked in fine characters of gold.[j] The figure was made in two halves, front and back, which could be fitted together to make one whole body.

[a] *Hsü Tzu Chih Thung Chien Chhang Phien*, ch. 105. Jen Ying-Chhiu (*1*), p. 47, says *shu thung*,[11] which would be brass (cf. *SCC*, Vol. 5, pt. 2, p. 208; Vol. 4, pt. 2, p. 145). That would not have been impossible, but it has no contemporary support.

[b] There has been a persistent tendency in the literature to call him Wei-Tê.[12] Sung Ta-Jen (*3*), p. 9, and many older authorities do this, possibly misled by a few lines in the *Sung Shih* (ch. 463, p. 8*b*) about a quite different person. So also the bibliography of that history misprints his name as Wei-I,[13] leading others astray. Wang Wei-I was Director of the Imperial Medical Service.

[c] Cf. Chhen Pang-Hsien (*1*), 2nd ed., p. 188.

[d] Particular efforts were made to help the weaker practitioners find the right spots, e.g. the *ssu hua hsüeh*[14] (VU 17, 19 and both VU 38); cf. *CCTC*, ch. 9, (pp. 289 ff.). The simple rules for this stemmed from Tshui Chih-Thi.

[e] Cf. Hsieh Li-Hêng (*1*), p. 31*b*; Jen Ying-Chhiu (*1*); Li Thao (*12*), p. 217.

[f] Cf. Chang Tsan-Chhen (*5*).

[g] Anon. (*90*), p. 24.

[h] Ch. 13, pp. 19*b* to 21*b*; quoted in *PWYF*, ch. 27, (p. 1403.1).

[i] None of the bronze figures surviving today has bronze viscera, removable or not, so far as we know. But in *SCC*, Vol. 6, we shall give details of the Buddhist statues in Japan with viscera of variegated cloths.

[j] Presumably by inlay rather than gilding, as they lasted so well.

1 王惟一 2 銅人 3 醫官院 4 仁濟殿 5 大相國寺
6 銅人腧穴鍼灸圖經 7 周密 8 齊東野語 9 章叔恭
10 精銅 11 熟銅 12 惟德 13 維一 14 四花穴

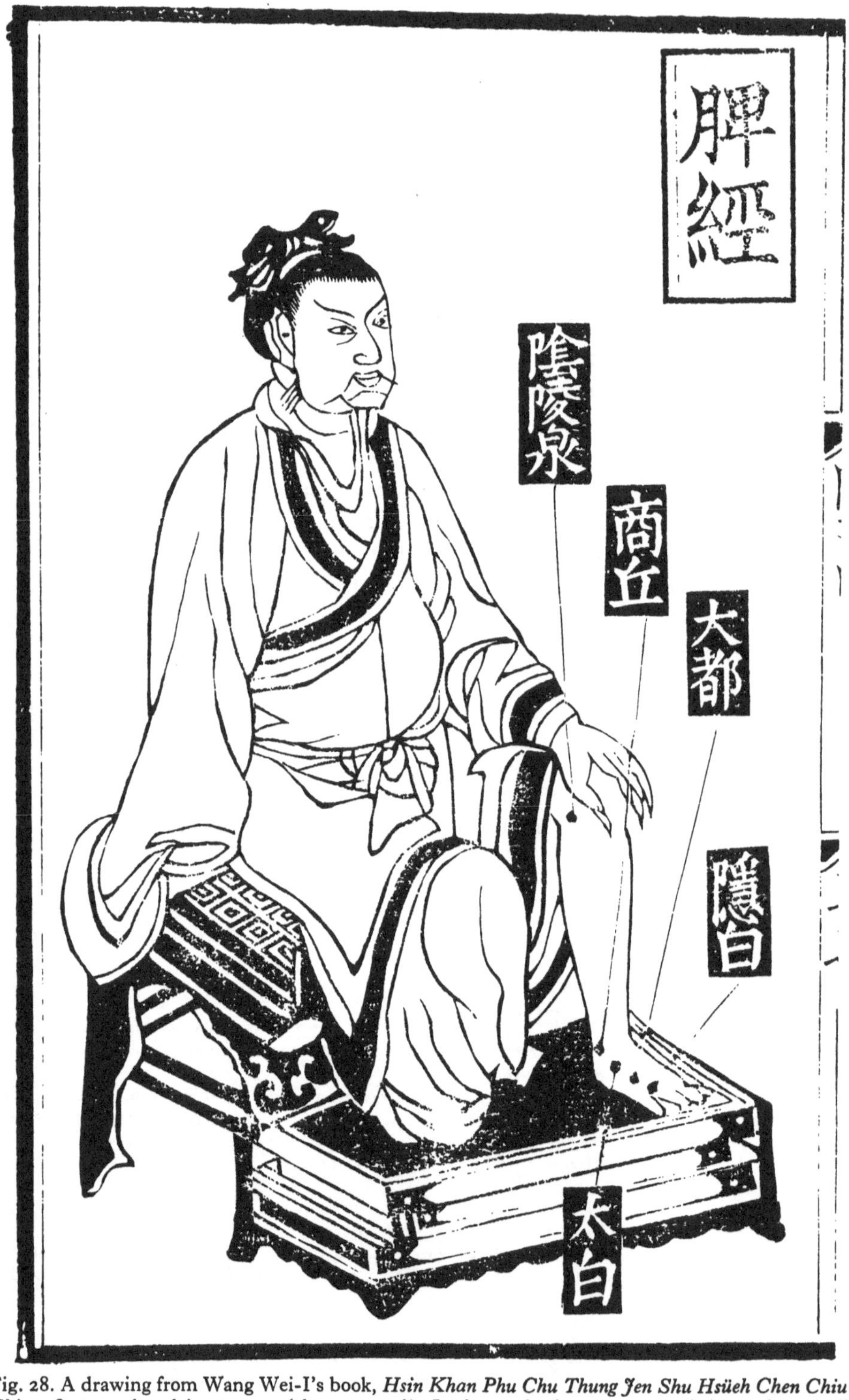

Fig. 28. A drawing from Wang Wei-I's book, *Hsin Khan Phu Chu Thung Jen Shu Hsüeh Chen Chiu Thu Ching*, first produced in +1027, (ch. 2, p. 17*b*). It shows the lower course of the podogenic lieno-pancreatic Thai-Yin acu-tract (cf. Table 4).

In old times this was used to examine the medical practitioners (*i chê*[1]); the body was covered with yellow wax and the inside filled up with water,[a] so that they could learn how to measure in terms of (relative) inches and tenths of an inch. In accordance with the diagnosis they were asked to insert their needles. When a needle was put in exactly at the acu-point, the water poured out, but if there was even a slight mistake, the needle could not penetrate at all. This was indeed an ingenious instrument.

Afterwards Chao Nan-Chung[2] returned the figure to the Palace. My uncle Chang Shu-Kung made two diagrams, and had them carved on wood blocks so that they might be reproduced by printing. Therefore I mention the matter here.

So important was the text of Wang Wei-I's book considered that a large part of it, if not the whole, was carved on tablets of stone before +1030 (Fig. 29). At the time of the fall of Khaifêng in +1126, or just afterwards, the Jurchen Chin authorities demanded the bronze figures as one of the conditions in a peace treaty, but it is not clear that they were handed over. However, when in the time of Chou Mi himself the Yuan emperor transferred the capital to Peking, the Pacification Commissioner Wang Chi[3] was ordered to move the statues and the stone tablets north and place them in the Shen Chi Tien[4] or Hall or Marvellous Mechanisms (of the Body) at the Imperial Medical College, Thai I Yuan.[5] This must have been done, because under the following dynasty, the Ming, when the Peking city-wall was being repaired about +1445, the stone tablets were buried within it, only to be revealed and described in our own time by Yü Kho (*1*).[b] In the meantime the Ming emperor in +1443 had ordered new stone tablets to be inscribed with the text of this veritable classic, and lodged in the Temple of the Medical Deities (Yao Wang Miao[6]) in the Thai I Yuan at the new capital, Nanking. A fresh wood-block edition of Wang Wei-I's work was also put in hand, and the Chêng-Thung emperor himself, Ying Tsung, added to it a preface of his own.

Four centuries earlier it had been the Sung emperor Jen Tsung, who, mindful of the dangers of careless needling, commissioned Wang Wei-I's famous task. But Wang was not the only eminent acupuncturist at that court, there was also Hsü Hsi,[7] who treated the emperor himself successfully. Since he replied, when asked, that his methods were those of the ancient medical sage Pien Chhio (p. 79 above), the emperor built a votive temple to that worthy. Hsü Hsi's book of +1034, *Shen Ying Chen Ching Yao Chüeh*[8] (Confidential Essentials of a Manual of Marvellously Effective Acupuncture), has come down to us, even if only partially, as another indication of the flourishing state of the art in the +11th century.[c]

Many more writings followed before its end. In spite of the efforts of Wang and Hsü, the nervousness about the dangers of acupuncture continued, as we see from a work of about +1050 by an author known to us only by his philosophical sobriquet, the *Hsi Fang Tzu Ming Thang Chiu Ching*[9] (Moxibustion Manual for the Micro-

[a] The text has *hung*, mercury, but that would surely have been impossible as an amalgam would have formed, and weakened the walls.

[b] See Fig. 29.

[c] See further *Sung Shih*, ch. 462, p. 5*b*; *SIC*, p. 283; Li Thao (*12*).

1 醫者 2 趙南中 3 王檝 4 神機殿 5 太醫院
6 藥王廟 7 許希 8 神應鍼經要訣 9 西方子明堂灸經

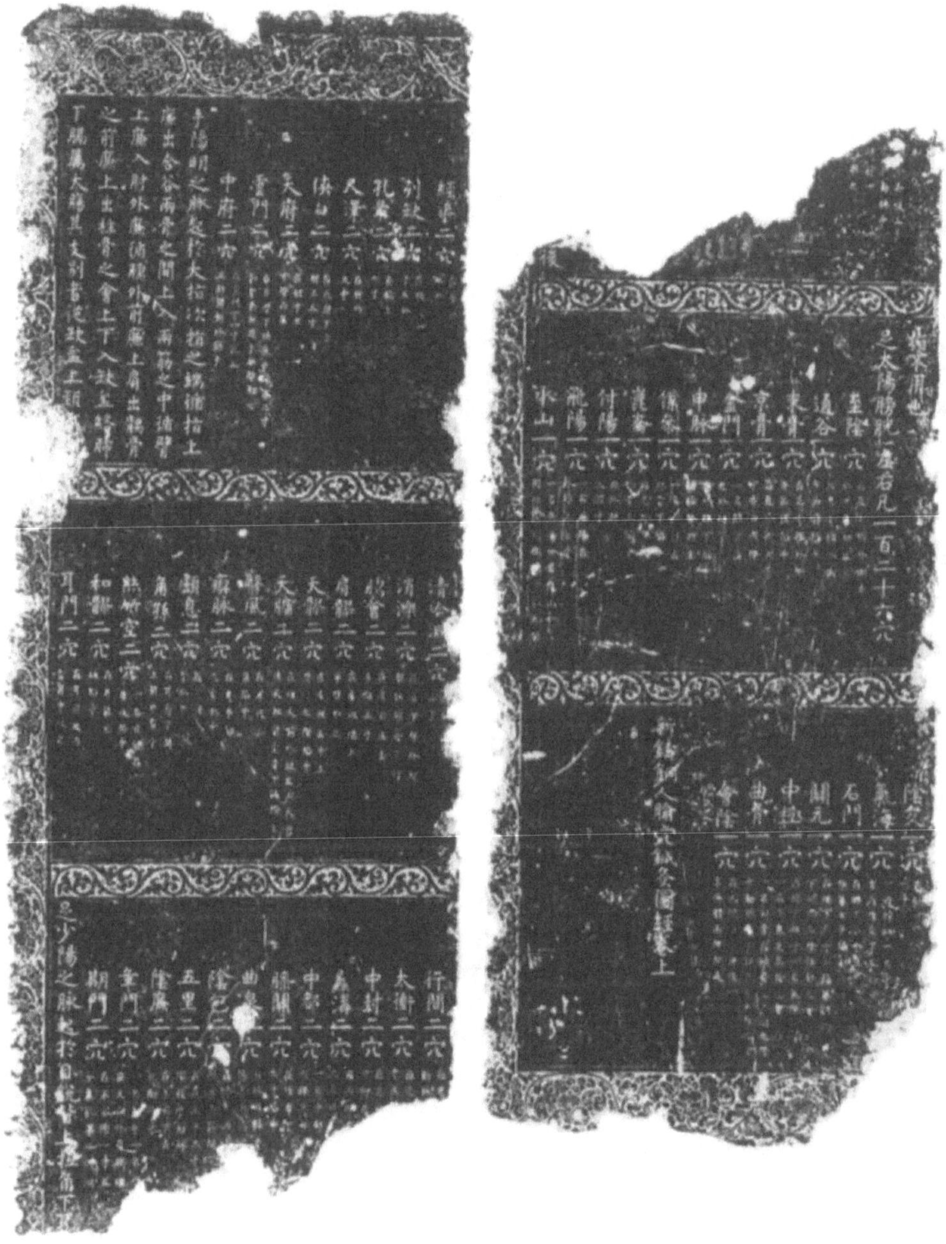

Fig. 29. The text of Wang Wei-I's book inscribed on tablets of stone before +1030, then at a later date, about +1445, immured in the Peking city-wall, and only brought to light in our own time. Description by Yü Kho (*1*); photo: National Historical Museum, Peking. The right-hand fragment enumerates acu-points on the podotelic vesical Thai-Yang tract, the left-hand one some of those on the cheirogenic tricoctive Shao-Yang tract (cf. Table 4). The small writing underneath each entry gives synonyms and exact locations.

cosm).[a] The Western-Direction Master followed Wang Wei-I's loci only partially, and used them purely for radiant heat therapy and cauterisation. Liu Yuan-Pin[1] about +1080 was less timid, however, and continued the full practice of the needle in his *Tung Thien Chen Chiu Ching*[2] (Penetrating Elucidation of Acupuncture and Moxa),[b] relying on transmitted manual skill and long experience (*chhüan phing shou shu yü shih yen*[3]). Another famous acupuncturist of this time was Phang An-Chhang,[4] who cured the poet Su Tung-Pho of a swollen hand by the use of a single needle in +1083.[c] Yet it is not difficult to understand why some physicians in all periods feared the technique, for not only was there the danger of piercing nerve-trunks and blood-vessels by careless or ignorant handling, but also the risk of infection, the unwitting inoculation of pathogenic bacteria. Nothing was known in those days about the necessity of sterilisation, and not all acupuncturists carried out systematically procedures which more or less amounted to it (cf. p. 104 above).

The life-size bronze figures became so renowned that a tendency arose to apply the term Thung Jen to books on acupuncture which had nothing to do with them. An important case of this is the work that bears the title *Thung Jen Chen Chiu Ching*.[5] As Chang Tsan-Chhen has shown,[d] this text differs considerably from that of Wang Wei-I, both in the names of loci and the selection of points for treating various diseases; it is indeed a different book, and seems to be the product of quite a different school (cf. Fig. 30).[e] Furthermore it must be of Thang or Wu Tai date, since it quotes from Chen Chhüan's *Chen Ching* of +620 or so, and is quoted by the *Thai-Phing Shêng Hui Fang*[6] of +992. It is thus a precious document which may be compared with the books of Sun Ssu-Mo and Wang Thao.

On various previous occasions we have remarked on the scientific, technological and Taoist interests of the court of Hui Tsung, who acceded in +1101 and reigned till the overthrow of the dynasty by the Jurchen Chin in +1126.[f] It is therefore the less surprising to find that a great imperial medical encyclopaedia was commissioned in +1111, and successfully completed under the chief editorship of Shen Fu[7] in +1118: the *Shêng Chi Tsung Lu*[8]—to this day an invaluable mine of information about Sung medical science.[g] Four chapters are devoted to acupuncture (out of some 200), not a large proportion, but enough to describe the tracts both regular and auxiliary, and to give directions for the treatment of many disease syndromes in this way.

Towards the latter part of the dynasty, between +1210 and +1225, a new work was compiled by Wang Chih-Chung,[9] the *Chen Chiu Tzu Shêng Ching*[10] (Manual of Acupuncture and Moxibustion Profitable for the Restoration of Health).[h] This was

[a] *ICK*, p. 320.
[b] *ICK*, p. 325.
[c] *Tung-Pho Chih Lin*, ch. 5, p. 10*b*.
[d] (*1*), p. 47 (*5*). Cf. *ICK*, p. 319.
[e] Cf. Hsieh Li-Hêng (*1*), p. 31*b*.
[f] See, for instance, *SCC*, Vol. 4, pt. 2, pp. 500 ff.
[g] It was reprinted under the Yuan in +1300.
[h] *ICK*, pp. 327 ff.

[1] 劉元賓 [2] 洞天鍼灸經 [3] 全憑手術與實驗 [4] 龐安常
[5] 銅人鍼灸經 [6] 太平聖惠方 [7] 申甫 [8] 聖濟總錄 [9] 王執中 [10] 鍼灸資生經

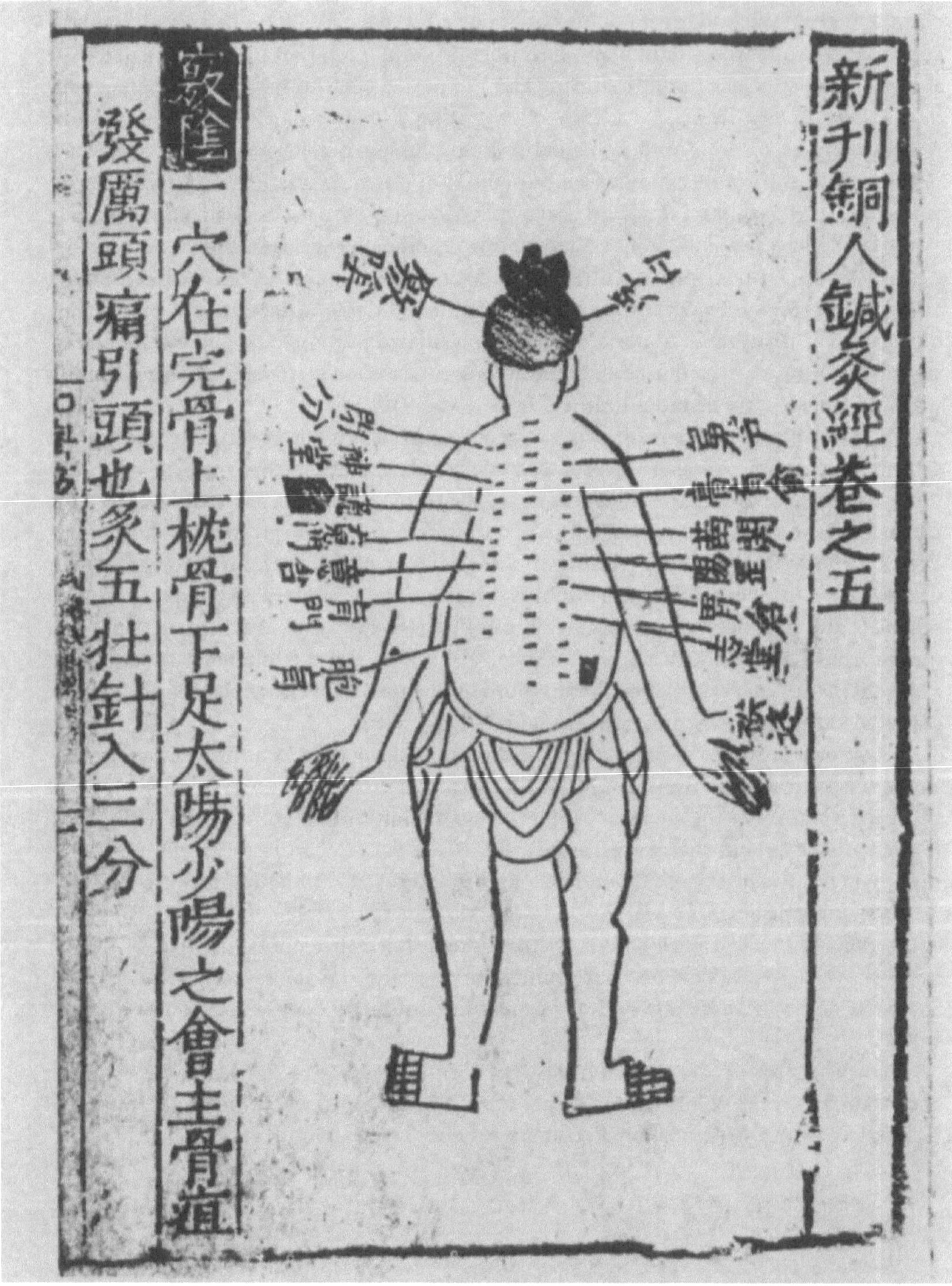

Fig. 30. A page from the *Hsin Khan Thung Jen Chen Chiu Ching* (ch. 5, p. 1*a*). The drawing, rather archaic in style, shows a number of acu-points on the back of the body belonging to the podotelic vesical Thai-Yang tract, and also two acu-points on the head, Fu-pai and Chhiao-yin, which belong to the podotelic felleic Shao-Yang tract (cf. Table 1). The text to the left begins a discussion of the Chhiao-yin point. This book is much older than that of Wang Wei-I, and must date back to Thang or Wu Tai times; the words 'bronze figure' must have been applied to it subsequently in error. On this see Chang Tsan- Chhen (5). In this Thang text, as also in the Sung one of Wang Wei-I himself, neither the exact acu-point names used, nor the order of their enumeration, always correspond exactly with the usages of the present day.

based on all the previous texts available,[a] and drew up a classification of 360 acu-points, not according to the tracts but anatomically whether on the back, front, head, trunk, extremities, and so on. Wang's clinical case-histories were particularly good, and he included an index of illnesses with the needle and moxa points suited for curing them.

(vi) *Circadian rhythms and cosmic cycles*

We have now to turn our attention to the northern part of the country and the work of Tou Han-Chhing[1].[b] Tou was renowned as a specialist in external medicine, and though we cannot surely fix the dates of his birth and death it is clear that the height of his activity in writing came at just about +1234, the time when the Jurchen Chin State was being taken over by the Mongolian power, later to become the Yuan dynasty of China. He acquired most fame perhaps for his *Piao Yu Fu*,[2] a mnemonic ode elucidating obscurities in acupuncture and moxibustion,[c] but this was only part of his *Chen Ching Chih Nan*,[3] or 'compass-bearings' for the acupuncture manuals, finished by +1241.[d] So valuable were these rhyming instructions considered that long afterwards, in the Chêng-Thung reign-period (+1436 to +1449), they were carved on stone tablets in Nanking—along with the immortal words of Wang Wei-I. The exact relationship of Tou Han-Chhing, not only with his teachers and his students, but with his contemporaries living down in the south under the Sung, remains very obscure, and recalls the puzzling question of the great mathematicians of exactly the same period, men like Li Yeh and Chhin Chiu-Shao, who seem to have worked independently, hardly having knowledge of each other at all.[e] Tou was also responsible for two other works, the *Tzu Wu Liu Chu*[4] and the *Tou Thai-Shih Hsien-sêng Liu Chu Fu*.[5] The former title might be englished as 'Noon and Midnight Differences in the Flowing of the Chhi',[f] and the latter as 'Master Doctor Tou Han-Chhing on the Circulation of the Chhi'.[g] But what was meant here was not the circulation of the blood and *chhi* round the human body, which, as we know, was reckoned at only sixty times less speed than that of the real Harveian circulation; it was rather a set of circu-

[a] Particularly valued at this time was the *Thai-Phing Hui Min Ho Chi Chü Fang*[6] of +1151 and the emendation of this was what started Wang Chih-Chung on his project. Moreover, he included textual materials from the books of Chen Chhüan and Hsü Hsi (pp. 122 and 133 above). A colleague of his active in these years was Wênjen Chhi-Nien,[7] who produced a popular book on moxa *Pei Chi Chiu Fa*[8] (Moxibustion for Emergencies). See Anon. (*83*), p. 73, and p. 178 below.

[b] We often write Tou Han-Chhing (*b*), to distinguish him from another physician of exactly the same name, who lived a couple of centuries earlier.

[c] A modern colloquial version with a commentary is given by Chhen Pi-Liu & Chêng Cho-Jen (*2*).

[d] The other two were: *Ting Pa Hsüeh Chih Nan*,[9] a mnemonic aid for finding the eight assembly points (cf. p. 61 above), and *Hsieh Chê Kung Thu*,[10] a help in treating the diseases which occurred in the northern winters (cf. *CCCY*, ch. 3, p. 207). On them see Kan Tsu-Wang (*1*); Chhêng Tan-An, Chhen Pi-Liu & Hsü Hsi-Nien (*1*), pp. 136ff., 190ff.

[e] See *SCC*, Vol. 3, p. 41, and more recently the valuable book of Libbrecht (1).

[f] It will be remembered that the noon and midnight double-hours (*wu* and *tzu*) straddled our noon and midnight points; cf. Needham, Wang & Price (1), p. 200.

[g] Only 66 acu-points were used in this, i.e. the 60 *shu hsüeh* and the 6 extra *yuan hsüeh*; see p. 65 above, as also *CCIF*, ch. 26, (p. 316.1).

1 竇漢卿 2 標幽賦 3 鍼經指南 4 子午流注
5 竇太師先生流注賦 6 太平惠民和劑局方 7 聞人耆年
8 備急灸法 9 定八穴指南 10 叶蟄宮圖

lations in the longer rhythms of day, month and season.[a] And thereby hangs a tale.

It has to do with a development of thought and experience which introduced many new conceptions into acupuncture and Chinese medicine in general. It was based on a conviction that it was no use giving treatment, and particularly acupuncture, unless one took account of what we should nowadays call diurnal or circadian rhythms (hence the 'noon and midnight' watch-word, *tzu-wu*[1]), longer cycles of flow such as the monthly period, where we might think of endocrine changes analogous with the lunation (hence the 'flowing and pouring round', *liu-chu*[2]), and thirdly, the cycle of the seasons of the year, widely differing in the illnesses that could be expected, and the courses which they would probably pursue.[b] All this was summarised in the expression *tzu-wu liu-chu fa* or technique, and presently it found its full theoretical panoply in a system called the *wu-yün liu-chhi*,[3] 'the cyclical motions of the Five Elements and the six Chhi'. We shall find that although it started with a deeply correct perception of the recurrent phases of human physiology in time, it petered out eventually in a repetitious formalism. The substance was true natural knowledge, but the structure became so complex that the ordinary practitioner could only learn it by rote and all was in the end arbitrary and mechanical.[c] Let us first see how far back this train of thought can be detected.

Tou Han-Chhing's two texts must have been written within the decade +1230 to +1240. The same time and some quite neighbouring place must have given birth to a similar writing, the *Liu Chu Chih Wei Fu*[4] (Ode on the Minutiae of the Circulations),[d] either by Ho Jo-Yü[5] or Tou Kuei-Fang.[6] There was very little background to these expositions, chiefly the *Tzu Wu Ching*[7] (Noon and Midnight Manual),[e] ascribed to high antiquity, but in fact mentioned in no bibliography before +1151, so the supposition would be that it was written not much earlier than that either. The ancestor of the genre would be a tractate in mnemonic verse with the title *Tzu Wu Liu Chu Cho Jih An Shih Ting Hsüeh Ko*[8],[f] on how to select loci for acupuncture or moxibustion according to the diurnal cycle, the day of the month and the season of the year, written by a Mr Hsü in the Wu Tai period about +930.[g] All considerations

[a] See p. 46 above. It will further be remembered that *tzu* and *wu* were symbolic of the winter and summer solstices respectively, and of course that they participated in the sixty-year cycle.

[b] Cf. the basic statement in *NCLS/MC*, ch. 7, (p. 964).

[c] This is well expressed by Porkert (1), pp. 105–6. But he rather over-estimates, we think, the antiquity of the *wu-yün liu-chhi* theory, which he calls 'phase energetics'. This conforms with his own system of interpretation and terminology, not closely followed by us (cf. the critique of Needham & Lu Gwei-Djen, 9).

[d] Cf. *SIC*, pp. 297–8. Part at least is preserved in *CCCY*, ch. 4A, (p. 229), but it is not rated so highly as the work of Tou Han-Chhing.

[e] *SIC*, p. 285; *ICK*, p. 306.

[f] Preserved in *CCCY*, ch. 4B, (p. 263).

[g] On this dating see Chhêng Tan-An, Chhen Pi-Liu & Hsü Hsi-Nien (*1*), p. 2; they identify him as Hsü Wên-Po.[9] This authorship may have been simply an attribution to the physician of the same name who lived in the Liu Chhao period (*fl.* +400 to +425) and wrote on pharmacy and gynaecology (see *ICK*, pp. 648, 1233; *SIC*, pp. 311, 753). His biography in *Nan Shih*, ch. 32, p. 14*b*, shows that he also knew acupuncture well.

1 子午　2 流注　3 五運六氣　4 流注指微賦　5 何若愚
6 竇桂芳　7 子午經　8 子午流注逐日按時定穴歌　9 徐文伯

point to the *tzi-wu liu-chu* concepts as arising in the Northern Sung, or at earliest in late Thang.[a]

In this case they would have been little in advance of the more theoretical and meteorological *wu-yün liu-chhi* system. The oldest treatment of this appears to have been contained in a work of +1099 (again in that brilliant age of the emperor Hui Tsung), the *Su Wên Ju Shih Yün Chhi Lun Ao*[1] (A Discussion of the Mysterious Pattern of the Cyclical Changes of the (Five Elements and the Six) Chhi in the 'Questions (and Answers) about Living Matter'),[b] by Liu Wên-Shu.[2] A hundred years later (but still before Tou Han-Chhing was born) came the *Nei Ching Yün Chhi Yao Chih Lun*[3] (A Discussion of the most important points about the Permutations of the (Five Elements and the Six) Chhi in the '(Yellow Emperor's) Manual of (Corporeal) Medicine'),[c] written by Liu Wan-Su[4].[d] The reason why these authors kept harking back to the classical *Nei Ching, Su Wên* was because the expressions *wu-yün* and *liu-chhi* do occur there, but never combined in one phrase.[e] Only in the 'doubtful' or 'inserted' chapters towards the end of the book is there an explicit discussion of the *wu-yün liu-chhi* lore of times and seasons, aetiological and therapeutic.[f] It is hard to believe that the fullness of the doctrine had been handed down only by oral tradition since the −2nd century, and it is sure enough that the elaborations came only towards the end of the Northern Sung.

This raises a piece of unsettled business. Scholars are not agreed about the origin of these systems.[g] The seven doubtful chapters of the *Huang Ti Nei Ching, Su Wên* (chs. 66 to 71, and ch. 74)[h] have been suspect for centuries, in fact since the Sung; they are much longer than the other chapters and written in a recognisably different style. There is no evidence for their existence earlier than the edition of Wang Ping,[5] presented to the throne in +762. Their titles appear neither in Chhüan Yuan-Chhi's[6] Liang edition, nor in the *Huang Ti Nei Ching, Thai Su* arranged during the Sui by Yang Shang-Shan;[7] nor does the extant text of the *Thai Su* say anything about *yün-chhi*. The *wu-yün liu-chhi* system is also totally absent from the writings of Chang Chung-Ching, Huangfu Mi (cf. p. 119), and even Sun Ssu-Mo (p. 121). On the other hand we cannot be at all sure that it was Wang Ping who inserted the chapters and

[a] The parallelism here with the time-phasing of alchemical procedures is quite remarkable. As we saw in *SCC*, Vol. 5, pt. 3, pp. 60ff., heating was regularly increased and decreased in cycles following the diurnal revolution and the lunation. Diagrams of commentators there reproduced (Figs. 1351, 1352, 1353) date between +947 and +1284, but the idea clearly goes back as far as Wei Po-Yang's book of +142, a millennium earlier, and this is uninterpretable without it.

[b] *ICK*, p. 1394. See also *SIC*, p. 94.

[c] *ICK*, pp. 1395ff.

[d] Another book of his, entitled *Su Wên Hsüan Chi Yuan Ping Shih*,[8] comes from about the same date; see *ICK*, pp. 830ff.

[e] *NCSW*, ch. 9, (p. 55).

[f] Indeed the full phrase occurs in *NCSW*, ch. 71, (p. 442).

[g] Among many discussions we may mention, besides Fan Hsing-Chun (*9*), the paper of Wang Shih-Fu (*1*), the brief summary of Yang Tho (*1*), pp. 206ff., on the doubtful chapters, and the Western-language exposés of Porkert (1), pp. 56ff.

[h] Two others, chs. 72 and 73, have long been missing, so there would have been nine interpolated chapters altogether.

1 素問入式運氣論奥 2 劉溫舒 3 內經運氣要旨論 4 劉完素
5 王冰 6 全元起 7 楊上善 8 素問玄機原病式

the theory. True, Lin I[1] and his co-editor Kao Pao-Hêng[2] between +1068 and +1077 suggested that Wang Ping incorporated in the *Su Wên* another Han writing, till then circulating independently and entitled *Yin Yang Ta Lun*[3] (Great Discourse on the Yin and Yang).[a] But this has not survived separately, and there is no evidence of its identity with any text of the same or similar name cited by Han medical writers.

Now Fan Hsing-Chun (*9*) thinks that the *liu-chhi* idea first took form in a non-medical context in the Wei apocrypha of the *I Ching* (Book of Changes) in the Han period, under the auspices of adepts and diviners like Ching Fang[4] (*fl.* −45).[b] The *wu-yün*, i.e. the permutations, or cyclical changes of the five elements, was originally quite a separate idea. Fan follows the development of the two step by step. The trouble with the view that it was Wang Ping who first put them together and then incorporated the seven relevant chapters into the *Su Wên* (possibly using some Han text, now lost, as a basis for his pastiche) is that they contain materials which Wang Ping could not have known about.[c] Fan suggests rather that it was Hsü Chi[5] (d. +936) in the late Thang and Wu Tai periods, and his group, who popularised the new theories. Hsü Chi's book *Chhi Hsüan Tzu Yuan Ho Chi Yung Ching*[6] (Manual of (Medical) Affairs in the Yuan-Ho reign-period (+806 to +820) by the Revealing-of-Mysteries Master), produced about +889, discusses *yün-chhi* a great deal, especially in the first of its three chapters. This was only 17 years before the close of the Thang dynasty. As Fan Hsing-Chun acutely noted, there is no mention of *wu-yün liu-chhi* in the *Thai-Phing Shêng Hui Fang* (+982 to +992), nor in the *I Hsin Fang* (+984). But by the time of the *Shêng Chi Tsung Lu* (+1117) it has become prominent, indeed the subject of the first six chapters.[d] And we find that scientifically-minded scholars such as Shen Kua[7] in the late +11th century were very interested in it. He discusses it in the *Mêng Chhi Pi Than*.[e] Finally, by +1144 Chhêng Wu-Chi[8] had fully incorporated *wu-yün liu-chhi* into his annotated edition of the classic *Shang Han Lun* (Treatise on Febrile Diseases).[f] As for the insertion of the chapters into the classic, it must presumably have taken place at some time during the Wu Tai or early Sung periods.

By the Ming time the system was generally accepted. Chu Hsiao's[9] *Phu Chi Fang*[10] (Practical Prescriptions for Everyman), in +1418, treated extensively of it; and later in the same century complexity reached its height with the *Summa* of Chhüan Hsün-I[11]

[a] Lin I's preface is reproduced in *ICK*, p. 20.

[b] Cf. *SCC*, Vol. 4, pt. 1, p. 218 and elsewhere. Several I Wei[12] have survived.

[c] It is true that a Taoist medical book, the *Hsüan Chu Mi Yü*[13] (Confidential Sayings of the Mysterious-Pearl Master), which deals with the *wu-yün liu-chhi* theories, was at one time attributed to Wang Ping, though as early as the Sung this authorship was decisively rejected on stylistic grounds. See *SKCS/TMTY*, ch. 110, p. 22*b*, as also *ICK*, pp. 1390–3 and *SIC*, pp. 49 ff. The book, which is not in the *Tao Tsang*, dates more probably from the +10th to the +12th centuries, between the times of Hsü Chi and Liu Wan-Su. Another title attributed to Wang Ping, and dealing with the same subject, was the *Thien Yuan Yü Tshê*,[14] on which see *SIC*, p. 92, and p. 144 below.

[d] Cf. Chhen Pang-Hsien (*1*), p. 180.

[e] *MCPT*, ch. 7, para. 18 ff. on pp. 12*b* ff.

[f] *Chu Chieh Shang Han Lun*.[15] See the special study by Hsü Jung-Chai (*1*).

1 林億 2 高保衡 3 陰陽大論 4 京房 5 許寂
6 啓玄子元和紀用經 7 沈括 8 成無已 9 朱橚 10 普濟方
11 全循義 12 易緯 13 玄珠密語 14 天元玉册 15 註解傷寒論

& Chin I-Sun[1] called *Chen Chiu Tsê Jih Phien*,[2] a guide to the choice of days (and times) for acupuncture and moxibustion (+1447).[a] On the ever-prevailing macrocosm–microcosm doctrine (*thien jen ho i*[3]), the act, and also the nature, of the needling or the moxa heat or cautery, must necessarily depend upon the hour of day or night, the position in the lunation, and the state of the season of the year. As Chin Li-Mêng[4] wrote, in his preface to the work of Chhüan & Chin:

> Therefore the classical manuals of acupuncture say that if you know the right time to apply it an illness is bound to be cured, but if you miss the hour, diseases are difficult to deal with. So there is nothing more important in acupuncture and moxibustion than to choose the right moment, the acceptable time.

How could one briefly describe the *wu-yün liu-chhi* system? It was essentially an apparatus of cycles the components of each of which coincided or resonated with those of the others from time to time, producing nodal moments which were felt to be significant of real natural causation. Several basic ideas were involved in this Science of the Yin–Yang Cycles (Yün Chhi Hsüeh,[5] as it was so often called). One was that no life, no growth, nor disease, nor recovery, could come about if the cooperation of ouranic and chthonic, heavenly and earthly, forces was lacking. The celestial (*thien*[6]) and the terrestrial (*ti*[7]) had to combine their powers; and in this system it is noteworthy that the five elements operated from the heavens while the six *chhi* were those of the earth. Another idea was that the affairs of health and sickness proceeded according to a number of subtle rhythms, which, for effective intervention, had to be caught at the right times and moments. Then again there was the conviction that man was not isolated from Nature, indeed mirrored in himself the whole, so that cyclic astronomical, meteorological, climatic and epidemiological factors mattered enormously for physiological and pathological processes; and there were conclusions to be drawn, and medical prognostications to be made, from situations when the weather proved inappropriate for the season.[b] The dominance of this proto-science after the Thang period was a turning-point in the history of Chinese medicine, for in it abstraction triumphed over empiricism and practical experience. The loss of much of the older literature in the Jurchen Chin invasions, and the rise of Neo-Confucian philosophy, all helped to make physicians more learned in theory than adept in the clinical arts.

The basic law of change underlying the *wu-yün liu-chhi* system was constituted by the age-old sexagesimal cycle of the ten 'celestial stems' (*thien kan*[8]) and the twelve 'terrestrial branches' (*ti chih*[9]), two sets of time-keeping characters, the original meanings of which were uncertain already in antiquity. The reader will be familiar with them from our earlier account,[c] where we said that they were like two enmeshing

[a] This was preserved only in Japan until it was reprinted in 1890.

[b] There is a relatively brief exposition of the theory by Jen Ying-Chhiu (*3*), a good historical account by Fan Hsing-Chun (*9*), and a descriptive analysis of it in English and German by Porkert (1). See also Anon. (*81*), pp. 151 ff.; Anon. (*98*), p. 38.

[c] In *SCC*, Vol. 3, pp. 396 ff.

1 金義孫 2 鍼灸擇日編 3 天人合一 4 金禮蒙 5 運氣學
6 天 7 地 8 天干 9 地支

cogwheels so that not until sixty combinations had been made would the cycle repeat. From the Shang period onwards they were used as a day-count, and from the Han onwards as a count of years. The *chih* served also as designations for the twelve months, the twelve azimuth compass-points, and the twelve double-hours of each day and night.

Next come the five *yün*,[1] Yang 'circumambulators', celestial in nature. These echo the five 'elements' (*hsing*[2]),[a] and their heavenly position here invites the speculation that in this system they originally derived from the five planets.[b] They run in the enumeration sequence EMwWF, which is the same as the Mutual Production Order (*hsiang shêng*[3]).[c] Each of these is associated with two of the *kan* (Table 17).[d]

Table 17. *Pairing of* yün *and* hsing *stems*

	normal pairing (*phei*[4]) used by the diviners and mutationists (*shu hsüeh chia*[5])			pairing used by the medical *chhi* cycle experts (*yün chhi hsüeh chia*[6])		
		Yang	Yin			
E	*wu chi*	戊	己	*chia chi*	甲	己
M	*kêng hsin*	庚	辛	*i kêng*	乙	庚
w	*jen kuei*	壬	癸	*ping hsin*	丙	辛
W	*chia i*	甲	乙	*ting jen*	丁	壬
F	*ping ting*	丙	丁	*wu kuei*	戊	癸

As the *Nei Ching* says: 'The five circumambulators, with theii (control of) Yin and Yang, form the eternal order of heaven and earth'.[e]

In the same way, on the earthly side, each of the six meterorological Chhi (or 'weather *pneumata*') is associated with two of the *chih*, again in pairs (*phei*[4]), and characterised by one or other of the six forms of Yin and Yang,[f] as well as by each of the five elements here made into six by means of the two forms of Fire.[g] These relationships can be tabulated easily enough, but before doing so we must consider what these six Chhi were.

Essentially they were very ancient. In one of the oldest records we have of nascent

[a] The unsatisfactoriness of this translation was made clear in *SCC*, Vol. 2, p. 244, but we can never bring ourselves to discard it. Porkert (1) uses 'evolutive phases'. Needham & Lu Gwei-Djen (9) point out the undesirability of this, and suggest possible entirely new coinages, such as 'metapheres' or 'methistemes'. The problem of common consent in translation remains.

[b] Which of course have borne, since high antiquity, the names of the five elements; cf. Vol. 2, p. 262, Vol. 3, p. 398.

[c] See Vol. 2, pp. 253 ff. In the more recondite elaborations of the present theory, however, the Mutual Conquest Order (*hsiang kho*[7] or *hsiang shêng*[8]) also plays an important part, especially in connection with the six Chhi.

[d] From *NCSW*, ch. 67, (p. 337); Jen Ying-Chhiu (3), pp. 6, 14.

[e] *Wu yün Yin Yang chê, thien ti chih Tao yeh*[9] (*NCSW*, ch. 66, (p. 329), one of the 'suspect' chapters, of course).

[f] Already familiar, if only from the naming of the acu-tracts.

[g] These we encountered already long ago, in Table 43 (*SCC*, Vol. 4, pt. 1, p. 65).

1 運　2 行　3 相生　4 配　5 數學家　6 運氣學家
7 相克　8 相勝　9 五運陰陽者天地之道也

Table 18. *The six-fold characterisation of pathogenesis*

The Chou system as expounded by I Ho (−540)							The Sung system (from *c.* +950 onwards)[a]				elements or circumambulators[b]
1	Yin	陰		*han*	寒	cold[c]	1	*han*	寒	cold	w
2	Yang	陽		*jê*	熱	heat[c]	2	*huo*	火	torrid heat	PF
							3	*sao*	燥	dryness, parching, scorching	M
							4	*shu*	暑	humid heat	MF
3	*fêng*	風	wind	*mo*	末	extremities[d]	5	*fêng*	風	wind	W
4	*yü*	雨	rain	*fu*	腹	abdomen[e]	6	*shih*	濕	damp moisture	E
5	*hui*	晦	darkness	*huo*	惑	doubt[f]					
6	*ming*	明	brightness	*hsin*	心	heart, mind[g]					

[a] The order in which the Chhi are given in this column brings out their parallelism with those of the most ancient system, but it is not an order of enumeration used in expositions of the Yün Chhi Hsüeh doctrine. There it follows other sequences, such as *han, shu* (*jê*), *sao, shih, fêng, huo* (*NCSW*, ch. 67, (pp. 337 ff.), cf. Jen Ying-Chhiu (*3*), p. 33).

[b] Symbols as in *SCC*, Vol. 2, p. 253. E for earth, M for metal, w for water, W for wood. As for the two forms of fire, PF, 'princely fire', stands for *chün huo*,[1] and MF, 'ministerial fire', for *hsiang huo*.[2]

[c] Identified with forms of pyrexia. These terms later became names of syndromes described in the *Shang Han Lun* (*c.* +200).

[d] Including the head (dizziness, headaches, etc.), as well as all troubles of the limbs.

[e] All diseases of the viscera, probably also some oedematous conditions, and ascites.

[f] 'Out of his wits'. Interpreted as delirium or cerebral abnormality.

[g] Considered to imply cardiac or psychological disease or malfunction.

[1] 君火 [2] 相火

Chinese medical thought, I Ho[1] the physician, sent by a Prince of Chhin to attend a Prince of Chin in −540, gives a prognosis that his illness, caused by excesses, is incurable, and then descants upon a kind of quasi-meteorological pathology.[a] Excess of Yin or Yang, or of four further external factors of a weather-like, diurnal or seasonal character, leads to six types of diseases (see Table 18). Of these the first two, for example, have always been understood as referring to different types of fever, the fifth indicates cerebral abnormality, and the sixth cardiac and psychological malfunctions. The fact that this is a table of sixes calls in itself for remark, because one has to emphasise repeatedly that from the beginning Chinese medical thought involved a sixfold characterisation, while the parallel natural philosophy involved fives.[b] By the time that we come to Liu Wên-Shu and Liu Wan-Su in the +12th century, the Sung period,[c] the technical terms for the sixfold types of disease, and doubtless their exact meanings also, have greatly changed, but they are still six (as in Table 18, col. 2), and these were the six Chhi of the *wu-yün liu-chhi* system, and all the other medical theories of those times.

One can therefore construct the following table (Table 19). From this and from Table 17 on p. 141 it will be noticed that the correlations of the *kan* and the *chih* are quite different in the Yün Chhi Hsüeh system from the usual paired relationships, in fact metamorphosed. This is because they have to fit in with the continuous diurnal and annual cyclical changes of the celestial elements (circumambulators, *thien yün*[2]) and the earthly meteorological conditions (*ti chhi*[3]). The different lists are given in an answer of Kuei Yü-Chhü[4] (one of the secondary interlocutors) to Huang Ti, and in a commentary of Wang Ping, both in suspect chapters of the *Nei Ching, Su Wên*.[d] The explanation lies in a strange and little-known system of natural philosophy contained in a lost book with the title *Thai-Shih Thien Yuan Tshê*[5],[e] a passage of which

[a] *Tso Chuan*, Duke Chao, 1st year; tr. Couvreur (1), vol. 3, pp. 35ff. See also the discussion in Needham (64), pp. 265, 266–7, from Needham & Lu Gwei-Djen (8).

[b] Cf. p. 42 above. The close synthesis made in Yün Chhi Hsüeh between the theories of the ancient Chinese philosophical schools and those of the medical thinkers is striking. Parallels with the familiar Aristotelian elements and the Galenic humours come constantly to mind, but the difference is great, for the fourfold pattern was never typical of indigenous Chinese ideology.

[c] We put it this way because the only enumeration and description of the six Chhi comes in a *Su Wên* chapter which is one of the suspect ones, quite possibly stemming from Wang Ping in the +8th century; *NCSW*, ch. 74, (p. 449), *NCSW/PH*, ch. 74, (p. 458), *NCSW/WMC*, ch. 74, (p. 776); cf. Fan Hsing-Chun (9); Hsieh Li-Hêng (2), vol. 1, p. 436. The passage is not in the *Nei Ching, Thai Su* of the +7th century. Again, in *NCSW*, chs. 66 and 67, (pp. 329ff.), also probably Thang, there are detailed correspondences between the six Chhi, the elements (or circumambulators), and their effects on the organs of the body. It is true that the expression *liu chhi*[6] occurs in *NCSW*, ch. 9, (p. 55), but only in connection with divisions of time, as six *chieh chhi*[7] (fortnightly periods, cf. *SCC*, Vol. 3, p. 405), or one quarter of the year—and even that chapter has sometimes been suspected of being an interpolation.

[d] The former is *NCSW*, ch. 67, (p. 337), the latter is ch. 66, (p. 336).

[e] The oldest reference to any such title is in the *Sung Shih* bibliography, which lists a *Thai-Shih Thien Yuan Yü Tshê Chieh Fa*[8] (ch. 207, *i wên chih* 6, p. 3*b*). The *Tao Tsang* once had three versions of this work, but all were lost, so they are listed only in Ong's catalogue, p. 57. One had a commentary attributed to Pien Chhio. They must therefore have been on medical philosophy, but without a real knowledge of their content it would be hazardous to translate their titles. Taken together, these facts indicate that the text and its system was not much earlier than the Sung, perhaps worked into the *Nei Ching* by Wang Ping himself, and also that it was Taoist in origin. Cf. the note on p. 140 above.

1 醫和 2 天運 3 地氣 4 鬼臾區 5 太始天元冊 6 六氣
7 節氣 8 太始天元玉冊截法

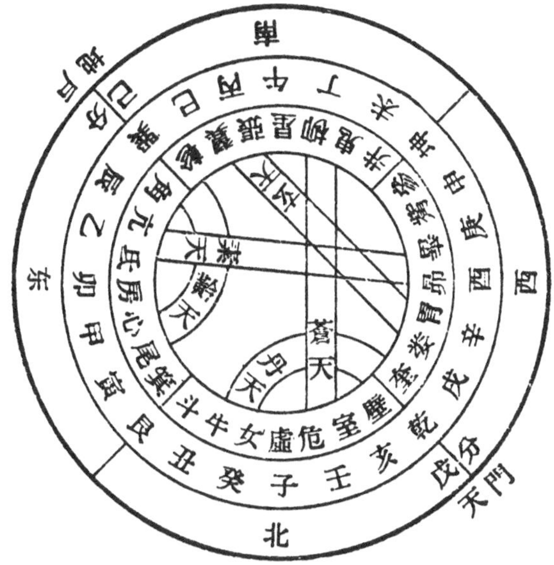

Fig. 31. Example of a diagram in the complicated mediaeval computus for determining optimal times for acupuncture and moxa in accordance with the recurrent cyclical changes in the human body (circadian rhythms) and the recurrent celestial-terrestrial permutations and combinations. This was the doctrine of *wu yün liu chhi*, the cyclical changes of the Five Elements and the Six Chhi. In the diagram the circles from outside inwards are: (*a*) 4 compass-points, south at the top; (*b*) 8 *kan* and 12 *chih* (cyclical characters, see *SCC*, Vol. 3, p. 396), plus 4 kua (see Vol. 2, p. 313), making 24 compass-points (see Vol. 4, pt. 1, pp. 297–8); (*c*) the 28 *hsiu* (lunar mansions). Connections are shown by the cross-linkages, looking like some of the old attempts to represent the rings of armillary spheres (see Vol. 3, p. 351); these are labelled as a series of heavens, from the lowest characters upwards successively—red, caerulean, yellow, white and black. It was into these five groups that the *hsiu* were unequally divided (see text). From Jen Ying-Chhiu (*3*), p. 15.

Chhi Po quotes to Huang Ti immediately afterwards.[a] In this pattern of things the twenty-eight lunar mansions (*hsiu*[1]) were divided into five groups according to the colours of the *chhi* of the heavens[b] (but not in a continuous round or sequence),[c] and these were then associated with an outer ring of twenty-four compass-points containing eight *kan* and twelve *chih*.[d] The arrangement is shown in Fig. 31.[e]

[a] *NCSW*, ch. 67, (p. 338).

[b] Red (*tan*[2]), yellow (*chin*[3]), caerulean (*tshang*[4]), white (*su*[5]), and black (*hsüan*[6]). These are not the ordinary terms for the colours of the four quarters and the centre, nor do they correspond with the usual correlations. For example, red can be associated with the north (as it is in the diagram of Fig. 31), not only with the south; and all the colours change their positions according to the diurnal and longer cycles. Could such things be explained, perhaps, by knowledge of celestial phenomena such as the aurora borealis? This set of colours also recalls that meteorological–mineralogical one in the *Huai Nan Tzu*, ch. 4, pp. 12*a*ff.; on which see *SCC*, Vol. 3, p. 640, and Vol. 5, pt. 4. Taoist traditions and speculations loom again through the mists.

[c] As the astronomical palaces were; cf. Vol. 3, pp. 234ff.

[d] The remaining four places were taken by *kua*; see Vol. 4, pt. 1, pp. 297–8. The *hsiu* at their culminations are of course in the south, and *vice versa*.

[e] Jen Ying-Chhiu (*3*), p. 15.

[1] 宿 [2] 丹 [3] 黅 [4] 蒼 [5] 素 [6] 玄

Table 19. *Correlations in the* Yün Chhi Hsüeh *system*[a]

Yin–Yang form		element			Chhi		*chih*; normal Yang–Yin pairing (*phie*[1])		*chih*; pairing (*phei*[1]) in the Yün Chhi Hsüeh system	
Shao Yin	少陰	*chün huo*	君火	PF	*huo*	火	*tzu wu*	子午	*wu ssu*	午巳
Thai Yin	太陰	*thu*	土	E	*shih*	濕	*chhou wei*	丑未	*chhen hsü* & *chhou wei*	辰戌 丑未
Shao Yang	少陽	*hsiang huo*	相火	MF	*shu*	暑	*yin shen*	寅申	*wu ssu*	午巳
Yang Ming	陽明	*chin*	金	M	*sao*	燥	*mao yu*	卯酉	*shen yu*	申酉
Thai Yang	太陽	*shui*	水	w	*han*	寒	*chhen hsü*	辰戌	*tzu hai*	子亥
Chüeh Yin	厥陰	*mu*	木	W	*fêng*	風	*ssu hai*	巳亥	*yin mao*	寅卯

The cycle started about a fortnight before the beginning of each year in the Chinese lunar calendar.[b] Every year had a dominant Yin (i.e. terrestrial) circumambulatory *chhi* (*chu yün*[2]), depending on what the *kan* for the year in the ten-year cycle (*ta yün*,[3] *chung yün*[4]), shown in col. 3 of Table 17 was. If it was a Yang one (*chia*, *ping*, *wu*, *kêng*, *jen*) the year was said to be 'superabundant' (*thai kuo*[5]); if it was a Yin one it was said to be 'insufficient' (*pu chi*[6]).[c] For example, the initial year of the series was a *chia* (Yang) one, and therefore its dominant would be E (*thu yün*[7]). At the same time there was also a 'visiting circumambulator' (*kho yün*[8]) from the celestial level,[d] and this was important because it was believed to dictate the pulse of patients and hence the acupuncture treatment which it was appropriate to give them.

Within each year the twelve months were divided into six periods (*pu*[9]), each characterised by one or other of the forms of Yin and Yang (col. 1 of Table 19),[e] and of the medical-meterological Chhi (col. 3 of Table 19). The former were also considered *chhi*, and the third position in their clockwise round necessarily corresponded to the South and the summer solstice. This position was called that of the 'heaven-governing *chhi*' (*ssu thien chih chhi*[10]). And correspondingly the meteorological Chhi associated with it (col. 3 of Table 19) was the 'dominant *chhi*' (*chu chhi*[11]). Conversely, the opposite position (i.e. the sixth and last of the year cycle) corresponded to the

[a] From *NCSW*, ch. 71, (p. 442), cf. Jen Ying-Chhiu (*3*), pp. 34–5, 44; Porkert (1), p. 65.

[b] The point was defined as 60 days and 87·5 quarters before the spring equinox (cf. Needham, Wang & Price (1), p. 199), i.e. starting with the Ta Han *chieh chhi* (cf. Vol. 3, p. 405) in the twelfth month. See Jen Ying-Chhiu (*3*), p. 38.

[c] In this context these terms had reference to the change-over point between the years, whether the Chüeh Yin started 13 days before Ta Han *chieh chhi* or 13 days later. Thus there was a continual alternation between Yang years and Yin years.

[d] The arrangements for identifying it were complicated, and reference should be made to *NCSW*, ch. 66, (p. 330) and Jen Ying-Chhiu (*3*), p.51.

[e] Not however in the same order; here it goes: Chüeh Yin, Shao Yin, Shao Yang, Thai Yin, Yang Ming, Thai Yang.

1 配 2 主運 3 大運 4 中運 5 太過 6 不及
7 土運 8 客運 9 步 10 司天之氣 11 主氣

North and the winter solstice, and this was called 'the *chhi* in the sources' (*tsai chhüan chih chhi*[1]). Each one of the six Yin–Yang forms or *chhi* took turns at occupying these two positions. The former fixed the quality of the 'rising' half of the year, just as the latter fixed it for the 'setting' half. Finally there was also a 'visiting *chhi*' (*kho chhi*[2]), i.e. the *chhi* which occupied the position two places behind the 'heaven-governing *chhi*'.[a]

A moment ago we spoke of alternating 'super-abundant' and 'insufficient' years. Were there never harmonious years? There were, and the technical term for them was *phing chhi*;[3] they came round when the consequences of their *kan* and *chih* in the sixty-year cycle balanced each other.[b] This happened only when both were of the same sign (Yang or Yin) and both indicated the same dominant circumambulator (*chu yün*[4]). For example, in a *kuei ssu*[5] year the *chu yün* would be F, yet both characters are Yin; and *kuei* will be in the north while *ssu* will occupy position three in the south, so that their *chhi* will compensate for each other. From what has now been said it can be seen that no year was ever quite the same in its characteristics, and when the permutations and combinations in the system repeated in full it was at very long intervals exceeding sixty years.

All these relationships were expounded in discoidal diagrams of much complexity from which it was possible to infer what the meterorological conditions of a particular time of year would be expected to be, and hence what illnesses were to be foreseen. But only too often the weather failed to correspond with this rather arbitrary prediction system, and in this case some of the technical terms already encountered were used in a different sense. If the factual phenomena went beyond the deduction (hotter or colder, rainier or drier) the situation was called 'over-vigorous' (*shêng*[6] or *thai kuo*[7]); if it failed to come up to expectation it was termed 'weak' or 'failing' (*shuai*[8] or *pu chi*[9]). Similarly, the term *phing chhi*[10] was used for situations in which the meteorological conditions fell out exactly as the pundits expected from the cyclical sequences. Thus Wang Ping (or whoever it was that wrote ch. 69 of the *Su Wên*) says that

> if in a given year Wood is super-abundant, the Wind Chhi will be roving and rampant, the Earth element (will be damaged)[c] and hence the spleen will be subject to heteropathies; the people will suffer from a kind of diarrhoea with flatulence, their appetite will decrease and they will be depressed and listless, with a heavy feeling in abdomen and extremities...[d]

Contrariwise:

> if in a given year Wood is insufficient, the Dryness Chhi will be on the march,[e] the life-giving Chhi will fail to resonate (with the season), plant growth will be retarded, and everything will be inhibited, frustrated and dried up...The people will have excessive appetite

[a] See Jen Ying-Chhiu (*3*), p. 40.
[b] Cf. the note on p. 148 below.
[c] Because W conquers E in the Mutual Conquest order.
[d] *NCSW*, ch. 69, (p. 366), *NCSW/PH*, ch. 69, (p. 380), tr. auct. adjuv. Porkert (1), p. 78.
[e] Because M conquers W in the Mutual Conquest order.

1 在泉之氣 2 客氣 3 平氣 4 主運 5 癸巳 6 盛
7 太過 8 衰 9 不及 10 平氣

without gaining weight, there will be pains in the thorax and lower abdomen, with flatulence and another kind of diarrhoea...[a]

And the text continues with similar statements for all the other elements or circumambulators.[b] Such was the complex algorithm by the light of which the learned physicians of the Sung decided exactly when, and where, to apply their acupuncture and other treatments.

To sum it up, the Yün Chhi Hsüeh system presents at first sight a certain similarity with the medical astrology of the Western Middle Ages, but the likeness does not go very far. The theories of the circumambulators and the Chhi were after all based on more or less regular seasonal phenomena and the rhythms of climate and weather, and in a way they had much more to do with the prediction of diseases and epidemics.[c] It was rather from the *tzu-wu liu-chu* system that the physician could draw conclusions about the ideal times for applying acupuncture and moxa to individual patients. The aim of the whole operation was the counter-balancing of the abnormal quality or quantity of *chhi* which was causing the pathological disturbance against the normal external macrocosmic *chhi*, which varied in both respects according to the double-hour, the day, the month, the season and the year.[d] This was the third significance of *phing chhi*,[1] 'harmonising the *pneumata*'.[e] If our exposition here has been rather lengthy we hope to be forgiven because the five circumambulators and the six Chhi were applied in Sung and Yuan times to the whole of medicine, including drug therapy as well, which in some of the books that have here been quoted plays an even more important part than acupuncture.

There can be no doubt that the Yün Chhi Hsüeh computus was a daunting edifice of *a priori* systematisation, 'by far the weakest link so far discerned in the correspondence system of Chinese medicine'.[f] Contrary to statements sometimes made, it did take considerable notice of geographical latitude and altitude,[g] but it was based on a body of meteorological knowledge essentially medieval in character. Indeed the great medical historian Li Thao has gone so far as to maintain that it inhibited the further progress of Chinese traditional medicine after the Sung;[h] it tended to be the

[a] *NCSW*, ch. 69, (p. 370), *NCSW/PH*, ch. 69, (p. 383), tr. auct. adjuv. Porkert (1), p. 79.

[b] Throughout these passages there are references to the planets, so an astrological element is not wholly absent, though we cannot go into it here.

[c] It will have been evident that much of the argumentation was based on the Mutual Production and Mutual Conquest theories of the five elements, especially in the relationships between *chu yün* and *kho yün* in a given year.

[d] The evocation of balancing here recalls the Arabic alchemical 'Theory of the Balance' ('Ilm al-Mīzān), typical of the +9th century, a not dissimilar age, on which see *SCC*, Vol. 5, pt. 4, pp. 459ff. Both this and the Yün Chhi Hsüeh aimed at the quantitative, but succeeded in attaining only the numerological.

[e] This again recalls another 'equalisation' technique, that of Sun Ên and his disciples, on which see *SCC*, Vol. 2, pp. 150–1. Their Taoist sexual liturgies, so interesting for the history of religion, which aimed to harmonise the Yin and Yang, were flourishing around +400, just about the date of Hsü Wên-Po (cf. p. 138 above).

[f] Porkert (1), p. 105.

[g] *NCSW*, ch. 70, (p. 395), ch. 71, (p. 441); Jen Ying-Chhiu (3), p. 74. 'There are high places and low places, and the *chhi* is warm or cool, cold on the heights and hot on the plains...These differences must be carefully attended to.'

[h] (*2*), pp. 10, 13. A similar judgment may be seen in Chhen Pang-Hsien (*1*), pp. 31, 179.

[1] 平氣

delight of men who were better scholars than practising physicians, and encouraged proto-scientific theory-making rather than empirical study and clinical recording. At the same time psychological factors can never be forgotten where medicine is concerned, and so complex a system, with its many diagrams and confident predictions, could have given great heart to many doctors working in tough conditions of poverty and plague. Not only so, but the patients themselves would have been very impressed – with good therapeutic results if only by suggestion – all the more because the advent of printing was contemporaneous with the Yün Chhi Hsüeh and brought it widely to public knowledge. Clearly no description of the history of acupuncture could omit some account of it, especially since it is still in use to this day by a certain number of traditional Chinese physicians.[a] Its period of doctrinal dominance came to an end, however, in the latter part of the Ming, when men such as Wang Chi[1] (*fl.* +1522 to +1567)[b] and Chang Chieh-Pin[2] (+1563 to +1640)[c] criticised it severely. The former deplored its mechanical application by physicians numerologically inclined, without any real understanding of the environmental background of epidemiology; and the latter felt that in his own legalistic use of it he had sometimes been like a frog surveying the world from the bottom of a well.[d] Both considered, however, that when fully understood and judiciously applied the system could still be a guide to practice.

Just how right the old Chinese bio-medical observers were in visualising regular cyclic changes in the function and composition of living bodies, especially those of human beings, can best be appreciated by those who are familiar with the researches of the last couple of decades on 'biological time-keeping'. A whole new department of the life sciences has opened. It has been established beyond doubt that there are a great number of inbuilt rhythms in organisms of all the phyla of the animal kingdom,[e] and beyond that, in many plant forms also; biological clocks, as it were, which govern motion, rest and sleep, feeding and excretion, the chemical composition and the internal relations of tissue fluids, glands and other organs.[f] The long known phenomena of plant photoperiodism may be a manifestation of such inbuilt rhythms. These may be of almost any length of time, but among the commonest are those which repeat every twenty-four hours, and these are called diurnal or circadian

[a] See Anon. (*81*), pp. 151–2; (*98*), pp. 38ff. Similarly, a modern practical account of ***tzu-wu liu-chu fa*** is given in Anon. (*90*), pp. 440ff.

[b] Author of the ***Pên Tshao Hui Pien***, on which see *SCC*, Vol. 6, pt. 1.

[c] Eminent physician and author of the *Lei Ching* (+1624). Both these are quoted by Jen Ying-Chhiu (*3*), pp. 75–6.

[d] A certain parallelism presents itself here between the systematised Yün Chhi Hsüeh and the highly simplified manuals produced today both in East and West, for the 'barefoot doctors' on the one hand, and for occidental clinical acupuncturists on the other (cf. p. 12 above). Lack of theoretical understanding is liable to produce failures, but for that acupuncture itself cannot be blamed.

[e] Reviews by Harker (3); Danilevsky (1); Withrow (1); Scheving (1).

[f] One reason for the great contemporary relevance of this is a development of which the old Chinese physicians could never have dreamed, the growth of rapid and world-wide air travel. Many human psycho-physiological rhythms are upset by the sudden transpositions which it imposes. For a good account of the problems see Nicholson (1).

[1] 王機 [2] 張介賓

rhythms.[a] Hence the significance of the *Tzu Wu Ching*, the 'Noon and Midnight Manual'.

Let us take a very brief *tour d'horizon* of this literature, which has brought to light some extraordinary facts. For example, the timing may be accurate to 0·1 % without external stimuli. Organisms are not always born or hatched with all the biological clocks ticking. Bird embryos, it seems, show some circadian rhythms while still in their eggs (e.g. the movements of the chick in developing hen's eggs). In the human infant, however, rhythms are established only after some weeks of post-natal life.[b]

	weeks after birth
skin, electrical resistance	1
urine excretion	2·5
body temperature	3
heart-beat, rate	6
K and Na excretion	8
sleep	16

Then circadian rhythms can persist through the complete anatomical dissolution and reconstruction of insect metamorphosis,[c] and also through long hibernation in mammals.[d] It may be possible to localise some biological clocks in particular organs, 'conductors of the physiological orchestra' as it were, for Harker (2) has shown that transplanting the sub-oesophageal ganglion into a headless cockroach induces circadian rhythms of donor amplitude in the previously arhythmic host.[e]

Among circadian rhythms in mammals there is one of nucleic acid synthesis, so fundamental for all cell-division, growth and repair. A minimum of desoxyribonucleic acid (DNA) synthesis in the liver of the mouse occurs at 04.00 hr but the minimum of ribonucleic acid (RNA) synthesis is at 16.00 hr, parallelling a cycle of activity of the adrenal glands.[f] Their largest corticosterone production occurs at 18.00 hr.[g] In man there is a marked circadian rise and fall in the urinary excretion of 17-OH corticosteroids, going along with potassium excretion and body temperature.[h] This last seems to be adrenal-controlled, like the day and night rhythm of oxygen-consumption, the fluctuation of liver glycogen and phospholipids, and the numbers of leucocytes in the blood.[i] Again, it is not generally known that the composition of

[a] Cf. the symposium proceedings edited by Aschoff (1).
[b] Cf. Halberg (1), and especially Hellbrügge (1).
[c] Harker (1), p. 20.
[d] St Girons (1); over months spontaneous arousals and activity in the garden dormouse (*Eliomys quercinus*) invariably occurred between about 17.00 and 04.00 hr.
[e] Cf. also Harker (3), pp. 12ff.
[f] Halberg (2); Halberg *et al.* (1).
[g] Halberg (1).
[h] Halberg (2); Lobban (1).
[i] Roberts (1).

human saliva is quite different at different times of day and night. Its sodium concentration and Na/K ratio is greatest in the early morning and falls to a minimum in the evening, resembling the course of aldosterone excretion.[a] And naturally pharmacology is not exempt from diurnal cycles; it has recently been found by Smith & Shearman (1) that the intra-amniotic effectiveness of prostaglandin $PGF_{2\alpha}$ in inducing abortion is greatest at 6 p.m. and much less effective at other times of day or night.

All these observations pose two distinct problems. First, to what extent are the diurnal rhythms evoked by external signals such as light and darkness, or even more subtle influences such as the magnetic field of the earth? Conversely, how far are the rhythms the manifestation of intra-cellular biological clocks which go on working even though the environment is changed to perpetual light or perpetual darkness, or otherwise uniformised? There are many results which can only be explained on the latter assumption. In Spitzbergen's 'white nights' the excretory rhythms of potassium and other ions in man would not adapt to constancy; they could be trained to as short an interval as 16 hr and to as long a one as 28 hr but not beyond those limits.[b] And secondly, what exactly are these internal biological clocks? As yet, no one knows.

Some of the observations which form the stimuli for these questions are as old as the pre-Socratics and the Warring States, but so far all the resources of modern science have not sufficed to solve the basic problem, and two contrasting views have crystallised.[c] The 'exogenous' view is that rhythmic geophysical forces provide living organisms with informational inputs which regulate the timing of their recurrent processes. The 'endogenous' view is that organisms possess internal autonomous biological clocks not immediately dependent on the external world, and constituting a self-sufficient timing mechanism. One can see that the insistence of the ancient Chinese physicians on the rhythmic character of physiological and pathological phenomena, both diurnal, monthly and annual,[d] brought them clearly into the main line of human knowledge of this strange microcosm–macrocosm relationship.

Among the most interesting of the oscillations, from our present point of view, are those which are to be seen in the pathological states of man. Every organ involved has its own cycle. Among clinicians it is well known that crises of cholecystitis tend to occur during the early hours of the morning; and patients with Parkinson's disease may show a complete cessation of the disabling symptoms between 21.00 and 24.00 hr each evening.[e] Asthma paroxysms are characteristically nocturnal, occurring as the adrenocortical activity drops to its nadir; and histamine-sensitivity is most acute at 23.00 hr, just when the blood levels of the 17-OH corticosteroids are lowest.[f] There

[a] Grad (1); Blair-West *et al.* (1), p. 641.

[b] Lewis & Lobban (1, 2). Lobban (1) considers many other forms of dissociation. Light is an important influence, but intrinsic factors are present as well.

[c] See especially the interesting debate in Brown, Hastings & Palmer (1). Cf. also Bennett (1); Lewin (1).

[d] On annual biological rhythms see the symposium edited by Pengelley (1). Phenomena to be remembered here are those of migration in birds and mammals, swarming in invertebrates, hibernation in mammals, and reproductive cycles in many phyla. There is even evidence that season of birth in man affects mental stability and schizophrenia; cf. Dalén (1).

[e] See Leonard (1); Richter (1).

[f] Reinberg (1).

is a diurnal rhythm in pain threshold;[a] and it is common knowledge that in fevers body temperatures increase in the evening. These are all circadian phenomena. But many cycles of longer phase have been found in medical records, as Richter (1) has shown. For example:

	av. time of cycle (days)
diencephalic lesion	2
intermittent hydrarthrosis	11
cyclic agranulocytosis	21
Hodgkin's disease	21
schizophrenic catatonia (fast-phased)	24
(natural ovulation)	28
schizophrenic catatonia (slow-phased)	36
duodenal ulcer	139

It will hardly be believed that a set of circadian rhythms in clinical experience is recorded in the *Nei Ching, Su Wên*. Yet in ch. 22 the characteristic times of crisis and remission (*hui*[1]) are set forth for each one of the horreal viscera (*tsang*[2]).[b] Thus we learn that in patients suffering from disease of the liver, there will be a remission of symptoms in the morning, the condition will grow worse in the afternoon, and quiet down again towards midnight.[c] Diseases of the spleen, however, will cause most suffering at sunrise and during the morning, calming down again in the afternoon and giving almost complete remission towards sunset. Naturally the confusion of many pathological conditions associated with one particular organ was a primitive trait, but it is quite remarkable enough to find such clinical observations systematically recorded at all.

From all this it is clear that the old Chinese idea of 'circulations of the *chhi*' profoundly affecting human beings in health and disease was a very justifiable one.[d] We have often had occasion to point out that of all ancient cultures, China was by far the most 'circulation-minded' (cf. p. 24 above).[e] After all, the apparent diurnal revolution of the heavens was very familiar, and the planetary revolution periods were sufficiently well known at quite an early date.[f] There was also the annual rhythm of the seasons. If this sort of thing was taking place in the macrocosm, why should one hesitate to accept the conclusion, strongly indicated as it was by clinical experience, that the microcosm was the theatre of rhythms too? The natural ovulation and menstruation

[a] References in Sauerbruch & Wenke (1), p. 19. This is relevant to the neurophysiology of acupuncture analgesia, on which see pp. 231 ff. below.

[b] *NCSW/WMC*, ch. 22, (pp. 234 ff.), tr. Porkert (1), pp. 120, 125, 131, 138 and 141.

[c] This has support from modern medicine, e.g. in jaundice, where the times from 16 to 20 hr are the worst.

[d] Almost the only writer who has appreciated this is Looney (2).

[e] Cf. Pagel (9, 19, 25) and Huard & Huang Kuang-Ming (1). Also *SCC*, Vol. 2, p. 483.

[f] Cf. Vol. 3, pp. 398 ff. and Table 33.

1 慧   2 臓

rhythm would always have given an incontestable paradigm.[a] Mention of celestial phenomena, however, reminds us that medieval European medicine was deeply under the spell of astrology. Exactly how this pseudo-science was used in clinical practice is not always very clear.[b] Conclusions could obviously be drawn from the patient's genethliacal horoscope, and the specific influences of planets and zodiacal constellations on organs and parts of the human body was a commonplace, while the state of the heavens at the time of the onset of the illness would naturally matter.[c] Comets and sttange new stars (novae) were also implicated in epidemics. But although the zodiacal signs rotated and the planets came and went, it does not appear that Western astrology suggested any rhythms intrinsic to the patient himself. This the Chinese system did, and the therapist, whether applying acupuncture or pharmacy, took great care to find and make use of the right, the acceptable, time. Unfortunately, lacking the methods of modern science, the Chinese physicians constructed an arbitrary and numerological, almost glyphomantic, scheme, from the flow of double-hours, days and months, expressed by the five elements, the two sets of cyclical characters (ten and twelve), and the twenty-eight lunar mansions. The systems were so complicated as to lead one to suspect that when a phsyician was choosing a suitable time to apply acupuncture he did so on the basis of his clinical experience, inherited from previous generations of teachers and acquired by himself in the course of practice, finding good reasons for his action afterwards from the interplay of the chronographic symbols. Pseudo-sciences are liable to work like that.[d] This one, used alone, gave the Chinese doctors little possibility of determining the best time for intervention, as we can do today when we want to, at least in some cases, but they probably hit the right mark anyway much of the time. And in so far as they did so, was it not in part precisely due to their well-justified intuition of cyclic changes in the bodies and minds of men, both in health and sickness? 'Truly there is a time for everything', says Nick Culpeper, in 'A Doctor of Medicine', 'and the physician must work with it — or miss his cure.'[e]

(vii) *Last phases of the tradition*

At this point we rejoin the historical account of acupuncture and moxa as techniques developing through the centuries. With the establishment of the Chin[1] Tartar State in the north in +1127 after the fall of Khaifêng, China was divided into two nations with the Southern Sung capital at Hangchow.[f] This situation lasted for just over a

[a] To what extent the ancients were profoundly impressed by this regularity can be seen in the history of embryology and generation theory (cf. Needham, 2).

[b] There is a chapter on it in Eisler (1), pp. 246ff.; and it enters in to every description of medieval European natural philosophy, cf. Singer (3, 16).

[c] The Library of Gonville and Caius College in Cambridge, where all the volumes of our work have been written or edited, conserves two astrolabes which were the property of our second founder, John Caius (d. +1573) and supposedly used by him in aiding diagnosis, therapy and prognosis by astrology. He was Archiater-Royal at the English court under three reigns.

[d] The classical exposition of this, in the form of a story, is Rudyard Kipling's 'A Doctor of Medicine', in his collection of 1910, *Rewards and Fairies*.

[e] Loc. cit., p. 269.

[f] *SCC*, Vol. 1, pp. 140ff.; Li Thao (2,6, *6*).

[1] 金

hundred years, but by +1234 the Mongols were strong enough to liquidate the Chin power and to turn their attention to the south, though the Sung dynasty could still survive for 49 years. The Tartars and Mongols in the north were much less cultured than the Chinese in the south,[a] and poverty prevailed on both sides of the frontiers, with military campaigns continuing year after year,[b] so none of the arts of peace (including medicine) could prosper. Such conditions throw into greater relief the achievements of four great physicians of those times, the Chin Yuan Ssu Ta Chia[1] as they are called. One of them, Liu Wan-Su,[2] we have already mentioned (p. 139 above), and the rest will be discussed in connection with other aspects of medicine.[c] Once the Yuan dynasty had fully established itself, conditions greatly improved, and a formerly unheard-of ease of communication with the Western world opened up. A Nestorian physician from Syria could practise medicine in Peking,[d] perhaps an Italian Franciscan friar also,[e] while some Chinese medical knowledge may have passed westwards with the two Uighur priests from North China who journeyed thither, one to become Catholicos of the whole Nestorian Church,[f] the other to sojourn in Rome and Bordeaux before returning to Mongolia.[g]

Meanwhile the making of bronze human figures for teaching or examination was going forward again in the Mongol capital. Some of the men just mentioned may well have been personally acquainted with a Nepalese master-craftsman named A-Ni-Ko,[3] who had gone to seek his fortune at the Yuan court. In the *Yuan Shih* we read:[h]

> During the Chung-Thung reign-period (+1260 to +1263) A-Ni-Ko, accompanied by an Imperial Tutor, had an audience with the emperor. Shih Tsu (Khubilai Khan) enquired of him, saying: 'What are your special skills?' He replied: 'Your subject takes his own intelligence as his teacher. He is well informed concerning the art of painting, modelling (Buddhist statues) and the casting of metal figures and images.' The emperor ordered the Bronze Microcosmic Statue for Acupuncture and Moxibustion Demonstration to be brought in and shown to him...The emperor said: 'It has been a long time since this one was

[a] But they steadily adopted Chinese customs and in the end became very much assimilated.

[b] Massacres of populations of captured cities were a regular feature of Mongolian 'frightfulness', but significantly all manner of artisans, and medical men, were in general spared.

[c] Their names: Chang Tzu-Ho,[4] Li Kao[5] and Chu Chen-Hêng.[6]

[d] This was Ai Hsüeh,[7] i.e. Īsa Tarjaman, i.e. the interpreter, whose original name was probably Jesus or Isaiah (+1226 to +1308). He rose high in the Mongolian service, because besides his medical skill he was also a master of pharmacy, astronomy and some aspects of engineering. He ended as a Han-Lin Academician and Astronomer-Royal.

[e] John of Montecorvino of course (+1247 to +1348), Archbishop of Khanbaliq (i.e. Peking). He reached China in +1289 and Peking in +1292. On his practice of medicine see Li Thao, op. cit.

[f] Marqos Bayniel (+1245 to +1316).

[g] Rabban Bar Sauma (*c.* +1225 to +1294). In +1285 he was sent to the Latin West on a diplomatic mission, and found a warmly friendly welcome at Rome and as far West as Bordeaux. On both these men see Wallis Budge (2). On the +13th- and +14th-century cluster of technological transmissions see Needham (64), pp. 200–1.

[h] Ch. 203, p. 12*a*, tr. auct., cf. Yü Kho (*1*), p. 24. Wang Jen-Chün (*1*) in his *Ko Chih Ku Wei* of 1896 (cf. *SCC*, Vol. 1, p. 48), paraphrased the passage (ch. 2, p. 28*a*,*b*), and added characteristically: 'Nowadays the Western medical schools have charts of the anatomy of the whole body—my opinion is that they all arose from this.' For a biography of A-Ni-Ko see Chu Chhi-Chhien & Liu Tun-Chên (*1*), p. 140. On A-Ni-Ko as an architect see Vol. 4, pt. 3, p. 75.

1 金元四大家 2 劉完素 3 阿尼哥 4 張子和 5 李杲
6 朱震亨 7 愛薛

made, and now it is incomplete and partly broken. Nobody here can repair it. Do you think that you could restore the thing, or even make a completely new one?' To which A-Ni-Ko answered: 'I have never made such a statue before, but I would like your august permission to try.'

The following year (+1265) a new bronze figure was completed, with all the necessary details of joints, diaphragm, and acupuncture loci. The metal-workers (of the court) sighed at his extreme skill and greatly admired him, not without regrets at their own inability to do such things.

This new push must have brought results, for as soon as the +14th century came in, useful books on acupuncture came out, one after the other. Appropriately, the first was by some Mongol or Muslim, the original form of whose name is uncertain, for in +1303 Hu-Thai-Pi-Lieh[1] (or Hu-Kung-Thai[2]) produced his *Chin Lan Hsün Ching Chhü Hsüeh Thu Chieh*[3] on how to find the acu-points in relation to the tracts.[a] To assist in the explanation of Tu Mo and Jen Mo[b] as well as the regular tracts, it contained anatomical diagrams of the viscera and charts of the male body, front and back. Thereupon, in +1329, an autochthonous Chinese, Wang Kuo-Jui[4] by name,[c] followed up with a 'jade dragon' manual instead of Hu-Kung-Thai's 'golden orchid'. This was the *Pien Chhio Shen Ying Chen Chiu Yü Lung Ching*,[5] based on the 'marvellously successful principles of Pien Chhio';[d] it was mainly composed of mnemonic verses.[e] Probably the literary expression 'jade dragon' only meant 'infinitely precious'. But a Thang writer of +863 records details of a beautifully carved jade dragon which belonged to Yang Kuang-Hsin[6] in +542; inside it was hollow and could be filled with water, the which, on being poured out, made sounds like music.[f] Another Thang book, of +855, tells a similar story about the emperor Ming Huang (r. +712 to +755); in this case the jade dragon brought beneficial responses when paraded at ceremonies of praying for rain.[g] Perhaps then the jade dragon was just a trope, but the phrase may well have been a conscious allusion to other images which had been filled with water long before the time of Wang Wei-I (p. 131 above). Meanwhile, in +1315, Tu Ssu-Ching[7] had edited a medical work of great value in 19 books, 3 of which were on acupuncture;[h] this is the *Chi Shêng Pa Sui*[8] (Selected

[a] *ICK*, pp. 334–5. The significance of the 'golden orchid' in the title is not clear to us.

[b] Cf. p. 49 above. These had been recognised already in the −1st-century *Nei Ching, Ling Shu*, but were not adopted to make the 'fourteen tracts' until Hua Shou's time (p. 156 below).

[c] He was a *ling i*, or wandering medical pedlar (see Needham (64), p. 265)

[d] *ICK*, p. 336. There was an earlier Yü Lung Ko by a Mr Yang,[9] and Wang Kuo-Jui incorporated it in his own work.

[e] Chhen Pi-Liu & Chêng Cho-Jen (*2*) give ten of these mnemonic stanzas, called *fu*[10] or *ko*.[11]

[f] *Yu-Yang Tsa Tsu*, ch. 10, p. 3*a*.

[g] *Ming Huang Tsa Lu*, cit. in *Lei Shuo*, ch. 16, (p. 1079).

[h] They included *Chen Ching Chieh Yao*,[12] *Chieh-Ku Yün Chhi Chen Fa*,[13] and *Chen Ching Tsê Ying Chi*.[14] Only the last was by Tu Ssu-Ching himself, in all probability; the first was by some unknown author though attributed to Huangfu Mi, and the second was by Chang Chieh-Ku[15] & Chang Pi,[16] written about +1235. In addition, this book reprinted the *Tou Thai-Shih Hsien-sêng Liu Chu Fu*, on which see p. 137 above.

[1] 忽泰必烈 [2] 忽公泰 [3] 金蘭循經取穴圖解 [4] 王國瑞
[5] 扁鵲神應鍼灸玉龍經 [6] 楊光欣 [7] 杜思敬 [8] 濟生拔粹
[9] 楊氏 [10] 賦 [11] 歌 [12] 鍼經節要 [13] 潔古雲岐鍼法
[14] 鍼經摘英集 [15] 張潔古 [16] 張璧

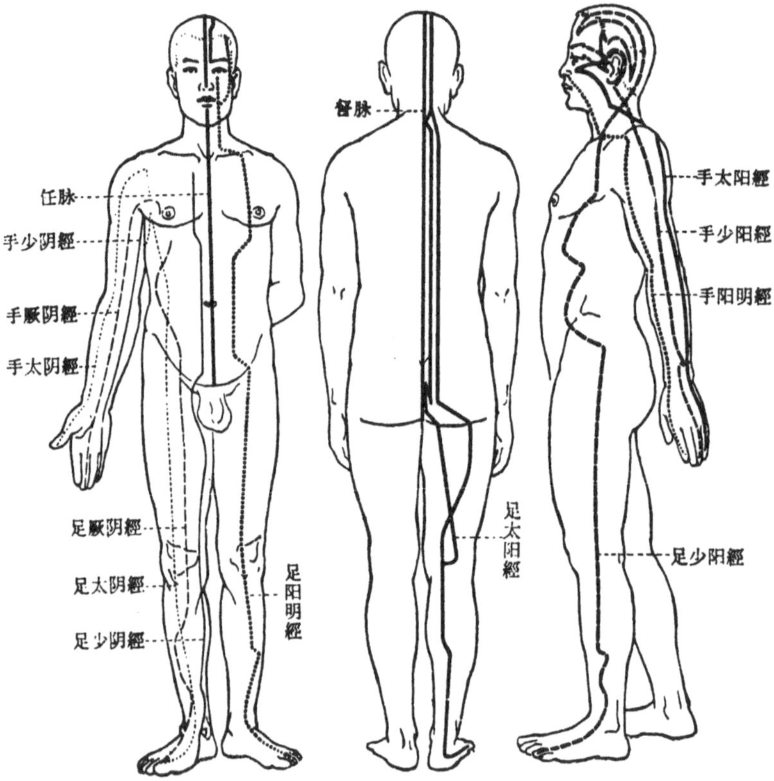

Fig. 32. The fourteen acu-tracts (twelve regular tracts plus Tu Mo and Jen Mo), as described in Hua Shou's book of +1341, *Shih-ssu Ching Fa Hui*. From Anon. (*91*), p. 6.

Materials for the Preservation of Health). He was essentially a traditionalist, but a clear and excellent writer very readable today.

The last great landmark in the Yuan period was the *Shih-Ssu Ching Fa Hui*[1] (Elucidation of the Fourteen Acu-Tracts), by Hua Shou[2] in +1341, an outstanding physician of the late Yuan period (Fig. 32). He was a brother of Liu Chi[3] but changed his name in order to practise medicine.[a] This gives us a link with other aspects of science and technology, for Liu Chi was a Chuko Liang-like figure, a successful military commander interested in astronomy, calendrical science, astrology and geomancy, but also significantly associated with some of the earliest books on gunpowder and gunnery. Hua Shou was the first to use the term *ching hsüeh*[4] instead of *chhi hsüeh*,[5] and he also spoke of *khung hsüeh*,[6] which was always the usual term in Japan.[b] He recognised 657 acu-points and emphasised still further the importance of

[a] Hua Shou was a *ju i* (see Needham, loc. cit.), or scholarly lettered physician. He was the student of Kao Tung-Yang,[7] a very renowned acupuncturist who never wrote a book.

[b] Cf. Yeh Ching-Chhiu (*1*), p. 46.

[1] 十四經發揮 [2] 滑壽 [3] 劉基 [4] 經穴 [5] 氣穴 [6] 孔穴
[7] 高洞陽

the median tracts Tu Mo and Jen Mo, which he saw were the only auxiliary tracts to have named loci of their own. Discussing the most fundamental aspects of the flow of the *chhi*, he spoke of the opening and closing (*khai ho*[1])[a] as it were of valves, along the inter-communicating and ever-branching channels. He also developed theories of reservoirs and spillways, thus once again pointing up the ancient mental connection between pneumatic physiology and hydraulic engineering.

During the Ming dynasty, from +1368 onwards, a certain kind of stratification of social classes tended to harden into two distinct schools or *phai*,[2] sometimes uncannily resembling in their differences the strife between the Fellows of the Royal College of Physicians in London and the unlicensed 'hedge-doctors' who roamed the country-side practising as and where they could.[b] In China these were called *tshao tsê ling i*,[3] the wandering medical pedlars who tinkled their bells on jingling staffs like Buddhists or Taoists as they passed through the village streets and hamlet paths. Their medical (and even surgical) knowledge was handed down within their families from father to son, and even if such a man rose to official rank as a medical official (*i kuan*[4]) he never lost the quality of the *ling i phai*.[5] This he retained even if a famous writer, as in the case of Wang Kuo-Jui, whose book of +1329 we have just mentioned. Another example could be the *Shen Ying Ching*[6] of Chhen Hui[7] & Liu Chin,[8] finished in +1425,[c] though this work had a preface by the great scientific Maecenas of the Ming, the prince Ning Hsien Wang,[9] whom we have met with in many connections in other places, and shall meet with again.[d] To this school also belonged the greatest acupuncture writer of any period, Yang Chi-Chou,[10] active during the last decades of the +16th century (p. 159 below). In general, however, the books of the 'practitioners' (*ling i phai*[5]) were not elegantly written, nor did they always say exactly the same thing, nor did they stick to the classics very closely — but every word of theirs was based directly on clinical experience, and therefore their works remain precious still.

The other school was that of the 'scholar-physicians' (*ju i*[11]). Hua Shou, for instance, with his book of +1341 (p. 156 above), was an imperial cousin even though he changed his name, and like all the other medical scholars, he depended greatly on the previous and the ancient literature—in his case on Sun Ssu-Mo and Wang Thao as well as the classics. The books of the scholarly men were generally clear and easy to understand, with subjects ranged in logical sequence, but they were weaker on the side of practical experience, so that when they made emendations in the received doctrines they were prone to do so according to intuition and not always with the background of first-

[a] These had been technical terms in some of the Warring States philosophies.

[b] Cf. Clark (2) on the history of the College and its competitors, continually suppressed but ever rising anew. We have just been thinking of the great herbalist Nicholas Culpepper (+1616 to +1654), on whom see Arber (3); and an excellent example would be Robert Talbot of Cambridge who secretly introduced quinine (see Duran-Reynals, 1).

[c] *ICK*, pp. 341–2. The *Ssu Khu Chhüan Shu* bibliographers were very superior about this book, saying that the writers were unknown men, talking wildly like Taoists.

[d] *SCC*, Vol. 1, p. 147, Vol. 3, pp. 512–13, Vol. 4, pt. 1, p. 167, pt. 3, pp. 493, 531, Vol. 5, pt. 3, pp. 210–11, Vol. 6, pt. 1.

1 開闔 2 派 3 草澤鈴醫 4 醫官 5 鈴醫派 6 神應經
7 陳會 8 劉瑾 9 寧獻王 10 楊繼洲 11 儒醫

hand personal knowledge.[a] The scholar-physicians flourished more and more as time went on. In the +16th century there was Kao Wu,[1] whose two books, *Chen Chiu Chü Ying*[2] (A Collection of Gems in Acupuncture..., +1529) and *Chen Chiu Chieh Yao*[3] (Important Essentials..., +1537) have conserved an excellent reputation to this day.[b] Kao Wu had a very modern spirit because he always gives rather exact sources for his statements and quotations—as does his contemporary the prince of pharmacists, Li Shih-Chen.[4] Then there was Wang Shih-Shan[5] with his 'Questions and Answers' book, the beautifully written *Chen Chiu Wên Tui*,[6] in +1532.[c] Wang was a scientifically-minded man, who strongly insisted on his ignorance of certain matters, having suffered much from people who pretended to know while in fact not knowing at all. Some of these scholars were close to the imperial court, like Hsü Fêng[7] in +1439, whose compendium of acupuncture and moxibustion, the *Hsü Shih Chen Chiu Ta Chhüan*,[8] was edited by the imperial physicians at the request of the emperor, Chu Chhi-Chen[9] (Ying Tsung[10]), who himself endowed it with a preface of his own.[d]

Here may be mentioned the activities of the Ming in the making of bronze acupuncture statues.[e] The old one of A-Ni-Ko was taken to the palace about +1370, and a new one cast in +1443, i.e. in the Chêng-Thung reign-period, when acupuncture texts were being carved on stone tablets at the capital (p. 133 above), and the emperor was himself composing prefaces for medical books.[f] Then in the following century statues were needed again, perhaps because of the spread of instruction and examination, so around +1537 or a little later Kao Wu organised the casting of three figures, a man, a woman and a boy.[g]

As we leave the +16th century, a word may be given to a much admired epitome of diseases and acu-points relative to them, entitled *Pai Chêng Fu*[11] (Ode on the Hundred Syndromes).[h] This was included by Kao Wu in his *Chen Chiu Chü Ying*, and most probably written by him.[i] Then comes a work of uncertain authorship, entitled *Hsün Ching Khao Hsüeh Pien*[12] (An Investigation of the Loci along the Tracts), probably by Yen Chen-Shih[13] and not before +1575 as it quotes no work later than the Wan-Li reign period. It is noteworthy for some very interesting diagrammatic pictures of the expanding or contracting module coordinate system discussed above (p. 124), cf. Fig. 33.[j] Lastly we come to the treatise still of the highest usefulness

[a] On the characterisation of the two schools here see further in Hsieh Li-Hêng (*1*), pp. 32*b* ff.

[b] See *ICK*, p. 345 and Anon. (*83*), p. 103. Kao Wu was active in the bronze figure field, too.

[c] *ICK*, pp. 344–5. Wang was representative of the view that acupuncture could cure plerotic diseases of excess very well, but not eremotic diseases of insufficiency. Further, it could supplement drugs and potions, reaching places which they could not. This contradicted a more obvious idea, and showed an appreciation of the role of the nervous system, as we should say.

[d] Cf. *ICK*, p. 351; Li Thao (*10*), p. 58; Chhêng Tan-An (*2*), p. 15.

[e] Li Yuan-Chi (*1*).

[f] A reproduction of this bronze statue is figured in Anon. (135), pl. 1.

[g] *TSCC*, *I shu tien*, *I pu*, ch. 532, in *tshê* 465, (p. 32.2).

[h] A modern explanation will be found in Chhen Pi-Liu & Chêng Cho-Jen (*2*), p. 128.

[i] Ch. 4A, (p. 241).

[j] Towards the end of vol. 2, (pp. 371 ff.).

1 高武 2 鍼灸聚英 3 鍼灸節要 4 李時珍 5 汪石山
6 鍼灸問對 7 徐鳳 8 徐氏鍼灸大全 9 朱祁鎮 10 英宗
11 百症賦 12 循經考穴編 13 嚴振識

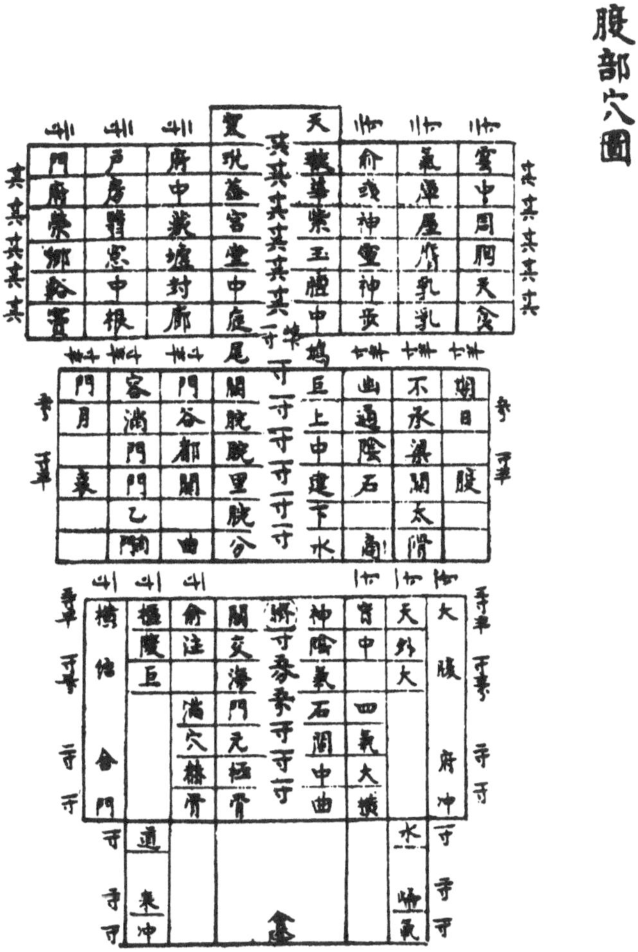

Fig. 33. Another module diagram from the *Hsün Ching Khao Hsüeh Pien* of *c.* +1580. The anterior aspect of the body, divided horizontally at the base of the sternum and at the umbilicus. Many measurements are given, e.g. horizontally (laterally) 2 ins., 1·5 ins. etc. and vertically 1·6 ins., 0·5 ins. and so on. These were the standard distances from which the relative inches were derived.

today, the *Chen Chiu Ta Chhêng*[1] of +1601, the work of Yang Chi-Chou[2].[a] This book, which had various other titles at different stages of its composition, parallels the *Pên Tshao Kang Mu* (+1596) as the acme of a tradition;[b] there was never anything as good later. Though Yang was a *ling i* rather than a *ju i*, he was fairly scrupulous in playing down his own personal discoveries, and on the stylistic side there was nothing for reproach; perhaps one could almost say that he synthesised the two schools or traditions in himself.

[a] Identical, we believe, with Yang Chi-Shih.[3] His grandfather had been a Thai I[4] or Director of the Imperial Medical Service, so there was a family tradition of medicine.

[b] Cf. Anon. (*83*), p. 104; *ICK*, pp. 351–2; Li Thao (*10*), p. 58. Massage is included in ch. 10.

[1] 鍼灸大成 [2] 楊繼洲 [3] 楊濟時 [4] 太醫

After this, the whole of the Chhing period constitutes nothing so much as an anti-climax in this field. When Hsü Ling-Thai[1] wrote his interesting survey of the history of Chinese medicine in +1757, he had to speak of acupuncture as rather a lost art, for there were then left very few experts in it, and young physicians were at a loss to find teachers who could instruct them in it. And yet it never died out altogether. Hsü Ling-Thai listed the many ways in which failures could have come about, insufficient attention to the proper time at which it should be done, carelessness in the selection of the acu-point to be used and its inexact localisation, finally inattention to the way the needle should be inserted and the hand-movements which should be applied to it. Moxibustion fared much better, and in the +18th century there were a good many practitioners using it,[a] but pharmacy and oral medication were overwhelmingly dominant at this time, and when scholars like Hsü surveyed the ancient and medieval literature they were astonished to see how great a part acupuncture had played in it. A number of reasons have been given for the decline of the art. Perhaps from the beginning of the Manchu régime onwards an upsurge of vulgar Confucianism encouraged a fear of doing damage to the sacred body bestowed on one by one's parents; and to this misplaced filial piety the same trend added a strangely Victorian prudery, since acupuncture and moxa required the baring of the body, and this was anathema to the ultra-Confucian moralists.[b] Perhaps these influences were something of a distorted nationalist reaction to the foreign-ness of the Manchu ruling classes. In any case the nadir was reached in 1822, when an edict forbade the teaching of these subjects in the Imperial Medical College, the Thai I Yuan,[2] because even the slightest exposure was 'an injury to propriety and refinement (*yu shang ta ya*[3])'.[c] Nevertheless there were always a few books on acupuncture during these times, for example the *Ming Thang Ta Tao Lu*[4] (Broad Outline of the Microcosm) by Hui Tung,[5] with which we may close our bibliography.

Finally, it would be in order here to review the successive bronze statues from the Sung onwards which in some sense recorded surface anatomy and the location of the acu-points. As we have seen, the tradition was started by Wang Wei-I in +1027, and

[a] Could not a parallel be drawn here perhaps between the gradual triumph of *nei tan*[6] over *wai tan*[7] alchemy? See *SCC*, Vol. 5, pt. 3, pp. 200–1, 206–7, 218–19.

[b] Hence also, of course, the prevalence of the little ivory statuettes on which a female patient could point out to the physician the site of her pain.

[c] Anon. (*90*), p. 20; Li Yuan-Chi (*1*), p. 4, repr. in Chhêng Tan-An (*3*). But the doctorate in acupuncture and moxa (*chen chiu po shih*[8]) had started in the Thang period (Lu Gwei-Djen & Needham (2), also in Needham (64), p. 388); and this speciality (*kho*[9]) had been one of nine in the +12th century, and one of thirteen in the +13th (Needham (64), p. 392). So great an inheritance, therefore, could not easily be abandoned, and once again, in 1908, on the orders of the Manchu statesman Tuan Fang,[10] acupuncture and moxa were excluded from the official medical examinations. Finally in 1922 the Kuomintang decreed (with total ineffectiveness) the abolition of all Chinese traditional medicine. This recalls the earlier official prohibition of Chinese traditional medicine in Japan in 1876, also very ineffective. In 1884 a further law restricted medical practice to those with modern-Western qualifications, but in the following year, as a response to strong professional and popular pressure, a licensing system for Chinese-traditional practitioners was established. In 1918, after a report by the Ministry of Education, acupuncture and moxibustion were declared officially rejected. Yet still the system did not die. Cf. Hashimoto Masae (*1*), p. 51; Homma Shōhaku (*1*), p. 4.

1 徐靈胎　2 太醫院　3 有傷大雅　4 明堂大道錄　5 惠棟
6 內丹　7 外丹　8 針灸博士　9 科　10 端方

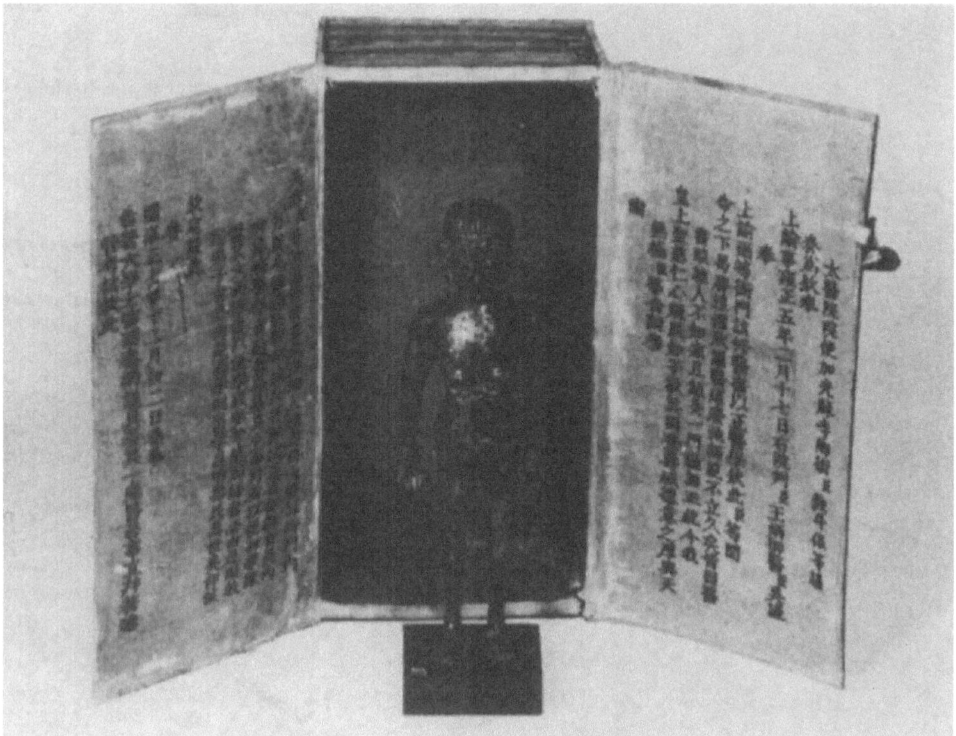

Fig. 34. Bronze acupuncture figure 10·25 ins. in height, with its box covered in yellow silk. This is one of a number made according to an imperial decree in +1727, the text of which is recorded within the two lids of the box, together with details of the court physicians who were to receive the figures. The Imperial Medical Administration (Thai I Yuan) was ordered to have the figures cast so as to promote the study of medicine and especially that branch of it known as acupuncture. Photo: Wellcome Medical Museum, London.

the location of both his figures at Khaifêng was recorded in almost contemporary sources. The Chin Tartars wanted one of these in +1128, if not both, but even if they got one it was recovered by Khubilai Khan (Shih Tsu) when he organised the removal of the capital to Peking around +1290. In the meantime, in +1265, he had had the Yuan statue cast by A-Ni-Ko, so that for a time at least there must have been three, for we hear of this last as still existing in +1370. During the Ming, another was added under Ying Tsung in +1443 (Fig. 27), and finally in or around +1537 Kao Wu arranged for three new ones, a man, a woman and a boy. In +1727 a series of small bronze models (Fig. 34) was made for the imperial physicians,[a] and about that time a full-size one was kept in the Yao Wang Miao[1] (Temple of Medical Deities) at Peking.

[a] Doctors of less exalted sort made do until quite recent times with jointed wooden puppets like dolls on which the acu-points and tracts were inscribed. One of these is described and figured by van Vloten (1), p. 15.

[1] 藥王廟

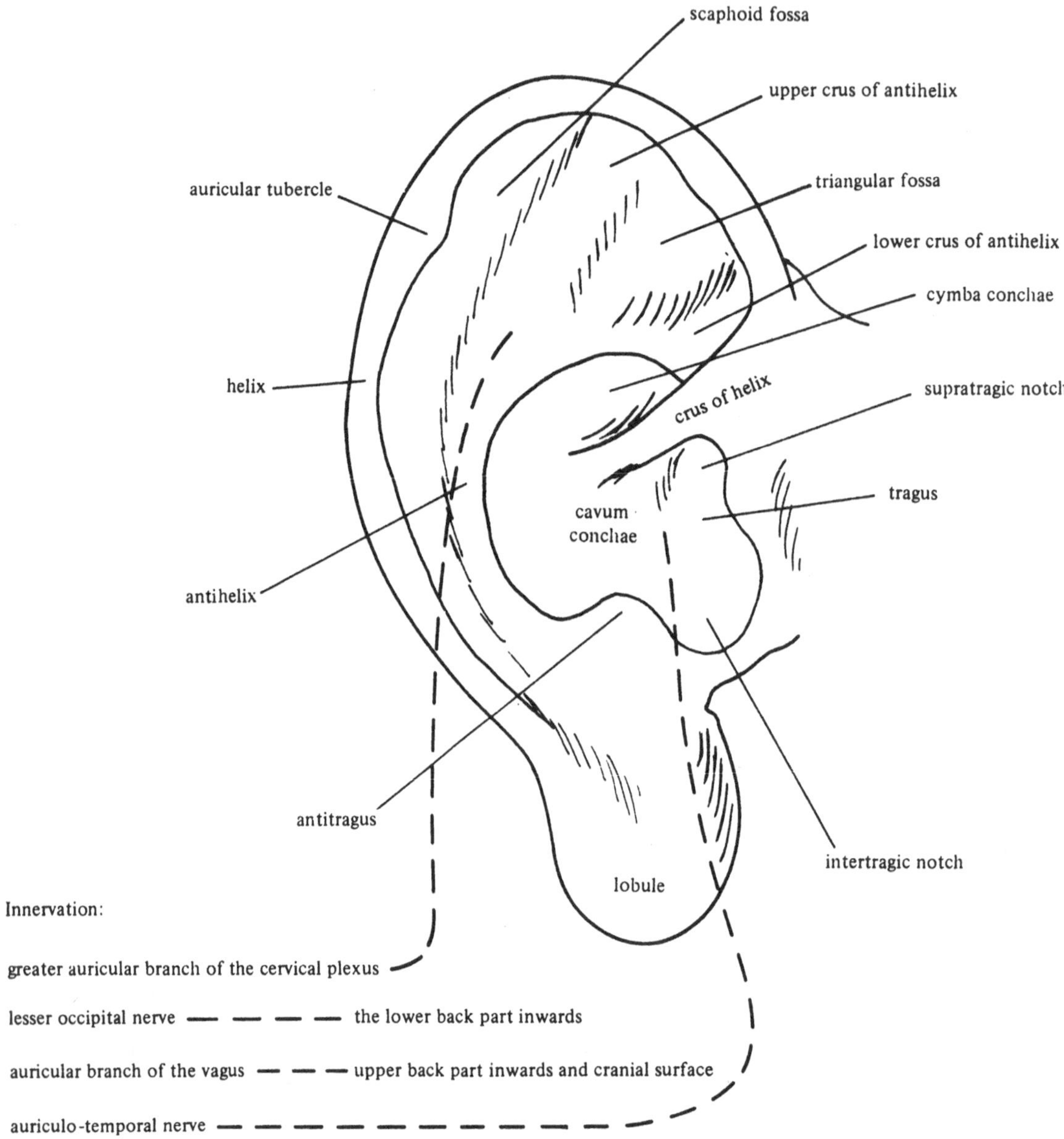

Fig. 35. Anatomical nomenclature of the auricula or external ear.

It is believed that later copies were made in Japan, notably in +1797 and again in 1934 and 1941.[a]

Opinions differ considerably on the present locations of all these historic examples of medical art. Hsieh Li-Hêng (*1*) saw one ancient-looking bronze figure in the Yen Tê Tien[1] hall of the Palace Museum in Peking in 1934. Although it was only 4 ft. high, it consisted of two castings joined along the edges, just as Wang Wei-I's was, but there was no sign of viscera models. Chhen Pang-Hsien believes that one of Wang's was lost in the +12th or +13th century, and the other taken to Japan during the upheavals of 1900.[b] Two Thung Jen are in the Tokyo Museum today, but the history of them is very confused. According to Chhen Tshun-Jen (*4*), who made a special study of the matter, the catalogue of the Pacific Science Congress of 1925 said that one was cast in +1663 and the other made in Japan and presented to the emperor in +1797. But there are no Chinese records of a casting in the former year. One of the figures is of rather thick bronze plate, empty inside, and consisting of ten segments joined together with fine copper wire, the positions of the points being engraved without holes. The other resembles in many ways what we know of Wang Wei-I's design. Could it be perhaps the original one from the Sung period?

In any case, such bronze acupuncture figures keep on turning up. In 1959 an old traditional physician, Shen Hsiao-Chai of Paoting, presented to the government a statuette of this kind which had been preserved in his family and was considered to be some five centuries old. In Kuomintang days it had been kept in a hollow wall, and during the Japanese occupation it had been buried. If the dating was anything like right, this figure must have been cast in the Ming period, and would therefore belong among those mentioned already on p. 133 above.[c]

As we end this historical sub-section the thought which comes most to mind is that China is a living civilisation, not a dead one, so that all her traditional arts and techniques are at this day in lively development; and acupuncture is by no means an exception. Here too, and in other domains of medicine, there has been an adoption of folk practices which never received much mention in the works of the learned,[d] side by side with entirely new devices hitherto unheard of. To begin with, there has been a considerable increase in the number of acu-points not on any of the tracts (the *chhi hsüeh*,[2] cf. p. 52 above). An authoritative contemporary source lists them now as follows:[e]

head and neck, esp. face	13 points
thorax and abdomen	3
lumbo-dorsal region	32
arms and hands	9
legs and feet	6
	63

[a] At the present day plastic is very widely used for making these figures, sometimes transparent for the medical schools, sometimes quite small-scale, for the use of the general Chinese population.

[b] (*1*), 2nd ed., pp. 188–9. The loss at this date is affirmed in the history of the Imperial Medical College, *Thai I Yuan Chih*.[3]

[c] Anon. (119), p. 104.

[d] One instance of this would be the various forms of finger pressure; cf. p. 212.

[e] Anon. (135), pp. 204 ff. Anon. (*123*) has many more.

[1] 延德殿 [2] 奇穴 [3] 太醫院誌

They have been found valuable in a great variety of diseases such as migraine, trigeminal neuralgia, glaucoma, thrush, epilepsy and various psycho-pathological disorders. Another advance has been the increased use of multiple-needle acupuncture.[a] Here five or seven needles are fixed into a light hammer head and tapped at one locus or another with varying degrees of strength or delicacy. Although the *mei hua chen*[1] (plum-blossom cluster) and the *chhi hsing chen*[2] (seven stars cluster) are not essentially new inventions, they have taken a more prominent position, and are widely used since 'most of the diseases which respond to acupuncture' can be treated in this way.[b] Then electro-acupuncture, the therapeutic use of weak currents instead of the manual motion of the needle by the acupuncturist, has entered into regular use.[c] And in some cases the needles are allowed to remain in position, stimulating the nerve-endings for as long as a week at a time; this intra-dermal embedding is accomplished by small devices something like drawing-pins.[d]

But the strangest and most spectacular development in therapeutic acupuncture of recent years has been the exploration of the auricula or external ear, both for therapy and diagnosis.[e] The claim is made, both in East and West, that the musculature of the outer ear has connections with all the other parts of the body, a somewhat distorted image of which can indeed be superimposed on its plan.[f] The usual anatomical nomenclature of the parts of the auricula is shown in Fig. 35; generally speaking the lay-out of sensitive points on its surface simulates the form of a foetus within the uterus, upside down, with the neck region below and the gluteal area and lower limbs at the top (Fig. 36*a*, *b*, *c*, *d*). The correlation is as follows (cf. Fig. 37*a*, *b*):

lobule	facial region, eyes, etc.
antitragus	head and neck
tragus	inner nose, throat, adrenal gland
supratragic notch	external ear
crus of helix	diaphragm
antihelix	spinal column, thorax, abdomen
upper crus of antihelix	lower limbs and feet
lower crus of antihelix	gluteal region
triangular fossa	genital organs
tubercle of helix	hand
scaphoid fossa	upper limbs and hands
intertragic notch	ovary
cymba conchae	liver, gall-bladder, spleen, kidney, bladder, pancreas
cavum conchae	heart, lungs, *san chiao*
grooves under crus of helix	intestinal tract
cranial surface of auricula	back

[a] See especially Anon. (*173*); Wu I-Chhing (*1*).

[b] Anon. (135), pp. 23 ff. Cf. p. 130.

[c] Anon. (135), pp. 26–7. We speak elsewhere of the beginnings of this (pp. 188, 214).

[d] Anon. (135), p. 27.

[e] The most succinct recent explanation in a Western language is that of Anon. (135), pp. 269 ff. See also Anon. (*123*), pp. 348 ff.

[f] No more so, however, than the sensory and motor 'homunculi' of Penfield & Rasmussen (1), reproduced in Clarke & Dewhurst (1), p. 128.

[1] 梅花針 [2] 七星針

Some 72 acu-points have been recognised all over the auricula; generically they are called *fan ying tien*[1] (resonance points), and most of them are named after the parts of the body to which they relate. Some have special names, however, such as Phing-chhuan,[2] the anti-asthma point on the antitragus, or the Shen-mên[3] of the ear at the tip of the triangular fossa. A few of them have strongly analgesic properties. For diagnosis the physician seeks the points of maximum pain when tested by a probe or pinhead, alternatively a probe-electrode may be used, taking readings on an ammeter (cf. p. 187). Thence conclusions may be drawn for combining with other observations to establish the nature of the illness.

At first sight it would seem incomprehensible how an apparently unimportant appendage could have such relations with all the other parts of the body. However, its innervation is exceptionally complicated, coming from four main sources—the greater auricular branch of the cervical plexus, the lesser occipital nerve, the auricular branch of the vagus, and the auriculo-temporal nerve. It may not be inconceivable, therefore, that the neurons in these trunks should have intra-cerebral connections with centres in several different parts of the brain, each directly related with even the more remote parts of the body.

The origins of the system are also a little obscure. It is true that in the *Nei Ching, Ling Shu* it is said that all the *mo* meet at the ear;[a] and both there[b] and in the *Nan Ching*[c] there are not a few references to acupuncture at or near the ears for deafness, tinnitus, and the like; but there is nothing approaching the elaboration of modern times. Similar recommendations occur in Thang and later texts.[d] The modern movement seems to have started almost simultaneously in China and Europe, for a French physician, Nogier (1, 2), began to work the system out around 1956,[e] and the Chinese development was not very much earlier.[f] The former seems to have been influenced by isolated empirical records of ancient and medieval surgeons,[g] while the latter drew inspiration no doubt from the Chinese medical classics.

It only remains to mention a few more techniques which have arisen in the Chinese practice of acupuncture, some derived perhaps in part from Western stimuli. For example there has grown up a practice of hypodermic injections at acu-points, often the *ah shih hsüeh*, or places where there is tenderness on palpation.[h] Among the solutions injected are placental extracts, vitamins, antibiotics, and various traditional Chinese plant drugs,[i] not omitting distilled water—which is very reminiscent of a

[a] *NCLS/MC*, ch. 28, (p. 1148).

[b] *NCLS*, chs. 4, 10, 16 and 28. So also *NCSW/PH*, ch. 63, (p. 338), mentioning IG 1, 4 and 19.

[c] Ch. 40.

[d] *Pei Chi Chhien Chin Yao Fang*, ch. 29, (p. 511); *Chhien Chin I Fang*, ch. 26 (p. 316).

[e] His first three German papers of 1957 were quickly translated into Chinese, by Yeh Hsiao-Lin (*1*). We now have his book on 'auriculo-therapy', Nogier (3). See also König (1).

[f] Among the best handbooks of it in Chinese are Anon. (*119*) and (*164*, *165*, *169*). A clinical report of 800 cases is given by Huang Hsien-Ming *et al.* (*1*).

[g] And not least by a rural healer in south-eastern France, who about 1950 cured many cases of sciatica by cautery applied to the external ear.

[h] See Anon. (135), pp. 280ff.

[i] Notably extracts of the flowers of *Carthamus tinctorius* (*hung hua*[4]), see Anon. (*110*), p. 260, pl. 151. Also the roots of angelica species: *A. dahuricus* (*pai chih*[5]), op. cit., p. 27, pl. 4; *A. pubescens* (*tu huo*[6]), p. 178, pl. 103; *A. polymorpha* = *sinensis* (*tang kuei*[7]), p. 395, pl. 177.

[1] 反應點 [2] 平喘 [3] 耳神門 [4] 紅花 [5] 白芷 [6] 獨活 [7] 當歸

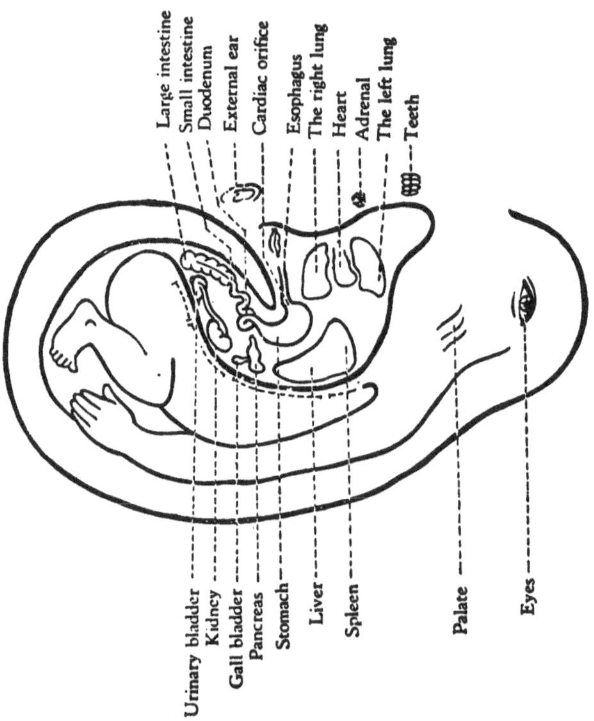

Fig. 36*b*. See legend on p. 167.

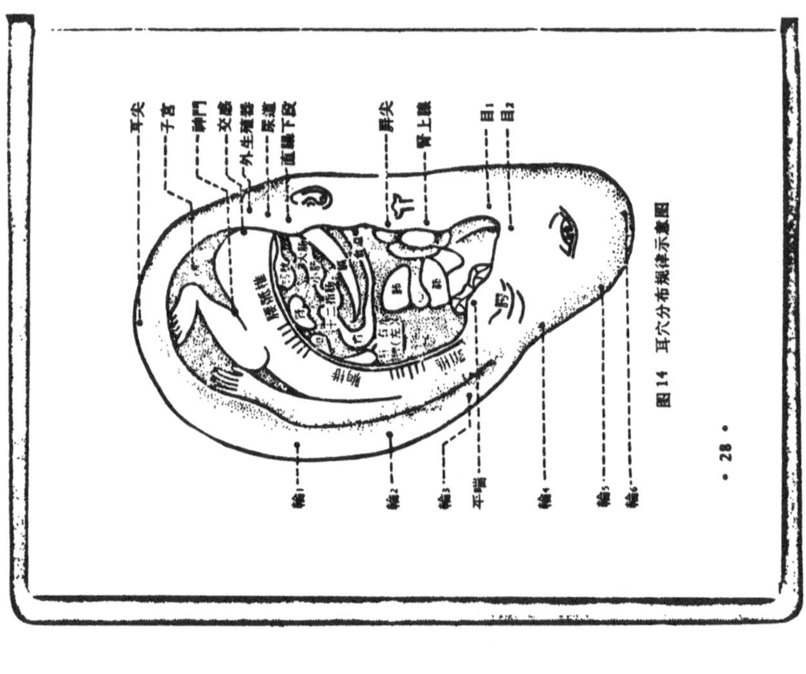

Fig. 36*a*. See legend on p. 167.

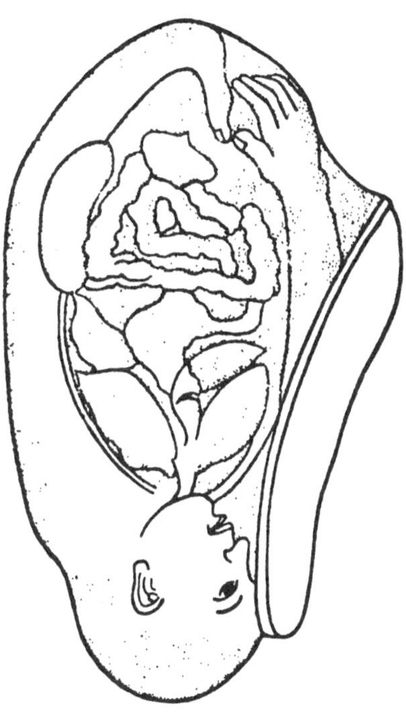

图16 耳背治疗示意图

Fig. 36*c*

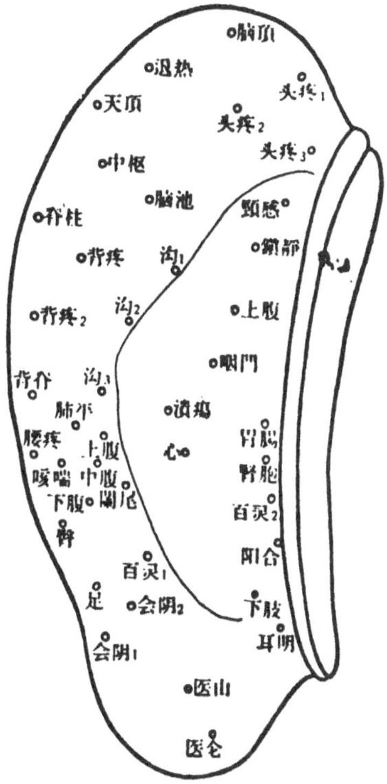

图 17 耳背穴位图

Fig. 36*d*

Fig. 36. (*a*) Front of external ear, showing some of the recently identified acu-points, and the inverted foetus simulacrum (Anon. *119*). (*b*) The same, with the corresponding parts of the body marked in English (Anon. 135). (*c*) The back of the auricula, showing the inverted foetus simulacrum (Anon. *119*). (*d*) Recently identified acu-points on the back of the external ear (Anon. *119*).

treatment which grew up in Europe earlier in the present century (cf. p. 209). Another new method consists of 'strong stimulation' at points where pain or tenderness is felt, extending to the actual 'massage' of principal peripheral nerves by forceps.[a] This is done under local anaesthesia, and is said to be effective in restoring voluntary motion after poliomyelitis and in post-meningitic paralysis. Lastly the old counter-irritation techniques of the West have been resumed in a new form in China by using sterilised catgut as a mild seton (cf. p. 244), especially at acu-points.[b] Western antecedents (barbarous though they were) are here acknowledged, and the procedure is said to be quite effective in gastric or duodenal ulcer, bronchial asthma, back and leg pain, etc. All in all, it is clear that acupuncture in China is very much alive, and even in a state of ferment quite apart from the remarkable story of acupuncture analgesia which we shall discuss in detail presently.

[a] Anon. (135), pp. 283 ff.

[b] Anon. (135), pp. 289 ff.

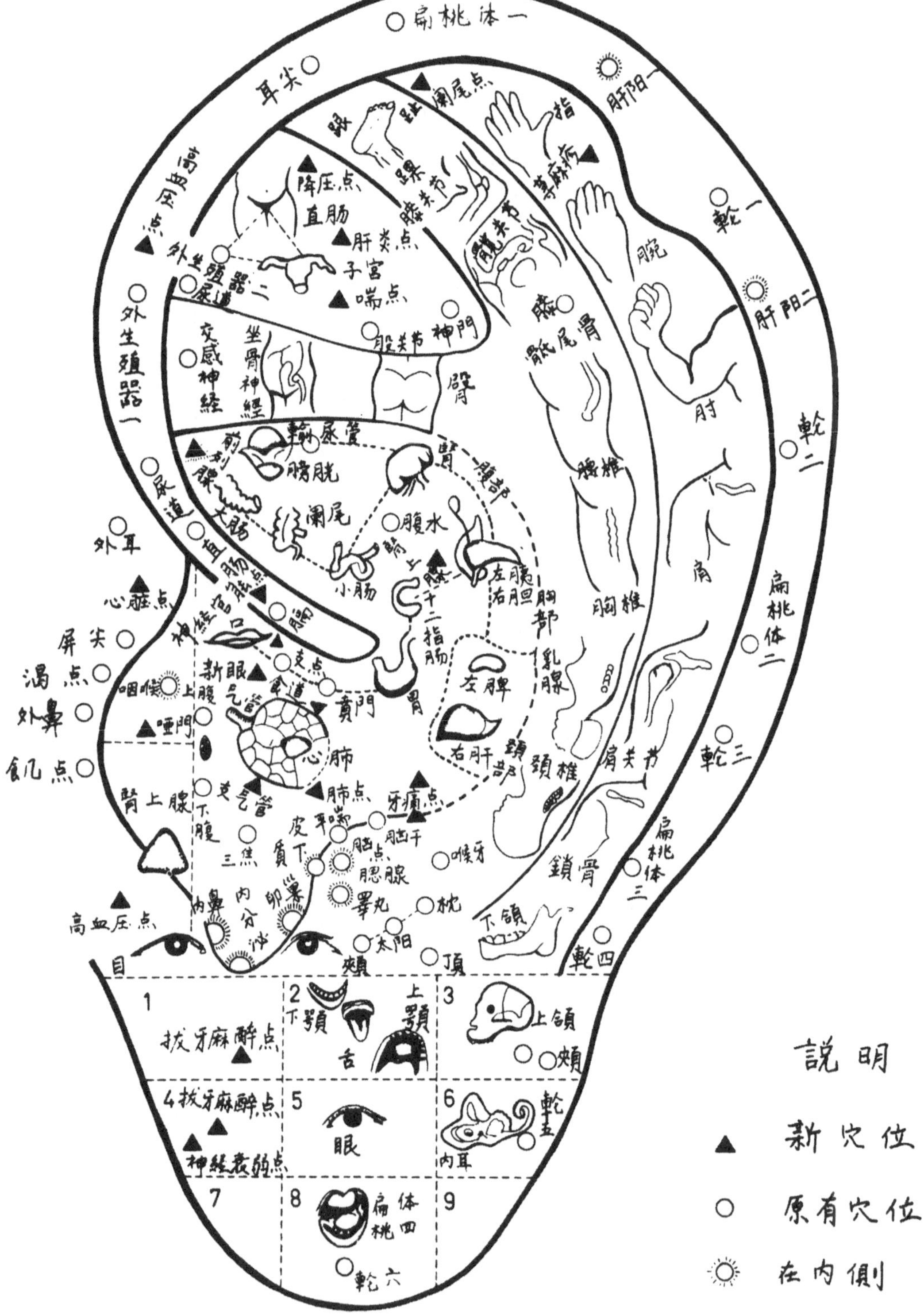

Fig. 37*a*. See legend on p. 169.

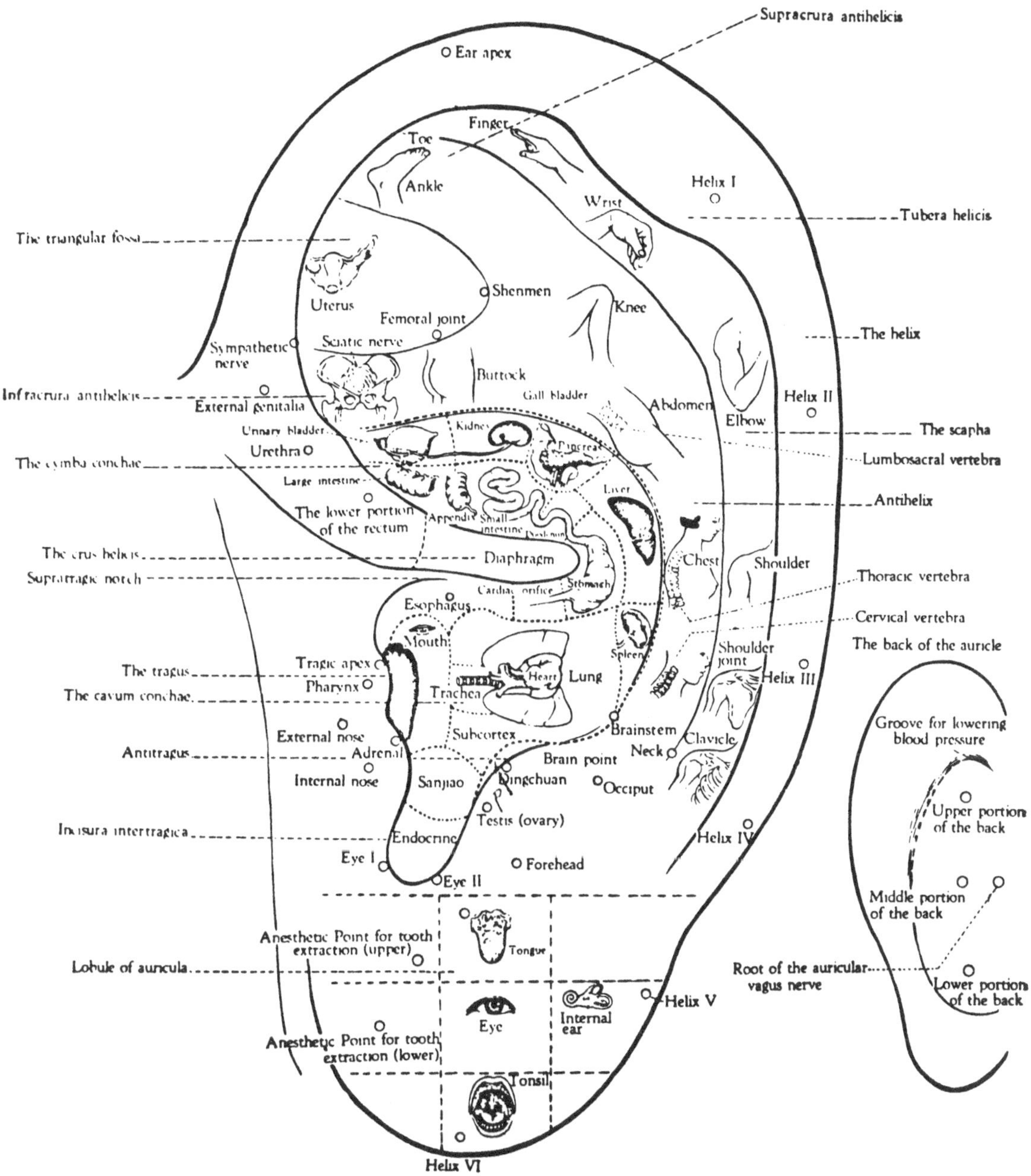

Fig. 37*b*

Fig. 37. (*a*) Front of external ear, with acu-points marked and indications of which part of the body they affect (photo: Prof. P. Lisowski, Dept of Anatomy, University of Hongkong). (*b*) Approximate translation of the preceding diagram (Anon. *135*).

(4) Moxibustion

The ancients said that a man who understands drugs but does not know acupuncture, or one who knows acupuncture but does not know moxa, can never make a real physician (*shang i*[1]). Truly moxibustion and acupuncture are the most important of the techniques.

So wrote Chin Li-Mêng,[2] the author of the preface to the *Chen Chiu Tsê Jih Pien*[3] (On the Choice of Days and Times for Acupuncture and Moxa) in +1447, and his judgment was that of most mainstream practitioners of Chinese medicine through the centuries. Here we recur to the very first page of this monograph, where a brief definition of moxa heat-treatment and cautery accompanied our explanation of what was meant by acupuncture. Moxibustion[a] is the burning of *Artemisia* tinder (*ai*[4]), generally shaped into cones, which may or may not be placed directly on the skin so as to give rise to an eschar, but also held in the form of cigar-like sticks some little distance away from the body surface, so that a mild treatment with radiant heat can be applied. The traditional term for the process was *ai jung chiu*[5].[b] As we shall see, the points of choice for moxa application usually coincided with acu-points, though not always; and moxa was regarded in general as most appropriate for chronic diseases while acupuncture was preferred for acute ones.

Moxibustion, or the burning of moxa, necessarily comes under the rubric of counter-irritation.[c] That it can relieve pain of nearly all kinds is relatively easy to understand, especially in the light of the facts and interpretations which we shall bring forward later on (pp. 244ff.) in the discussion of the physiology and neurophysiology of acupuncture, both for therapy and for analgesia; and if the cortical recognition of pain is inhibited then many reflex reactions to it will be inhibited also, thereby perhaps affording the natural healing powers of the body an opportunity for acting upon the pathogenic agent or the malfunction which is causing the pain. The induction of slight inflammation, too, may stimulate phagocytosis; and the small running sores produced by moxa may activate the ACTH axis and raise the cortisone levels of the blood.[d]

Let us now say something of the classical doctrine of the preparation and properties

[a] The etymology of the word moxa will be discussed presently in connection with the early transmission of these techniques to Europe (p. 291 below).

[b] Lexicographers give *chiao*,[6] but one never encounters it in the medical literature. Originally it meant a torch, and the glowing rod also which the diviners applied to the oracle-bones (cf. *SCC*, Vol. 1, p. 84).

[c] Cf. Brockbank (1), pp. 105ff.

[d] A great deal of research on the physiology of moxibustion, following the lead of Miura Kinnosuke, has been done in Japanese (and to a lesser extent, Chinese) laboratories in recent years, but the results have not as yet been very conclusive. Effects on red and white blood corpuscle counts, agglutinin titres, antibody formation, the onset and arrest of inflammation and suppuration, etc., etc., have all been measured and reported. Full accounts of the findings can be found in Hara Shimetarō (*1*); Chang Shih-Piao (*1*); and Chhêng Tan-An (*1*), pp. 44ff.; Anon. (*123*), pp. 399ff. We have not come across any notable résumé of this field of work in a Western language.

1 上醫 2 金禮蒙 3 針灸擇日編 4 艾 5 艾絨灸
6 燋

of moxa.[a] *Chhi ai*,[1] i.e. *Artemisia* spp.,[b] from Chhichow in Hupei (Li Shih-Chen's birthplace, incidentally), was generally considered to be the best, collected during the fifth month of the Chinese calendar and thoroughly dried.[c] The leaves were then ground to a fine powdery material, fibrous because of the white hairs on their under surface, greyish in colour and resembling cotton floss — this is the *ai jung*[2] or *shu ai*.[3] Since the leaves contain a yellowish-green oil, it is necessary to expose the tinder to strong sunlight for several days so that the oil evaporates; if this were not done the moxa would be consumed too fast and would cause more pain to the patient. The tinder is kept in dry air-tight containers for as long as possible before use. The unanimous testimony of moxibustionists is that although pain is produced when the tinder burns down to the skin, it is not a really unpleasant pain, and indeed leaves the subject with a deep glowing sensation (*chhang khuai*,[4] *khuai kan*[5]), a feeling of well-being, analogous to the subjective responses characteristic of acupuncture (cf. p. 192). This cannot bo reproduced with burning tobacco, wood, cotton or similar substances, nor by localised application of steam heat or electrical devices. Sakamoto Mitsugi and other Japanese experts are inclined to think that some active principle is absorbed from the burning moxa, just as we know that doses of nicotine are absorbed from glowing cigarettes or cigars even though most of the alkaloid must be lost in the ash of the glowing tip. At any rate no other substance will give the pleasant feeling of relief which is given by moxa. As for the eschars produced, all the Chinese books provide prescriptions for washing lotions and plasters to take care of the burns if they prove troublesome to heal.

The moxa can be as large as a cigar or as small as a grain of millet. But often it was desired to apply the stimulus of a heat treatment only, without actual cautery, and this was called *wên chiu*[6] (warming moxibustion), or formerly *wu pan hên chiu*,[7] i.e. moxa that left no scar on the skin.[d] The classical way of doing this was to use a layer of some vegetable substance between the skin and the burning incense-like cone.[e] One technique was to have it burn down on a layer of soya-bean paste (*tou chiang chiu*[8]); or else a slice of garlic, or a slice of ginger (*ko suan chiu*,[9] *kong chia chiu*[10]), could be interposed.[f] Such heat treatment would supposedly first constrict and then dilate the

[a] One of the best accounts of this is to be found in Chhêng Tan-An (*1*), pp. 33 ff. Cf. Morohashi dict., vol. 9, p. 516.

[b] In *SCC*, Vol. 1, Fig. 29, opp. p. 164, we reproduced the drawing of *Artemisia alba* (*pai ai*[11]) from Li Shih-Chen's *Pên Tshao Kang Mu*. The modern name is *A. argyi* (Anon. (*109*), Vol. 4, p. 541). *A. vulgaris, var. indica* (R 9; Khung Chhing-Lai *et al.* (*1*), p. 298; CC 17; BII/77, 429) is another abandoned specific name. The mugwort is mentioned in some of the oldest Chinese texts, such as the *Shih Ching* (Book of Odes), I, (6), viii, 3 (cf. Legge (8), vol. 1, p. 120; Waley (1), p. 48; Karlgren (14), p. 49; Mao no. 72) but not in a specifically medical context.

[c] *PTKM*, ch. 15, (p. 7), cites various authorities as prescribing either the third day of the third month or the fifth of the fifth.

[d] Good modern descriptions are in Chang Shih-Piao (*1*), ch. 4, pp. 8, 9 and Chu Lien (*1*), ch. 3, pp. 67–9.

[e] Cf. *CCTC*, ch. 9, (p. 291.2) which, at the end of the +16th century, recommends a dried paste made of flour and the ground seeds of *Croton tiglium*.

[f] Anon. (*201*), a collection of 'hedge-doctor' practices, reports the use of layers of a certain kind of paper.

[1] 蘄艾 [2] 艾絨 [3] 熟艾 [4] 暢快 [5] 快感 [6] 溫灸
[7] 無瘢痕灸 [8] 豆醬灸 [9] 隔蒜灸 [10] 隔薑灸 [11] 白艾

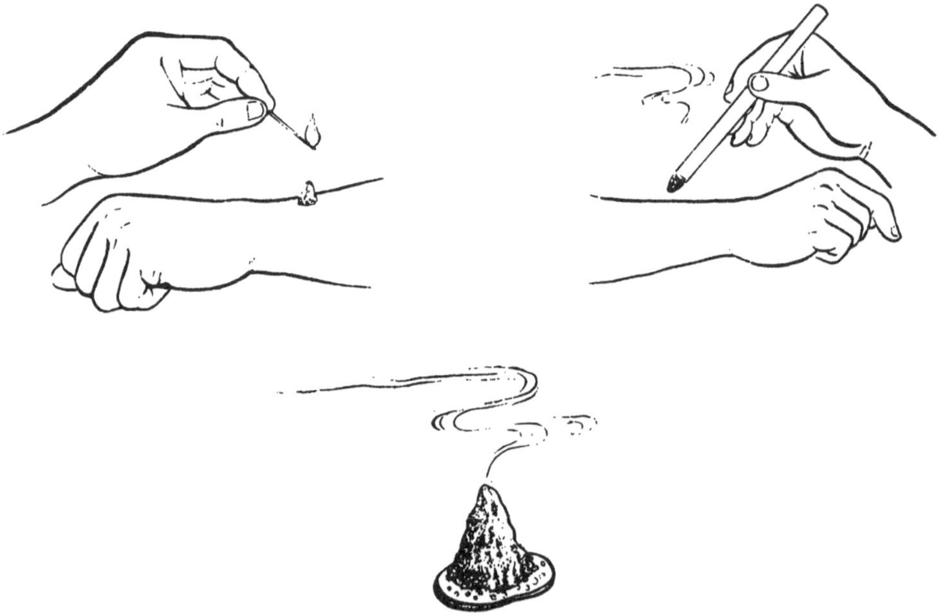

Fig. 38. Techniques of direct and indirect moxibustion (from Anon. *135*). (*a*) Direct moxibustion with an *Artemisia* tinder cone. In scarring moxa the cone was allowed to burn down to the skin, raising a blister or pustule and leaving a scar. In non-scarring moxa the cone is removed as soon as the patient experiences slight scorching pain, and the process is repeated (top left). (*b*) Indirect moxa with a layer of ginger, garlic or other vegetable tissue interposed between the cone and the skin (bottom). A layer of salt is also sometimes used. (*c*) Indirect moxa with the cylindrical moxa stick (top right). With these different methods moxa can vary from cautery to mild heat treatment.

blood-vessels, act as a stimulus to numb or paralysed regions, exert a tranquillising effect on irritated nerve-endings, and protect against bacterial infection. These were medieval procedures, but during the nineteenth century the practice grew up of burning the moxa within a paper covering like an elongated cheroot, and making passes with this over the area to be treated (Fig. 38); this is known as *ya chiu*,[1] and is widely used today.[a] The old books contain some curious traditions about the way in which moxa cones should be lighted,[b] best from a burning-glass or burning-mirror held in the sun's rays,[c] alternatively by the aid of a moxa stalk itself lit from a flame of sesame oil, or else by that of a wax candle; splints of pine, cypress and other woods were not recommended.

Although moxibustion was considered to need less skill than acupuncture,[d] it was

[a] Cf. Chu Lien (*1*), p. 69.

[b] *CCCY*, ch. 3, (pp. 201–2); *CCTC*, ch. 9, (p. 293.2). Both quote an ancient book with the title: *Ming Thang Hsia Ching*.[2]

[c] Cf. *SCC*, Vol. 4, pt. 1, pp. 87 ff. One of the synonyms of *Artemisia* moxa is *ping thai*,[3] nicely explained by statements in *PTKM*, ch. 15, (p. 7), that the ancients ignited the tinder with the use of rays concentrated through a burning-glass made of ice.

[d] See Hsieh Li-Hêng (*1*), p. 32*a*.

[1] 押灸 [2] 明堂下經 [3] 冰臺

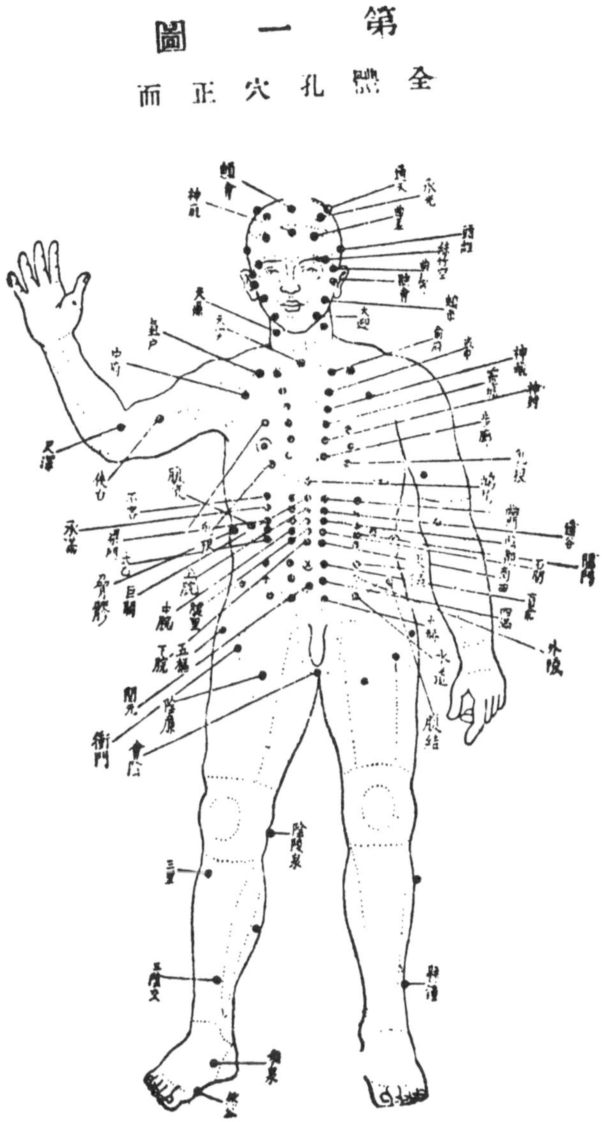

Fig. 39. Moxa spot diagram for the front of the body, from Chang Shih-Piao (*1*), ch. 4, p. 13.

essential that the cautery or thermal treatment should be applied at the right loci.[a] These were not all the same as the classical acu-points, though the great majority of them were. Figs. 39, 40 show the distribution of moxa points on the front and back of the body, as used in recent times.[b] And just as there were 'forbidden points' for

[a] *Chhien Chin Yao Fang*, ch. 29, (p. 518.2) in +655; *Chi Shêng Pa Sui*, ch. 3, p. 2*a* in +1315.
[b] From Chang Shih-Piao (*1*), phien 4, pp. 13, 14.

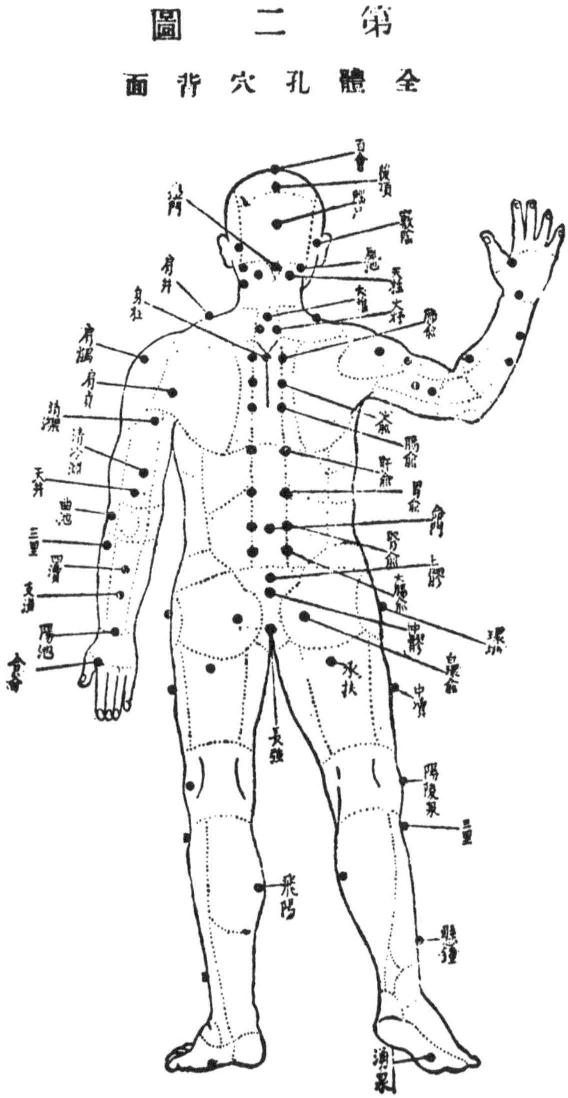

Fig. 40. Moxa spot diagram for the back of the body, from Chang Shih-Piao (*1*), ch. 4, p. 14.

acupuncture (p. 68 above) so also there were some for moxa.[a] With the growth of practice and experience many of the prohibited acu-points and moxa points have now come into use, but others are still considered inadvisable.[b] One of the commonest untoward happenings was fainting (*yün chen*[1]), and this was equally likely to occur at

[a] Cf. *CIC*, ch. 5, (pp. 107–12); *Chi Shêng Pa Sui*, ch. 2, p. 9*a* (in *Tou Thai-Shih Liu Chu Chih Yao Fu*); and, for a modern reference, Anon. (*123*), pp. 19ff.

[b] One can find mnemonic rhymes in modern books, e.g. Anon. (*91*), p. 362, both for needles and moxa.

[1] 暈鍼

certain loci with moxa, but methods of revival have always been given in the texts.[a] The moxibustionists also made use of points where pain was felt acutely, the *ah shih hsüeh*[1] (pp. 52 above, and p. 211 below); and in some cases, though by no means in all, they prescribed accompanying medication per os. Anciently only one locus, either for needling or moxa, was used at one time, and they were never applied simultaneously;[b] furthermore there were those, as we shall see, who looked askance at one or the other of the treatments, the hesitations varying from time to time through the historical periods.

History indeed is what we come to now, and an interesting one it is. Of course, a great many books which have moxa in their titles and their contents have already been described during our survey of the literature on acupuncture, but there was a distinct, if subsidiary, tradition of writings which specialised in moxibustion and said little or nothing about acupuncture. There has been a tendency among historians of medicine to suppose that moxa-burning went back far into the mists of antiquity, even into neolithic times,[c] but this may not be anything more than an echo of the tradition about 'stone needles' which we have dealt with already (p. 70). The *Shih Ching* (Book of Odes, *c.* −7th century) has a reference to the gathering of mugwort, as we have seen (p. 171), but no indication of what it was used for. One of the earliest medical references occurs in the *Mêng Tzu*[2] book, datable about −300. Mencius is saying that if one of the feudal princes were really to love and serve the people they would all flock to him, and he would not be able to avoid becoming the hegemon (the successor of the Chou High Kings) even if he did not want that great position.

> But now [he goes on] the ambitions of some of the present (feudal) princes to mount the throne are like a man seeking for mugwort three years old in order to cure a seven-years' illness. If it has not been kept in store beforehand, the patient may well die without ever getting it. If the princes fail to set their minds (here and now) on the love and service of the people, they will (far from attaining the leadership of the States) meet with sorrow and disgrace, and go down in the end to ruin and death.[d]

In other words, if they do not now, well in advance of any opportunities, take to heart the good doctrine, 'old, but true', needed to cure their selfishness, they can never have any hope of the leadership. Although there is here an indubitable medical reference, it makes no direct mention of moxa cautery, so some other properties of the *Artemisia* genus, most likely the important anthelminthics which some species of it contain, could have been in Mencius' mind. But Li Shih-Chen[e] certainly regarded

[a] *CCCY*, ch. 3, (p. 193). See also a modern paramedical handbook, Anon. (*172*), pp. 72–3, Eng. tr., pp. 96–7.

[b] Yeh Ching-Chhiu (*1*), p. 15.

[c] Wang Chi-Min & Wu Lien-Tê (1), pp. 2, 25, 45, for example. The conviction of the great antiquity of moxibustion is now much reinforced by the manuscripts recently unearthed from the Ma-wang-tui tomb and discussed on p. 111 above. It may well turn out to be more ancient than acupuncture, so that the tracts were first codified for cautery rather than for needling.

[d] *Mêng Tzu*, IV, (1), ix, 5, tr. auct., adjuv. Legge (3), p. 177; Ware (6), p. 102.

[e] *PTKM*, ch. 15, (p. 7). Chhêng Tan-An (*1*), p. 33, also believes that moxibustion was in use by the late Chou and Chhin time.

[1] 阿是穴 [2] 孟子

this as a clear reference to the necessity of sunning, drying and storing *Artemisia* tinder for a long time before application as a counter-irritant.

That there was a *Chiu Ching*[1] (Moxibustion Manual) in Han times, and probably more than one, is very likely, but they have all been lost for many centuries; indeed the title listed in the *Sui Shu* bibliography (+656)[a] is marked as having disappeared already by the end of the Liang dynasty (+556). The title comes again, however, in the bibliography of the *Chiu Thang Shu* (+945),[b] so either an ancient text had been recovered or it was some later work that took the same simple name; and that in its turn has failed to come down to us. The situation about Han writings on moxa is complicated by the fact that *ai*[2] (*Artemisia* spp.) does not figure at all in the oldest of the pharmaceutical natural histories, the *Shen Nung Pên Tshao Ching*[3] of the −2nd and −1st centuries. But it is treated of in some detail in the *Ming I Pieh Lu*[4] (Additional Records of Famous Physicians),[c] which says that as moxa it cures a multitude of diseases, and gives instructions for the sunning and drying, as well as reciting a number of its internal pharmaceutical actions. That work was a disentanglement, made between +523 and +618, of the contributions of Li Tang-Chih[5] (*c.* +225) and Wu Phu[6] (*c.* +235), and the commentaries of Thao Hung-Ching[7] (+492), from the text of the *Pên Ching* itself. This would suggest that the oldest extant descriptions of *Artemisia* moxa were written either in the Three Kingdoms period (+3rd century) or towards the end of the +5th, when Thao Hung-Ching was studying alchemy, medicine and natural history at Mao Shan under the Chhi and the Liang.[d]

These centuries were quite prolific in moxibustion literature, as we know from further entries in the *Sui Shu* bibliography, though none of the texts has survived. For example there was a *Chhi-Po Chiu Ching*[8] (Master Chhi-Po's Moxa Manual),[e] claiming high antiquity because of the ascription to the Yellow Emperor's interlocutor (cf. p. 90 above); with a *Tshao Shih Chiu Fang*[9],[f] and a *Lei Shih Chiu Fang*[10] (Mr Tshao's, and Mr Lei's, Moxa Recipes, respectively).[g] Particularly interesting is the fact that two of these pre-Sui works were illustrated, as one can see from their titles—an anonymous *Chen Chiu Thu Ching*[11] (Manual of Acupuncture and Moxibustion with Diagrams and Pictures), and a *Chen Chiu Thu Yao Chüeh*[12] (Important Essentials of Acupuncture and Moxa with Illustrations).[h] One cannot date any of these with assurance, but some of them may have been at least as old as the +3rd century, the

[a] Ch. 34, p. 28*a*, under the *Huang Ti Pa-shih-i Nan Ching*.[13] Cf. *ICK*, p. 312.
[b] Ch. 47, p. 9*b*.
[c] Cit. *PTKM*, ch. 15, (pp. 7–8).
[d] See *SCC*, Vol. 5, pt. 3, pp. 119–20.
[e] *Hsin Thang Shu* bibliography, ch. 59, p. 19*b*. Cf. *NCSW/WMC*, ch. 12, (p. 132).
[f] *Sui Shu* bibliography, ch. 34, p. 32*a*.
[g] Mr Lei appears in the *Hsin Thang Shu* bibliography, ch. 59, p. 19*b*. One wonders whether he could have been the Venerable Master Lei (Lei Kung,[14] Lei Hsiao[15]), responsible for a number of books on medicine and pharmacy about +470 (cf. *SCC*, Vol. 5, pt. 2, pp. 336–7).
[h] Both are to be found in the *Sui Shu* bibliography, ch. 34, p. 32*a*.

1 灸經　2 艾　3 神農本草經　4 名醫別錄　5 李當之
6 吳普　7 陶弘景　8 歧伯灸經　9 曹氏灸方　10 雷氏灸方
11 針灸圖經　12 針灸圖要訣　13 黃帝八十一難經
14 雷公　15 雷斆

time of Huangfu Mi's *Chen Chiu Chia I Ching* (*c.* +280, cf. p. 119 above), which alone would suffice to show how widespread moxibustion was towards the end of the Han. And here would be the place to recall the activities of Pao Ku,[1] the wife of the great alchemical writer Ko Hung,[a] and a woman physician renowned in her time (*c.* +300) for skill as a moxa specialist.[b] Still keeping within this period we may also mention the lost work of Chhin Chhêng-Tsu,[2] written about +460, entitled *Yen Tshê Tsa Chen Chiu Ching*[3] (Manual of Acupuncture and Moxibustion Loci seen on the Lateral Recumbent Figure).[c] An eminent physician of the Liu Sung, he also wrote on clinical diagnosis, sphygmology, pharmacy and natural history.[d]

With the Thang period came the time of more specialised books on moxibustion which have successfully come down to us. About +670 Tshui Chih-Thi,[4] a high official (Vice-President of the Imperial Secretariat) who had a deep interest in medicine, wrote a treatise on the cure of tuberculosis-like diseases by moxa, the *Ku Chêng Ping Chiu Fang*[5].[e] It had four diagrams and gave minute instructions for finding the most relevant acu-points (VU 17 and 19 on the back) in what became known as Tshui's *ssu hua chiu fa*[6].[f] Afterwards VU 15 was added in the classical *chiu lao fa*,[7] the method of moxa for tubercle.[g] In the +7th century there was also a *Ming Thang Chiu Ching*[8] (Manual of Moxa for all Parts of the Body) by an unknown author.[h] This could have been written before the Thang, but its exact date is doubtful; at any rate it was included by Wang Huai-Yin[9] in the *Thai-Phing Shêng Hui Fang*[10] (Prescriptions Collected by Imperial Benevolence during the Thai-Phing reign-period) of +992,[i] and enlarged for the subsequent edition of +1311.[j] Sui and Thang times saw a considerable polarisation of feeling as between acupuncturists and moxibustionists. As we saw at an earlier stage (p. 127), Wang Thao[11] spoke strongly against the dangers of needling in his *Wai Thai Pi Yao*[12] of +752 (Important Formulae and Prescriptions revealed by the Governor of a Distant Province), and he included only moxa and heat-treatments, eschewing acupuncture, so that his could be regarded as the first great textbook on moxibustion. Sun Ssu-Mo[13] in the Sui and early Thang had at first been of the same opinion, but changed his mind as his experience grew, and

a See Vol. 5, pt. 3, pp. 75 ff., and p. 121 above.

b P. 129 above. There is a special study of her by Sung Ta-Jen (*5*). It is interesting that later on we shall find, in connection with the first transmission of moxa knowledge to Europe, that it was a woman physician who cured Hermann Buschof of his gout in Batavia in the +17th century (p. 292).

c *Sui Shu* bibliography, ch. 34, p. 28*a*; it did not survive the Liang.

d See *SIC*, pp. 163, 229, 255, 749, 1352. His biography is given in *I Shuo*,[14] ch. 1, and we have met him before, in *SCC*, Vol. 5, pt. 3, p. 45. His work in the present field has cropped up already, p. 121.

e It was much emphasised by Wang Thao in *WTPY*, ch. 13, (pp. 351, 353).

f *CCTC*, ch. 9, (p. 289.2).

g *CCCY*, ch. 2, (p. 142). This indeed was given as the title of Tshui's book in the *Sung Shih* bibliography, ch. 207, p. 21*a*. Cf. *ICK*, p. 316. Tshui's methods were so highly regarded that an account of them was inscribed on a stone stele at Khun-ling Chün; cf. *Su Shen Liang Fang*, ch. 1, (p. 22).

h Cf. *ICK*, p. 319.

i Ch. 100.

j See Hsieh Li-Hêng (*1*), p. 32, who says the additions were mostly from Wang Wei-I[15] (p. 131 above).

1 鮑姑 2 秦承祖 3 偃側雜針灸經 4 崔知悌 5 骨蒸病灸方
6 四花灸法 7 灸勞法 8 明堂灸經 9 王懷隱 10 太平聖惠方
11 王燾 12 外臺秘要 13 孫思邈 14 醫說 15 王惟一

in later writings gave as much attention to acupuncture as to moxa.[a] Of course moxibustion had always had its critics, and at the end of the Han Chang Chung-Ching[1] had been nervous of the powerful internal reactions caused by cautery, saying that it was sometimes difficult to recover the proper balance of *chhi* and *hsüeh* (*pneuma* and blood) after its use.[b]

Another important book on moxa followed in the Sung, the *Hsi Fang Tzu Ming Thang Chiu Ching*[2] (Moxibustion Manual of the Microcosm, i.e. the Human Body, by the Western-Direction Master).[c] This was printed about +1050, forming a kind of companion to Wang Wei-I's book on the life-size bronze figure (p. 131 above), and issued first, as that had been, from Phingyang in Shansi. The Master of the Western Quarter, whoever he was, included diagrams of moxa points for the front and back of the body, and also the two sides, right and left. Then in +1128, a few years after the fall of the Northern Sung capital, Khaifêng, to the Chin Tartars, Chuang Cho[3] published his famous tractate *Kao Huang Chiu Fa*[4] (On Moxibustion at the Kao-huang Acu-point, VU 38).[d] This is a locus near the scapula (Fig. 41),[e] and its name stems from that very ancient passage which we read on p. 78, where in a *Tso Chuan* consultation about −580 a disease was said to be incurable because it had ensconced itself 'between the heart and the diaphragm'. During the wars against the Tartars (from +1067 onwards) Chuang Cho suffered many hardships, contracting what seem to have been malaria, beri-beri, and many ailments more; but none of the physicians wandering among the refugees could do him any good. Eventually, in +1107, he met one named Chhen Liao-Ong[5] who used this acu-point and gave him three hundred moxa cauteries at it, after which all his symptoms cleared up and his health was restored. Perhaps also he found more salubrious living conditions at some refuge in the south. But he was anxious that everyone should know of the value of the locus, and himself measured it out in people of different body builds, giving diagrams and directions at the end of his book to ensure its exact identification. This Kao-huang point, and its related acu-points VU 17 and 19 (beside the 8th and the 11th thoracic vertebrae respectively),[f] are still today regarded as important for moxa, and used in pulmonary tuberculosis,[g] bronchitis, pleurisy, 'neurasthenia' and general weakness.[h]

Lastly there were two more important books on moxa alone during the Southern Sung. In +1226 Wênjen Chhi-Nien[6] finished his *Pei Chi Chiu Fa*[7] (Moxibustion Methods for Use in Emergencies), a treatise provided with excellent illustrations (Figs. 24, 42).[i] This deals with 23 diseases, including malaria, appendicitis, boils,

[a] See p. 127 above.
[b] See Yeh Ching-Chhiu (*1*), p. 15.
[c] *ICK*, p. 320.
[d] *ICK*, pp. 326, 266, 142.
[e] VU 43 in some reckonings; cf. Anon. (*107*), p. 140.
[f] *CCTC*, ch. 9, p. 48*a* (pp. 289.2, 290.1) with picture, and a quotation from *I Hsüeh Ju Mên*.
[g] It is interesting that as late as 1822 Larrey (1), the eminent French military surgeon (cf. p. 300 below), regarded moxa as a sovereign remedy in phthisis. Cf. Brockbank (1), pp. 127–8.
[h] Anon. (135), p. 150.
[i] Cf. *ICK*, p. 329, *SIC*, p. 294.

[1] 張仲景 [2] 西方子明堂灸經 [3] 莊綽 [4] 膏肓灸法 [5] 陳了翁
[6] 聞人耆年 [7] 備急灸法

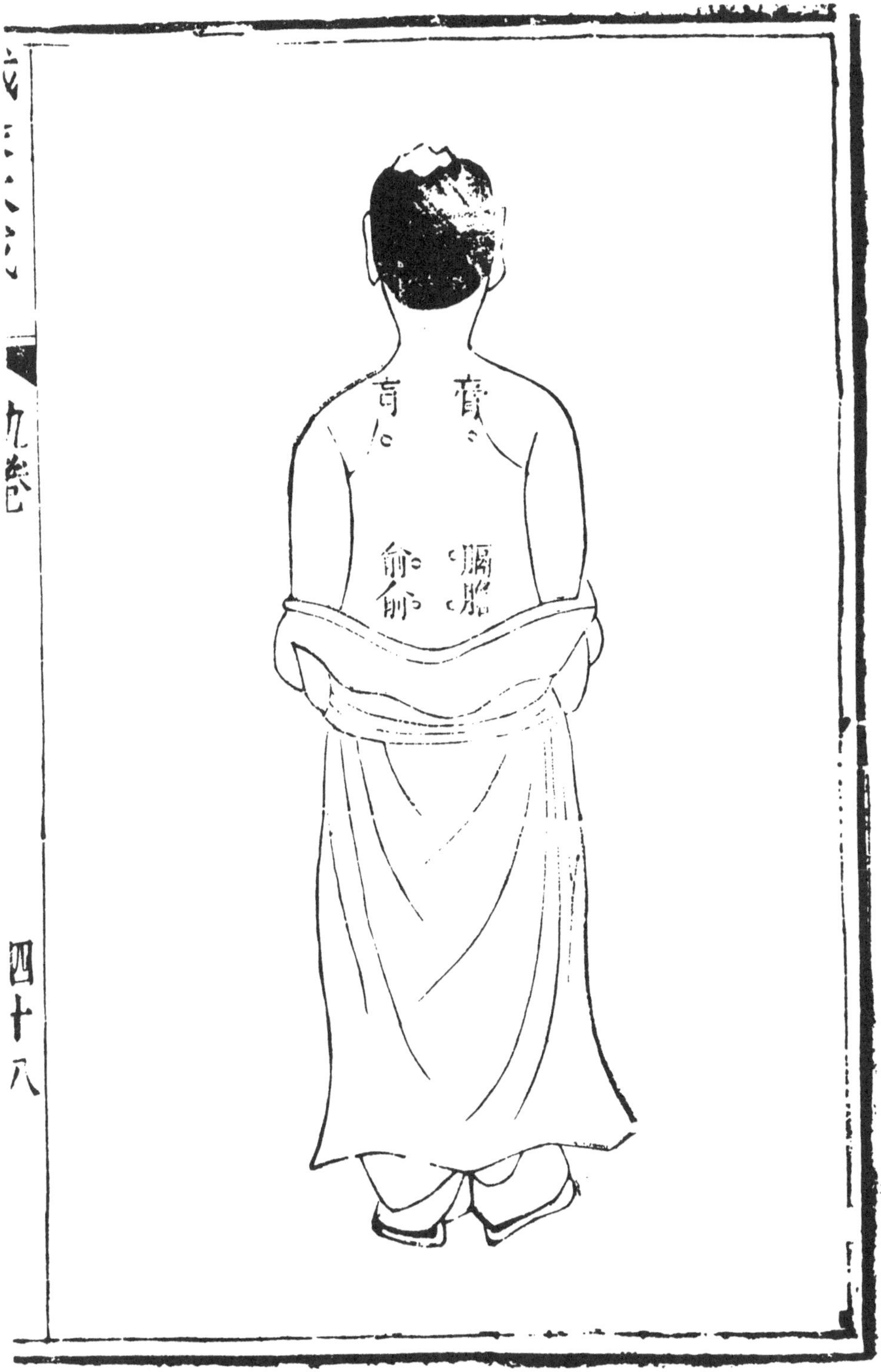

Fig. 41. The acu-points Kao-huang, Ko-shu and Tan-shu, depicted in *Chen Chiu Ta Chhêng* (+1601), ch. 9, p. 48*a*.

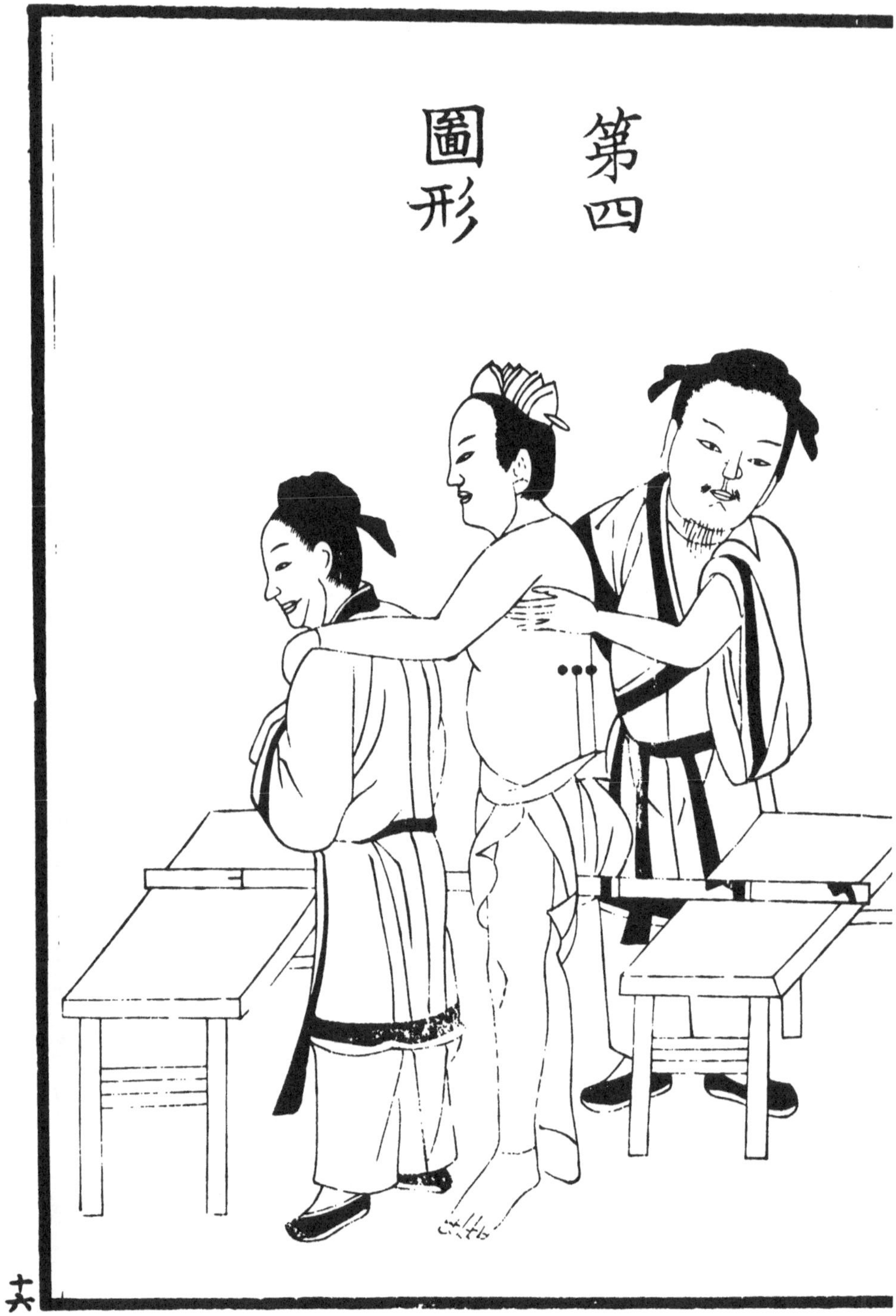

Fig. 42. The astride position for moxa at the Kao-huang acu-point, *chhi chu ma chiu fa*; a drawing in the *Pei Chi Chiu Fa* of +1226 (p. 16*b*). Possible reasons for the adoption of this technique are discussed in the text.

ulcers, carbuncles and some psychological troubles.[a] At the beginning of the illustrations there is a particularly good one showing the module system for the location of points for acupuncture or moxa (cf. p. 125). Wênjen Chhi-Nien based his accounts on two earlier books written between +1100 and +1126 by Chang Huan[1] and not extant now, nor would his own text and pictures have been available to us if they had not been safely preserved in Japan until 1890. Wênjen's book is generally bound up with a later tractate of +1447 which also survived only in Japan,[b] the *Chen Chiu Tsê Jih Phien*[2] (On the Choice of Days and Times for Acupuncture and Moxibustion)[c] written by Chhüan Hsün-I[3] & Chin I-Sun.[4] This links up with much which has already been said about the diurnal and other rhythms in man, and the lore which the Chinese accumulated about the optimum times for moxa and acupuncture (pp. 137ff. above).

It only now remains to mention a few of the special uses of moxibustion which present uncommon interest. First, then, it was employed in the Middle Ages, rather surprisingly perhaps, as a prophylactic. Officials travelling to Wu and Shu, wrote Sun Ssu-Mo in the +7th century, generally arrange to have two or three unhealed moxa spots on their bodies, for in this way they will be protected against malaria (*nio*[5]), epidemics (*wên*[6]), pestilences (*chang*[7]) and infectious ulcerating sores (*li*[8]).[d] There was a proverb which said: 'if you wish to be safe, never allow the San-li acu-points to become dry'.[e] And moxa tinder was one of the most important components of first-aid kits whenever people went on journeys. Even at home, a careful scholar would apply moxa at three or more points on the body after each ten-day period of good health.[f] The practice continued down to the +17th century, a thousand years later, at least, for Wu Khung-Chia,[9] in his preface of +1640 to a reprint of Wang Thao's +8th-century *Wai Thai Pi Yao*, wrote that 'the use of three-year-old moxa tinder can ensure that no illness will follow it'.[g]

Secondly, one finds in the moxa books some strange procedures for getting the maximum effect from the cautery or heat-treatment applied. One of these was called *Chhi chu ma chiu fa*,[10] the setting of moxa on the back while the patient rides 'a-cock horse' on a bamboo pole supported by friends or assistants on each side.[h] The excel-

[a] The author wanted to propagate moxibustion because drugs were so expensive, and he felt it was by far the best treatment for the poor. This reminds us of a famous Sung painting of moxa being applied to a peasant farmer (Fig. 43). However, Wênjen Chhi-Nien did include a number of drug prescriptions in his book, notably some containing alcoholic extracts of *Lonicera japonica*. Like so many other Chinese scholars, he had originally become interested in medicine because of the illness of his own mother.

[b] Both were rediscovered and reprinted by Lo Chia-Chieh in 1890.

[c] Cf. *ICK*, p. 320.

[d] *CCYF*, ch. 29, (p. 519.2). Cf. Chu Lien (*1*), p. 69.

[e] This was quoted, for example, by Wang Chih-Chung about +1220 (see p. 135 above), and he added the Tan-thien acu-point as well; cf. *Tongŭi Pogam*, ch. 23, (p. 779.2).

[f] *CCYF*, ch. 27, (p. 481.1). Cf. Yeh Ching-Chhiu (*1*), p. 15.

[g] Pp. 16–17.

[h] *Pei Chi Chiu Fa*, sect. 2, pp. 13aff., ill., p. 16b; *Chen Chiu Ta Chhêng*, ch. 9, p. 49a (p. 290), attributed to a Mr Yang[11] from a *Shen Ying Ching*,[12] not otherwise known. Cf. p. 159 above.

1 張渙 2 鍼灸擇日編 3 全循義 4 金義孫 5 瘧 6 瘟
7 瘴 8 癘 9 吳孔嘉 10 騎竹馬灸法 11 楊氏 12 神應經

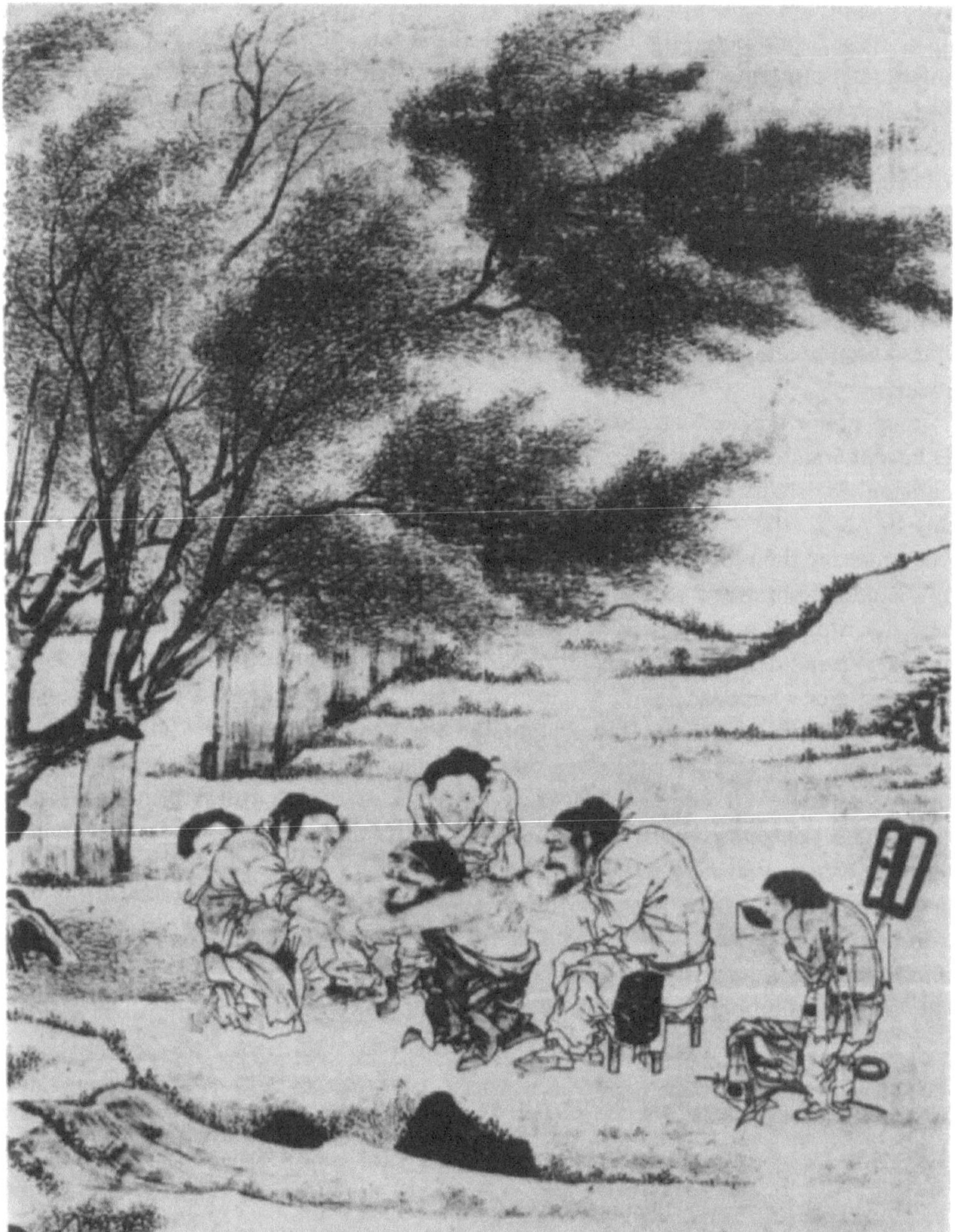

Fig. 43. A scroll-painting of moxibustion by a rural physician; his boy stands ready on the right with a soothing plaster, but the old farmer is not enjoying it. The artist was Li Thang of the Southern Sung (+12th or +13th century, probably *c.* +1150). *Chiu Ai Thu*, from Anon. (*32*).

lent illustration from the *Pei Chi Chiu Fa* is reproduced in Fig. 42. The two Kao-huang acu-points here at issue (VU 38) are, we know, about half-way down the scapula. The +13th-century explanation was that all the circulation passes through them, and its current can be blocked or overflowing,[a] so that the moxa restores the flow to normality, healing the boils or oedemas (*yung chü*[1]) which are infections (*tu chhi*[2]) due to malfunctions of the nutritional process (*ying wei*[3]). But why riding on a bamboo? Because the coccyx (*wei-lü*[4])[b] is lifted, and gates are opened for the pouring *chhi* and *hsüeh* (*liu chu*[5]);[c] then the perineal regions and external genitalia feel hot as if steamed, the sensation of heat descends to the sole of the foot (lit. the Yang-chhüan acu-point, R 1), and finally passes all round the whole body. Interpreting this in modern terms might mean that the moxa must stimulate certain posterior primary rami of the thoracic nerves (probably Th. 3, 4 and 5), and that others will not do. So the function of the astride position might be an adjustment of the skin of the back in such a way as to produce exactly the effect desired.[d]

Another important traditional use of moxa was in cases of snake-bite. In the *Thai-Phing Kuang Chi*,[6] a vast collection of anecdotes, mirabilia and memorabilia assembled in +978, Chao Yen-Hsi[7] is quoted as saying that if a person is bitten by large, dangerous venomous snakes (*o shê*[8]), specifically the *fu shê*[9],[e] or the *hui*[10],[f] moxa should be burnt immediately upon the spot.[g] This will give instant relief of the pain, and if it is not done death will follow; the marks of the teeth will show where the cautery is to be given. No doubt in Arabic and European medicine also cautery was customary in such cases, and it does not seem unreasonable to think that if a little delay occurred in the absorption of the venom into the circulation, destruction of the epithelial layers at the point of entry could save the patient.

Finally, Chinese physicians are experimenting with moxa to this day. A very recent report (Anon. *174*) has studied the responses of patients with influenza, chronic bronchitis and other infections of the respiratory tract to fumigation with an incense composed of *Artemisia* tinder and the powder of *Atractylis ovata*.[h] The inhalation

[a] Cf. what was earlier said (p. 22) on the hydraulic engineering background of Chinese circulation physiology.

[b] This expression had far-ranging significances in Chinese scientific and proto-scientific language, see *SCC*, Vol. 4, pt. 3, pp. 548–9.

[c] Cf. the account on pp. 137 ff. above.

[d] It may be remembered that the medial cutaneous branches of the posterior primary rami of the thoracic nerves descend for some distance close to the vertebrae before reaching the skin, while the lateral branches may travel down as much as the breadth of four ribs before they become superficial.

[e] This is the pit-viper, *Agkistrodon* spp., cf. R 120.

[f] Either *Trimeresurus* spp., according to R 121, or *Trigonocephalus Blomhoffii*, according to Tu Ya-Chhüan *et al.* (*1*), pp. 1964.2, 1965.1.

[g] Ch. 220, p. 4*b* (p. 857); quoted in *Li Tai Ming I Mêng Chhiu*[11] (Brief Lives of the Famous Physicians of All Ages), by Chou Shou-Chung,[12] ch. 1, (p. 6). Completed in +1220, this book must be one of the oldest histories of medicine in the world.

[h] *Tshang shu*,[13] a thistle-like composite, cf. R 14; CC 34; B II/8, B III/12; Khung *et al.* (*1*), p. 1273. Now known as *Atractylodes japonica* (Anon. (*109*), vol. 4, p. 601). The dried roots have been used in medicine for centuries, they contain at least one alkaloid, atractylon, and when powdered are burned in smokes for their insect-repellent and antiseptic properties. Anciently the plant was much prized by

[1] 癰疽 [2] 毒氣 [3] 營衛 [4] 尾閭 [5] 流注 [6] 太平廣記
[7] 趙延禧 [8] 惡蛇 [9] 蝮蛇 [10] 虺 [11] 歷代名醫蒙求
[12] 周守忠 [13] 蒼朮

mixture was composed of 10% of the former and 40% of the latter, the rest being made up of the dust of various woods. Beneficial effects were found in some 4000 cases, checked by diminution or disappearance of symptoms but also by agglutinin tests and other objective criteria. Since chronic bronchitis is one of the commonest diseases in contemporary China, any techniques which will combat it successfully are eagerly sought for.

(5) Therapy and Analgesia; Physiological Interpretations

The time has come at last to consider the whole acupuncture complex in terms of modern scientific knolwedge. Something can now really be said about this, though only a few decades ago it would have been much more speculative. The subject differs, however, in several ways from most of those which we have had to treat of in our volumes—in geology or mechanical engineering, for instance, the concepts and practices of traditional China were essentially identical with those pertaining in the rest of the world, here they were characteristic and different, requiring specific explanation in terms of physiology and pathology. The subject is also still in some ways a controversial one, and currently in rapid development, much more so than our subjects usually are. There is a vast literature on it too,[a] from which we can only choose for mention a few books and papers, sometimes because of their typical nature, sometimes because they seem particularly illuminating.[b] Readers with little physiological background will need some parallel reference books for adequate understanding, general introductions to the history of neuro-physiology perhaps,[c] a basic work on the anatomy of the central and peripheral nervous systems,[d] and introductory accounts of their functions in relation to body and mind.[e]

Of course, it would still be possible to find certain people in the world opposed to any attempt to explain acupuncture — or any other branch of Chinese medical technology for that matter — in terms of modern science. Some practising Chinese physicians of the old style, learned in the millennial literature which we have already surveyed, would be likely to take this view. And indeed during our conferences in many hospitals and medical schools in China in 1964 and 1972 we had ample opportunities of observing how difficult it was for the traditional medical men to deviate from the classical ways of thinking, even with the best will in the world for cooperation with the modern-Western-trained physicians and surgeons, so clearly does the body of Chinese medical philosophy as a whole supply a kind of trellis-work on which to

Taoists in pursuit of elixirs of longevity and material immortality; cf. *SCC*, Vol. 5, pt. 3, p. 11 *et passim*.

[a] Bulging bibliographies are constantly being produced, as from the National Medical Library at Bethesda, Md., cf. Nowak (1). But the subject has always been dogged in the West by the low scientific level of most of the literature.

[b] There are innumerable semi-popular introductions to be consulted—among the best, those of Ho Ping-Yü (17); Bowers (2); Štovičková (1); Lisowski (1).

[c] See Poynter (3); Clarke & Dewhurst (1).

[d] Barr (1).

[e] Nathan (1); Rose (1); Luria (1).

hang the accumulated clinical experience of more than two thousand years. For this difficulty there is no easy solution.[a]

It may be well to notice, too, that it is one thing to interpret in terms of the modern sciences what Chinese medicine actually did, but another thing to interpret in similar terms what the Chinese physicians thought they were doing. The second of these ventures is much more problematic than the first. It may be that in the philosophy of science there is simply no way of incorporating earlier conceptual paradigms in terms of later ones; how can one give an equivalent for 'black bile', or *anathumiasis*,[b] or *modus violentus*,[c] in terms of chólic acid or fumaroles or aerodynamics—even though the pragmatic knowledge of humanity goes steadily on? Hence the reluctance felt by some to accept the systematic attempt of Porkert (1) to explain the different kinds of *chhi* in the ancient medical philosophy in terms of energy.[d] Khoubesserian (1), representing one group of French acupuncture practitioners, had already stressed the danger of applying our modern concept of energy to the classical *chhi* circulation (cf. p. 14 above), especially in the many facile analogies with biophysical electric currents, impedances, etc.; and he had characterised the old Chinese system (not unjustly) as archaic, medieval, indeed essentially scholastic, even though its day might not yet be quite over. The Yin and Yang, he urged, were intrinsically pre-Renaissance ideas, in that they could be made to explain anything,[e] and the Five Elements were as unacceptable today as Aristotle's four—yet in spite of this many Western physicians practising acupuncture showed an 'illuminisme' which had no need of laboratory tests or modern diagnostic procedures. 'If we wish', he wrote, 'to be taken seriously, and not to be confused with bone-setters and faith-healers, we must abandon the whole more or less Chinese mass of philosophy, cosmogony and mythology in which we have been entangled these forty years past. Let us clear the decks, and look at our problems without preconceived ideas. The study of the anatomy and physiology of the skin, and of the central and sympathetic nervous systems, the investigation of the physico-chemical and enzymic reactions in the body, all these should provide us with the means of solving the problem of what acupuncture really is and does.'[f] Though a rather extreme statement, this has the interest of coming from

[a] Cf. the judicious piece of 'thinking aloud' by Huard & Huang Kuang-Ming (13). As an example of the desperate attempts made by some to integrate classical and traditional Chinese medical theory with modern science one may glance at the book of Fujita Rokurō (*1*).

[b] Cf. *SCC*, Vol. 3, p. 469.

[c] Cf. Vol. 4, pt. 1, p. 57.

[d] See our critique of his interesting and thought-provoking work; Needham & Lu Gwei-Djen (9; as also p. 16 above).

[e] Our account of Yin and Yang in Vol. 3, and indeed in many other places throughout our work, is of course distinctively historical, elucidating the role they played in Chinese thinking down the ages. The difference here is that for the first time we find these concepts in earnest use related to practical actions today, though what was rational and progressive in the Han and Thang may no longer be so. The role of Yin and Yang in world-outlooks of spiritual wisdom is something else again.

[f] 'Si nous voulons vraiment être pris au sérieux, et ne pas être confondus avec les rebouteux et les guérisseurs, il faut que nous renoncions à tout le fatras philosophique, cosmogonique, mythologique plus ou moins Chinois dans lequel nous nous empêtrons depuis quarante ans. Faisons table rase, et abordons nos problèmes sans idées préconçues. L'étude de l'anatomie et de la physiologie de la peau, des systèmes nerveux et sympathiques, des réactions physiques, chimiques et enzymatiques dans

a Western acupuncture physician, and many of his colleagues in China would agree with him. For ourselves, we retain reservations, but the interpretative task is what we must turn our minds to in this chapter.

Here, then, we must first discuss the question of whether any histological structures correspond with the acu-tracts, acu-junctions, branch channels, acu-points, etc., which traditional Chinese medicine traced out diagrammatically on the body's surface. If not, can they be identified in any other way? After this the exposition must divide sharply into two parts, first the therapeutic use of acupuncture in accordance with the many centuries of its practice, and secondly the analgesic use of it which permits major surgery, a development only of the past two decades. After speaking of the therapeutic aspect something will be said of the possible origins of the system in ancient insight and correct observation, and then in turn its possible mode of operation in the light of modern knowledge of immunology and endocrinology. The second part will take us into the fascinating subject of the neuro-physiology of pain, the modern comprehension of which, though still far from complete, has enabled a fairly high degree of rationality to be achieved regarding the indubitable phenomenon of acupuncture analgesia, much more solidly based indeed than anything we can surmise about the therapeutic practice. Finally something must be said about the relation between the acu-points of the Chinese system and the loci of especial sensitivity or danger known to forensic medicine as well as to the traditional exponents of the military arts of East Asia.

There has been but one attempt in recent times to demonstrate a gross physical or sub-anatomical substratum for the *ching-lo* system. In 1963 Kim Bonghan (1, *1*) and his Korean group of histologists published accounts of certain corpuscles, both deep and superficial, and thin ducts or conduits in connection with them, both intra-vascular and extra-vascular. These microscopical discoveries were welcomed with varying degrees of caution,[a] and checked during the succeeding years by histologists in various countries, with the result that no confirmation of the findings could ever be obtained.[b] Kellner (1) produced some evidence that the subcutaneous tissue under the acu-points is better supplied with nerve-endings than other locations,[c] but could find no evidence for Kim's structures.[d] Follicles of hairs and vibrissae, especially when damaged pathologically, have much resemblance to his pictures. In the skin particularly, small blood-vessels may often be injured and go out of use, so that they fill with fibrin clot or loose connective tissue, and this could have given the impression

l'organisme, doit nous fournir des moyens d'investigations pour aboutir à une explication scientifique de l'acupuncture.'

[a] Cf. Rall (4, 5); Han Su-Yin (1).

[b] In 1964 we were informed by distinguished members of Academia Sinica in Peking that a special team of Chinese histologists visited Pyongyang to study Kim Bonghan's methods and results, but the upshot was entirely negative.

[c] Paradoxically, because the experience is commonly reported that at acu-points there is a distinctly decreased sensation from pin-prick than at other areas of skin, cf. Brown, Ulett & Stern (2); Plummer & Chhiu Yin-Chhing (private comm.). Here might be mentioned the curious parallel drawn by Mann (1), 1st ed. only, pp. 141ff., between the sense organs of the lateral line in teleostean fishes and the VF acu-tract in man. He no longer entertains it (11), but it still affords some food for meditation.

[d] And this was published in the German acupuncture journal

of fibrils running inside blood-vessels.[a] The Vater-Pacini corpuscles (sensory nerve-endings) may also have been misinterpreted.[b] The histology of the skin and subcutaneous tissues has now been so well known for so long that it is highly unlikely that any structures connected with the *ching-lo* system yet hitherto unrecognised will come to light. What about more subtle characteristics?

Much work has been devoted to the possible identification of acu-points by electrical methods, mostly by measuring skin resistance, impedance or potential.[c] Various forms of apparatus (*tshê ting i*[1]) have been invented both in West and East, as for example by Niboyet (2) and Brunet & Grenier (1), or in Japan by Manaka,[d] and also in China as well.[e] A great many papers have affirmed a lowered electrical resistance at the acu-points,[f] but there have been continued expressions of scepticism,[g] and it does not seem that any assured conclusions have as yet been reached. Indeed, the most critical studies have failed to confirm the differences reported in such measurements, suggesting that one can get any value by suitable manipulation and that self-deception is only too easy.[h] Nevertheless, electrical 'palpation' is used in China for detecting sensitive diagnostic points on the auricula or external ear (*erh hsüeh chen tuan*[2]).[i]

The reserves expressed in the preceding paragraph are still justified, but since it was written one of us (J.N.) has experienced a convincing demonstration of the apparent possibility of identifying the acu-points by electrical methods. At the Smythe Pain Clinic of the Toronto General Hospital Dr Raymond Evans has for some time past been experimenting with a Japanese-made apparatus measuring the electrical resistance of the skin.[j] The subject holds one electrode while the other, with a blunt end, is lightly touched on the skin at one place after another—when an acu-point is found the apparatus gives a buzzing or rattling like a Geiger counter, while at other locations only an occasional bleep or click is heard. At the same time a deep but

[a] Cf. Maximow & Bloom (1), pp. 325 ff. (skin), 333 ff. (hairs), 338 ff. (sebaceous glands). We are much indebted to Prof. E. N. Willmer for advice on this subject.

[b] A suggestion of Prof. Hans Selye, in conversation. Description in Barr (1), p. 33.

[c] Brown, Ulett & Stern (1) have obtained positive results with this last technique.

[d] See Grall (1). Several forms of apparatus have been placed on the market, and some are probably still used by clinicians seeking to locate exact points for acupuncture.

[e] Anon. (119). Cf. Husson (1) and Anon. (*123*), pp. 94 ff.; Anon. (*161*), pp. 154 ff.; Anon. (*162*), pp. 123 ff., for descriptions of the work of Hsiao Yu-Shan, Chang Hsieh-Ho and Than Shu-Thien. There is also a claim that acu-points along certain tracts have a very slight temperature difference from the rest of the skin (Anon. (*161*), pp. 150 ff.).

[f] Cf. Lavier (4); Niboyet & Mery (1); Niboyet (3); Bratu, Stoicescu & Prodescu (2); Kracmar (1).

[g] Especially de la Fuye (2), and Mann (1), rev. 2nd ed., p. 228.

[h] Even when all the precautions laid down by some workers are observed. See Noordergraaf & Silage (1); Burger, Noordergraaf & Vonken (1).

[i] Anon. (*114*), p. 307; Anon. (135), p. 279.

[j] The product of the Neuro-Medical Industry Works, designed by Nakatani Yoshio, it is termed a '*ryodoraku*[3] diagnostic machine'. It delivers a small amperage at 6 to 24 volts ranging around 40 pulses per min. Cf. Hashimoto Masae (*1*), p. 79; Sun Chin-Chhing (*1*), p. 152. Nakatani originally located about 370 points with his apparatus, mostly identical with the classical acu-points lying on the fourteen tracts.

[1] 測定儀 [2] 耳穴診斷 [3] 良導絡

painless pricking like a slight electric shock is felt in the underlying tissues.[a] Ho-ku and Tsu-san-li were thus easily demonstrable, but the tests have been made repeatedly on all the known acu-points of the body, and in a double-blind system too, where neither the subject nor the experimenter knew their location. Under such conditions the *pei shu hsüeh*, for example (p. 66), would all reveal themselves clearly. In spite of the negative histological observations already referred to, the thought arises that some connection with electrolyte distribution in the skin and subcutaneous tissues would be most likely, so that perhaps sweat-glands might be involved, not more numerous but more efficient than in other places.[b] Yet this would be hard to reconcile with another fact also established by Dr Evans, namely that the effect can be demonstrated on cadavers up to 5 hours after death.[c] And the puzzle remains: how on earth can these loci have been identified by the Chinese physicians two millennia ago?

Quite distinct from all these efforts at identification[d] is the practice of electro-acupuncture (*tien chen chih liao*[1]), i.e. the sending in of electric currents by means of acupuncture needles either at the traditional acu-points or other loci on the skin between the tracts.[e] The early history of this may well be European, beginning with the Chevalier Sarlandière in 1825,[f] but though the idea did not catch on much there it recurred in China with the modern revival of traditional medicine and is now the basis of certain forms of treatment.[g] In 1958 we had the opportunity of visiting the Electro-acupuncture Clinic of the Neurological Hospital in Sian, and saw the beginnings of a process (Figs. 44, 45) which since then has spread quite widely.[h] The needle electrodes carried current of about 1 milliamp at 0·004 volts, enough to cause intermittent twitching of the subcutaneous muscles and to stimulate many nerve-endings leading to different spinal and sympathetic paths. As is now generally accepted, valuable results can be achieved in many different types[i] of disease—hypertension,

[a] All this agrees closely with observations reported by Frost & Orkin (1); Reichmanis, Marino & Becker (1, 2). Professor Murray Gell-Mann has told us that he experienced very similar effects with a skin resistance apparatus constructed by the eminent electrical engineer, Vladimir Zworykin (priv. comm. 1977).

[b] This was a suggestion made by Prof. Hans Selye in conversation. Though very reasonable it would be rather difficult to prove.

[c] We had already learnt of this from Dr Janet Plummer and Dr Chhiu Yin-Chhing in Hongkong, who were using a Chinese-made apparatus, Sui-Wei 626; but we did not give it the attention it deserved because personal demonstrations on one of us (J.N.) at that time were not very successful. On this apparatus see Babich (1).

[d] Though some of the forms of apparatus just referred to were designed for electrical stimulation as well as for recording resistances. Cf. Lavier (4).

[e] Anon. (*114*), pp. 295ff.; Chu Lung-Yü (*1*).

[f] See Vergier (1).

[g] More perhaps for analgesia today than for therapy; see pp. 219ff. below.

[h] We should like to express our gratitude to Dr Chu Lung-Yü and his colleagues Wang Kho-Ming, Sun Chao-Jui and Wei Ching-Shun for the warm welcome they gave us (G.D.L. and J.N.) on that occasion. At first we thought that their work had something to do with the rather barbaric electric shock treatment for depression or schizophrenia so frequently used in the West, but this was far off the mark. Among the publications of this group are Anon. (*163*).

[i] The Sian group counted some seventy conditions. Dupuytren's disease was arrested without vitamin E, and tics and torticollis greatly alleviated.

[1] 電針治療

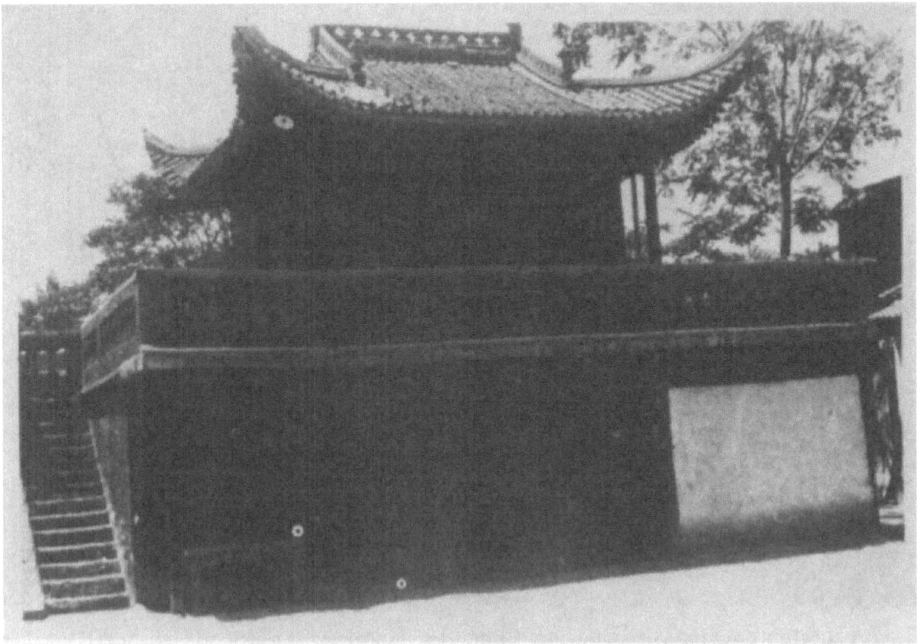

Fig. 44. Old buildings and courtyards in Hung-fu Lu, Sian, used in 1958 by the Electro-acupuncture Clinic of the North-western Neurological Hospital, and its biochemical laboratory. Here in that year we witnessed some of the earliest modern experiments with electro-acupuncture, which subsequently spread so widely, especially for acupuncture analgesia. Orig. photograph.

gynaecological disorders, light or incipient epilepsy,[a] neuralgias, labyrinthitis, paralytic states, even neuroses[b] and some paranoid psychoses,[c] together with a number of skin diseases.[d] Sometimes the Sian workers used the traditional acu-points, but as often as not they chose their implantation loci away from the tracts in accordance with modern knowledge of the nervous system and the dermatomes (p. 207 below); in most contemporary Chinese therapeutic electro-acupuncture this is still the procedure.[e] The Sian group were also responsible for some animal experiments of much interest.[f]

[a] The more recent study of Fêng Ying-Khun *et al.* (1), done with EEG (electro-encephalograph) recording, confirms that after six years of the disease no effects are obtained, but in earlier stages the needles induce both synchronisation and desynchronisation, suggesting a cortical plasticity which could explain the therapeutic responses.

[b] Both obsessional and anxiety states (*khung chü chêng*[1]).

[c] Cf. Kaada *et al.* (1), pp. 439 ff.

[d] Notably a fungus infection just known as *mei chün ping*,[2] common in NW China.

[e] Depths of insertion (up to 10 cm. when near plexuses) and strengths of current used varied much, and still do.

[f] After tying the sciatic nerve in rabbits there follows what seems like a sterile ulceration of the foot, with degeneration of the toes, so that the phalanges protrude; under electro-acupuncture for half an hour on alternate days this condition heals up completely. Must not this be a strengthening of the trophic action of the nerve-supply of the extremities? Again, using typhoid or paratyphoid antigens, also in rabbits, the serum antibody titre was doubled or quadrupled with ordinary acupuncture, but

[1] 恐懼症 [2] 黴菌病

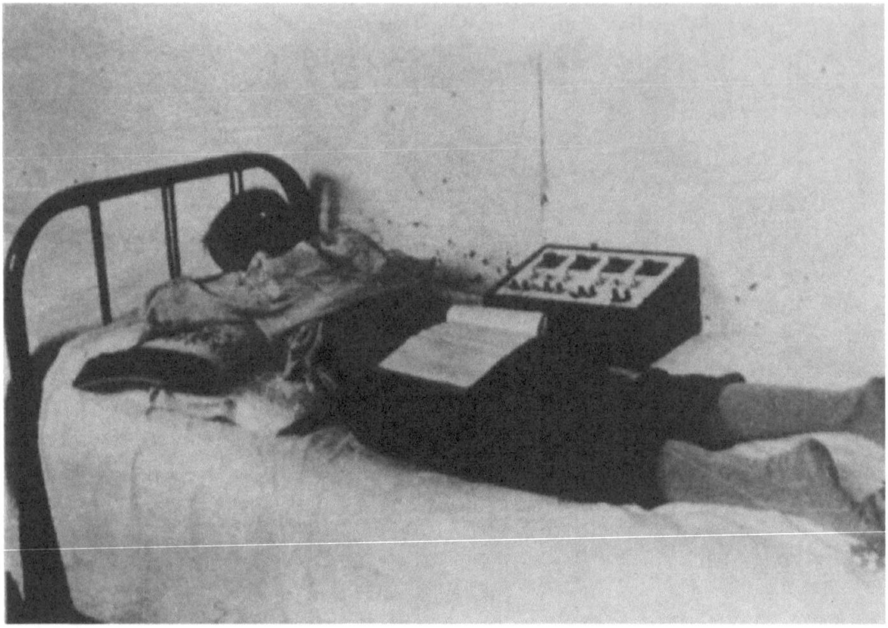

Fig. 45. A patient in the Electro-acupuncture Clinic at Sian in 1958. Electric pulses applied through needles inserted in the back. Orig. photograph.

Our record of this visit contains the note that 'electro-acupuncture does seem to reduce post-operative pain'. This is very significant today, for 1958 was in fact the year when Chinese physicians and anaesthesiologists began to apply acupuncture for analgesia in major surgery (*chen tzhu ma tsui*[1]). As we shall presently see (p. 230), it was not long before electrical stimulation was found more convenient and effective in many cases than manual or mechanical manipulation, and this is now in wide use today (*tien chen ma tsui*[2]).[a] Thus electro-physiology at this level touches acupuncture at three points, first the rather dubious domain of explorations of skin impedance and other properties, secondly the use of the needles as electrodes for stimulating nerve-endings and nerves in therapy, and thirdly their application in this way for analgesia, especially during surgical operations. But we must now return to our cogitations about possible objective correlates of the traditional acu-points and tracts.

Of course it is not necessary to restrict the mechanism of stimulus of the peripheral nociceptors to the electrical and the mechanical, for chemical structure and function may well intervene. The skin and the subcutaneous tissue are very rich in acid muco-

with electro-acupuncture a sixfold increase was obtained. Would this not mean a nervous (perhaps neuro-humoral) action on the reticulo-endothelial cells? Little evidence of any effects on inorganic blood constituents or blood-sugar was forthcoming, but electro-acupuncture could greatly accelerate the return of blood-sugar to normal after insulin, suggesting some kind of enhanced reaction to a physiological emergency. Speed of recovery from alloxan-induced diabetes confirmed this. The Sian group were extending their studies on electro-acupuncture to surgical shock states. In all this there is obviously a connection with the stress syndromes of Selye (p. 215 below).

[a] Meanwhile see especially Anon. (*114*), pp. 295 ff., (*131*).

[1] 針刺麻醉 [2] 電針麻醉

polysaccharides, hyaluronic acid and collagen, and it has been shown that elongated molecules of these kinds are the transducers which generate electric current in the auditory nerves from the pressure of sound waves in the ear and the consequent molecular deformation.[a] In the same way, rhodopsin is the primary chemical receptor in the retina of the eye, the nervous input being consequent upon its changes. Histologists speak of a muco-polysaccharide-protein 'sponge-work' in the connective tissue underlying the skin, and the properties of this need far more examination before it could be assumed that no physico-chemical reality underlies the traditional acu-points.[b] Histo-chemistry may have something important to contribute here.[c] Inglis too has done well to remind us[d] of the far-reaching cytological effects obtained in the classical technique of inducing artificial fertilisation in the eggs of amphibia and echinoderms by the prick of a fine needle.[e]

Indeed the whole approach to the interpretation of acu-tracts and acu-points so far has been insufficiently subtle. It was altogether too simple-minded to expect to find hitherto undescribed microscopical structures;[f] the real basis might be ultra-microscopic, or even dependent on totally unexpected knowledge which the electron microscope alone may reveal.[g] Even if no correlations of this kind turn out to be possible, it may still remain that the acu-tracts have a certain reality (as already suggested) as lines of equivalent physiological action.[h] There is a long way yet to go, and we should not put ourselves in the position of the distinguished astronomer who opined that 'space travel is bunk' only to find men walking on the surface of the moon a few years later. It might well turn out that we ought to be looking for biochemical and ultramicro-morphological characteristics of cells at the acu-points and along the acu-tracts. As yet we just do not know.

It is of course possible to defend the classical tradition while regarding it as a useful construct without any material substrate at all, as for example does Sun Chin-Chhing (*1*). Perhaps this has nowhere been more succinctly summarised than by Sugihara Noriyuki as follows:[i]

> Acupuncture and moxa are just using the Yin–Yang doctrine and the acu-tract/pulse linkage to build a consistent body of theory...The *ching-mo* (tract and vessel) system is

[a] Cf. Christiansen (1, 2); Vilstrup & Jensen (1).

[b] In considering the results of Raymond Evans referred to above (p. 187), Prof. Ursula Franklin of Toronto drew attention to phenomena such as those of superconductivity in metal crystals, and suggested that some particular type of bonding of the long molecules might underlie the properties of the acu-points. Lehrenbecher (1) voices similar ideas.

[c] On these subjects we are grateful for the opportunity of conversations with Dr Janet Plummer and Dr Chhiu Yin-Chhing in Hongkong. Cf. Chhiu & Plummer (1, 2).

[d] (1), pp. 123 ff.

[e] This parthenogenetic activation was first discovered by Bataillon (1, 2) in 1910 for frog and toad eggs. Subsequent reviews by Loeb (1); Parmenter (1) and Rostand (1) show how astonished everyone was at the potentialities of the unfertilised egg on its own thus revealed; cf. Needham (12), p. 352. As we should say nowadays, the maternal DNA alone is quite competent to produce a new adult organism having purely maternal characteristics.

[f] In the histological study of the 'micro-wounds' made by acupuncture needles a beginning has been made by Kellner & Feucht (1).

[g] At present speculations along these lines invite the epithet 'wild', as in the interesting paper of Haveroff (1), but such 'way-out' ideas have a habit now and then of being justified by time. Cf. Darras (1).

[h] Or even 'information transfer' (Greguss, 1).

[i] (*1*), pp. 33–4

simply the means whereby the Yin and Yang influences received both congenitally and nutritionally are carried to the specific parts of the body that require them...Conversely, when a person cannot carry out this function, the abnormalities of the pulse will reveal the diseased condition of an acu-tract. Acupuncture and moxa can cure this.

The modern scientific mind, however, has an insuperable repugnance to thinking in purely abstract terms, and the general tendency therefore is to believe that the multifarious nerve-endings and receptors in the skin and subcutaneous tissues are the anatomical entities responsible for mediating the effects of the acupuncture needles and the various forms of moxibustion.

Another approach to the nature of the acu-points is the study of the subjective sensations reported by those on whom acupuncture is performed. From time immemorial it has been customary in Chinese medicine to take note of what the patient says that he or she experiences, and according to universal consent the acupuncture procedure will do no good if none of the sensations makes its appearance. A positive result is termed *tê chhi*[1] (obtaining the *chhi*) or *chen kan*[2] (responding to the needle). The typical responses are four in number: *suan*,[3] *ma*,[4] *chang*[5,6] and *chung*.[7] The last three of these are easily explained. *Ma* is essentially a feeling of numbness, *chang* is one of distention, extension or fullness, rather as if the part concerned were oedematous or puffy. *Chung* is simply a feeling of heaviness.[a] *Suan* (implying 'sour')[b] is the most difficult to describe, but it can be thought of as an ache, something like a feeling of muscular fatigue or overstrain such as may be experienced after slightly excessive exercise in walking, climbing or playing athletic games. Presumably a few thousand muscle cells might be destroyed or injured as in the common experience of having 'strained a muscle'. One has to distinguish also between a quick primary response, which may be registered immediately, and a later secondary or prolonged response. Thus *suan* is likely to come on after *ma* has been felt, while *chung* is likely to ensue after *ma* or *chang*.[c]

The typical subjective responses are felt not only at or near the site of the acupuncture, but sometimes seem to travel slowly up or down the limbs or the trunk.[d]

[a] But it may also involve a characteristic ache (*thung*[8]), and sometimes a feeling of warmth (*jê*[9]). The latter may even express itself visibly as a superficial redness or vaso-dilation. Cf. Anon. (135), pp. 15–16.

[b] The word may also be written *suan*,[10] which means literally 'acid'. This uses the 'wine' radical (no. 164) instead of the 'disease' radical (no. 104).

[c] We are grateful to Dr Li Ta-Li of Chhêngtu for carrying out some acupuncture experimentally on one of us (J.N.) in 1972. The Tsu-san-li point (V 36) was used, one that has been widely employed in acupuncture analgesia. I felt no pain or other sensation on insertion, but then a curious feeling of numbness came on, as if running downward along the bones as far as the upper surface of the foot from the acu-point on the front of the leg below the knee. Manual manipulation of the needle reinforced the sensation from time to time. On changing the needle insertion so that it pointed upwards (*hsieh*, see immediately below) the feeling went up above the knee and was again reinforced by twiddling. When the needle was removed and I stood up, the leg felt as if slightly overstrained by exercise, and one did not want to put one's weight on it. There was still a definite ache (*suan*) an hour afterwards, and it spread to the gastrocnemius muscle behind. On the following morning the ache persisted, and could be intensified by flexing and extending the foot, but by mid-day it was gone. Thus *ma* had been followed by *suan*.

[d] Cf. Mann (11), pp. 42–3.

1 得氣　2 針感　3 痠　4 痲　5 痮　6 脹　7 重
8 痛　9 熱　10 酸

Innumerable patients have felt this, and we have a good statement of it from the *Chi Shêng Pa Sui*[1] of +1315. Speaking of the cure of headache, the text says.[a]

> Ask the subject to cough, then insert the needle at Ho-ku (IG4) on both sides to a depth of 5 *fên*,[b] and turn it counter-clockwise while the patient inhales three times, then clockwise again for three deep breaths. Repeat the counter-clockwise turning only this time for five inhalations, and the contrary one again in the same way. Then the patient will feel the sensation (*suan*[2]) rising slowly from the hands right up to the shoulders like a thread. Finally ask the patient to take one more deep breath, and withdraw the needle.

This strongly suggests that the conception of the acu-tracts may have arisen, at least in part, from the subjective sensations of those who were undergoing acupuncture. It would have been natural enough to envisage thread-like lines of communication after such experiences and what more reasonable than to suppose that the almost indefinable *chhi* flowed along them? This phenomenon, together with the many manifestations of referred pain (cf. pp. 205ff. below), may go a considerable way towards explaining how the whole acu-tract system came into being in the first place.

Are there any specific relations between sensations and acu-points? Not in general; the subjective responses are practically unpredictable, but *chang* tends to be more intense in the trunk regions, and all the sensations in the arms and legs are liable to last longer. In the extremities *ma* is sometimes followed by *chang* or *chung*, or again *chang* may precede *ma*. All the sensations, but especially *ma*, are commonly felt as spreading along a line or lines, and this is especially true of acupuncture in the back, but these are not necessarily the lines of the acu-tracts themselves, though they quite often are.[c] Inserting the needles in the sedative or antidromic direction (*hsieh*[3]) sends the sensation upwards, while inserting them in the tonic or syndromic direction (*pu*[4]) sends it downwards.[d]

Besides the feelings reported by the patient, there are also phenomena which can be experienced by the physician. He may notice a certain feeling of resistance or palpable motion of the needle, almost as if it was being caught or sucked into the tissues, indeed a kind of sphincter-like muscular contraction which opposes a certain difficulty to the withdrawal of the needle. This is called *chih chung kan*[5] (obstruction sensation) or nowadays *shou hsia kan*[6] (what is felt under the hand).[e] This muscle reaction has attracted the attention of physiologists who have compared the electromyogram (EMG) with the subjective reporting (Anon. *145*). Using IG 4 and 11, and V 36, they could find quite a reasonable correlation as follows (see p. 194):

[a] Ch. 3, pp. 2*b*, 3*a*, tr. auct.
[b] Tenths of an inch, and the inch in Yuan times was 3·07 cm. as against our 2·54.
[c] This observation might go far to explain the historical origin of the *ching-lo* system.
[d] We have here in mind a tract such as the Gastric Podotelic Yang-Ming Tract (V) just mentioned. There are many subtleties in these techniques, on which see Anon. (135), pp. 13ff.
[e] This effect was obtained experimentally in one of us (J. N.) at Kunming in 1972 with a rather deeper penetration at V 36, by Dr Liu Hêng-Fêng, to whom warm thanks are also due. In this case there was the same sequence of *ma* and *suan*.

1 濟生拔粹 2 酸 3 瀉 4 補 5 滯重感 6 手下感

	heavy	moderate	light or zero
objective sensation (*shou hsia kan*) } EMG, % of max.	79	41	20
subjective sensation (*chen kan*) } EMG, % of max.	85	41	23

Since the entire effects disappear under lumbar anaesthesia, and since almost nothing of them is left after intravenous pentothal, it is concluded that they must be due to simple spinal cord reflexes, showing that the nerve pathways are involved and functioning. It was thus of much interest to examine the situation in diseases of the nervous system, and this was done in another investigation (Anon. *146*). In conditions involving some degeneration of muscles or spinal motor neurons (such as amyotrophic lateral sclerosis, myasthenia gravis, and the sequelae of infantile paralysis), the subjects could experience *tê chhi* and give EMG graphs provided the general sensory functions in the limbs were not impaired. In syringomyelia and tabes dorsalis, where pain and temperature sensations were greatly reduced, little or no *tê chhi* or EMG could be obtained. Only in myodystrophy did the correlation fail, for no EMG could be elicited though the *tê chhi* sensations were still present. In general the results suggested that the conduction pathways of acupuncture sensations in the spinal cord were closely related to those for pain and temperature.

(i) *The therapeutic range*

We pass now to the types of disease which were classically treated by acupuncture (Fig. 46). It would be going too far to say that there were no limits to its use in traditional Chinese medicine, but there can be no question that it was employed in many illnesses due to the invasion of pathogenic organisms well known today, as well as for those arising from malfunctions of various parts of the body. It would also be desirable to make a distinction between the uses of acupuncture and moxibustion in traditional China, going back to the Middle Ages and beyond, and those recommended by physicians practising today (*a*) in East Asia, and (*b*) in Europe and the West; but unfortunately no real consensus of opinion has yet emerged, so that the comparison cannot be readily made. We may have a better picture of the situation if we attempt a little classification of diseases as follows:

(1) Diseases due to pathogenic organisms (bacteria, viruses, protozoa, fungi). Infectious or contagious.

(2) Diseases of dietary or toxicological origin—dietary deficiencies, lathyrism, heavy metal poisoning, perhaps coronary thrombosis.

(3) Allergic conditions.

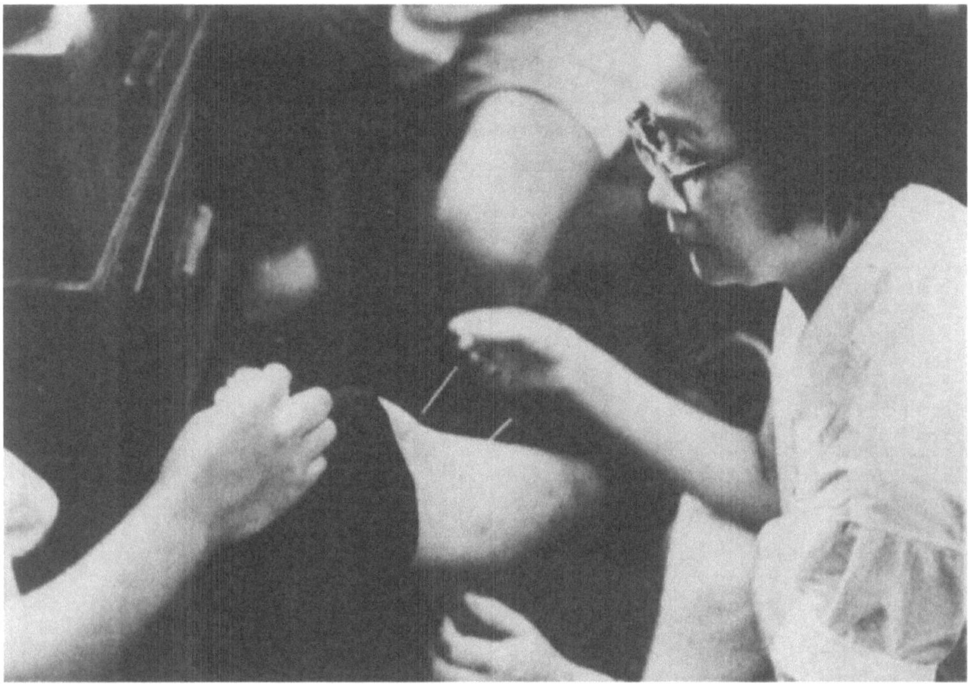

Fig. 46. Therapeutic acupuncture; treatment of the right leg of a patient in the clinic of the First of July Commune near Shanghai in 1971. Photo: Durham.

(4) Malfunctions, endocrine or traumatic, biochemical or biophysical. Sometimes congenital.

(5) Gerontological conditions, such as rheumatism, poly-arthritis, cerebral haemorrhage, or nummular eczema.

This aid to thought is elaborated in Table 20, where a wide variety of examples of affections still treated by acupuncture are mustered under the different categories. There it can be seen that the largest number of disease entities fall under the head of malfunction, whether in origin endogenous or exogenous. Such diseases as typhus, typhoid, cerebro-spinal meningitis, the various forms of encephalitis, or malaria or schistosomiasis, were certainly treated by acupuncture in pre-modern times; but it must always be remembered that the medieval physicians of China had a remarkable armamentarium of drugs with active principles at their disposal,[a] and acupuncture or moxibustion was rarely used alone. Anciently, acupuncture was probably applied in cataract, for neoplasmic growths, and for the intractable pain of malignancy, situations where it is hardly used at all today, but this would be because the weight of clinical experience over the centuries supplied to some extent the lack of solid statisti-

[a] One outstanding case comes to mind; it may well be that the Chinese were the only medieval people who had a genuine anti-malarial drug-plant (*Dichroa febrifuga*) at their disposal. We discuss this in *SCC*, Sects. 38 and 45.

Table 20. *Categories of diseases and pathological conditions in which acupuncture has been habitually used*

1 (pathogenic organisms)	2 (dietary or toxic)	3 (allergies)	4 (malfunctions)	5 (geriatric conditions)
bacillary dysentery[a] cholera[c] ethmoidal sinusitis chronic colitis hepatitis appendicitis[f] post-herpetic neuralgia post-poliomyelitic paralysis psoriasis tuberculous glands deaf-mutism (due to degeneration of auditory nerve)[i] other auditory disorders[i] tonsillitis[j] bronchitis conjunctivitis laryngitis acne eczema	beri-beri	asthma[b] hay-fever other allergies	gastric and duodenal ulcer nephritis hepatitis lumbago fibrositis sciatica[g] migraine[d] trigeminal neuralgia[d] haemorrhoids varicose veins[h] gout hypertension traumatic spinal injuries Bell's palsy[j] urolithiasis cholecystitis glaucoma dysmenorrhoea[k] cervical spondylosis 'slipped disc' Parkinson's disease goitre epistaxis haemoptysis haematemesis haematuria melaena[l] insomnia[m] tachycardia bradycardia renal colic jaundice[n] Paget's disease (osteitis deformans)[o]	rheumatism arthritis[d] hemiplegia[e] prostatitis cerebral haemorrhage

General References: Anon. (135); Mann, Whitaker *et al.* (1); Kaada *et al.* (1), p. 438; Nakayama (1); Woodley (1); McLeod *et al.* (1); Baruch (1); Vogralik (2); Basu (1); Said (1), p. 286; Bachmann (3); Chu Fu-Thang (1); Jalil (1); Bonica (2); Bischko (2); Gunn, Milbrandt *et al.* (1).

On general orientation we wish to acknowledge the help of many conversations with acupuncture physicians in China and Japan, as also with Chang Chien-Ying (Helen Cheung) and Hsiao Yung-Tshai (Y. C. Siow).

cal information. There are a number of ideas of a general nature current in the literature which need to be carefully noted as typical of this kind of cumulative medical wisdom. For example it has been said that everything which is physiologically reversible can be treated by acupuncture,[a] a definition not quite the same as the distinction between organic and functional pathologies. This distinction also has been commonly used to specify the limits of acupuncture techniques, though its applicability is equally often contested.[b] Again, it may be considered that acupuncture works best where severe pain is involved in the syndrome,[c] or that chronic affections respond better than acute ones. There is little doubt that in some cases the results can be extremely dramatic.[d] As for the psycho-somatic aspects of illness, one must never forget that it was a cardinal principle of Chinese medicine throughout the ages to treat the patient as a whole, with regard to all the circumstances of the case, mental

Notes to Table 20.

[a] Anon. (120).

[b] See Fujita & Minami (1); Mery (1); Gillet & Pinet (1) using tachypneumograph tracings; Wên Hsiang-Lai & Chau (1).

[c] One of us (G.D.L.) has vivid recollections of her mother's cholera in 1909 surmounting the crisis by the aid of acupuncture.

[d] Baruch (1) found the *wu hu hsüeh fa*[1] particularly effective; points on the hands at the tips of the fingers; cf. Hsieh Li-Hêng (*2*), p. 390. See also Mann (10); Yü Hsiung-Hung & Than Kuang-Chüan (1).

[e] We saw a number of patients being treated for these and similar conditions in China in 1972. See text.

[f] See Anon. (124, 125, 126); Krack (1). Our own experiences in Shanghai in 1964 we discuss in the text.

[g] Huang Chu-Chai *et al.* (*1*), a report of 100 cases, with 97·9 % successes. See also Leung Soon-Jack (1); McLeod *et al.* (1), pp. 40ff.

[h] Valory (1); Prunier (2).

[i] Anon. (127, 130); de la Fuye (4); Kao (1); Kao, Baker & Leung (1); Anon. (*169*); Fang Yu-An (*1*); Shih Liu & Ssu Chi (1). This has been one of the more controversial subjects. McLeod *et al.* (1) after study in China, felt that the effects had not yet been scientifically established. Mann (9) expresses scepticism but reports positive results in vertigo, tinnitus and labyrinthitis. Acupuncture for deafness is usually thought of as a recent Chinese development, but it was described already in the +14th century. The *Chi Shêng Pa Sui* (+1315), ch. 3, p. 5*a*, recommends SC 17 on both sides followed by acupuncture at VF 2, and for tinnitus, too, and blocked Eustachian tubes.

[j] Basu (1); Anon. (129). But McLeod *et al.* (1) doubt if the high spontaneous recovery rate in Bell's palsy has been allowed for.

[k] Lin Chhiao-Chih (1).

[l] This and the preceding four types of bleeding, of course symptomatic, were controlled by de la Fuye (1), presumably because of the vaso-constrictive effect of acupuncture.

[m] Especially by injecting lidocaine at acu-points on the auricula; Li Tsun-Nin (1).

[n] Nguyen Van Nghi (2).

[o] De la Farge (1).

---

[a] Mann (1–5, 11); Mann, Whitaker *et al.* (1). Possibly relevant here is the routine 66% success in the induction of labour in pregnancy reported by Yip, Pang & Sung (1).

[b] As by Broujean (1), who treated successfully bone lesions from wounds, cyphoskoliosis, disseminated encephalo-myelitis, bilateral coxarthria, arthritic ankyloses, etc. Guillaume (1) too, described how in many cases of ulcerations, salpingitis, etc., there can be *restitutio ad integrum* effected by acupuncture.

[c] Kaada *et al.* (1), p. 438; de la Fuye (3).

[d] Cf. Schmidt (1) for severe traumatic muscular pain; or Bachmann (2) reporting a case of subiliac ulcerative colitis with obstruction, intestinal vomiting and colic. Putensen (1) described an immediate recovery of the sense of smell, which had been lost for some years. Cf. Laforet (1).

[1] 五虎穴法

as well as physical.[a] For illnesses primarily psychiatric acupuncture is certainly still used in China today, though on the whole adjuvant to group therapy and the social approach rather than psychotherapy.[b] On the borderline here, remarkable results are being reported for the cure of drug addiction.[c]

The universal reproach directed against therapeutic acupuncture by modern scientific medicine is the lack of statistical evidence which would remove it from the sphere of folk-belief and suggestion. The absence of adequate clinical control experiments, the existence of the 'placebo effect' (cf. pp. 239, 261 below), and the relative paucity of quantitative remission and follow-up data even in contemporary China, is indeed a hindrance to many in taking therapeutic acupuncture seriously. So long as this lasts, both the affirmations[d] and the sceptical denials[e] by Westerners seem insufficiently based. But let no one say that the Chinese were unaware of the possibility of spontaneous recoveries and remissions. There is a passage in the *Chou Li* particularly interesting in this connection and worth giving here; it occurs in the section on the physicians of the imperial government.[f]

> The I Shih[1] is in charge of the medical administration (of the country). He collects all efficacious drugs (*tu yao*[2]) for the purpose of healing diseases. All those suffering from external maladies, whether of the head or the body, are treated separately by the appropriate specialists.
>
> At the end of the year he uses the records of each physician to decide on his rank and salary. Those who have cured 100% of their patients are graded in the first class, those who have had 90% successes are of the second class, those who have been 80% successful are placed third, those who have cured 70% are considered fourth-class, and the lowest grade of all contains those who could not cure more than 60%.
>
> [Comm. The reason why those who failed with four out of ten patients were placed in the lowest grade was because half the cases might well have recovered anyway, even without any treatment at all (*huo pu chih tzu yü*[3]).]

Thus the text itself, perhaps of the −2nd century, implies very clearly the keeping of clinical records, and the comment of Chêng Khang-Chhêng in the +2nd century

[a] This was perhaps an uncovenanted mercy arising from the resolute refusal of Chinese natural philosophers to make a sharp distinction between matter and spirit. Cf. *SCC*, Vol. 5, pt. 2, pp. 86, 92–3, and Needham (78).

[b] Kaada *et al.* (1), p. 440; Ratnavale (1); Anon. (*149*); J. J. Kao (1). It is said that acupuncture has replaced electro-convulsive therapy in Chinese psychiatric hospitals.

[c] Wên Hsiang-Lai & Cheung (1); Ng, Nguyen *et al.* (1); Bourne (1); similar control of tobacco addiction has been reported by Thoret (1). McLeod *et al.* (1), not usually given to easy acceptance of acupuncture claims, were particularly impressed with the results of the Hongkong group (p. 166). As Patterson (1) shows, in her interesting monograph, it is particularly the withdrawal symptoms which electro-acupuncture can keep at bay, allowing the patient to build up defences against the craving. Gregory Chhen (1) has meanwhile made the connection, obvious as soon as pointed out, between this addiction-therapy and the natural opioid peptides, the enkephalins and endorphins (probably deeply implicated in acupuncture analgesia), on which see p. 260 below.

[d] E.g. Niboyet & Bourdiol (1); de Morant (2, 3).

[e] E.g. McLeod *et al.* (1).

[f] Tr. auct., adjuv. Biot (1), vol. 1, p. 93. Attention was drawn to the passage by Veith (2), p. 163, but the essential point escaped both her and Wang An-Shih, whose interpretations she was studying. For a classical history of medical statistics see Greenwood (1).

[1] 醫師 [2] 毒藥 [3] 或不治自愈

is an admirable example of the scepticism and critical mentality of the scholars of ancient China. Such was the background of the clinical experience accumulated by the Chinese physicians concerning acupuncture as well as other treatments through the centuries. We may recall here a whole genre of medical literature, the *i an*,[1] or books of case histories, which spanned the centuries from Shunyü I in the Early Han (−2nd century) to the late Chhing time, rising to a crescendo after Hsü Shu-Wei[2] (*fl.* +1132).[a] There has been too little study of this critical and objective literature.

While it is true that the lack of sophisticated statistical analysis dogs all attempts to estimate the real value of therapeutic acupuncture, it would not be right to say that no statistics are available at all.[b] For example a group of ten qualified medical men in London reported on 1000 cases treated by acupuncture, the age of the patients ranging from 3 weeks to 92 years.[c] There was cure or great improvement in 439 cases, and moderate improvement or considerable alleviation in a further 290, so that one could say that 72·9 % showed marked responses to the treatment. Acupuncture was the principal therapy used in all these instances, chosen rather conservatively among the painful malfunctions. A more extensive set of figures for treatments given in the Soviet Union during the five years before 1962 covered 10,721 patients. Here the results, reported by Vogralik (3), were as follows:

	no. of cases	percentage
Cure or very significant relief with long remission	3505	32·7
Marked relief, with shorter remission	3986	37·1
Milder relief	2045	19·1
No effect	1185	11·1

Thus the sum of the two first grades came to 69·8 %, quite close to the figure obtained by the group in London. In this series also the conditions were mainly malfunctions such as gastric ulcer, hypertension, stenocardia and incipient glaucoma, or allergic affections such as bronchial asthma. Finally about the same time Canas (1), describing 122 cases in private practice in Paris, reported 85·7 % for the sum of the two first grades, and 68 % for the first grade alone. His cases included lumbago, sciatica, torticollis, sprains, hydrarthrosis, sinusitis, acute laryngitis, epistaxis and ulcerating varicose veins.[d]

[a] See Hsieh Li-Hêng (*1*), pp. 52*b*, 53*a*.

[b] A great number of papers containing statistical data have been published in China especially since 1960; see the collection in Anon. (*148*) and the bibliography in Anon. (*149*).

[c] Mann, Whitaker *et al.* (1).

[d] More recently, a series of some 660 cases treated in Miami, Florida, has been reported with statistical analyses (Anon. 151). Not unexpectedly, in view of their saecular tradition, rather higher percentages have been published from China. For example, Chu Lien (1) reported a series of 9513 patients with over 90 % responding satisfactorily to treatment, and more than 40 % experiencing complete cure.

[1] 醫案 [2] 許叔微

If we put together all these figures we obtain the following table.

			% in Grades					
place	ref.	approx. no. of cases	I cure or great relief	II marked relief	I+II	III slight relief	IV no effect	III+IV
U.K.	Mann, Whitaker *et al.*(1)	1000	43·9	29·0	72·9	—	—	27·1
U.S.S.R.	Vogralik (3)	10,700	32·7	37·1	69·8	19·1	11·1	30·2
France	Canas (1)	120	68·0	17·7	85·7	—	—	14·3
U.S.A.	Anon. (151)	660	55·7	16·4	72·1	13·8	14·1	27·9
	av.		50·7	25·05	75·05	—	—	2·49
	av. omitting the small French series		44·1	27·5	71·6	—	—	28·4

We shall recur to this pattern presently in a comparison between acupuncture therapy and acupuncture analgesia (p. 224).

A very different type of morbidity was tackled by a group of Chinese physicians who reported on 63 cases of bacillary dysentery.[a] Somewhat to their surprise, acupuncture and moxibustion proved to be more effective than either sulpha-guanidine, phage or the traditional Chinese drugs:

	acupuncture and moxa	sulpha-guanidine	phage	Chinese drugs
days to subsidence of symptoms	3·2	3·6	4·6	9·5
days before return of faeces to normality	4·6	6·2	6·0	9·3

All the patients were cured (which, whatever the spontaneity, would have given them high marks by the idealists of the *Chou Li*), there were no relapses during the following two years, and the treatment was adopted as standard.[b]

Here of course we can give only a very few examples of statistical studies of acupuncture therapy, but one well worth examining is the experience of hospitals in Shanghai, Canton and Kirin with appendicitis.[c] Broadly speaking, treatment with

[a] Anon. (120).

[b] Acu-points used were JM 4, 6, 8, 10 and V 25, 36. It was noticeable that the stimulus of the needle, mediated through the nervous system, would immediately inhibit the irresistible urge to defaecate.

[c] The first results were reported from 1959 onwards, Anon. (*170*, 124, 126), and in 1964 we were able to see the work at first hand in the Chungshan Hospital at Shanghai and obtain the figures in Table 21. Our thanks are due to Dr Li Chieh-Ying and Dr Hsiung Ju-Chhêng for their kindness on that occasion.

Table 21. *Appendicitis treated with acupuncture at the Chungshan Hospital, Shanghai*

					follow-up within 1·5 years			
	no. of cases	cured	improved	no effect	no. of cases	no recurrence	chronic symptoms	recurrence
simple uncomplicated	500	323 (64·6 %)	139 (27·8 %)	38 (7·6 %)	391	118 (30·2 %)	108 (27·6 %)	165 (42·2 %)
with local peritonitis	78	28 (35·9 %)	17 (21·8 %)	33 (42·3 %)	40	17 (42·5 %)	9 (28·5 %)	14 (35·0 %)
with appendicular abscess	12	5	6	1	11	5	1	5
						follow-up within 4 years (1530 cases)		
						20·3 %	38·4 %	41·3 %

acupuncture[a] would bring recoveries or remissions in about 92% of the uncomplicated cases, but inflammation would be likely to recur in 42% necessitating appendectomies ultimately.[b] With the needles kept in for half an hour two or three times a day there was almost always quick relief of pain and fall of temperature and most patients were free of symptoms after six days.[c] Recurrences, if not too severe, could also again be treated by acupuncture.[d] But the great interest of the Shanghai studies was that they included experimental appendicitis in dogs. The tip of the caecum was tied off and a mixed culture of staphylococci and streptococci injected into it; then acupuncture treatment was given, and the tissues of both treated and control animals removed for histological analysis on the fourth day. Inflammation was very heavy in the latter, and light to medium in the former. Particularly interesting was the fact that if the dorsal sympathetic ganglia and the trunk with its roots was cut on both sides between the 5th and the 12th segments the protective effect of the acupuncture was completely inhibited. In conjunction with this, it was significant that while the phagocytosis index (staph.) was increased in the treated animals by only 11·5%, the hydrocortisone level of the blood was increased by as much as 99%. We shall shortly return to this point (p. 213).

Let us add a few more examples of practical acupuncture therapy. Taking first the Chinese side, there is little in the scientific literature before 1949, previous writers having been interested only in the occasional accidents due to ignorant acupuncturists without proper medical training.[e] But once traditional medicine was restored to honour, many investigations were published. In pulmonary tuberculosis, acupuncture was found to be rather effective for neuro-functional ataxia (night sweating, thoracodynia, anorexia, moderate haemoptysis and insomnia), not so much so for calming the coughing, and not at all for the pyrexia.[f] Of course no radical cure could be effected, but the reduction of symptoms was marked in some 75% of the cases, with complete disappearance in 61%. In biliary ascariasis, a series of 48 cases was completely cured by acupuncture combined with the traditional prescription called *wu mei thang*,[1] the needles removing the pain while the plant drugs promoted expulsion.[g] Even in schistosomiasis, acupuncture brought about a disappearance of the clinical symptoms, while the number of parasite eggs in the faeces steadily decreased.[h] Such results could hardly be explained in any other way than by an increase in corticosteroids and an enhancement of antibody production.

[a] In some studies very favourable results were also obtained with traditional Chinese plant drugs (Anon. 125), some of which probably contain antibiotics.

[b] It was then usually found that stercoliths had been present.

[c] The leucocyte count would fall to normal levels within three days. Tenderness and abdominal pain would disappear in four days. The treatment was just as successful with children as with adults. In the Shanghai experience no traditional or modern drugs were given.

[d] For a personal account by a Western observer who participated in these studies, see Gregoir (1).

[e] See for instance Yin (1) and similar accounts in the *Chinese Medical Journal*.

[f] Chhen Kuo-Liang & Li Chhuan-Chung (1).

[g] Thung Shang-Thai & Chou Tê-I (1). *Wu mei* is the smoked unripe fruits of *Prunus mume*; cf. Chhen Tshun-Jen (*1*), vol. 2, pp. 1006 ff.; Anon. (*110*), p. 369 and fig. 213. It is the chief ingredient in this prescription, which has been shown by Wang Kuang-Chhien (*1*) to have considerable antibacterial activity in cases of chronic dysentery.

[h] Anon. (131), 54 cases.

[1] 烏梅湯

The drawback of the European acupuncture literature since about 1950, essentially 'anecdotal', is that the reports tend to describe only isolated cases.[a] But Krack (1) confirmed the effect in sub-acute appendicitis, as well as the customary conditions such as asthma,[b] herpes, erythema nodosum, colitis and chronic skin diseases. Ulcerating varicose veins were greatly helped,[c] as also Paget's disease (osteitis deformans)[d] and the tremors of Parkinson's disease.[e] One recurring observation, interesting in view of the common impression that acupuncture analgesia cannot be induced in children and infants, is that infantile affections may respond very well to acupuncture therapy, e.g. convulsions[f] and diarrhoea.[g] Alberti described a rather dramatic case of a 3-month-old baby with opisthotonus, contractures of the lower limbs, mydriasis, tetanus of the back muscles and general rigidity, which was restored to complete normality in a couple of months. The trouble about all such specific clinical reports is that one never knows whether the condition would have cleared up anyway, but the general impression one gains from the literature is that acupuncture can bring about a marked increase in the body's own resistance and healing power, together with direct effects on the nervous system in the case of neurological abnormalities. As Alberti himself pointed out, positive effects in infants have the significance that suggestion can be excluded.

Lumbago (cf. Table 20) has long been one of those conditions generally allowed as highly responsive to acupuncture treatment. Though it does not substitute for a statistical analysis, the following passage from the pen of one of the most distinguished physicians of modern times will be read with much interest. In his 'Principles and Practice of Medicine', William Osler wrote:[h]

> For lumbago, acupuncture is, in acute cases, the most efficient treatment. Needles of from three to four inches in length (ordinary bonnet needles, sterilised, will do) are thrust into the lumbar muscles at the seat of pain,[i] and withdrawn after five or ten minutes. In many instances the relief of pain is immediate, and I can corroborate the statements of Ringer, who taught me this practice, as to its extraordinary and prompt effect in many instances. The constant current, too, is sometimes very beneficial.

This must have been an inheritance from the acupuncturists of the early nineteenth century whom we discuss elsewhere (p. 297).

[a] Drawback perhaps, but we should always remember the spirited defence of the 'anecdote', i.e. the 'previously unpublished item of individual first-hand experience', by Nathan (5). Single cases may have much to teach.

[b] Confirmed by Gillet & Pinet (1) using tachypneumograph tracings.

[c] Cf. Valory (1); Prunier (2).

[d] De la Farge (1). Here anti-inflammatory corticosteroids also work well (Henneman, Dull, Avioli *et al.*, 1).

[e] Teboul & Teboul-Wiart (1).

[f] Prunier (1); Alberti (1).

[g] Betz (1).

[h] (1), p. 1131. For this reference we are much indebted to our old teacher, Sir Rudolph Peters. The exploits of Sir William Osler in that direction were not always successful, however, as in the celebrated case of Peter Redpath, the Montreal merchant and philanthropic benefactor of McGill University, described by Cushing (1), p. 177, and Fransiszyn (2). On the other hand, Morse (4) tells us that Sir James Cantlie (1851–1926), the surgeon and teacher of Sun Yat-Sen in Hongkong, and the man who saved him when detained in the (Manchu) Chinese embassy in London, habitually used acupuncture for sprains and chronic rheumatism with good results.

[i] On this see p. 211 below.

In 1972 we had the opportunity of studying personally the treatment of hemiplegia and similar conditions at the outpatient department of the Lung-Hua Hospital in Shanghai.[a] One patient with paraplegia after a spinal injury had been completely paralysed but could now walk unaided.[b] Needles were placed at eight acu-points in the back and stimulated electrically with pulses at 6 volts DC in such a way that he could himself control the strength and frequency of stimulus so as to get as much as possible without undue discomfort. Another was doing the same after an operation for vertebral fracture; originally his lower extremities had been anaesthesic as well as paralysed but he could now walk with the help of crutches. Two other patients were having heat treatment with moxa burning at the ends of 4 or 5 needles[c] in the back of the neck;[d] one after a stroke which had given slight general paralysis with aphasia, but she could now speak again; the other after hypertrophy of the cervical vertebrae with compression of the nerve roots.[e] Cupping was still in use for this, and also a needle-roller which drew a little capillary blood. Moxa cones were burning to the skin for asthma and chronic bronchitis;[f] this treatment leaves permanent marks, but the small scars are relieved with plasters made from medicinal plants. Acupuncture was also being employed on children, with good effects, for myopia, retinitis and degeneration of the optic nerve after high fevers. Such were some of the interesting procedures in this large general hospital, which deals with 2000 outpatients a day.

(ii) *Head Zones, dermatomes and referred pain*

The moment now has come to see what light modern neuro-physiology can throw on the ancient origins of the *ching-lo* and acupuncture system,what further light we can get from it, moreover, on the probable mode of action of the nerve impulses initiated by the peripheral stimuli of the needles. Here we have to think first of a cluster of phenomena not easily separable—'referred' pain, the 'Head Zones', the dermatomes (cutaneous areas supplied by the different segmental nerves of the spinal cord), and the spots or regions of surface tenderness caused by malfunctions or diseases of the viscera. In this way we may come to regard the doctrine of the connection of the main acupuncture tracts (*chêng ching*,[1] p. 44) with the internal organs as a most striking discovery or insight of ancient Chinese medical physiology, empirical no doubt but none the less extraordinary for that. Many of us must have had the common experience of sudden severe pain in some part of the body which disappears instantly as soon as a local pressure of gas is released in one or other part of the intestinal tract.[g] Correla-

[a] Our grateful thanks are due to Dr Chang Ling-Chen and Dr Huang Wên-Thung for the warm welcome which they gave us.

[b] We have seen a similar case in Cambridge, that of an Irish girl who had had three cerebral haemorrhages after falls from horses, with concussion; acupuncture had restored to her the capacity of walking without crutches.

[c] This is the *wên chen*[2] technique, cf. p. 104 above.

[d] These needles were made of silver. On the different metals that have been used see p. 74 above.

[e] This condition occurs relatively often in China (Dr Chang Hsiang-Thung, priv. comm.).

[f] This too is very frequently met with in China, and constitutes one of the biggest problems of medical practice.

[g] Referred pain can be extremely distant from the true site of origin. Especially after unilateral or bilateral cordotomy pin-pricks applied to analgesic parts of the body such as the leg brought pain

[1] 正經 [2] 溫針

tions of this kind, registered over many years in the clinical experience of the ancient physicians, must have been what convinced them that particular areas of the skin were connected with particular viscera.

And indeed they are. The peculiarity of visceral pain, triggered by malfunction or infection, as opposed to somatic pain, is that its localisation is very diffuse and it radiates into, i.e. is referred to, cutaneous areas.[a] The reference zone for a particular internal organ coincides with the segmental distribution of the somatic sensory nerve-fibres entering the cord at the same level as the fibres coming from the organ (*tsang*[1] or *fu*,[2] p. 22) in question. Thus for example cardiac pain is referred to the left side of the chest and the inner aspect of the left arm, because the sensory neurons from the heart as well as from these superficial tissue areas enter the thoracic spinal segments on the left side. Similarly pain from the gall-bladder or bile ducts is felt in the upper quadrant of the abdomen and the infrascapular region of the back on the right; kidney and ureter signals are reflected to the loins and inguinal regions.[b] Appendicitis pain starts at the umbilicus, but moves to the lower right quadrant of the abdomen as the inflammation reaches the adjacent peritoneum; this is the celebrated McBurney's point[c] important in diagnosis. So consistent and valuable are these cutaneous signs that atlases of pain patterns are now in general use.[d]

But the phenomenon of referred pain is not yet entirely understood. At first it was thought that there were nerve-cells with branched axons reaching both to the skin and to a particular internal organ, thus transmitting a mixed signal so that the brain could not localise the site of the injury. Another explanation suggested spinal reflexes, set off by the afferent visceral fibres homing in a particular segment, and causing peripheral vaso-constriction or other processes which would stimulate the cutaneous pain nerve-endings and so transmit signals which the brain would interpret as surface pain. Or again there might be common tract cells in the spinal grey matter so excited by impulses of visceral origin that they would respond to normally subliminal cutaneous stimuli. Perhaps the most probable explanation is misinterpretation by the thalamus in the diencephalon, at the base of the brain, and hence by the cortex, of the afferent inputs; pain of cutaneous origin being a much more common experience than internal pain.

sensations as far away as the shoulders or the abdomen; Nathan (2). In the instance given above, fingers, knuckles, ankles, toes can all be involved because their nerve-supply comes within the thoracic and lumbar dermatomes, segmentally connected with stomach and intestines through sympathetic ganglia.

[a] Excellent accounts of referred pain are to be found in Barr (1), pp. 334ff.; Melzack (1), pp. 172ff., 183ff.; Kuntz (1), pp. 438ff. Visceral afferent fibres all traverse autonomic ganglia and plexuses. The viscera are insensitive to touch, cutting and temperature, but very sensitive to stretching, as also to disturbed cell conditions such as changes of pH or abnormal metabolic processes. Useful books on the autonomic nervous system are those of Kuntz (1), who describes the anatomical and physiological features, and Burn (1), more chemical and pharmacological.

[b] Because in the first case the neurons from both sensory regions enter the cord through the seventh and eighth thoracic dorsal roots, while in the second case the first and second lumbar segments are involved.

[c] Generally identified with V 26.

[d] For example, that of Smith, Christensen *et al.* (1).

[1] 臟 [2] 腑

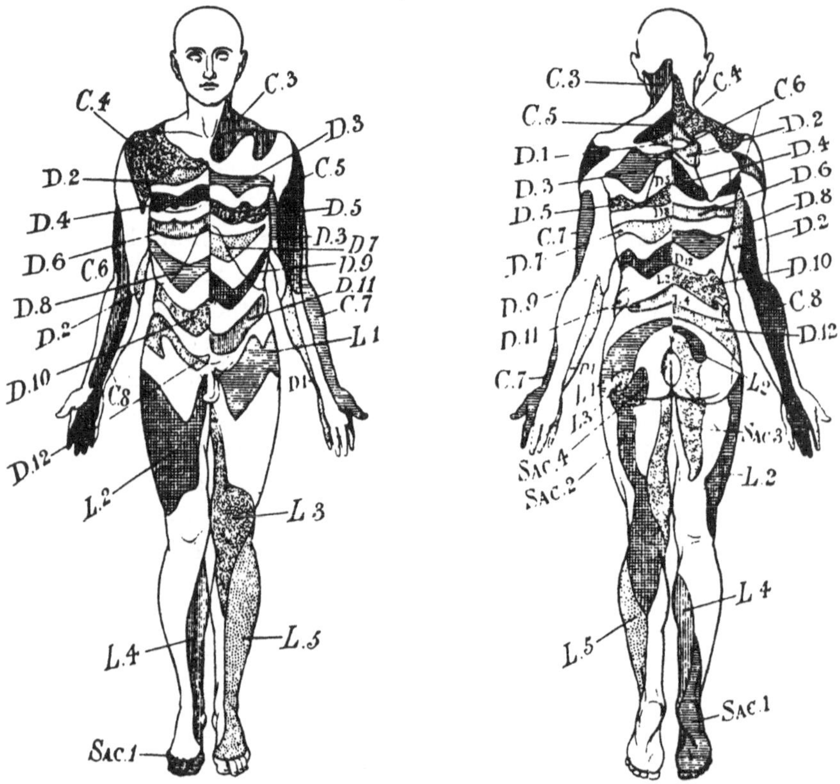

Fig. 47. Chart of the 'Head Zones', or areas of innervation of the peripheral surface of the body by the principal segmental spinal nerves (after Keegan & Garrett, 1). Henry Head elucidated these from 1893 onwards, demonstrating the cutaneous–visceral connections, and published drawings of this kind.

Modern physiological knowledge relates to the acupuncture system in many ways. For example, reverting to cardiac pain, it has been found that most patients with heart disease show a consistent pattern of 'trigger points' or areas in the shoulders and the chest.[a] If one or other of these is smartly pressed, intense pain lasting for hours may be induced. But there is something here beyond pathology, for in normal subjects the application of pressure at these points can produce marked discomfort of several minutes' duration and even liable to intensify after removal of the pressure. In most of the referred pain zones, too, there are one or more small trigger areas, pressure on which will intensify the pain both internal and external;[b] and if these are injected with anaesthetics like novocaine the pain is removed not only from the subcutaneous area but from the internal organ as well. The frequency of attacks of pain may greatly decrease after one such injection, or even permanently disappear.[c] All this is but an aspect of a considerable body of knowledge on painful trigger areas associated with the muscles and the fibrous fascia covering them, and we must return to it in a few moments; but one can see already that the traditional Chinese acu-

[a] Kennard & Haugen (1). [b] Travell & Rinzler (1, 2) [c] See Travell & Rinzler (1).

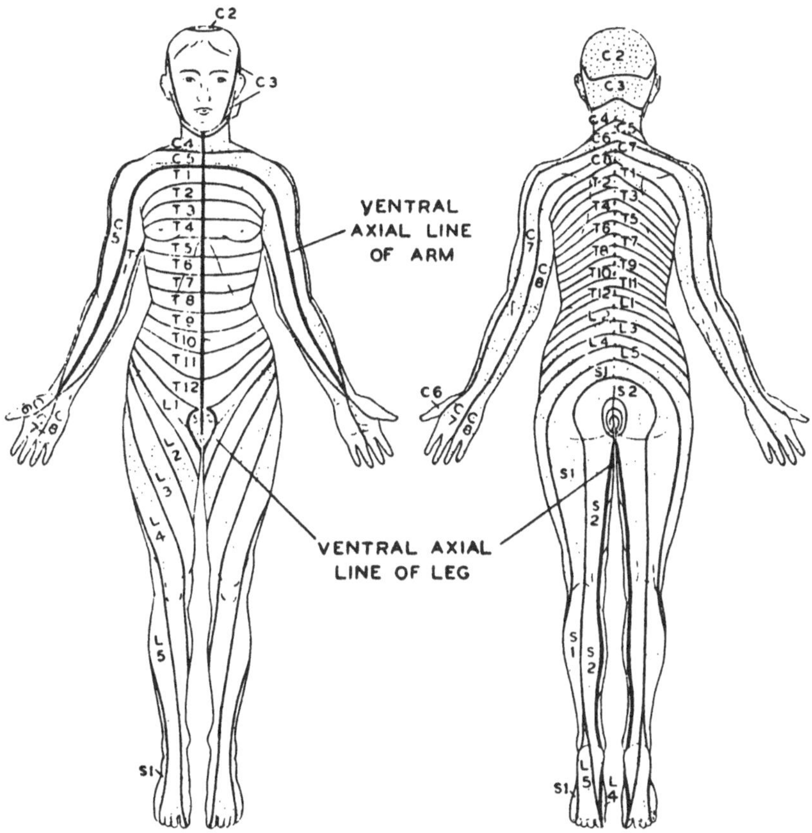

Fig. 48. The Head Zones, now called dermatomes, with their boundaries refined by more recent research (after Keegan & Garrett, 1). The patterns in the extremities continue in serial sequence from the spine, so one can see how the acu-tracts on the limbs course for long distances within the same dermatome (see text). In acupuncture analgesia it has become more and more evident that the needles must be in the same dermatome as the surgical intervention.

points, with their presumed visceral connections, were far from being entirely a figment of the imagination. On the contrary, clinical observations of referred pain might go a long way to account for how they came to be developed in the first place.

Knowledge of the cutaneous-visceral connections took great steps forwards in the last decade of the last century. In 1892 McKenzie (1) was pursuing the cutaneous tenderness associated with the pain of various visceral diseases, but the elaborate work of Henry Head published in the ensuing years (1) became classical for its subtlety and originality.[a] He studied not only the areas of cutaneous tenderness, but also those charted out by the distribution of herpes eruptions (a virus which travels along the nerves), as well as the limits of analgesia found in specific organic diseases of the central nervous system.[b] The result was the chart of 'Head Zones' seen in

[a] Cf. Cross *et al.* (1).

[b] He emphasised that only pain, and exaggerated heat and cold sensations, were affected, never touch.

Fig. 47.[a] They are now called dermatomes, and their topography has been much refined in more recent researches;[b] the chart of Keegan & Garrett (1) is shown in Fig. 48. Here it is instructive to note how the segmental character of the nerve distributions on the trunk—reminiscent indeed of an insect larva—is drawn out into extended longitudinal areas on all four extremities. This means that the acupuncture tracts on the arms and legs course for long distances within the same dermatome.[c] So also the auxiliary tract Tai Mo[1] (p. 45) cinctures the body along the last thoracic and the first lumbar dermatomes.[d] So also, as has been demonstrated in Anon. (128), the *pei shu hsüeh*[2] points on regular tract VU (p. 66) are each one on the same dermatome level as the segmental nerve supply of the organs after which they are named.[e] And this must give equal importance to the median line acu-points on the regulative auxiliary tracts Tu Mo[3] and Jen Mo[4] (cf. pp. 49, 50).[f] In contemporary Chinese medicine and acupuncture there is of course a full consciousness of the Head Zones and the dermatomes.[g] That they must have a great bearing on the phenomena of acupuncture is undoubted, but much neuro-physiological work remains to be done before all is clear; different acu-points may have different actions within the same dermatome, there may be influences radiating to neighbouring dermatomes, or even skipping one or two, and long inter-segmental Sherrington reflexes probably play a considerable part as well.

There can be no question that traditional Chinese medicine deeply appreciated the complex viscero-cutaneous relationships.[h] Much physiological work has now been done on them. In the forties it was found that stimulation of the dorsal skin in rats or rabbits brings about immediate changes in the intestinal tract, marked vaso-constriction or dilation according to the dermatomes used.[i] Stimulation of the epigastrial skin greatly affects the gastric muscles and the pyloric sphincter, causes also hyperaemia of the colon.[j] Peristaltic movements of the small intestine of the dog are strongly influenced by acupuncture at V 36, 37, increased if slow and reduced if fast.[k] Cardiac action in dogs is affected by acupuncture, perhaps because of a decrease in vagal

[a] Their modern use may be followed in works such as that of Cyriax (1).

[b] Cf. Keegan (1); Hansen (1); Hansen & Schliak (1). Kellgren (1, 2), interested in the control of muscular and rheumatic pain, and using saline injections, has also made new charts of the viscero-cutaneous zones.

[c] For example, P, SC, IG and IT on the arms, VF, G, LP on the legs (cf. Figs. 6, 7).

[d] Cf. Anon. (*162*), p. 58.

[e] Cf. Anon. (*162*), p. 37.

[f] Again Anon. (*162*), pp. 52, 54. And Chhung Mo[5] also, op. cit. p. 56.

[g] See for example Anon. (*114*), pp. 45–6; Anon. (*123*), pp. 92–3; and Ho Tsung-Yü (1), who says that the work of McKenzie and Head was slightly anticipated by G. A. Zacharin. For the West see also Mann (1), rev. 2nd ed., pp. 10ff.

[h] Anon. (128). We include cutaneo-visceral under this rubric.

[i] Cf. Kuntz (2); Kuntz & Hazelwood (1); Richins & Brizzee (1).

[j] Freude & Ruhemann (1).

[k] Li Chieh-Ying (priv. comm. Shanghai, 1964); and this is commonly seen in human patients undergoing laparotomies. So also gastric and intestinal motility can be greatly increased both in patients and in experimental animals by acupuncture and electro-acupuncture; Matsumoto, Ambruso & Hayes (1).

1 帶脉 2 背腧穴 3 督脉 4 任脉 5 衝脉

tone.[a] There is a shortening of the cardiac cycle and the P–R interval, a decrease in amplitude of the R-wave, and a decrease, extinction or inversion of the T-wave. The reflex arc could be blocked by lumbar anaesthesia, morphine, atropine, or vagus section. Similarly, moxa or acupuncture applied at TM 25 in dogs brings about a striking increase in cardiac output and stroke volume lasting for two hours, together with a significant decrease in total peripheral resistance.[b] Finally, decapitated fishes offer an interesting material because the contraction or expansion of the melanophores in the skin is such an evident response; here stimulation of the rectum, intestines, gall-bladder or spleen, whether electrical or chemical, causes a powerful contraction of the pigment-cells, the reflex passing through the sympathetic chain.[c] Conversely, stimulation of the skin with silver nitrate would give vaso-constriction of the appropriate part of the intestines, stimulation electrically would cause ischaemia of stomach or gut. But if the cord was intact, a spinal reflex takes precedence, and vaso-dilation occurs instead. These are simply repeatable laboratory demonstrations of the close neuronic connections between inner organs and superficial cutaneous areas of the body.[d] Surely the ancient Chinese discovery of such relationships was as brilliant as anything that we owe to Hippocratic medicine or Alexandrian physiology.[e]

Many aspects of these phenomena can be found described in the *Huang Ti Nei Ching* of the −1st and −2nd centuries. For example, speaking of the *pei shu hsüeh*[1] on the back, the *Ling Shu* says:[f] 'When one wants to determine an acu-point exactly, one should press hard with a finger at one spot after another, then if it is the right one, the patient will feel a relief of his pain (or at least a lesser degree of it).' And the text goes on to recommend the radiant heat of moxibustion, saying that if acupuncture is used the depth of the needling should be shallow. Such points were called *fan ying tien*[2] (stimulus-and-response points), or *ya thung tien*[3] (pain-pressure points). Moreover, beside the remote effects conclusions could be drawn from the specific tenderness in certain places reported by the subject. 'When internal organs are suffering abnormal conditions, certain small areas on the surface of the body exhibit hypersensitive reactions to pressure on the acu-points.'[g]

In the first months of 1947 one of us (J.N.) was staying, as so often, with Charles Singer at his home in Cornwall, and learnt that he had been having treatment for lumbago, fibrositis or back-ache, by the injection of local anaesthetics. But it had been found experimentally that injection of distilled water would sometimes do just as well,

[a] Wei Pao-Ling & Chang Hsi-Hsien (*1*), using ECG recordings and V 36.
[b] Lee Dochil, Lee Myung-o & Clifford (1, 2).
[c] Wernøe (1).
[d] Further researches on cutaneo-visceral and viscero-cutaneous reflexes are reviewed by Mann (11), pp. 3 ff., 10 ff.
[e] As Kretzschmar (1), p. 534, was so good as to say: 'It seems that the ancient Chinese discovered the connection between certain spots on the body surface and certain viscera many centuries before Head, McKenzie and the modern investigators.' He felt too that the Chinese acupuncture-tract charts, 'though shrouded in mysticism' (not perhaps exactly the *mot juste*), showed a striking similarity to contemporary charts of hyperalgic spots, trigger areas, tenderness zones, etc.
[f] *NCLS/PH*, ch. 51, (p. 373), *NCLS/MC*, ch. 51, (p. 1230).
[g] Anon. (*123*), p. 12.

[1] 背俞穴 [2] 反應點 [3] 壓痛點

or even the prick of the hypodermic needle without the injection of anything at all. I therefore wrote to Singer's consultant, Gilbert Causey, saying that if this were really so it approximated to the ancient Chinese practice of acupuncture, and asking for further details. Causey replied that his interest in such techniques had been awakened first by a member of the French school, J. J. Forestier, whom he had heard lecture in 1929. Causey's custom was to inject all types of fluid—novocaine, water,[a] osteocalcin, camphrosalyl—with equally satisfactory results. Naturally he was uncertain how far these effects had a true physiological basis, but the proportion of subjects relieved or cured was much higher than could be expected on the basis of the placebo effect (p. 239). Where a palpable fibrositic nodule was present, the relief might come, Causey thought, from the possibility of free muscular movements granted by the local anaesthetic, movements which would remove or spread the exudate and promote the resorption of the adventitious connective-tissue fibres. Such methods were already commonly used in the twenties.[b]

This brings us back to the study of painful trigger areas in muscle tissue and in the fibrous fascia between it and the skin.[c] The fibrositic nodules, their foci, may develop after virus infections or other fevers,[d] inflammatory processes,[e] or muscular strains and stresses.[f] They are liable to show local changes such as increased blood-flow, more sweating, and increased temperature. However they arise, they produce almost continuous volleys of impulses entering the spinal cord, and these could interact, either by summation or by jamming inhibition,[g] with inputs from abnormal viscera. Summation would lead to referral of the internal pain to larger skin zones surrounding the trigger areas. Cutaneous anaesthesia (as we have seen) abolishes both, and stimulation of non-pain nerve-endings or deep subcutaneous receptors, as in acupuncture, could prevent any of the pain impulses getting through to the cerebral cortex. There is a great deal of evidence that 'brief, mildly painful, stimulation is capable of bringing about substantial relief of more severe pathological pain for durations that long outlast the period of stimulation'.[h] And referred pain is undoubtedly eased by intense stimulation at the trigger areas; Travell & Rinzler (2), studying phenomena like those seen by Causey, could abolish myofascial pain not only by injecting local anaesthetics, but also by 'dry needling' of the area, without any injection at all.[i] Intense cold locally applied can also, they found, be effective, presumably by pain-impulse inhibi-

[a] Injection of distilled water (*shui chen*[1]) is also practised in contemporary China, cf. Anon. (*114*), p. 254.

[b] As by Sicard (1), vol. 2, and Feiling (1). Leriche (1) was one of the originators. The eminent anthropologist, Margaret Mead, relates in her autobiography (2), p. 112, how she was cured of a bad 'neuritis' in New York about 1920, when Janet Travell inserted dry hypodermic needles at the 'trigger points', a procedure 'so reminiscent of the Chinese method of acupuncture'.

[c] Cf. Cyriax (2); Copeman (1).

[d] Kennard & Haugen (1).

[e] Copeman & Ackerman (1).

[f] Korr, Thomas & Wright (1). Cf. Melzack (1), p. 174.

[g] See below, p. 231; the gating theory of Melzack & Wall (1).

[h] Melzack (1), p. 183.

[i] So also Kibler (1); Kretzschmar (1), p. 536.

[1] 水針

tion or gating due to hyper-activity of the heat–cold pathways. Techniques similar to these have had much success in the very difficult problems of agonising intractable pain—phantom limb pain after amputations, causalgia (burning pain due to violent deformation of nerves in bullet-wounds and the like), and the neuralgias.[a] Injection of hypertonic saline into the stump or the back gives sharp brief pain followed by prolonged relief,[b] and there are a number of reports that acupuncture will do the same.[c] On the other hand the physico-chemical stimulus of hypertonic saline injected into the cerebro-spinal fluid has been found to give prolonged relief in cancer pain,[d] though this is the one type of pain which acupuncturists have never been very confident that they can overcome, whether in China or the West.[e]

Clinical and physiological facts of this kind led to the appearance of several schools of therapeutics during the past fifty years. Huneke (1) led a movement of *neural-therapie* or 'curative anaesthesia' which involved injecting local anaesthetics[f] mainly at trigger points, hyperalgic or myalgic spots (the *irritations-zentrum*) but also into the peritonsillar tissues, the gums, and any healed scars on the body.[g] Sometimes the results were immediate and dramatic (the flash effect or *sekunden-phänomen*).[h] Huneke himself made the mental connection with acupuncture,[i] occasionally using dry needles himself, and it was even more strongly brought out in a book of Stiefvater (1).[j] Parallel with all this was the influence of Moss (1) in England, who laid great emphasis on trigger spots of hyperalgia while at the same time using and teaching classical acupuncture; and his lead was followed by a number of others in various parts of Europe.[k]

But it may be objected, and it has been, that the implantation of needles or hypodermics *in loco dolenti* is not true acupuncture, because in the classical Chinese system, the needling almost always takes place at a considerable distance from the site of the local symptoms. This is the distinction found in modern French acupuncture literature between proper acupuncture and 'aiguillo-therapie'. But the word 'almost' has wide connotation here, for in fact implantation at hyperalgic spots has been quite usual in China at least since the +7th century, when Sun Ssu-Mo[1] developed the knowledge of the *ah shih hsüeh*,[2] acu-points outside any regular or

[a] Melzack (1), pp. 57–8, 60ff., 65ff.; Beritashvili (1), pp. 187ff.

[b] Feinstein, Luce & Langton (1); Nathan (priv. comm. in Melzack (1), p. 58).

[c] Labrousse (1); Labrousse & Duron (1); Khoubesserian & Martiny (1); Benichou (1); de la Fuye (3); Mann, Bowsher, Mumford, Lipton & Miles (1).

[d] Hitchcock (1); Collins, Juras, Houton & Spruell (1).

[e] Even here there have been some encouraging case-histories; see Mann's postscript to the paper of Mann, Bowsher, Mumford *et al.* (1).

[f] Generally a product named impletol, containing 2% procaine hydrochloride in physiological saline solution, with 1·42% of caffeine. In the U.K. it was called procafin.

[g] The best exposition of the practices of the school in English is that of Kretzschmar (1). Good (1) gives an atlas of the typical myalgic spots in non-articular rheumatism.

[h] We have seen (pp. 197, 203 above) that the same can be said of acupuncture.

[i] (1), p. 114.

[j] Kretzschmar (1), p. 534, was very conscious of the relation of 'neural therapy' to old counter-irritation methods (cf. p. 244), and to moxibustion and acupuncture.

[k] Eraud (1); Rintzler (2).

[1] 孫思邈 [2] 阿是穴

auxiliary tract (cf. pp. 52, 127 above).[a] So here again we find practices introduced in modern medicine as something new having many centuries of unappreciated Chinese medical antecedents behind them. If indeed the *ah shih hsüeh* go back to the *Nei Ching*, *Ling Shu* and *Su Wên* these centuries would number as many as twenty.[b]

This might be the place to refer to the work of A. Weihe (1840–88), a homoeopathic physician of Stuttgart who has often been said to have re-discovered independently the Chinese acu-points. He believed that all diseases give premonitions during a latency period, and then declare themselves still more clearly, by producing hyperalgic points on the body surface, tender to finger pressure.[c] He defined 195 of these points, and thought that each one corresponded with a homoeopathic drug which should be given in very small doses.[d] Schoeler (1), who wrote a book on Weihe's system, combined it with that of Huneke by injecting these drugs at the appropriate spots. In 1929 Ferreyrolles & de Morant (1) noticed coincidences between 16 Weihe points and the traditional acu-points, but later a much more far-reaching correspondence was established by de la Fuye (5).[e]

The question of finger pressure and strong pinching or compression of folds of skin needs pursuing a little further. Neural inputs effected in these ways are a special technique in Japanese medicine, *shiatsu*[1],[f] and severe pinching to produce bruises occurs in Vietnamese folk-medicine, *bat-gio*;[g] while in Slavonic (Polish and Russian) folk-medicine there is a way of heavy massaging beside specific vertebrae for specific visceral malfunctions. Reminiscent of the *pei shu hsüeh* points, this is known as *kręgarstwo*.[h] In China it has been found, as we shall see in connection with acupuncture analgesia, that strong pinching of the Achilles tendon in mammals acts on pain impulses in the spinal cord in the same way as acupuncture at points known to raise pain thresholds (cf. p. 253 below). Probably belonging here also is the now long for-

[a] Especially in the *Chhien Chin Yao Fang* (+652), ch. 29, and the *Chhien Chih I Fang* (about +670). The technical term was introduced by him. Since the points were not necessarily on any tracts, they were also called *pu ting hsüeh*.[2] Cf. Anon. (*123*), p. 104.

[b] Cf. *NCLS/PH*, ch. 13, (p. 163).

[c] Like the McBurney point in appendicitis, to cite only the best known.

[d] According to Rousseau (1), Marshall Hall in 1841 was the first to observe pain points connected with visceral malfunctions (referred pain), but Schoeler (1) finds very similar ideas and statements in writings of the Swedish gymnastic expert P. H. Ling in 1834. On Ling we recall *SCC*, Vol. 5, pt. 5; cf. Westerblad (3), p. 36; Georgii (1, 2). The Griffin brothers in 1834 and 1843 (1), cf. (2), pp. 49ff., 57, seem more directly in the line of discovery. But the Chinese conviction of cutaneo-visceral links far antedates any of these.

[e] Of the 195 Weihe points, 132 (or at least 90) are closely identical with acu-points, 15 are on the tracts but not exactly at *hsüeh* loci, and 48 are extraneous to the tracts like *ah shih hsüeh*. It is strange that Weihe re-invented tracts too; his 'parasternal' is very like R, his 'mammary' like V, and his 'paraxillary' like P and VF. To VU correspond his 'paravertebral' and 'external oblique', both on the back. He also recognised Tu Mo and Jen Mo, though apparently never knowing them by their ancient names.

[f] See Namikoshi Tokujiro (1); Omura Yoshiaki (1), p. 88; Blate (1); Cerney (1); Ohashi (1); de Langre (1); Irwin & Wagenvoord (1).

[g] Described by Sterman (1) before he lost his life as a devoted army doctor in the Franco-Vietnamese war.

[h] Priv. comm. from the late Prof. Jerzy Konorski and his colleagues Stefan Soltysek and Ivan Divac at Zakopane in 1965.

[1] 指壓 [2] 不定穴

gotten 'zone therapy' for the relief of tooth pains, described by Ryan & Bowers[a] in 1921. This consisted in exerting strong pressures on the finger joints, either by means of spiral steel springs (called 'therapy zones') or by thick rubber bands amounting to tourniquets. It was found that pressure on the thumb would relieve pain in the incisors, the fore-finger was associated with the cuspids, the mid-finger with the bicuspids and the ring finger with the molars. Facial neuralgia was also greatly calmed, it was said, by similar pressure. Perhaps all this was just another way of stimulating the deep receptor nerve-endings in the hand—after all there are on the fingers no less than 16 tract acu-points and at least 4 non-tract points, while the hand as a whole has 26 and 22 respectively. When one remembers the prominence of the hand regions in the sensory cortex,[b] it may not be so surprising that its receptors can readily generate inhibitions.

(iii) *Corticosteroids and antibodies*

So far we have been talking mainly about the actions of acupuncture in terms of central and autonomic nervous conduction,[c] but this is undoubtedly not the whole story, for neuro-humoral effects must also enter in. It has been shown that they do this even in the analgesic effects of acupunctural peripheral stimuli, as we shall shortly see (p. 255); but we believe that they have a still more important part to play in the therapeutic effects. This means essentially, so far as we can see, the arousal to greater activity of (*a*) the cells of the suprarenal cortex which produce cortisone and related steroids, and (*b*) those of the reticulo-endothelial system, largely in the spleen, which can generate clones of cells producing antibodies against almost any foreign protein molecules. Thoughtful acupuncture physicians in the early fifties already saw fairly clearly that these must be the two main ways in which the 'natural healing power of the body' could be intensified.[d] Both effects would be brought about either directly by autonomic neural stimuli reaching the suprarenal-cortical and gonadic-interstitial cells,[e] or indirectly by neural activation of the hypothalamus and pituitary, followed by hormonal stimuli. At the present time a good deal of research on these subjects is going on, largely in China and Japan, though unfortunately we are not able to document it as fully as could be wished because of the difficulty of gaining access to the relevant publications.[f]

We have already mentioned (p. 202) the work of the unit at the Chungshan Hospital

[a] (1), pp. 186ff. This was the time when conditions such as long-standing sciatica were found to bed strikingly relieved by tooth extractions, 'the removal of foci of infection', a procedure which later became perhaps over-fashionable, and which again has now declined. Ryan & Bowers described such a case (p. 194).

[b] Cf. the 'sensory homunculus' of Penfield & Rasmussen (1).

[c] Schemes of possible pathways will be found in Vogralik (1, 2). Tung Chhêng-Thung & Li Yün-Shan (*1*) have reported regular increases of subordination motor chronaxia after acupuncture; this they interpret as indicating changes in the dynamic processes of excitation and inhibition in the central nervous system.

[d] See Agadjanian (1); Tiers (1), as also the Sian group under Chu Lung-Yü and the Shanghai group under Li Chieh-Ying.

[e] Cf. p. 216 below.

[f] For example, we believe that there is not a single complete run of the *Journal of Traditional Chinese Medicine* (*Chung I Tsa Chih*) in any European library. It contains a number of papers on laboratory experiments of the kind here envisaged, but we have not been able to consult it.

in Shanghai which found increases of the order of 100% in the hydrocortisone content of the blood after acupuncture at V 36 and other points.[a] Chang Hsiang-Thung's group and others have also found increases of 17-keto-steroid excretion after acupuncture.[b] Similar, and even larger, effects have been reported by Omura Yoshiaki.[c] This is supported by some Romanian work on the decrease of eosinophile leucocytes after acupuncture; Bratu, Stoicescu & Prodescu (1) found an average of −57% just as happens after injection of the adreno-cortico-tropic hormone.[d] In another series, they compared acupuncture with ACTH injection on the same patients, obtaining average decreases of −45% for the former and −40·2% for the latter.[e] Quite a lot has been done on changes in the total leucocyte count after acupuncture, and marked increases found, both in China,[f] Japan[g] and the West.[h] The increase is of the order of 40 to 60%, relatively transient, occurring whether or not the implantation sites were classical acu-points, and more marked after electro-acupuncture than manual. This phenomenon, if further confirmed, would relate rather to the second of the two main actions, antibody production and enhanced phagocytosis, especially as Bratu and his collaborators have found the increase to be greatest in the mononuclear leucocytes, which are especially connected with the reticulo-endothelial system.[i]

Again, we have already mentioned (p. 188) the work of the Sian Neurological Hospital unit which established a four-fold increase in typhoid and paratyphoid antibodies in rabbits after acupuncture, and a six-fold increase after electro-acupuncture. Li Cho-Lu reports an authoritative statement from Chou Kuan-Hua in 1972, summarising the work of a number of laboratories in China, that acupuncture causes prolonged increases in the antibody titre of the blood, both in human patients and experimental animals.[j] One of the most convincing papers on this is probably that of Chhen Kho-Chhin (*1*), who could demonstrate a conspicuous increase using *B. pertussis* antigen, especially after electro-acupuncture. Serum complement was also markedly raised as compared with the controls. Direct evidence of a similar kind has been provided by

[a] Human patients, estimations by the Kenneth–Silber method. Similar work is being continued by Dr Lin Hsü-Kao and his colleagues in Canton, who find that patients who respond well to acupuncture have high adrenocorticoid levels, while those who do not have low levels. Experimental atrophy of the suprarenal gland, and adrenalectomy, reduce the analgesic effect; activation of the ACTH axis increases it considerably (private communication from Dr Keith Betteridge and Prof. Peter Lisowski, 1975).

[b] Private communication to McLeod *et al.* (1), p. 127.

[c] (1), p. 82.

[d] The range varied from 24 to 95%.

[e] Bratu, Prodescu, Georgescu *et al.* (1).

[f] See Anon. (*129*) and Jen Khang-Thung (*1*).

[g] If Nakayama (1) is right that moxibustion increases the haemoglobin content of the blood, and the erythrocyte count too, that might be another defence mechanism against the stress of malfunction or bacterial attack.

[h] Cf. Craciun & Toma (1); Craciun, Toma & Turdeanu (1); Brown, Ulett & Stern (2).

[i] Bratu, Prodescu, Georgescu, Nitescu *et al.* (1).

[j] (1), pp. 62, 189. Cf. Chu Yang-Ming & Affronti (1), p. 161. In Anon. (*123*), pp. 399ff., we can find a full review of work done in Chinese laboratories during the past few decades on the effects of acupuncture and moxa on the digestive system (peristalsis, etc.), the circulatory system (including blood-pressure), the respiratory system, excretion, secretion (e.g. of bile), immune reactions and resistance against infection, and neurological phenomena. Another good review is in Chhêng Tan-An (*1*), pp. 24ff.

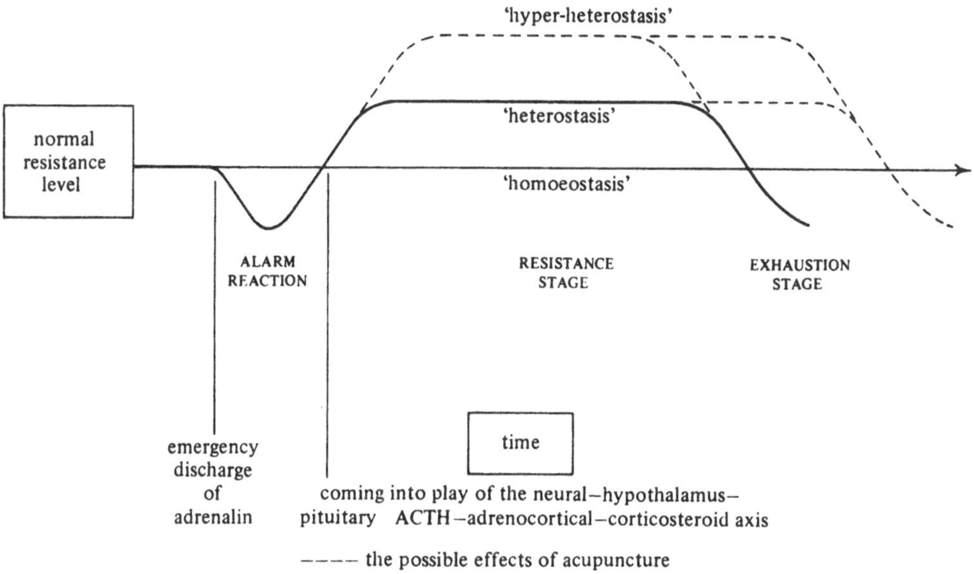

Fig. 49. Diagram to explain the theory of the Selye 'general adaptation syndrome'. Acupuncture may conceivably raise the level of heterostasis in the resistance stage, or postpone the advent of the exhaustion stage.

Chu Yang-Ming & Affronti (1) who found that acupuncture at certain loci prolonged the production of serum haemagglutinin in rabbits injected with sheep erythrocytes. In some conditions it would also exert an inhibitory effect on the progress of experimental allergic encephalomyelitis in guinea-pigs.

Finally it is evident that the whole subject needs to be brought into relation with the interesting work of the school of Hans Selye at Montreal on 'stress' and what he has called since 1936 the 'general adaptation syndrome'.[a] This has centred round the study of the entirely general aspects of physiological stress, i.e. the non-specific responses of the psycho-somatic organism to any unusual demands made upon it. Selye and his collaborators long ago established that any stress state, such as the entry of a pathogen, or the malfunction of a psycho-physiological system, induces first an 'alarm reaction', followed by a stage of increased resistance, and finally by a stage of exhaustion (cf. Fig. 49).

The alarm reaction to the stressor, initial and rapid, was first described in the classical work of W. B. Cannon in 1915 on 'bodily changes in pain, hunger, fear and rage'; it floods the circulation with adrenaline from the suprarenal medulla, raises the blood-pressure, constricts the peripheral circulation, speeds the heart, dilates the

[a] See Selye (1, 2, 3) and other writings. These paragraphs were much assisted by a conversation with Professor Hans Selye at Montreal in May 1975. He told us that for more than twenty years past he had spoken in favour of acupuncture as a method of enhancing the body's resistance to stressors. It might be described, he said, as a form of 'mini-shock therapy', far less blunderbuss in character than the flogging of the insane, insulin convulsions, or metrazole, or the pyrexia techniques introduced by Wagner von Jauregg about 1900. ECT *a fortiori*.

bronchi, mobilises liver glycogen, and activates the whole sympathetic (adrenergic) nervous system.[a] But at the same time the resistance of the body temporarily declines. Then follows the process of general adaptation. The stressor excites the hypothalamus, by way of neural paths not yet fully identified, to produce the substance that stimulates the pituitary gland to liberate the adreno-cortico-tropic hormone (ACTH); and this in turn causes a liberation of steroids such as cortisone and cortisol from the suprarenal cortex. These cortico-steroids have many effects—they elicit shrinkage of the thymus and atrophy of lymph glands, they inhibit inflammatory reactions, they continue the mobilisation of liver glycogen, they lower the number of eosinophile leucocytes in the blood, and they induce gastric and duodenal ulcers by causing contractions of the stomach and intestinal walls. The upshot of these effects is the stage of increased resistance (Fig. 49), a 're-setting of the thermostat' at a higher level (heterostasis); but as the 'adaptation energy' is finite, a stage of exhaustion eventually ensues.[b] The relevance of all this to acupuncture is that by intensifying the neural signals to the hypothalamus it could potentiate the pituitary–ACTH–adrenocorticoid axis, either raising the resistance to an even higher heterostatic level, or prolonging the stage of resistance, or both. Perhaps too it could act more directly upon the suprarenal cortex by way of the splanchnic nerves through the coeliac and renal autonomic plexuses.

In his later thought Selye distinguished between the 'syntoxic' and the 'catatoxic' response. This probably arose from the seemingly paradoxical circumstance that corticosteroids (and their synthetic derivatives) are anti-inflammatory,[c] though inflammation is of course the process of creating a barricade of connective tissue to oppose the invasion by the pathogenic stressor. Their function is therefore syntoxic, i.e. pacifying, tolerating and tranquillising, seeking a co-existence with the pathogen until it runs its course and dies a natural death. Accordingly they depress immune reactions, even against foreign grafts. On the other hand, a catatoxic response is as it were an incitement to combat, involving the enhancement of antibody formation, the synthesis of destructive enzymes, and the localisation of irritants by inflammation.[d] Some hormones accomplish this, especially the androgens secreted by the interstitial tissues of the sex glands, but certain synthetic compounds (especially pregneneolone-16α-carbonitrile) do it more effectively still. Correspondingly acupuncture could work in a parallel manner, either by increasing the output of gonad-stimulating hormones (GSH) from the pituitary gland, or perhaps directly through the pelvic splanchnic nerve-supply of testis and ovary via their appropriate autonomic plexuses.[e]

[a] See further in Cannon (1).

[b] This is probably not due to the suprarenal cortex; the failure lies rather in the brain, where the hypothalamus gives up the struggle and stimulates the pituitary no more.

[c] As for joints, eyes, the respiratory system, allergies, stings, venoms, etc.

[d] Many biochemical mechanisms are also naturally involved. For example, the fact that injury reaction as measured by protein metabolism in animals is not proportional to the extent of the injury (Cuthbertson, 1, 2). Or the fact that increased nitrogen catabolism continues for an unexpectedly long time after trauma (Flear & Clarke, 1).

[e] There has been some evidence for a long time past that the autonomic nervous system can exert regulatory effects on immunity and resistance, not necessarily through the gonads. See the review of Frei (1), and the discussion in Kuntz (1), pp. 492 ff.

Selye was always concerned to defend Pasteur and the great fathers of bacteriology from too narrow an insistence on the invading organism, for he felt that most of them had realised very clearly the equal importance of the 'terrain' on which the battle was to be fought.[a] 'Heterostasis', he said, 'depends upon treatment with artificial remedies which have no direct curative action, but which can teach the body to produce unusually high amounts of its own natural catatoxic or syntoxic agents so as to achieve fixity of the *milieu intérieur*, despite abnormally high demands that could not be met without help from outside.'[b] Heterostasis is a matter of strengthening the body's natural non-specific defences.[c] And in another place Selye wrote: 'Research on stress will be most fruitful if it is guided by the theory that we must learn to imitate, and if necessary to correct and complement, the body's own auto-pharmacological efforts to combat the stress factor in disease.'[d] This might almost be taken as an epigram for what therapeutic acupuncture may always have been doing.[e]

As one illustration of the kind of effect that acupuncture can have upon conditions of extreme stress, reference may be made to recent work on surgical shock in cats (Anon. *143*). After severe experimental losses of blood, acupuncture at the philtrum (TM 25, 26) delayed by half the time taken for the blood-pressure to fall to 50 mm Hg. The following table summarises this and other effects.

	acupuncture	controls
time taken for b.p. to fall to 50 mm Hg	15·2 min.	6·9 min.
blood loss to shock	21·8 ml/kilo	15·8 ml/kilo
blood transfusion needed	12·7 ml/kilo	32·7 ml/kilo
mortality in 3 hr.	25%	100%

Thus the onset of haemorrhagic shock was much delayed, and the experimental animals were capable of losing more blood than the controls.[f] Since the administration of phenobarbital completely abolished the effect, it must necessarily be mediated through the nervous system, as would be expected, though the exact mechanisms remain obscure and must be complex.

Just now, in defining 'stress', we included the 'malfunction of a psycho-physiological system', not only the invasion of pathogenic organisms or the action of toxic chemicals. Similarly, at the outset of this discussion (p. 8), we mentioned the ancient medical concept, as much Chinese as Greek, of *krasis*, i.e. the optimum mixture, balance or syntony of the major forces and processes in the body. Such

[a] At the end of his life, Pasteur is said to have remarked, perhaps with over-emphasis: 'Claude Bernard was right—the microbe is nothing, the terrain is everything!' (Inglis (1), p. 140).

[b] (4), p. 55.

[c] Op. cit. p. 57.

[d] (2), p. 12.

[e] Acupuncture physicians such as Bischko (1) saw long ago the relevance of Selye's conceptions for the traditional Chinese practices.

[f] One is almost tempted to suggest that acupuncture might be a valuable adjunct for ambulance units facing traumas with severe haemorrhage, along with all our other more modern aids.

a dynamic equilibrium of Yin and Yang was tantamount to health in the eyes of many an ancient and traditional physician. It is necessary therefore to take cognisance now of a form of imbalance which has been recognised by many medical scientists in modern times, even though somewhat difficult to pin down precisely—we refer to the idea of 'autonomic imbalance'.[a] All the viscera, and many other parts of the body as well, are innervated by both the sympathetic and parasympathetic nervous systems, the former essentially thoraco-lumbar in distribution and working mainly through adrenergic nerve-endings,[b] the latter essentially cranial and sacral, issuing its messages by means of nerve-endings that are mainly cholinergic.[c] Normally the two systems are synergistic in action, maintaining a functional balance like flexor and extensor muscles which never get in each other's way, but in various forms of malfunction and illness disturbances of the balance can occur. There can be an exaggerated tonus of either system, or both can be increased or else diminished.[d] The original conception of the autonomic balance was introduced by Eppinger & Hess (1, 2) in 1909, and it has been a part of general medical theory ever since. In approximately normal people there is usually some dominance of either the sympathetic or the parasympathetic, changing spontaneously in phasic or chronic ways, and centering upon a statistical point of balance.[e] There have not been lacking those who were willing to analogise this notion with the classical Yin–Yang balance of traditional Chinese medicine,[f] and it does chime in with an observation which has often been mentioned by Chinese surgeons and anaesthetists, if not so far discussed and studied as such, namely that during the course of acupuncture analgesia for major surgery there is a tendency for hypertensive patients to return to a normal level of blood-pressure, while those with hypotension show a rise to the normal level. After the analgesia has worn off the pressures rise or fall again to the abnormal levels characteristic of those patients, unless of course the surgical intervention has radically altered their physiological condition.

(iv) *Acupuncture and major surgery*

In July 1972 we found ourselves in the surgical department of the Second General Hospital of Chungshan Medical College at Canton,[g] about to join the growing and by now very large number of Western surgeons, physicians and men of science, who have personally witnessed major operations done under acupuncture analgesia.[h] The first case was that of a sailor aged 57 with a stone located high in the ureter. Four needles were used. One was implanted above the incision dorsally and one below it ventrally, both being stimulated throughout the induction and operation period by

[a] See the discussion of Kuntz (1), pp. 441 ff.
[b] I.e. those which transmit the neural stimulus by the secretion of nor-adrenalin.
[c] I.e. those which secrete acetyl-choline as transmitter. On all this see Burn (1).
[d] First established by Petren & Thorling (1).
[e] See Wenger (1).
[f] Cf. Looney (1). See also Bonica (2), p. 1549; Toyama & Nishizawa (1).
[g] This is a hospital of 550 beds, some 2500 out-patients, and about 750 staff members. We are most grateful to Prof. Ho Thien-Chhi for his explanations, and to the administrator, Ms Mo Tê-I, for information on the acu-points used.
[h] With us at this time was Dr Dorothy Needham, FRS.

a 9-volt direct current at 0·5 milliamps; one could see distinctly the subcutaneous contractions of the muscles.[a] Besides these there was one needle inserted in Ho-ku (IG 4), in the intercarpal space between the thumb and the first finger, a classical locus for the relief of pain, while the fourth was at Thai-chhung (H 3) on the upper surface of the foot.[b] The first of these two needles was continuously moved about by the anaesthetist the whole time, doubtless in order to keep the deep nerve receptors adequately stimulated. Throughout the operation the patient was awake and calm, able to speak with those in the theatre, and to make any movements which the surgeon requested; there was no wincing on the first incision or at any later time, nor any sign of pain or deep malaise.[c] After a while the inch-long stone was removed, a drainage-tube inserted, and the wound sutured.[d]

The second operation was a Caesarean section on a country girl aged 24, a primipara overdue on account of an abnormal foetal position, double uterus and contracted pelvis. She lay on her back throughout the procedure perfectly calm and impassive, not wincing or showing any signs of pain even during the extraction of the infant. Her own analgesia had no effect at all on the condition of the male baby, which cried as soon as normal breathing had been induced. In this case the acu-points were different. The Tai Mo auxiliary tract points (cf. pp. 45, 51 above) on each side were used, coinciding with those of the felleic tract VF 26, 27 and 28, the first-named being the most important. Then on the left leg San-yin-chiao (LP 6) was needled, and on the right leg the celebrated anodyne point Tsu-san-li in front of the knee (V 36).[e] Towards the end of the operation two further points were used, both in the concha of the external ear—Fei hsüeh[1] and Phi hsüeh,[2] the lung and the spleen point respectively. Later we met an ambulant patient who had had a pulmonary lobectomy under acupuncture analgesia a week or two before; he had felt no pain and was enjoying a good appetite.[f] The staff at Canton emphasised that there was relatively little psychological preparation beforehand, they simply explained everything and got the cooperation of the patients.[g] Only mild pharmaceutical sedation was used prior to the induction of the analgesia by acupuncture. The staff traced the beginnings of modern acupuncture analgesia[h] to Shanghai in 1958, where on the basis of its long-

[a] Signer & Galston (1) about this time reported other similar current characteristics; we return to the point on p. 230 below.

[b] Cf. Anon. (*114*), p. 207.

[c] Dr Huang Ta-Hsiang said that it takes from five to thirty minutes to induce analgesia adequate for such operations, and that afterwards it may last for several hours. Blood-pressure is carefully watched, since it may drop and corrective action become necessary, but in general, as we have noted, acupuncture seems to have a normalising effect on blood-pressure, reducing hypertension and increasing the pressure if low.

[d] The ureter itself need not be sutured, only dressed, as healing takes place quickly.

[e] This point is very close to the peroneal nerve and its branches.

[f] This was of special interest to one of us (G.D.L.) who had herself undergone a similar operation the previous year.

[g] No technique remotely resembling hypnosis was used.

[h] We write 'modern', but there is little reason to think that the technique could not have been known to Hua Tho and Huangfu Mi (cf. pp. 117, 119). They could perhaps have kept it as a professional secret. Others have also envisaged this, notably Jen Khang-Thung (*1*).

[1] 肺穴 [2] 脾穴

known power to help conditions such as migraine and arthritis, as well as the excruciating effects of some types of toothache, it was employed to relieve the pain of changing surgical dressings,[a] then extended to tonsillectomies, and finally with surprising success to operations on all parts of the body.

This may be a suitable moment to annotate the classical evidence for pain relief in ancient texts. The *Huang Ti Nei Ching*, *Su Wên* speaks many times of the use of acupuncture for this purpose.[b] So does the *Huang Ti Nei Ching*, *Ling Shu*, where the references are more scattered.[c] There is mention of toothache, backaches, rheumatic pains, various types of abdominal pain, and cardiac pain. Particular kinds of needles are prescribed, e.g. *fan chen*,[1] a term not usually found among the famous nine (cf. Table 16 above)[d] but which obviously indicates one of the techniques of heated or burning needles, and indeed is regarded as equivalent to *huo chen*[2] and *ta chen*[3] (no. 9).[e] Analgesic acupuncture is also recommended at *ah shih hsüeh* points, i.e. *in loco dolenti*, near where the pain is located.[f]

Further personal experiences followed at the Department of Oral, Facial and Maxillary Surgery of the Dental School and teaching hospital of the Szechuan College of Medicine, which occupies the campus of the former West China Union University at Chhêngtu.[g] Here we were present at a hare-lip operation, the repair of a thyroid cyst, and the resection of a mandibular adenoma. For the hare-lip procedure, which was completed in some 45 minutes, Ssu-pai (V 5) beside the nose was used, together with one of the new points on the auricula, Phi-chih-hsia,[4] in the conchal cavity just posterior to the antitragus; each of these, of course, bilaterally.[h] A current of 9 volts at 50 milliamps DC was used with 1000 pulses/min., and half an hour was required to get maximum analgesia, with the result that the patient was perfectly relaxed throughout, giving no movement whatever on incision, which he said felt like a pencil being drawn across the skin. Next came the neck operation, the removal of a congenital thyroid cyst and fistula. In this case the needles were implanted on both sides at

[a] Anon. (*129*). According to other reports it was the relief of post-tonsillectomy sore throats that led to the break-through (McLeod *et al.*).

[b] Especially in ch. 41; see *NCSW*, (p. 203), *NCSW/WMC*, (p. 373).

[c] See *NCLS/MC*, ch. 4, (pp. 930ff.), ch. 10A, (pp. 984ff.), ch. 13, (p. 1052), ch. 24, (p. 1124), ch. 27, etc.

[d] A synonym is *tshui chen*,[5] another *khuei chen*.[6] Cf. Yeh Ching-Chhiu (*1*), p. 46.

[e] See *CCTC*, ch. 4, (pp. 87–8), ch. 5, (p. 114); and *NCSW/PH*, ch. 62, (p. 330).

[f] Modern textbooks of acupuncture, for example Anon. (*123*), continue fully the ancient tradition, adding other applications such as trigeminal neuralgia, ischial and costal pains, testis pain and dysmenorrhoea. As we have seen (pp. 211, 245), acupuncture has been found useful even in phantom limb pain, one of the most intractable.

All this has been accepted, too, by even the more sceptical of Western observers, e.g. McLeod *et al.* (1), pp. 40ff., 44ff. Sciatica, back pain, cervical spondylosis, post-herpetic neuralgia and all kinds of painful conditions could be greatly relieved or cured by acupuncture, always excepting the intractable pain of malignancy. Cf. p. 235 below.

[g] This is a hospital of 100 beds, 90 dental chairs and 600 out-patients daily. We record our grateful thanks to Director Wang Han-Chang for the warm welcome he and his staff gave us.

[h] The simultaneous use of tract acu-points and auricular points for analgesia is now general, cf. Anon (*114*), pp. 146ff.; Anon. (*119*), pp. 40ff. The most effective acu-points are listed in many places, e.g. Anon. (*161*), p. 89. Evidently points in the fields of the trigeminal and upper cervical nerves must be used for all operations on the head and neck.

[1] 燔鍼 [2] 火鍼 [3] 大鍼 [4] 皮質下 [5] 焠鍼 [6] 恢鍼

Hsia-kuan (V 2) and Fu-thu (IG 18), and the electrical stimulation was the same. The patient was comfortable and gave no sign of motion, malaise or restlessness at any time. But the most impressive operation was that for a man of 40 with an osseo-adenoma; here a length of the mandible extending from the second bicuspid from left to right had to be removed,[a] and it was most striking to see the bone being sawn through with a thread-saw, while the patient was conscious, relaxed and immobile, showing no pain or discomfort. The same acu-points were used as in the previous case, but the cycles of electrical stimulation were stepped up to 1500/min. None of these three patients had received pharmaceutical sedatives or muscle relaxants beforehand.[b]

Such were our personal experiences. What then can be said about the development and present practice of acupuncture analgesia[c] in general? After the first successes in 1958, surgeons throughout China experimented with many different types of operation,[d] and ten years later a peak was reached when acupuncture analgesia was attempted in some 60 % of all surgical operations done.[e] As always, chemical anaesthetics were held available in case of failure, and with the passage of time it became clear that acupuncture had a distinct and limited range of effectivity, so that today the technique has become the method of choice in from 15 to 30 % of all cases.[f] These are, of course, average figures for the whole country, and the real frequency varies much from one centre to another depending on the specialities and the experiences. But when one looks at the total success achieved it is striking to reflect that at the present time something like a million painless operations have been performed under acupuncture.[g] Moreover, in selected cases and subjects the success rate can often be well over 90 %.

[a] For about a year the piece would be replaced by a plastic substitute, and after that a second operation would graft in bone from the 7th rib. If the condition had been left unattended the adenoma, though benign, could have grown to several kilos in weight, resulting in a disfigurement like those in the oil paintings at Guy's Hospital dating from the early years of modern medical practice in China and described by Brooks (1).

[b] By 1972 it was becoming the general practice in this hospital to use acupuncture analgesia in all forms of chair dentistry, such as fillings and extractions, instead of local anaesthetics, in most cases.

[c] As will be seen, we retain the term analgesia, though common usage, especially in Chinese foreign-language publishing, calls it anaesthesia. Etymologically this is quite justified, but since the introduction of chemical anaesthesia in the forties of the last century (cf. Prescott (1), pp. 16ff.), the term (coined, it seems, by Oliver Wendell Holmes) has universally come to imply total unconsciousness. Local anaesthesia has always therefore been a misnomer. Furthermore, since there is doubt whether an absolutely painless condition can be attained by acupuncture alone (i.e. without the prior use of a chemical sedative and some psychological preparation) hypo-algesia would be even more correct, if perhaps pedantic. On this see Anon. (*114*), p. 8. Among the many accounts, that of Kaada *et al.* (1) is the most balanced and informative, though we supplement it by others mentioned as they occur. It resulted from a study-tour of Norwegian physicians and surgeons in China in 1973.

[d] Hui Wên & Fu Wei-Kang (1); Anon. (*129*, *130*).

[e] Tobimatsu *et al.* (1).

[f] Gingras & Geekie (1); Kaada *et al.* (1). Kaada (2) and Burgess, Casey, Chapman *et al.* (1) give lower figures, 10 % or under, but much depends on what is taken as the total for all surgical interventions. Some sources give a million operations with acupuncture analgesia in 1974 alone (Anon., 149). Furthermore, other new methods, each with their own advantages, such as pharmacological anaesthesia, have in the meantime arisen.

[g] The literature has become very large, and we can only mention a few of the more important contributions that we have been able to use.

Among the earliest published accounts in China were those of Shêng Lü-Chhien & Chang Tao-

The method is most effective in the surgery of the head (including craniotomies and all dental operations), the neck, and the thorax (including pulmonary lobectomies and open heart operations; Fig. 50).[a] It is also good for Caesarean sections and perineal interventions,[b] less so for abdominal operations as such (laparotomies), mainly because the muscles of the wall do not adequately relax,[c] and because traction or stretching of the viscera and their membranes causes deep malaise or quasi-pain which the needle stimuli do not exclude.[d] Acupuncture is also being used a good deal in bone surgery, though again it does not give its best results in amputations or other operations on the limbs. In the great majority of operations acupuncture alone seems not to give a sufficiently deep level of analgesia,[e] and it is generally supplemented therefore by pharmacological pre-medication.[f] Phenobarbital may be given in a small dose the night before, or pethidine intramuscularly or intravenously about half an hour before entering the theatre. Local infiltration with procaine may be added, but it has been

Hsieh (1) and Han Fêng-Yen, Lin Ju-Hêng, Chhen Kho-Chhin & Sun Jung-Khun (1). Both reported successes with acupuncture analgesia in oral and dental surgery, and both dealt with work done in 1959.

Further articles in Western languages from China were those of Hsin Yu-Ling (1); Hui Wên & Fu Wei-Khang (1); as also Anon. (121, 122, 123).

The first important publications in Chinese took the form of a series of articles in *Hung Chhi*, and these were reprinted in growing numbers in successive collections: Anon. (*129, 130, 131*).

Besides this, there have appeared authoritative expositions in book form, e.g. Anon. (*114*), esp. pp. 4ff.; (*123*), esp. pp. 419ff.; Anon. (*135*).

Among the numerous publications by Western medical men, surgeons and physiologists, mainly, though not exclusively, on the basis of personal studies in China, we may cite: Dimond (1); P. E. Brown (1); Melzack (3); Wall (2); Smithers *et al.* (1); Woodley (1); Maillet (1); Hamilton, Brown, Hollington & Rutherford (1); Capperauld, Cooper & Saltoun (1); McLeod *et al.* (1); Bowers (2); Bischko (2); Burgess, Casey, Chapman *et al.* (1).

Outside China acupuncture analgesia for major surgery has been attempted in several parts of the world. From Hongkong there are the favourable reports of Chêng & Ting (1); Wên Hsiang-Lai (1); Wên, Cheung & Mehal (1). From France there is an account of 50 operations by Nguyen Van Nghi (1), which gave 64 % results in Grade I, 86 % in Grades I and II combined, with 14 % in Grade IV. From America, Ho & Chhen (1) have reported very satisfactory results in a tonsillectomy and the treatment of an infected salivary calculus. From Austria, much work will be found in the papers of Benzer & Pauser (1); Benzer, Mayrhofer, Pauser & Thoma (1); Majer & Bischko (1) were markedly successful with tonsillectomies.

Most of the work in the Western world has been concerned with dentistry. Nygaard-Østby (in Kaada *et al.* (1), p. 433) on returning to Norway had the extraction of an upper molar done on himself with acupuncture analgesia with complete success; he could feel the severance of the periodontal fibres yet no pain whatever. Brunet (1) used electro-analgesia with success in dentistry, i.e. the application of electrodes to acu-points but no needle insertions. Variable results have been reported by Mann (6, 7), and research is continuing. See also Bresler (1); Petricek (1).

Probably the only treatise on acupuncture analgesia in a Western language so far is the book of Nguyen Van Nghi, Mai Van Dong & Lanza (1). But Anon. (*114*) has been translated into English at the National Institutes of Health at Bethesda, Maryland.

---

[a] Dimond (1); Anon. (*123*); Richter, Baum, Kunkel *et al.* (1).

[b] Hyodo & Gega (1) report much success with acupuncture analgesia in normal childbirth, especially for multiparae.

[c] Even with succinyl-choline. But this position may change if the new muscle relaxant alkaloid isolated from *Stephania tetrandra* (*shih chhan su*[1]) proves of great value (cf. Anon. (*109*), vol. 1, p. 784.2; Anon. (*110*), p. 149, fig. 84).

[d] Cf. Anon. (*123*), p. 421.

[e] This comes out well from the report on eight hundred partial resections of the stomach and duodenum for the removal of persistent ulcers (Anon. *175*). But it has been a very general experience.

[f] Cf. Anon. (*114*), pp. 74ff.

[1] 石蟾蜍

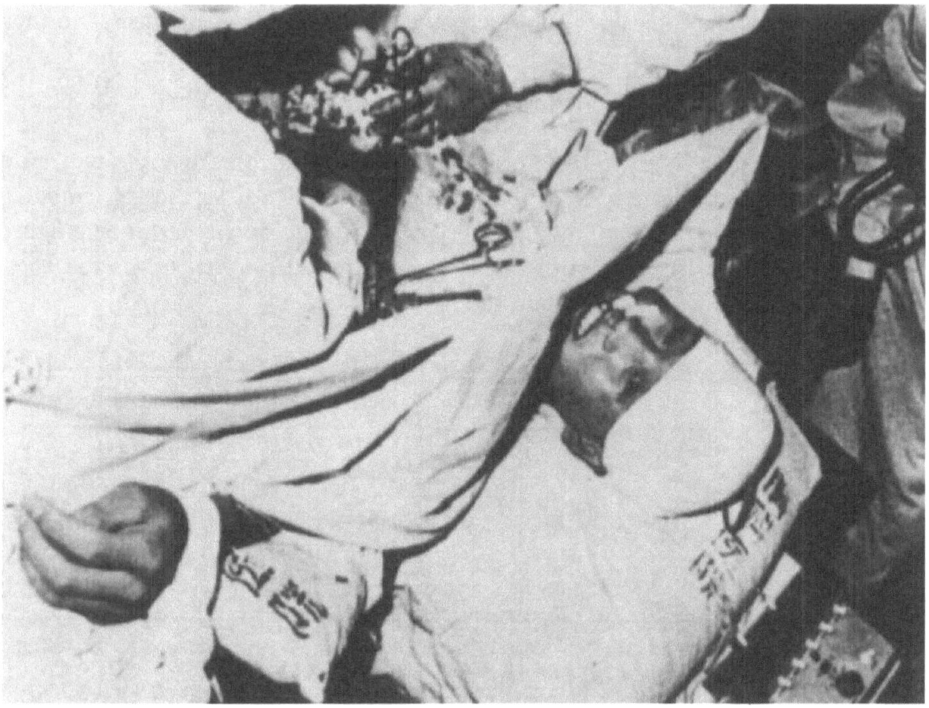

Fig. 50. An open-heart operation under acupuncture analgesia (Kaada *et al.* (1), p. 434); commissurotomy for mitral stenosis at the Shanghai Chest Hospital, 1974. Three electro-acupuncture needles were inserted in the lower left arm, and one subcutaneously in the left chest in a paramedian position. The electro-stimulator is seen in the lower right corner of the photograph. The surgeon has his right index finger inside the exposed heart. The patient is conscious, with his eyes open, and capable of responding to any request from the surgeon.

the almost universal opinion of the many modern-Western medical men who have followed the procedures in China that all the pre-medication would be far from sufficient alone to permit the surgery.[a]

The effectiveness of acupuncture analgesia has been rated by four grades (cf. Table 22). Grade I denotes an excellent analgesic effect. The patient is calm and feels only slight pain during a few of the surgical steps; blood-pressure, pulse-rate and respiratory rate are normal or practically so. In Grade II the analgesic effect is described as good, though the patient may groan occasionally as if with dull pain, while there are slight changes in the physiological data just mentioned. A small amount of local chemical analgesic may be used. Grade III implies cases where the analgesia is fair but the patient evidently feels some pain, not enough however to need the interruption of the surgery or to require more pethidine, though more local anaesthetic may be given at certain points. Finally, Group IV patients show a poor degree of

[a] Since the advent of acupuncture analgesia, Chinese surgeons have modified their technique in various ways, notably by increasing the speed of individual incisions. This is what is called the *fei tao*[1] (flying knife) procedure. Cf. Chêng & Ting (1); Woodley (1).

[1] 飛刀

analgesia, with marked changes in the physiological functions so that recourse has to be had to chemical anaesthesia.[a] Table 22 gives the percentages of success in more than 80,000 operations carried out in Shanghai hospitals down to the end of May 1973.[b] The figures speak for themselves, and demonstrate beyond a doubt that acupuncture analgesia is a real phenomenon.

It does not seem to have been pointed out so far by anyone that the pattern of statistical success and failure with acupuncture analgesia is rather closely similar to that which is emerging for acupuncture therapy. If we digest the percentage figures in Table 22 and compare them with those which have been given on p. 200 above for therapeutic acupuncture, we obtain the following table:[c]

	Grades					
	I	II	I+II	III	IV	III+IV
acupuncture analgesia	37·3	38.15	75·45	17.0	7.8	24.8[d]
therapeutic acupuncture	44.1	27.5	71.6	(16.4)	(12.6)	28.4

To what extent this might point to a community of mechanism between the two applications remains an open question. Could it possibly be a measure of some sort of efficiency within that immensely complicated electro-chemical telephone exchange, the central and autonomic nervous system?

Pre-medication by small doses of analgesic drugs has already been mentioned, but there is also unquestionably a psychological factor. It has been a general experience that acupuncture analgesia is more difficult to bring about in tense, anxious or apprehensive patients, and their reaction is improvable by tranquillisers.[e] Experimental studies on the rise in pain threshold in healthy subjects have confirmed the existence of considerable individual variations in response to acupuncture;[f] for

[a] Chemical anaesthesia is now not the only alternative, for pharmacological anaesthesia is being re-introduced in China. Scopolamine from *Datura metel* (*yang chin hua*,[1] Anon (*109*), vol. 3, p. 729.1; Anon. (*110*), p. 392, fig. 226) is combined with the new alkaloid anisodine from *Anisodus tanguticus* (*kan chhing sai lang-tang*,[2] Anon. (*109*), vol. 3, p. 711.1) and gives excellent anaesthesia after induction by chlorpromazine, promethazine or dolantin, and ketamine if necessary, luminal being used for pre-medication. Physostigmine is used as an analeptic to awaken the patient, for both induction and recovery periods are rather long. We ourselves have long suspected the presence of effective anaesthetic plant-drugs in the Chinese pharmacopoeia, and their probable use as early as the Han.

[b] Anon. (134). Preliminary figures were given in Kaada *et al.* (1).

[c] The figures in brackets derive from the Russian and American statistics only, and the relatively small French series is not embodied here.

[d] Of the 48 major operations studied by a party of American anaesthesiologists in China in 1974, the first two grades accounted for 73 % and the second two 27 %—a proportion extremely similar to that given here. See Burgess, Casey, Chapman *et al.* (1), p. 26.

[e] Chang Hsiang-Thung (1); Hyperthyroidism also reduces the effect.

[f] Anon. (128) (*128*).

[1] 洋金花　　[2] 甘青賽莨菪

Table 22. *Effectiveness of acupuncture analgesia (80,000 surgical operations carried out in Shanghai hospitals to the end of May 1973).*

	Percentages			
	Grade I	Grades I & II	Grades I, II & III	Grade IV
craniotomy[a]	35	71	97	3
retinal detachment	32	73	80	20
thyroidectomy[b]	54	85	95	5
total laryngectomy	54	84	93	7
pulmonary resection	18	44	97	3
mitral commissurotomy	32	73	94	6
open heart surgery with extra-corporeal cardio-pulmonary circulation[c]	12	77	87	13
sub-total gastrectomy	17	62	96	4
abdominal hysterectomy	34	74	85	15
internal fixation of fractures with three-flanged nails	52	90	96	4
Caesarean section[d]	—	—	97	3
dental extraction[e]	70	97	—	3
Veterinary operations (horse, donkey, mule, buffalo, pig)				
(head, neck, chest, abdomen, limbs)	30	70	95	5

example 20% of Swedish volunteers failed to react.[f] Many factors are no doubt involved; in China it has become the practice to test patients on the previous day so as to ascertain their *tê chhi* intensity (cf. p. 192 above), for those who have it most markedly will respond best to the acupuncture.[g] It is now fairly common to monitor the patient's physiological responses associated with pain during the course of operations, particularly the galvanic skin response (GSR), pulse amplitude and type of respiration, so that the anaesthetist can increase the stimulation or give additional drugs. A point which has not so far been made in discussions of this subject is that the classical Chinese medical literature as far back as the Han contains repeated

[a] E.g. meningiomas, pituitary tumours, etc. 482 successful cases are reported and discussed in Anon. (*138*).

[b] See the account of 700 cases in Anon. (*140*).

[c] See the detailed report on 107 cases in Anon. (136).

[d] Peking Hospital of Gynaecology and Obstetrics (J. Setekleiv, in Kaada *et al.* (1), p. 436).

[e] Han Fêng-Yen *et al.* (1).

[f] Andersson, Ericson, Holmgren & Lindqvist (1); Andersson, Ericson & Holmgren (1). We shall return to this question in connection with the physiological mechanism of acupuncture analgesia (p. 261 below).

[g] Chiang Chen-Yü, Chiang Chhing-Tshai, Chu Hsiu-Ling & Yang Lien-Fang (1); Anon. (*129*, *130*); Anon. (*142*), 818 cases.

statements that anyone who does not believe that acupuncture will do him good should not have it—we shall give the text below (p. 241). But whether there is any justification for regarding this confidence of the patient in the doctors and the method as partaking of the nature of hypnosis, as has been proposed from time to time,[a] we shall discuss there also. We do not know of any attempt to apply tests for suggestibility used in experimental psychology either to prospective surgical patients or to healthy volunteers, either in China or the West. What is certain is that under acupuncture analgesia a patient shows none of the trance-like or somnambulistic states characteristic of hypnosis;[b] he is alert to a normal or almost normal degree, he can co-operate actively with the surgeon[c] and converse with the anaesthetist, he can ingest liquids for refreshment or medication, eat and swallow, he can tell those around him exactly what he is feeling, and finally at the conclusion of the operation he can in many cases get off the table unaided and walk back to his bed.[d]

A number of factors are taken into account in the selection of patients for acupuncture analgesia. For example, age matters. Acupuncture is not ineffective in children, as has often been suggested in the West,[e] but they are liable to show lack of cooperation and may therefore be excluded, as is the case with the very old, albeit that in some geriatric cases chemical anaesthesia may not be desirable and acupuncture then comes to the surgeon's relief. The type of operation envisaged is also an important consideration. If deep analgesia and full muscular relaxation is required, chemical anaesthesia is to be preferred, as also in operations on the limbs. Acupuncture analgesia is seldom used for operations necessitating more than 3 hours, though it has been successful up to 6 hours.[f] On the physical condition of the patient practice has differed, for sometimes acupuncture analgesia has been avoided in situations of shock and severe blood loss, yet other accounts have reported good success in all

[a] This was the view of Wall (1), but after a study-tour in China he retracted it in Wall (2). Others have also favoured this interpretation, e.g. Kroger (2); Chisholm (1); McRobert (1). Among them was Dr M. K. Rajakumar of Kuala Lumpur, whose opinion we could not share, but to whom we are much indebted for valuable references on hypno-anaesthesia (cf. p. 237 below), the reality of which is also indubitable. But the vast majority of observers find very little in common between acupuncture analgesia and hypnosis, e.g. Smithers *et al.* (1); McLeod *et al.* (1).

[b] Dr Ronald Katz (in Jenerick (1), p. 109) has written: 'I have assisted at four operations under acupuncture analgesia and many more than that under hypnosis. The patients behave differently. Those under hypnosis are in a tight, self-contained world, seemingly totally unaware of what is going on about them. Patients under acupuncture were part of the team; joking, laughing, and commenting freely. One of the latter was also experienced in hypnosis, and he said that so far as he was concerned, the two were entirely different.'

[c] Cooperation with the surgeons had a particularly important consequence when a thoracotomy was undertaken on a male patient who had long practised Taoist breath-control exercises (cf. *SCC*, Vol. 5, pt. 5). The essential diaphragmatic breathing on the non-operated side could indeed be achieved under acupuncture analgesia, and a new use was thus found for an ancient technique of physiological alchemy. It is now taught to all patients beforehand, and replaces the positive pressures of oxygen and nitrous oxide necessary in chemical anaesthesia.

[d] One might add that many patients take an active interest in the progress of the operation. A man may examine the organ or piece of tissue which has just been removed from his body. A woman may look lovingly at the baby which only a few moments before has been delivered by Caesarean section.

[e] E.g. Wall (1). But Anon. (*132*) gives us a report on 1308 children of ages ranging from 1 day to 14 years operated on successfully to a rate of 81 % with acupuncture analgesia. Anon. (137) extends this to 1474 cases. See also Anon. (*114*), pp. 223ff.

[f] Dimond (1).

kinds of haemorrhagic, toxic and traumatic shock.[a] Finally, the patient's state of mind is an important consideration, and it seems that many more patients opt for acupuncture analgesia than are judged suitable for it.[b]

The advantages of acupuncture analgesia are numerous, and have been summarised as follows.[c] First, it is very safe, for no deaths or serious complications have ever been reported for it, which is more than can be said of chemical general anaesthesia.[d] Secondly, there is little or no interference with physiological functions such as circulation, respiration, digestion, or fluid and electrolyte balance. Post-operative nausea rarely occurs, nor any of the other complications such as pleurisy or later infections of the respiratory tract, pneumonia, bronchitis, etc., or urinary retention, constipation or abdominal distension; and never any symptoms of mental abnormality. Anyone familiar with the frequency of these sequelae of chemical anaesthesia will be deeply impressed by their absence after acupuncture. Obviously the method is particularly suitable for weak or debilitated patients, and especially for those with cardiac, hepatic, renal and pulmonary malfunctions. Occasional hypersensitivity to chemical anaesthetics must also be remembered, and since the analgesic effect outlasts the active stimulation by periods as long as 24 hours, and always 2 or 3, post-operative pain, medication and nursing are alleviated. Again, the patient is definitely awake, and can therefore respond to the requests of the surgeon to perform movements from time to time or to report his reactions; this can be particularly useful in such operations as those for the correction of strabismus, or where nerve-trunks may be affected,[e] or in laryngectomy, thyroidectomy and Caesarean section. Lastly, the method is simple, convenient and cheap; for example in the remote depths of the country far from well-equipped operating theatres, where auxiliary medical personnel ('barefoot doctors', *chhih chiao i shêng*[1]) might be doing minor surgery—and, by the same token, for conditions that might pertain in war.

What, it may be asked, are the principal acu-points used for the induction of analgesia? The practice of the first explorers was to use a great many, and in a lung resection for instance more than forty were employed.[f] But it soon became evident that the number could be greatly reduced, and at the present time such resections are accomplished with the use of only three needles at most. Four are not uncommon, but one would rarely find more than five. Originally the acu-points were selected according to traditional theory along the tracts, but it has become more and more general to select points essentially according to the segmental distribution of the spinal and cranial nerves, and not to worry too much about their relation to the tracts.

[a] Anon. (*133*); 86% success, blood pressure was restored to normal faster, and less transfusion blood was required. Cf. the animal experiments mentioned on p. 217 above.

[b] As many as 90%, according to P. E. Brown (1).

[c] Cf. Kaada *et al.* (1); Anon. (*114*), p. 6; Hsin Yu-Ling (1); Jen Khang-Thung (*1*).

[d] And also more than can be said of therapeutic acupuncture; cf. Peacher (1).

[e] For example in facial operations where areas supplied by branches of the trigeminal nerve are concerned.

[f] See Anon. (128); Hsin Yu-Ling (1); Anon. (*129*, *130*).

[1] 赤脚醫生

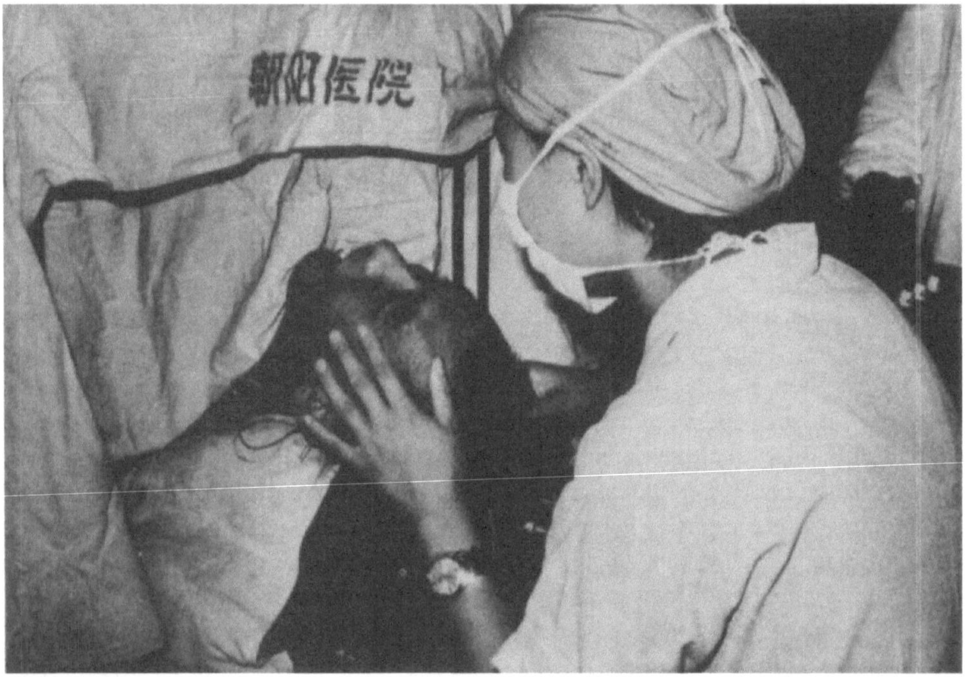

Fig. 51. A gastric operation at Chhaoyang Hospital (1971) showing the use of auricula acu-points for surgical analgesia. Photo: Durham.

The relation of the points most generally used to the dermatomes is given in Table 23;[a] from this it can be seen how the choice for particular operations would be made. Pain threshold experiments show that it is generally raised all over the body, though to different extents in different regions, so that there is considerable specificity.[b] Thus with stimulation at Ho-ku (IG 4) in the hand, a place served by the cervical nerves C 6, 7, the rise in pain threshold was greater for the trigeminal and cervical areas than for thoracic and abdominal regions, though by no means lacking there. The general results indicate that although the analgesic effect is wide-spread, it is most complete in the same dermatome as that which is stimulated, and in neighbouring dermatomes.[c] A consequence of the great elongation of the dermatomes along the limbs is that although many acupuncture analgesia points seem to be far removed from the area of the operation, they actually belong to the same segmental innervation field. But in addition to the points on the body, it has become normal to use the new

[a] See also Table 4 in Anon. (*123*), pp. 419ff.; and especially Anon. (*114*), pp. 78ff.; Anon. (135), pp. 296ff. About 30 acu-points have become well known for their analgesic properties. A tribute should be paid to the many volunteers who contributed to the gaining of this knowledge in the early stages.

[b] For example, Chiang Chen-Yü, Chiang Chhing-Tshai, Chu Hsiu-Ling & Yang Lien-Fang (1); Anon. (128).

[c] This effect was strikingly observed by Chapman, Chhen Chao-Nan & Bonica (1) in their study of the perception of induced dental pain. Acu-points on the head were much more effective than points of acu-tracts on the body or limbs.

Table 23. *Acu-points commonly used for acupuncture analgesia in relation to the dermatomes in which they are sited*

Region of body	Name (cf. Table 4)	Denomination	Dermatome
inner surface of arm, and axilla	Ta-ling Chhi-mên[a] Chou-jung	HC 7 HC 4 LP 20	C 7 C 5 T 2
outer surface of arm	San-yang-lo Chih-kou Ho-ku Pei-nao[b]	SC 8 SC 6 IG 4 IG 14	C 7 C 7 C 6, 7 C 6
anterior surface of leg	Tsu-san-li Shang-chü-hsü San-yin-chiao Hsien-ku	V 36 V 37 LP 6 V 43	L 4 L 4 L 4 L 5
head and neck	Chhüan-liao[c] Hsia-kuan Thien-jung Ta-ying Fu-thu Chien-ching	IT 18 V 2 IT 17 V 8 IG 18 VF 21	V ii[d] V iii[d] C 2, 3 C 2, 3 C 2, 3 C 4
external ear (auricula)	Chiao-kan-shen-ching[1] [e] Shen-mên[2] [g]	— —	—[f] —[f]

acu-points on the external ear, the auricula, either alone or in combination with the former (Fig. 51).

One of the most extraordinary recent developments in acupuncture has been the discovery that every part of the body has been found to have its representative area on the auricula.[h] Some of these points, especially the two incorporated in Table 23, have been found to have a generalised sedative and analgesic effect on the body as a

[a] Kaada *et al.* (1) name this Chhêng-chin.

[b] Particularly important for pulmonary resections (Anon. *141*), with 611 cases.

[c] The great analgesic value of this point for spinal cord operations and brain tumours is emphasised in Anon. (*139*) analysing 619 cases.

[d] Branches of the trigeminal nerve, (i) ophthalmic nerve, (ii) maxillary nerve, (iii) mandibular nerve.

[e] Called by Kaada *et al.* (1) 'sympathicus'. It is on the ridge between the triangular fossa and the concha, just under the beginning of the helix.

[f] The sensory innervation of the auricula is complex, see p. 162.

[g] Just at the tip of the triangular fossa.

[h] Anon. (*119*, *164*, *165*). Cf. Nogier (1, 2, 3); Huang Hsien-Ming *et al.* (*1*); König (1). The innervation of the auricula is fourfold; (*a*) the greater auricular branch of the cervical plexus, (*b*) the lesser occipital nerve, (*c*) the auricular branch of the vagus, and (*d*) the auriculo-temporal nerve. Presumably this can only mean that sensory fibres passing through all these nerves communicate somewhere in the brain with centres corresponding to many different parts of the body. Cf. p. 164.

1 交感神經 2 神門

whole, hence their constant use in surgery. They bring about greater relaxation of the abdominal wall muscles,[a] and all these effects have also been obtained by implanting needles at certain new acu-points on the nose.[b] It can hardly be irrelevant that animal experiments have shown that stimulation of the nose and the concha of the external ear can produce an immediate and widespread inhibition of spontaneous muscle potentials of the trunk and limbs, as well as of respiratory movements and pulse rate.[c]

Last of all, the methods of stimulation. Most traditional is the purely manual. After a quick and painless insertion to a depth of up to 0·5 to 1·0 cm., the needle is rotated and given push-and-pull movements two or three times a second. In some operations this 'twiddling' may be continued throughout, in others it may be stopped as soon as the *tê chhi* feeling is reported, and the needles simply left *in situ*. For a certain time small mechanical manipulators electrically driven were in use, but later this was almost entirely given up in favour of electro-acupuncture, the coupling of a pulsed stimulator to the implanted needles. Batteries give a DC current of from 3 to 9 volts from which biphasic pulses of 0·3 to 1 m/sec. duration at 80 to 100 volts but very small milli-amperage are delivered to the needles, the frequency varying from 1 pulse every 2 sec. to several hundred per sec.[d] Intensity is increased until contractions of subcutaneous muscles appear or the patient's tolerance level is reached. Sometimes the slower 1 pulse per sec. has been found more effective than 35 or so.[e] Whether the stimulation is manual or electrical, it must start from 20 to 30 minutes before the initial incision. Electrical stimulation has also been tried with the use of unimplanted electrodes, and this can be effective too.[f] Another analgesia method, used occasionally in China, has been called hypodermic acupuncture; here 3–10 ml. of fluid are injected into an acu-point instead of implanting a needle, but for ear points a good deal less is used (0·2 ml.).[g] Probably the local distension of the subcutaneous tissues has the same effect as the needles of stimulating mechanically the deep pressure receptor nerve-endings.[h] Finally, very strong finger pressure on certain acu-points may induce considerable degrees of analgesia useful for minor operations; for example at the Ho-ku point, or at the Achilles tendon between VU 60 (Khun-lun) and R 6 (Chao-hai).[i]

[a] Hence their special value in splenectomies and other laparotomies.
[b] See Anon. (*133*, *134*).
[c] Andersen (1); Frankenhauser & Lundervold (1); Kaada *et al.* (1).
[d] Naturally there is considerable variation in the details. See Kaada *et al.* (1); Melzack (3); McLeod *et al.* (1). In 1973 the commonest technique was 80 to 120 per sec.; Jenerick (1), p. 67.
[e] Anon. (128). But this is now little used (1973); Jenerick (1), p. 67.
[f] Cf. Andersson, Ericson & Holmgren (1); Brunet (1).
[g] Tobimatsu *et al.* (1). Almost any solution is effective—distilled water, saline, 5 % glucose, vitamin B or various plant drugs. But what is difficult to understand is that the effect is reported also upon injection of pethidine or procaine, which would be expected to inhibit the nervous input. Cf. p. 247 below.
[h] This is a curious development, the converse of what happened in the West (p. 210 above), where 'dry needling' arose naturally and independently out of injections of local anaesthetics for rheumatoid conditions, fibrositic nodules etc.
[i] Already (p. 212 above) we have seen various forms of the 'pinch' therapy in various parts of the world. And below (p. 253) we shall see that it has been used in studying the neurophysiology of acupuncture analgesia. Obviously it has a relation with certain physiotherapeutic procedures, especially 'connective-tissue massage'.

(v) *The neuro-physiology of acupuncture analgesia*

Acupuncture analgesia cannot be understood without an examination of the physiology of pain, taking into account the clinical and psychological phenomena which are associated with it.[a] Perhaps the first thing to do is to realise that the bodies of men (and all the higher animals) are composed, as it were, of centres and circumferences. The 'centre' is the region of the highest centres of the brain, i.e. the cerebral cortex, and the 'circumference' is the surface of the body from which the peripheral nerve-endings, the somatic sensory receptors, are constantly sending inwards and upwards messages and reports about the state of the local defences or activities. Thus one has an upward or afferent ascending flow of neuronal information, but at the same time there is also all the time a downward or efferent descending flow of modulating instructions. One could almost visualise the state of affairs in the image of a tidal river, especially with a periodical bore, for now the waters of the incoming sea are triumphant, boiling and bubbling against the fresh water and driving it inland, while at another time the sea water withdraws and the river is dominant far down the estuary. So in the same way the sensory input is sometimes beating against the centre, at other times the centre, when the conditions are right, can modulate or even inhibit, or 'pay no attention to', the urgent messages from the periphery.[b] The fact is that pain comes into consciousness only as the result of many influences working in different directions; it is certainly the product of the alarm firing of the peripheral nociceptive nerve-endings, but it is also affected by cultural learning, past experience, the significance of the situation, the concentration or attention of the mind, and other cognitive factors. Thus the physiology of pain raises many difficult and complicated questions. Biologically there can be no doubt that pain is primarily a signal that some of the tissues of the body are being injured, yet there are circumstances in which it need not be felt at all, even though there has been no suppression of consciousness by chemical or pharmacological anaesthesia. Pain too may continue for years after tissues have healed and damaged nerves have fully regenerated, or even after that part of the body which was causing the pain has been totally removed by amputation. Whatever can be going on in the central nervous system to allow such a strong cognitive control of the somatic sensory input, and to operate what has been called the cognitive-evaluative mechanism?

The answer most relevant to our present problem is provided by the theory of 'gating', namely the view, for which there is much experimental evidence, that there are at various levels of the central nervous system, whether in the successive segments of the spinal cord or in the mid-brain, centres where there are junctions between the sensory neurons and other nerve-fibres. If one sensory input can inhibit another at

[a] Here we shall be following in the main the lucid descriptions and discussions of Melzack (1). Specific applications of pain theory to acupuncture analgesia will be found also in Melzack (3, 4, 5); Melzack & Jeans (1). A comprehensive bibliography of the subject down to the end of 1974 has been prepared by Graystone & James (1). Cf. also Nathan (4, 6).

[b] *Khang thung*,[1] in the words of Jen Khang-Thung (*1*).

[1] 抗痛

such a gate, it can be seen that there are ways in which pain impulses can be prevented from reaching the cortical cells, and this we can call ascending or afferent inhibition.[a] Similarly, there appear to be ways in which the gates can be closed by signals coming from above, and this we may call descending or efferent inhibition.[b] The most obvious analogy is that of a telephone exchange in which incoming messages of one kind can occupy the lines and jam the further transmission of messages of another kind; conversely instructions may be sent down from above to ignore the incoming messages which it is not the intention of the control room to take cognisance of.[c] Hence we shall divide our exposition into five parts, first a sketch of the physical means for the transmission of pain impulses, secondly a brief account of the gate-control theory, thirdly a study of the forms of efferent inhibition to the gate (or gates), fourthly some notes on the experimental imitation or reproduction of efferent inhibition, and last a study of the forms of afferent inhibition to the gate.

A burn, an incision or wound, a sprain, or a local inflammation, is signalled inwards by a code of electrical impulses originating from nociceptive nerve-endings at the periphery of the body. These receptors are widely branching bushy networks of fibres which lie in skin areas overlapping with one another. Thus a pattern of nerve impulses moving at different speeds and with different frequencies enters the dorsal horn[d] of the spinal cord at one or other segmental level, passing through a region called the substantia gelatinosa where the neurons are very densely packed and diffusely interconnected. The impulses then begin the ascent of the spinal cord (Fig. 52) along three main pathways. Some pass across the cord towards the anterior or ventral side and go upwards in the spino-thalamic tract to the thalamus[e] or thalamic nuclei in the brain, whence they are relayed to the overlying cortex regions. Others continue up on the dorsal side in the dorso-lateral tract, crossing over to the ventral side only at a higher level, cervical perhaps instead of thoracic. Others again continue still further dorsally as far as the lower medulla and pass through the medial lemniscus in the mid-brain to join all the others in the thalamus. Just above the lemniscus on each side is a part of the brain known as the reticular formation, a tangled thicket of short neurons with innumerable interconnections forming the central core of this level. From this region there radiate many pathways taking the incoming sensory stimuli to a great variety of other points in and below the cortex itself. It is not certain that

[a] Jen Khang-Thung's *shang hsing i chih.*[1]

[b] Equally his *hsia hsing i chih.*[2]

[c] This double control was already adumbrated by Sauerbruch & Wenke (1) in 1936 when they wrote that the sensation of pain may be modified 'in the brain and spinal cord by the intensification or inhibition of excitations stemming from pain receptors by excitations of a different origin, or by centrifugal impulses which originate in the central nervous system and influence the pain-conducting pathways' (1963 ed., p. 46).

[d] A word on this technical term. As seen in transverse section of any part of the spinal cord, the central grey matter has a roughly H-shaped or butterfly-like outline, surrounded by the white matter. The two dorsal horns of the H are the receptive or sensory (afferent) parts, while the two ventral horns are the instructional or motor (efferent) parts. Cf. Barr (1), pp. 59ff.

[e] This is a walnut-sized data-processing centre within the forebrain underneath the cortical canopy. Cf. Barr (1), pp. 169ff.

[1] 上性抑制 [2] 下性抑制

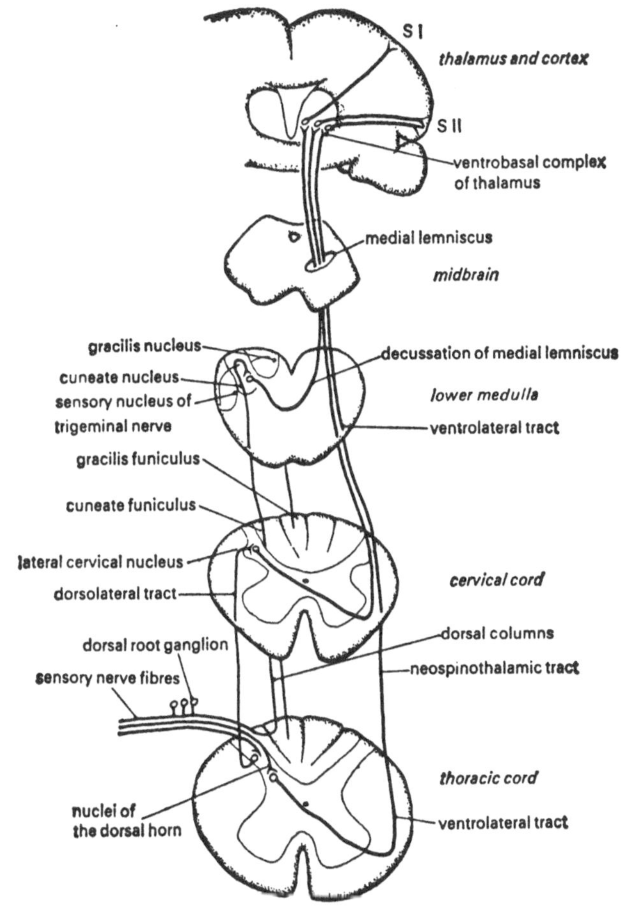

Fig. 52. Ascending pain nerve tracts in the spinal cord. The three main rapidly-conducting somato-sensory pathways are (*a*) the dorsal-column medial-lemniscal route, (*b*) the dorso-lateral tract of Morin, and (*c*) the neo-spinothalamic tract. The lower cross-sections are shown on a scale larger than that of the upper ones. From Milner (1970) after Melzack (1), p. 87.

the cortex, however, is the final conning tower or destination for pain, since there is evidence that after processing the information received it transmits it to deeper centres the nature and position of which are not yet clear. Nevertheless the cortex is intimately associated with consciousness, while the reticular formation, in what has been called the centrencephalic area, is its *sine qua non.*[a]

In order to understand the gate-control theory of pain, proposed by Melzack & Wall (1) in 1965, and now widely accepted, if in more generalised form,[b] it is necessary to understand that nerve-fibres come in very different diameters, like cables fatter or thinner, with or without coats of that insulating material known as myelin, and conducting the nervous impulse at very different speeds. The myelinated fibres

[a] Dr Wilder Penfield, in discussion at Montreal.
[b] See the critical review of Nathan (3).

convey it relatively fast, the unmyelinated ones much more slowly. The largest of the myelinated type are called A-fibres and classed according to size as α, β, γ and δ; they provide many of the afferent somatic routes and all the efferent somatic ones. Thinner than the Aδ fibres are the B-fibres, still myelinated but slow; these are the visceral afferent pathways and also the pre-ganglionic visceral efferent ones. Thinnest, smallest and slowest of all are the C-fibres, having no insulating myelin sheath; these perform the function of somatic afferent lines for pain, light touch and temperature signals, as well as the extremely slow post-ganglionic visceral efferent lines.[a] To give an idea of the sizes and speeds involved, one need only say that the largest and fastest Aα fibres are as thick as 20μ in diameter and conduct at a speed of up to 120 m./sec., which is really like a flash, but the slow Aδ fibres are no more than 2μ in diameter and the impulse passes no faster than 5 m./sec. Important for us also are the Aβ fibres, intermediate in character, some 15μ in diameter, and transmitting at something like 100 m./sec. Lastly, the C-fibres are no more than 1μ in diameter or a little over, and their normal speed of transmission is no more than 1 m./sec., if occasionally a little higher, never exceeding 2 m./sec.[b]

With such a variety of communication wires and cables (and only the barest outline has been given) it is easy to understand that all kinds of mutual competitions, enhancements and inhibitions are possible. For example it is clear that the fibres which carry pain impulses are the thin slow ones of the Aδ and C types, while those of larger size, especially the fast Aβ types, carry sensations of other kinds.[c] This helps to explain differences in sensibility which have been known for a very long time but not comprehended. Thus we can now see that the difference between these fast and slow fibres corresponds with the classical distinction made by Head (2) between epicritic and protopathic sensation, based originally on the phenomena observed during the regeneration of severed nerves.[d] The distinction between the speeds was first appreciated by Zotterman (3);[e] and a relation between the situation now and the course of its evolutionary development has been established by Bishop (1), for the fast myelinated fibre system responsible for epicritic sensibility can be shown to be phylogenetically new, while the largely unmyelinated system responsible for pain and protopathic sensibility is phylogenetically old.

With this background in mind we are ready to appreciate the conclusion of Melzack & Wall, built on a wealth of experimental data, that the more rapidly conducting fibres inhibit synaptic transmission in the more slowly conducting fibre system that carries the pain signals.[f] Under pathological conditions the ancient slow system can

[a] Cf. Barr (1), pp. 29, 268 ff. These are the only fibres involved in the classical dorsal horn gating theory of Melzack & Wall (p. 235). The Aδ ('fast pain') fibres are pure nociceptors and connect directly into the lateral spino-thalamic ascending tract.

[b] There is in fact a linear relation between the conduction rate and the diameter of mammalian myelinated nerve fibres; cf. Ruch & Fulton (1), fig. 29.

[c] Noordenbos (1). Cf. Foerster (1); Zotterman (1, 2).

[d] There has been much refinement of these ideas more recently. We have to differentiate between two pains, two warms, two colds and three touches (Bishop, 1). Of the 'two pains' the C-fibres are more likely to be involved in spinal gating, the Aδ ones, perhaps, in central gating.

[e] In 1933, then independently by Lewis & Pochin five years later; cf. Lewis (1).

[f] (1), pp. 973 ff.

establish a kind of dominance over the more recent fast one, giving rise to slow or diffuse burning pain[a] or hyperalgesia,[b] in fact the protopathic complex. But conversely under physiological conditions it is possible for the fast afferent system to dominate over the slow one, closing the gate and inhibiting the further transmission of pain impulses. Here the effective inhibitory influence is exerted by the large fibres of the $A\beta$ type, coming not from pain receptors but rather from nerve-endings concerned with pressure and stretch recognition, or possibly from those proprioceptive sensors which report the position of the body and its parts in space. Thus broadly speaking it may be said that the impulses in the small slow pain fibres tend to open the gate and transmit their messages to the higher centres, while those coming in over the large fast afferent fibres tend to close it. The significance of this for acupuncture analgesia will at once be obvious, for the counter-stimulation of non-pain receptors would clearly have the effect of jamming the exchanges and preventing the pain impulses from making their way up the cord to the cerebral cortex. At the same time it has always to be remembered that other descending efferent impulses in the cord may also have the effect of closing the gates and preventing the signalling of pain into consciousness.

Something further will need to be said on the exact location of the gating mechanisms, but for Melzack & Wall they were primarily in the dorsal horns of the cord segments, indeed in the substantia gelatinosa already mentioned.[c] As for the way in which the inhibitory influence is exerted, it could be either pre-synaptic or post-synaptic. In the former case it would be a matter of blocking the impulse at the terminal synapse or by decreasing the amount of transmitter substance secreted by its dendrites and normally passed on to the next cell. In the latter it would be a question of increasing or decreasing the level of excitability to stimulation of the neuron following in the chain. At first the emphasis was laid on the former, but it is now fairly sure that both kinds of effect play a part.[d]

(vi) *Efferent inhibition*

Let us now look first at the control from above, the descending influences,[e] or what we may call the efferent inhibition exercised at the gates. This is particularly important for the evaluation of acupuncture analgesia if only because of the fact that Western observers have been so ready to ascribe it uncritically to 'hypnosis'. There can be no question but that cognitive processes in the higher centres are capable of exerting powerful effects on the perception of pain. Attention, anxiety, anticipation and past experience work like this by means of descending efferent fibres in the brain and spinal cord which influence afferent conduction at the lowest synaptic points of the

[a] Lewis (1).

[b] Noordenbos (1).

[c] Cf. Melzack (1), pp. 156–7. Here, however, and in later papers (3, 4, 5) full recognition was also given to the role of the reticular formation in the brain-stem, and other high-level sites.

[d] Op. cit., p. 158.

[e] Melzack (1), p. 160. Serotonin axons descending from the raphe nucleus in the brain stem to the spinal cord are certainly involved here (cf. p. 243). The enkephalins (see pp. 259ff. below) may well act on these raphe cells.

incoming information pathways; hence the modulation of pain perception.[a] To begin with, there are factors which one could describe as cultural.[b] Religious exaltation or political excitement are capable of extraordinary inhibitions of pain perception. There are many well-known examples, from the hook-hanging of India[c] to the sun-dance self-torture ceremonies of the Amerindians of the Northern Plains,[d] and it is probable that the scourging of the ephebes in ancient Sparta was of the same character. Indeed we do not need to go beyond the East Asian culture-areas to find the same thing, as in the phenomena of Chhêng Huang Miao[1] (city-god) processions, or certain ceremonial usages among Buddhists and Taoists, notably too, if more mildly, in the ascetic practices of folk-Buddhism in Japan. Furthermore there is a distinct ethnic element in pain perception threshold and pain tolerance level, for it has been shown experimentally that there are marked cultural components in responses to pain, measurable contrasts between Amerindians, Northern Europeans, Jews, Chinese and Mediterranean peoples.[e]

Past experience also plays a part in what the higher centres instruct the gates to do. Dogs reared in isolation and deprived of the normal environmental stimuli do not respond normally to stimuli usually felt as pain.[f] Reflex movements made in response to fire or pin-prick showed that something was registered in the nervous system, but the emotional disturbance was so small that curiosity impelled the animals to experience the tissue damage again, and the perception of this damage was simply not registered. Here we are in presence of the semantic element in perception, what the mind interprets from neural experience. There is much evidence that the meaning attached to pain-producing situations greatly affects the kind and intensity of the pain perceived. One of the most famous observations in this field is that of Beecher (1) that at the battle of the Anzio beach-head during the second world war soldiers severely wounded were so delighted that they were at last out of the firing-line that they felt little pain, and only 30% needed morphine at the dressing-station though 80% of civilians in ordinary life with similar traumatic injuries would require it. The soldiers were not in shock states for they would complain like anyone else at a change of dressings or an inept venous puncture, but their psychological condition was capable of operating the gate inhibition from above.[g] Yet another example of this comes from the celebrated work of Pavlov (1, 2) who found that noxious stimuli in dogs, such as electric shocks, intense pressure or heat, which normally caused a violent reaction, could be accepted imperturbably if the animals were conditioned by the immediate presentation of food. The pain signal was now interpreted as the herald of a pleasure. So it is clear that a peripheral stimulus is localised, identified and evaluated before

[a] Melzack (2).
[b] Melzack (1), pp. 21 ff.
[c] Description by Kosambi (2).
[d] Description by Wissler (1).
[e] See Zborowski (1), on the psychological side, and several physiological studies cited in Melzack (1), p. 25. One of the best and earliest papers was that of Josey & Miller (1).
[f] Experiments of Melzack & Scott (1).
[g] Cf. Beecher (2, 3).

[1] 城皇廟

it produces perceptual reaction and the corresponding behaviour. And probably all of us have had the experience of finding a dreadful toothache disappear as soon as we have entered our dentist's waiting-room.

Next comes a wide group of factors definable as attention, anxiety, anticipation, distraction and suggestion. Athletic injuries are often sustained during exciting games, yet not registered until the player has walked off the field. One would not call this hypnosis, but the manipulation of attention, together with powerful suggestion, are certainly important elements in the induction of the hypnotic state.[a] This is not sleep, though it has aspects somewhat resembling sleep.[b] The word 'trance', so often used, is probably inappropriate.[c] But it is certainly true that analgesia can accompany hypnosis, for with appropriate suggestion the subject can be pricked, cut or burned without experiencing pain.[d] Hypno-anaesthesia for major surgery is therefore not only a possibility but a fact. Reports are many,[e] but the most classical are those of Esdaile (1–4) who in the middle of the last century found himself in India as a surgeon of the East India Company, and carried out hundreds of severe operations under hypnosis in public hospitals in that country.[f] But since the hypnotic state is sleep-like the patients were not alert enough to co-operate with the surgeon. A further feature of hypno-anaesthesia is that only some 15–20% at most are sufficiently suggestible to respond to it successfully;[g] and it is interesting that when Esdaile returned to his native Scotland his successes became dramatically less.This percentage contrasts with the much higher proportion of people in China who have come through surgery well under acupuncture analgesia,[h] and the equally high percentage of those in European or Western countries who have shown a pain threshold rise with acupuncture.[i] Moreover hypno-anaesthesia requires a considerable period of previous training, which is

[a] There is a vast literature on this, but here may be mentioned only Chertok (1); Kroger (1); Barber (1) and Fromm & Shor (1). On the history of hypnosis, from Anton Mesmer (+1734 to 1815) onwards, there are good papers by Ackerknecht (1); Galdston (1); Rosen (1) and Kaech (1). James Braid (+1795 to 1866) was the first to abandon the idea of 'animal magnetism' for hypnosis—'nervous sleep' or 'mono-ideism', what we should now call suggestion.

[b] Chertok (1), p. 97; F. J. Evans (1). Nor does it resemble physiologically the diverse kind of meditation states (Bowers & Bowers, 1).

[c] As urged impressively by Barber (2).

[d] Hence attempts to use hypnosis in intractable pain; Hollander (1); Sauerbruch & Wenke (1), p. 63.

[e] Prescott (1), pp. 40ff.; Barber (2); for Caesarean section and hysterectomy Kroger & de Lee (1); for cardiac surgery Marmer (1); for appendectomy Owen-Flood (1). The first recorded use of 'mesmerism' for major surgery as the sole anaesthetic medium was by Decamier & Dupatet in Paris in 1821.

[f] Cf. the comments of Chisholm (1); McRobert (1). The operations included amputations, resections of facial cancer, and removal of scrotal tumours. John Elliotson (+1791 to 1868) also employed hypno-anaesthesia for a time at University College Hospital in London (1837 onwards) but it was not wholly a success, and he was much persecuted for his interest in such phenomena. See Fromm & Shor (1), pp. 16ff.

[g] Le Cron (1); Le Cron & Bordeaux (1); Kroger & de Lee (1); Mason (1); Kroger (1), pp. 183ff. and Evans (2) rate it no higher than 10%. It is interesting that the percentage of hypnotisable subjects can be increased by light doses of narcotics such as barbiturate or pentothal, according to Chertok (1), p. ix. This recalls the pre-medication in acupuncture analgesia though the mental state is quite different. In another study, Shibutani Kin-ichi (1) compared hypnotisability with response to therapeutic acupuncture for chronic pain, and found no correlation. Some patients of very non-suggestible type responded to acupuncture most successfully. This is confirmed by Omura Yoshiaki (1), p. 94.

[h] Cf. P. E. Brown (1); Dimond (1); Signer & Galston (1).

[i] Cf. Andersson *et al.* (1); Man & Baragar (1); Mann (8); Mann, Bowsher *et al.* (1). See p. 249 below.

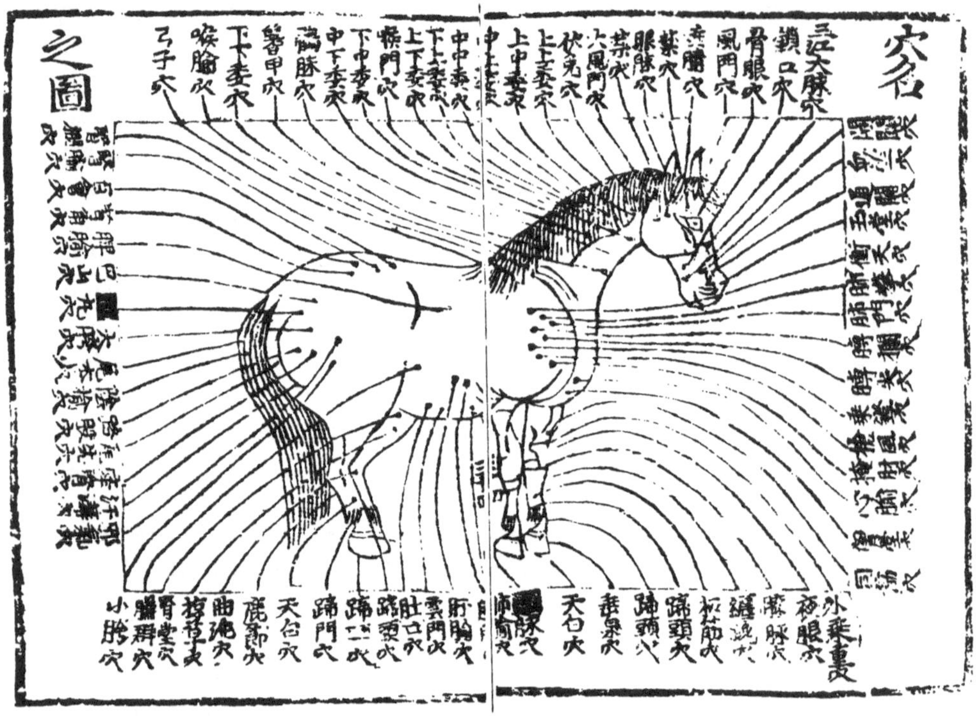

Fig. 53. Veterinary acupuncture; points on the body of the horse. A drawing from the *Ma Niu I Fang* of +1399.

not the case with acupuncture analgesia, though of course for this there has to be some psycho-physiological preparation (cf. pp. 222, 224).

An interesting point arises here. It is well known that people cannot be hypnotised against their own will; one must be prepared to co-operate with the hypnotist and accept freely his suggestions.[a] On the other hand when a barbiturate is injected no amount of will-power can succeed in preventing the anaesthesia that will result. Where acupuncture analgesia stands in this context is rather obscure, for we do not know of any psycho-physiological experiments set up to determine whether the exercise of strong will-power in an antagonistic direction could prevent or delay the onset of the effect. The only observation relevant seems to be that of Woodley (1), an Australian anaesthesiologist, who when in China and Hongkong had himself prepared by electro-acupuncture as for a molar extraction. The result was an area of oral numbness not at all unlike that produced by novocaine injection into the gums, as is normally done for extractions.[b] Further exploration of this area would be well worth while, for there has been so much concentration on making acupuncture

[a] Chertok (1), p. x; Fromm & Shor (1), pp. 527 ff. This is the reason why the hypnotic subject can be made to do strange or even embarrassing things during or after the 'trance' period, but not anti-social or autonocive things—the superego always remains in control.

[b] Hsin Yu-Ling (1) also says that acupuncture analgesia is independent of the will, but considerably enhanced by confidence. Prof. Patrick Wall when in China also had himself prepared for surgical intervention, and though highly objective, not to say reasonably sceptical, experienced *tê chhi* sensations and rise of pain threshold. Cf. Wall (2).

analgesia work, and so much attention to the psycho-cortical preparation necessary, that the limits of possible resistance have hardly been made clear.

Those who contest the relevance of hypnosis in acupuncture analgesia, or even suggestion regarded as its most fundamental element, naturally call upon the witness of children and animals. At various points in the preceding pages we have mentioned that contrary to a prevailing impression in the West, acupuncture analgesia does succeed with children and infants, with whom indeed it has been used therapeutically for hundreds of years (pp. 158, 203–4, 226). But the same holds true for animals, especially the domesticated mammals, which have been given acupuncture at least as far back as the great veterinary manuals of the Yuan period (+14th century; cf. Fig. 53);[a] and since the discovery of acupuncture analgesia in recent years a whole volume of surgical operations has been done on them with its aid. Kaada's group reported that 95% of all such operations are now carried out under acupuncture, and 80% in abdominal surgery.[b] Following the classification used in Table 22 (p. 225 above), the success of the results was as follows:

Grade	I	I and II	I, II and III	IV
%	30	70	95	5

This is not quite so good as in some of the categories of surgery on man, but still rather impressive. However, the problem of hypnosis was bound to come up again, for ever since Athanasius Kircher placed the beak of his hen on the line of white chalk in +1646, controversy and discussion have centred round 'animal hypnosis', a term the very justification of which is not sure.[c] There is no doubt that many animals are given to 'playing 'possum' in the presence of danger, entering a state of immobility and reduced responsiveness to external stimulation, but whether this 'still reaction', as it is sometimes called, has anything to do with human hypnosis is to this day much debated. In spite of some similarities, the most generally held view at present is that there is little connection between them.[d]

Of great importance in this connection are the facts which have been established about the placebo effect. This is an old medical term going back to Chaucer which denotes the giving of a 'non-medicine' to a patient to induce a beneficial psychological state within the psycho-somatic entity.[e] According to universal clinical experience,

[a] For a modern practical treatise see Anon. (*171*), and for charts Anon. (*160*). Tsou Chieh-Chêng (*1*) has pushed further back, in a study of the veterinary use of acupuncture and cautery in the Thang period.

[b] (1), pp. 429, 437.

[c] It is certain, as Melzack points out (3, 4), that animals cannot be hypnotised in the usual sense.

[d] Cf. Ratner (1) in Gordon (1), pp. 530ff.

[e] The word 'placebo' originally referred to the Vespers in the Latin Office for the Dead, since it was the first word of the first antiphon, taken from Ps. cxvi, 9. The oldest literary mention is of +1225. Hence, perhaps because of the tag *de mortuis nil nisi bonum*, it came to mean flattering and flattery. The first use in this sense comes in +1340, and Chaucer wrote in +1386: 'Flatterers be the Devil's Chaplains that sing ever Placebo'. This continued till the end of the +17th century, after which the word was adopted into pharmacy and medicine, as one can see from the 'Medical Dictionary' of Hooper in 1811, where it is defined as 'an epithet given to any medicine adapted more to please than benefit the patient'. To what extent physicians before the +18th century realised that remarkable effects could follow the administration of pharmacalogically inactive substances remains an open question.

severe pain, often post-surgical, can be relieved in some 35% of Euro-American populations by giving the patient a placebo, i.e. an inactive coloured solution of salt or sugar, instead of morphine or some other genuine analgesic drug.[a] When one considers that morphine, even in considerable amounts, will relieve severe pain in only about 75% of patients, other analgesics then being needed, one comes to the astonishing conclusion that as much as half of the morphine effect may not be truly pharmacological.[b] These facts must evidently be borne in mind in considering not only acupuncture but all therapeutic and analgesic techniques whatsoever.[c]

The case of 'audio-analgesia' is instructive in this connection. In 1959 Gardner & Licklider (1) discovered that intense auditory stimulation could suppress the pain of dental drilling or extraction in many subjects; the input was named 'white noise' and delivered through earphones. But the technique often failed, and there were difficulties in demonstrating experimentally any influence of noise-distraction on pain threshold. The situation was elucidated by Melzack, Weisz & Sprague (1) in an interesting paper which showed that the auditory stimulus plus suggestion would do what neither alone could perform.[d] The groups were as follows:

Control		establishment of base-line for pain-tolerance duration
Group 1	auditory stimulus with no prior suggestion or information	no increase
Group 2	auditory stimulus with strong prior suggestion	marked increase
Group 3	a placebo hum with strong prior suggestion	no increase

This showed that the auditory distraction alone would not do, and also that the suggestion alone would not do, but the combination of suggestion with the central nervous distraction would really give in average normal subjects a considerable measure of analgesia. In Melzack's words, the device did not fail (though much less used in practice today), because it was 'a stratagem to modulate pain tolerance'. This example is particularly instructive in connection with acupuncture analgesia because it shows

[a] Beecher (1).

[b] Melzack (1), p. 33. But see p. 261 below, where the work of Levine *et al.* (1) is discussed. It is now known that the placebo effect arises from the endogenous production of morphine-analogues.

[c] Evans (2) found no significant relationship between suggestibility or hypnotic susceptibility and pain reduction by placebo. It seemed to be greater for pain threshold than for pain tolerance. Commenting on the work of Smith, Chiang, Kitz & Antoon (1) who (in a rather small series) found a certain correlation between high hypnotisability and successful acupuncture analgesia in experimentally induced ischaemic pain, Evans pointed out that response to acupuncture could be predicted only from one end of the distribution of hypnotisability. Poorly hypnotisable subjects will similarly be poor placebo-reactors, but highly hypnotisable ones may or may not be.

[d] See also the account in Melzack (1), pp. 34ff.

how effectively the gating mechanism, wherever it is, can be operated at the same time both from below and from above. Anxiety is one of the most important factors here.[a] The mere anticipation of pain is enough to raise the anxiety level and consequently the intensity of the pain felt. Hill, Kornetsky *et al.* (1, 2) have shown that if anxiety is psychologically dispelled, a given level of nociceptive input is perceived as significantly less painful than the same stimulus under intense anxiety. Hence the circumstance so much insisted upon by all those who have studied acupuncture analgesia in China that there is always an instilling of confidence into patients by a careful explanation of what is to be expected beforehand. There is calming, assurance, allaying of apprehension, and the induction of an emotionally anti-traumatic mentality. This is what the basic documents call the 'dual dynamic forces' (*liang-ko chi chi hsing*[1]),[b] the suggestion acting efferently on the one hand, and the counter-stimulation acting afferently on the other.

Probably few realise how far back in Chinese medical history the condition of psychological confidence in acupuncture is to be found — the efferent component, as we should say in this neurological discussion. We promised earlier (p. 226) a good quotation from the Han period, and here it is. The *Huang Ti Nei Ching*, *Su Wên* says that a good physician should take into account the background of his patient's thought when making a choice of treatment. For example:

> when dealing with a person who believes in ghosts and spirits[c] it is not much use to tell him about the effectiveness of (rational) medicine. When consulted by someone who cannot bear the idea of acupuncture (and moxibustion) it will not help to expatiate to him on the successes of skill in those techniques. When a patient refuses a particular way of treatment his illness will never be cured by it, and in the end no success will be achieved.[d]

Thus one may say that the factor of suggestion, or auto-suggestion, if we may so term the patient's confidence in the methods of the physician, was rather fully appreciated already at the dawn of rational medicine in China. For acupuncture analgesia this is surely of great significance.

A few words now on the experimental reproduction of efferent inhibition. Anatomically there is every support for the idea that the cortex can send down instructions to the gating points in the dorsal horn of the cord, or wherever else they are, at all lower levels. Fibres from the cortex, especially its frontal part, connect with the reticular formation and thence downwards through the reticulo-spinal system; and there are large fast neuron chains in the pyramidal tract, the cortico-spinal fibres, as they are called, which join the cortex to every segment of the cord.[e] Attention, past experience, and all kinds of cognitive conditions can therefore exert influence on what goes on below. Many neuro-physiological experiments acquire significance in the light of this.

[a] Melzack (1), pp. 31 ff.
[b] Anon. (*129*). This is quite close to the standpoint of Wall (2) who speaks in terms of distraction plus suggestion plus tranquillisation.
[c] I.e. in apotropaic medicine, the placation of the spirits of the dead, or of various gods and deities.
[d] *NCSW/PH*, ch. 11, (p. 70).
[e] Cf. Barr (1), pp. 73–4.

[1] 两個積極性

For example, if an afferent nerve entering the spinal cord is stimulated, the signal going up to the brain can be recorded electrically on a tracing; but if at the same time some higher centre, such as the cerebellum or part of the cortex, is also stimulated, the ascending afferent signal is almost completely suppressed—as if the nervous system now had something else on its mind.[a] Melzack & Wall were therefore led to develop the idea of a 'central control trigger',[b] activating the selective function of the brain which maintains control over the sensory input. It is as if signals from the body's periphery have to be identified and evaluated in terms of past experience, localised and perhaps inhibited, before the systems responsible for pain perception and subsequent motor activity are brought into play.[c] In a way, pain is something that has to be learned.[d] This information-processing pattern can be illustrated by a simple example; if one picks up a very hot cup of tea in what we know to be a very precious or expensive cup, one will probably not drop the cup but replace it awkwardly on the table and only then nurse one's hand.[e]

But the cortex need not be involved, for there are groups of cells within the brain-stem which can exert the most powerful inhibitory or adjuvant effects on the transmission of pain signals. For example, it is known that lesions of the central tegmental tract in cats produce a marked hyperalgesia,[f] something like the Déjèrine–Roussy syndrome in man. Conversely, electrical stimulation of many points in and near this tract can produce profound analgesia in rats.[g] Morphine may act, at least in part, by exciting fibres in these regions that have strong inhibitory effects on somatic sensory input, for its effects on the transmission of afferent impulses within the cord are abolished if this is transected below the brain-stem.[h] Again, stimulation of the reticular formation and the tegmental tract gives rise to a massive cortical secretion of γ-amino-butyric acid (GABA), one of the chemical transmitters released by inhibitory neurons.[i] It seems sure that ultimately the physiology of pain signal transmission will involve neuro-humoral as well as neural factors. Work done recently in China demonstrates both of these. On the one hand physiologists in Shanghai have recorded potentials from the caudate nucleus[j] of rabbits in response to electro-

[a] Hagberth & Kerr (1).

[b] Melzack (1), p. 161; Melzack & Wall (1), p. 976. Related conceptions described by Melzack are those of a 'central intensity monitor' and a 'central biassing mechanism'.

[c] Loc. cit.

[d] This is probably why intractable pain is very seldom met with in children (Dr Raymond Evans of Toronto, in conversation).

[e] Melzack, op. cit., pp. 165–6.

[f] Melzack, Stotler & Livingston (1). This is part of the reticular formation in the mid-brain. Cf. Barr (1), pp. 94, 101.

[g] Reynolds (1); Mayer, Wolfle, Akil *et al.* (1); Liebeskind, Guilbaud, Besson *et al.* (1). There is no paralysis or 'trance', the animals are just pain-free with all the other sensory and motor functions intact.

[h] Sato & Takagi (1). This means that the descending efferent inhibitory fibres can no longer function, and the gates are left open without the higher control.

[i] Melzack (1), p. 166. This observation is of interest in connection with the Chinese cross-circulation experiments shortly to be mentioned.

[j] This is in the corpus striatum, one of the basal ganglia of the telencephalon or fore-brain, a grey mass embedded in the white matter of the lower part of each cerebral hemisphere. Cf. Barr (1), pp. 198–9.

acupuncture at Ho-ku (IG 4) and Tsu-san-li (V 36). Electrical stimulation of the same caudate area gave a rise in pain threshold like that found with acupuncture itself, and augmented the analgesic effect of needling, while conversely its destruction reduced or abolished the effect.[a] Here we are still in the realm of a purely neural descending inhibition. But on the other hand there may be an intervention of serotonin.[b] The drug reserpine increases and prolongs the analgesia effect of acupuncture in rabbits,[c] and one of the most important actions of reserpine is the liberation of serotonin from the pre-synaptic terminals of descending mono-aminergic tracts. Now the analgesic effect of mid-brain reticular stimulation in rats mentioned above is blocked by inhibitors of serotonin synthesis.[d] Therefore it looks as if serotonin, passing down through the central canal in the raphe of the spinal cord along with the cerebrospinal fluid, and diffusing out at various levels to the gates, may also be exerting a block on ascending pain impulses. Of course such an effect would be very much slower in action than any direct neural transmissions.[e] But this might be relevant to acupuncture analgesia, the duration of which often lasts quite long after the stimulation of the needles has ended.[f]

Similar evidence comes forward in the work being carried out by Thang Pei-Chin (1). In decerebrate or lightly anaesthetised animals nociceptive stimulation can elicit mimetic reflex movements (both somatic and autonomic) that simulate expressions of cortically-registered pain. These are the 'pseudo-affective reflexes' of Sherrington. In dogs anaesthetised with chloralose and given bradykinin injections as nociceptive stimuli the vocalisation and respiratory reflexes could be suppressed and reduced respectively by electro-acupuncture. But not until 50 minutes after the cessation of the acupuncture did the vocalisation reflex reappear. This could hardly be accounted for otherwise than by the action of a chemical transmitter diffusing relatively slowly.

The fact is that analgesic and hyperalgesic centres are scattered close together all through the reticular formation in the mid-brain, and their topographic location is now actively proceeding.[g] The action of the analgesic centres in the cat, for example, is quite dramatic, for all kinds of stimuli normally painful[h] cease shortly to elicit any reaction; at the same time the spontaneous respiratory rate drops to half the normal level as in most types of chemical anaesthesia. The centres do not switch on and off

[a] Kaada *et al.* (1), p. 427. Parallel confirmatory experiments have been reported by Lineberry & Vierck (1); Delgado, Obrador & Martin-Rodriguez (1).

[b] I.e. 5-hydroxy-tryptamine; Burn (1), pp. 90ff.

[c] Private communication to Kaada *et al.*, pp. 424, 427, from Hsiang Man-Chin & Hsin Yu-Lin, cf. Anon. (118).

[d] Akil & Mayer (1).

[e] Serotonin could explain the effects of CSF exchanges (p. 256 below) but not the cross-circulation experiments, because it does not pass the blood-brain barrier. Some precursor or breakdown-product could of course be involved. But the enkephalins and endorphins (pp. 259ff. below) do pass to some extent, however. And serotonin action could be fast if it energised axons emanating from the raphe nucleus, as it seems to be able to do (cf. p. 235 above). Cf. Kaada (2), pp. 738ff.

[f] Cf. p. 219 above. Bresler (1) found post-acupuncture analgesia for oral surgery lasting as long as 12 hours after cessation of the stimulus.

[g] These paragraphs owe much to conversations with Prof. Ronald Melzack, Mr Warren Soper, Mr George Nieman and Dr Elizabeth Fox at Montreal in May 1975.

[h] E.g., clamping the external ear, injection of formol or histamine into the paw, piercing the abdominal wall, etc. In the rat, painful heat stimuli no longer bring any response.

with great speed; the analgesia they cause develops only gradually over a period of about 5 minutes, and lasts for at least 2 or 3 minutes after the cessation of stimulation.[a] These centres, it may be noted, are not at all the same as either the 'pleasure centres' or the 'aversive centres' discovered by Olds & Milner in 1953 in the median forebrain bundle,[b] hypothalamus and mid-brain.[c] Later we shall consider (p. 255) whether the analgesia centres are not part of the mechanism of efferent (though not cortical or cognitive) inhibition in acupuncture for surgery.

(vii) *Afferent inhibition*

And now at last we must think about the afferent or ascending inhibitory effect at the gate or gates, the direct peripheral physiological effect rather than any influences coming down from above. One way to classify this action of acupuncture would be under the general head of 'counter-irritation', a concept extremely old in medicine both in West and East. Its history in Europe has been traced by Brockbank, who has enumerated the methods traditionally used.[d] The mustard plasters familiar to all of us are but one among many agents — inflammatory plants,[e] blistering mixtures, cantharides,[f] and wet or dry cupping,[g] which go back at least as far as Aretaeus in the +2nd century. Setons,[h] issues or fontanelles,[i] cautery and eschars,[j] can be traced

[a] Melzack & Melinkoff (1). The close parallel here with acupuncture analgesia will be apparent. It even suggests that the diffusion of some neuro-chemical agent, and its attainment of some critical concentration, may be involved. On the other hand the time may be required for the recruitment of a critical number of active neurons. But both Akil *et al.* (1) and Oliveras *et al.* (1) have shown that naloxone can prevent the induction of analgesia caused by electrical stimulation of these centres in the mesencephalic central grey tissue. The neuro-chemical significance of this will be apparent a few pages below (p. 260).

[b] Cf. Barr (1), pp. 186–7.

[c] Olds (1, 2). Brief accounts will be found in Nathan (1), pp. 192ff.; Melzack (1), p. 101; Rose (1), pp. 234ff. These pleasure centres are potentiated by the modern anti-depressive drugs. If a chemical substance could be found which would stimulate exclusively the analgesic centres it would be a great advance in anaesthesiology.

[d] (1), pp. 105ff.

[e] For example, thapsia, pellitory and mezereon. The first is mentioned in Pliny (*Nat. Hist.* XIII, xliii, 124–6); it is *Thapsia Asclepium* (= *garganica*), an umbelliferous plant. Cf. Lenz (2), p. 568. The second is Spanish pellitory, *Anthemis Pyrethrum* of the compositae, described by Woodville (1), vol. 2, p. 286; cf. Lenz (2), p. 471; Clapham, Tutin & Warburg (1), p. 848. The third is *Daphne Mezereum* of the Thymelaeceae, described by Woodville (1), vol. 1, p. 68; cf. Lenz (2), p. 461; Clapham, Tutin & Warburg (1), p. 467.

[f] Cf. *SCC*, Vol. 5, pt. 2, p. 290. The 'Spanish fly' or 'blistering beetle', *Cantharis vesicatoria*; cf. Brandt & Ratzenburg (1), vol. 2, pl. 18. The old Chinese physicians used a related genus, *Mylabris*.

[g] Cf. Vol. 6, Sect. 44. See also Brockbank, op. cit., pp. 67ff.

[h] A seton was a running sore deliberately made by threading through and under the skin strands of silk or twine and leaving them there indefinitely. The word means a bristle, and indeed this was one of the earliest types of foreign body to be used. Horse hairs were also employed. Techniques of this kind are now being tried again at selected acu-points in China, especially for chronic bronchitis (Kao, 2).

[i] An issue or 'little fountain' (fontanelle) was similar to a seton but using a more bulky foreign body to keep the wound open, for example a little ball of gold or silver.

[j] An eschar was a sore or ulcer artificially produced by severe cauterisation with an instrument of red-hot iron. This was analogous to the moxibustion of China, but since the glowing moxa was by no means always allowed to burn the skin, and since acupuncture was often relatively painless, it must be allowed that traditional Chinese practice was rather more civilised than that of ancient, medieval, and even eighteenth-century Europe. Indeed in +1712 Engelbert Kaempfer said precisely this. 'Nam primus ignem fundit, cedit alter metalli aciem; aciem vero, non ferocis chalybis sanguinantis, nec ignem quosque candentis ferri; quo utroque trux supra humanitatem chirurgia Occidentis in mortalium saevire

back to Paul of Aegina in the +7th century. Often dismissed as folk-medicine, all these have been extremely widely used, and successfully, for the relief of pain by what may be termed hyper-stimulation analgesia.[a] A recent study by Elliott (1) has considered the more sophisticated modern descendants of these techniques—rubefacient creams, methyl nicotinate, capsicum,[b] nonylic acid vanillylamide, etc. — interpreting their action in terms of erythema (increased capillary blood supply) spreading the bradykinin produced by the sweat glands to stimulate strongly the local afferent nerve-endings. Counter-irritation is quite real. Even brief successive applications of cold or heat produce significant decreases in some kinds of pain.[c] And of course the Chinese parallel is the entire moxibustion story, together with its derivatives in the West in and after the +17th century, which we describe more fully elsewhere.[d] As expressed in contemporary China, the brain 'confronts an antithesis'(or contradiction, *mao tun*[1]), and in the competition of stimuli there are 'two sensations contending' (*hsiang tou chêng*[2]).[e]

Many modern techniques have relations with these phenomena. For example, strong saline solutions injected into the stump of an amputated extremity will give transitory sharp pain but will relieve severe phantom limb pain for long periods of time.[f] Acupuncture here will also give relief.[g] Painful low temperatures applied to the skin can raise the pain threshold elsewhere by 30%.[h] Stimulation of peripheral nerves by low-intensity electric shocks can abolish neuralgic pain for a long while afterwards, and the effect can be enhanced by pharmacological analgesics.[i] Electrodes

membra jubet, opera detestabili iis, quorum humana mollities et mansuetudo praecordia occupat; sed ignem gratiosum, et non verendum magis, quam quo sibi litari hoc caelo Dii ipsi amant, nimirum remisse gliscentem turundam, volutam ex herba Regii nominis Artemisia' (*Amoenitates Exoticae*, pp. 584–5). Fransiszyn (1) did well to notice this. A translation might read: '(Of the two sources of surgery of the Koreans, Chinese and Japanese) the first was heat, the second the sharpness of metal, sharpness, I say, but not those ferocious bloody cauteries of iron, nor yet the flaming of red-hot brands, with which our Western surgery commands the atrocious ravaging of the limbs of mortals, beyond the dictates of humanity, in works detestable to all those who have any kindness and gentleness left in their hearts; and as for the heat, it is a grateful warmth no more to be feared than that which the gods themselves enjoy as it rises from their sacrifices, a warmth from glowing cakes which have been rolled from a dried plant with a royal name, *Artemisia*.' Similar translations, one from Kaempfer's inaugural dissertation of +1694, are given by Bowers & Carrubba (1, 2).

[a] Melzack (1), pp. 183ff., 199. Another example, well known to all who have lived in East and Southeast Asia, is the Chinese mentholated ointment known as 'tiger balm'.

[b] The chili plant, *Capsicum annuum* (*Piper indicum = nigrum*), containing the blistering agent capsaicin, an outstanding irritant. See Burkill (1), vol. 1, p. 446; Woodville (1), vol. 3, pl 391; Lenz (2), p. 541.

[c] This we know from the careful study of Gammon & Starr (1), one of the few modern investigations of counter-irritation. All its uses are most successful when applied to the same dermatome as the source of pain, evoking the many viscero-cutaneous reflexes.

[d] Pp. 170, 291.

[e] Anon. (*129*).

[f] Feinstein *et al.* (1); Melzack (1), pp. 49ff., 57–8. The effect is most reproducible, but in practice it has been replaced by anti-depressant drugs in many clinics (Dr Raymond Evans, Toronto, in conversation).

[g] Cf. Labrousse (1); Labrousse & Duron (1); Khoubesserian & Martiny (1); Benichon (1); Mann, Bowsher *et al.* (1); Miles & Lipton (1).

[h] Parsons & Goetzl (1).

[i] White & Sweet (1); Wall & Sweet (1); Picaza *et al.* (1).

[1] 矛盾 [2] 相鬬爭

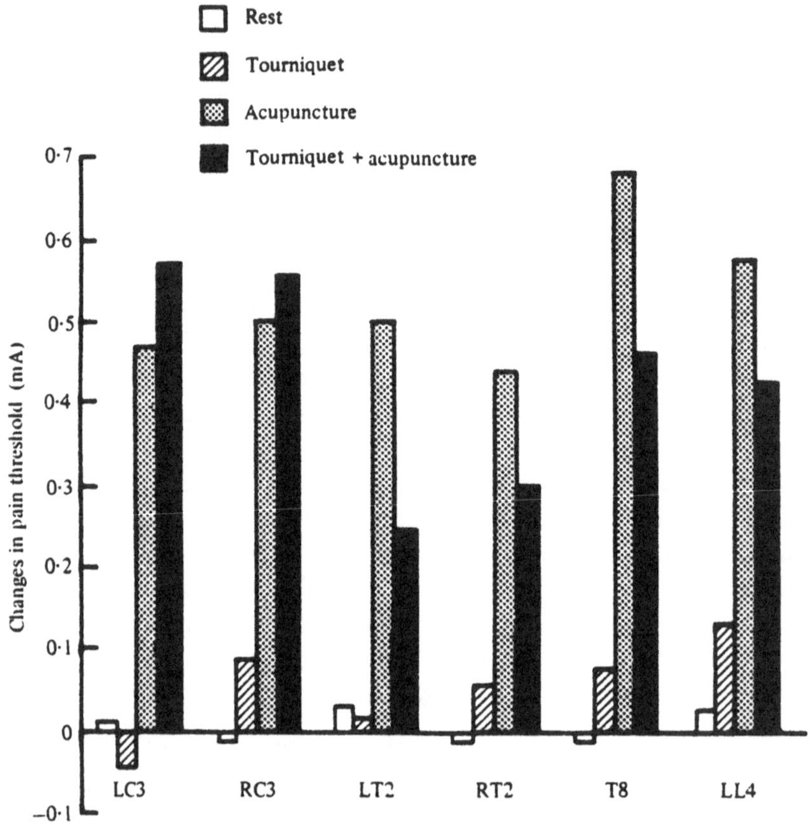

Fig. 54. Changes in pain threshold at different cutaneous points under conditions of rest, tourniquet, acupuncture, and acupuncture following tourniquet (Chiang Chen-Yü, Chiang Chhing-Tshai *et al.*, 1). C, T, L, cervical, thoracic and lumbar segments, L, R, left or right. The acupuncture effect is still present after vascular occlusion of the left forearm. Chinese subjects.

can be implanted near the dorsal columns of the spinal cord in patients with traumatic or pathological pain, with arrangements enabling them to control their own rate of stimulation; this produces painless tingling feelings and in the majority of cases the pain itself is effectually relieved.[a]

What then is the situation with acupuncture? First of all, its primarily neural mediation has been proved in interesting experiments. Vascular occlusion of the upper arm does not stop the acupuncture analgesia effect. Chiang Chen-Yü, Chiang Chhing-Tshai *et al.* (1) measured the pain threshold in a number of volunteers at six different points on the skin in four different dermatomes[b] after a quarter of an hour of (*a*) rest, (*b*) manual acupuncture of two points on the left forearm,[c] (*c*) complete vascular occlusion by means of a tourniquet,[d] (*d*) the same acupuncture under

[a] Nashold & Friedman (1); Shealy *et al.* (1).

[b] C_3, T_2, T_8 and L_4.

[c] C_5, C_{6-7}.

[d] The effectiveness of this was checked by injections of radioactive isotopic iodine; only after the release of the tourniquet was any uptake by the thyroid gland detectable.

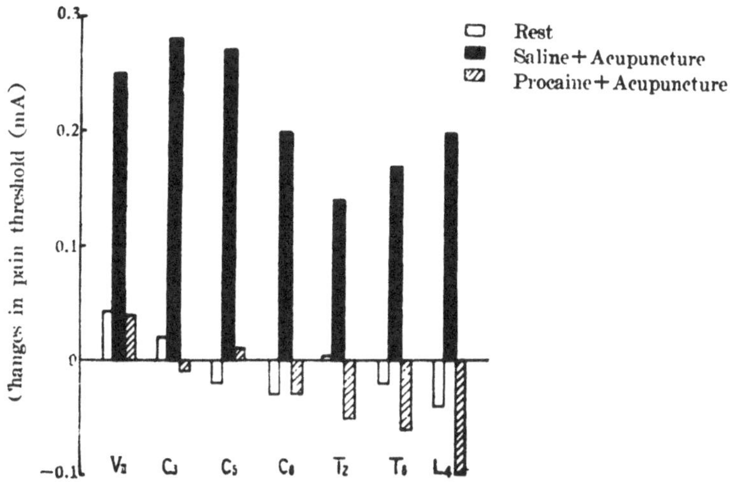

Fig. 55. Changes in pain threshold at different cutaneous points under conditions of rest, acupuncture following injection of normal saline, and acupuncture after injection of 2 % procaine solution, into the needled point (Chiang Chen-Yü, Chiang Chhing-Tshai *et al.* 1). Symbols as in the preceding diagram V, a point supplied by the maxillary branch of the trigeminal nerve. The local anaesthetic abolishes the acupuncture effect. Chinese subjects.

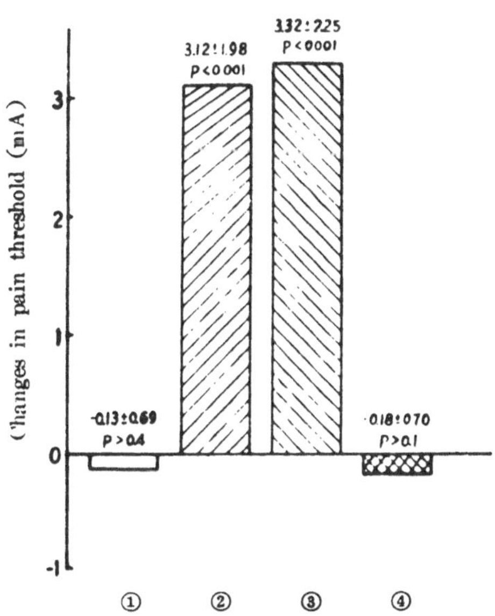

Fig. 56. Changes in pain threshold at different cutaneous points under conditions of (1) rest, (2) acupuncture, (3) acupuncture following blockade of cutaneous nerves supplying the skin over the needling point, and (4) acupuncture following blockade of the muscular nerves supplying the deep tissues underlying the needling point (Chiang Chen-Yü, Chiang Chhing-Tshai *et al.* 1). The needles thus stimulate the deeper receptors rather than the nerve-endings immediately under the skin surface. Chinese subjects.

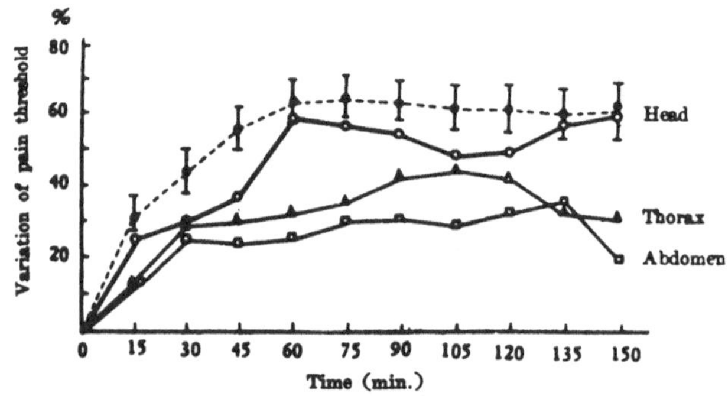

Fig. 57. The rise of pain threshold, and its persistence, as measured by a potassium ion algometer, in response to continuous acupuncture at Ho-ku (IG 4), at different regions of head and trunk. The dotted line represents the average pain threshold in all regions during intermittent acupuncture. Since Ho-ku is in dermatome C 6–7, it is interesting that the effect was higher in the trigeminal and cervical areas than for the thoracic and abdominal segments. Anon. (*128*), Chinese subjects.

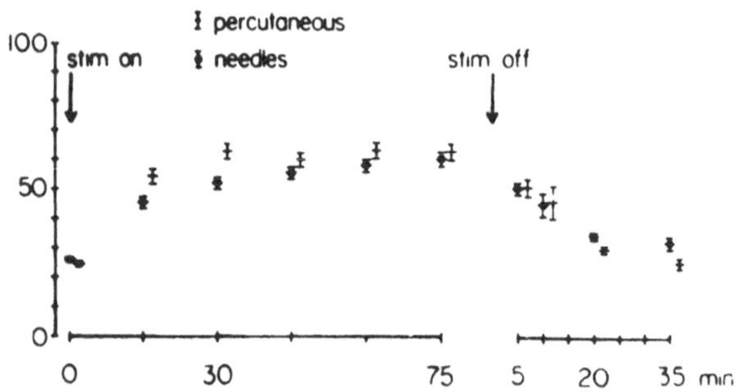

Fig. 58. Rise, and persistence of pain threshold rise, measured in terms of the current necessary to produce pain when applied to dental surfaces; mean values and standard errors. Percutaneous stimulation, i.e. by surface electrodes, was very slightly more effective than the acupuncture itself in these experiments; and it is indeed used in some Chinese hospitals. Andersson *et al.* (1), Swedish subjects.

these conditions. As Fig. 54 shows, there was a marked and general rise in pain threshold at various sites, and this action was completely unaffected by the interference with the circulation.[a] On the other hand, the same authors found (Fig. 55) that infiltration of procaine or novocaine into the deep subcutaneous tissues did abolish the phenomenon.[b] Light local anaesthesia of the skin surface, however, had

[a] Such a result would hardly be consistent with an interpretation of the pain threshold rise as a placebo-like phenomenon.

[b] So also Anon. (*128*, *129*, *130*); (128); Jen Khang-Thung (*1*). Placebo injections of saline have no effect.

no effect on it (Fig. 56).[a] Such observations go far to prove that the acupuncture needles stimulate deep receptors, and that they act fundamentally through the peripheral sensory nervous system.

A considerable amount of experimental work has now been done on pain threshold variations induced by acupuncture, with results somewhat variable, but many positive. For example, Fig. 57 shows the rise in pain threshold, as measured by the potassium iontophoresis algometer method,[b] in response to continuous acupuncture at Ho-ku (IG 4), in normal Chinese volunteers.[c] Fig. 58 shows the results of a similar experiment in Sweden, also on volunteers, measured in terms of the electric current needed to produce pain when applied to dental surfaces.[d] On the other hand, experiments at Toronto have not been so impressive. Using a Wolff–Hardy–Goodell focused electric heat beam, acupuncture not at the recognised points produced a small effect, hardly greater than that of a placebo narcotic injection, while the insertion of needles at regular acu-points produced a larger effect, though not very large. In contrast to this the injection of morphine gave an effect about four times greater, yet with the curious feature that it did not necessarily work for all sites on the body.[e] The same apparatus has been used to measure accurately the latency of a voluntary terminating response to painful stimulus in medical student volunteers at Dalhousie University, with stronger effects both for acu-points and other loci, the former more than double the latter, and the latter well above the controls.[f] Other Canadian work has yielded still more positive results. In a Winnipeg study it was found that when acupuncture was done on leg sites corresponding to dermatomes L_3 and L_5 as many as 92·5% of the volunteers had markedly diminished pain sensation after five minutes. The analgesia lasted for 20 minutes and normal pain sensation was recovered in about a quarter of an hour (Fig. 59).[g] Of particular interest was another investigation, with technique based on sensory decision theory, in which it was found that the pain of dental stimulation was significantly reduced by acupuncture, and to an extent approximately paralleling the effect of 33% nitrous oxide.[h] This in itself would be insufficient for surgery if not reinforced by cognitive factors and tranquillising premedication. Finally, there has been a careful study by Stewart, Thomson & Oswald

[a] Chiang Chen-Yü *et al.* (1). Cf. Wall (2). These facts apply both to tract acu-points and to others chosen for segmental dermatome reasons. Furthermore the *tê chhi* effect corresponds; with superficial nerve-block you get it still, but deep block stops it.

[b] Benjamin & Helvey (1). On dolorimetry in general see Beecher (4).

[c] Anon. (*128*), (128). Cf. Wall (2).

[d] Andersson, Ericson & Holmgren (1); Andersson, Ericson, Holmgren & Lindqvist (1); Stacher, Wancura *et al.* (1).

[e] Personal communication from Dr Raymond Evans of the Smythe Pain Clinic at the Toronto General Hospital. It will be remembered that this was the laboratory which could successfully identify classical acu-points by means of skin electrical resistance measurements. Cf. Brennan, Veldhuis & Chu (1).

[f] Berlin, Bartlett & Black (1). Here Wai-kuan (SC 5, not HC 6 as they thought) was used as well as Ho-ku.

[g] Man & Baragar (1). The pain sensation here was subjective recording of pin-prick. There were only slight changes in sensations of heat and vibration, none at all for cold and the two touches, light and dull. Cf. Mumford & Bowsher (1).

[h] Chapman, Gehrig & Wilson (1). Curiously, the acupuncture was more effective than anaesthetic gas for medium and strong stimuli, and rather less so for the weak stimuli.

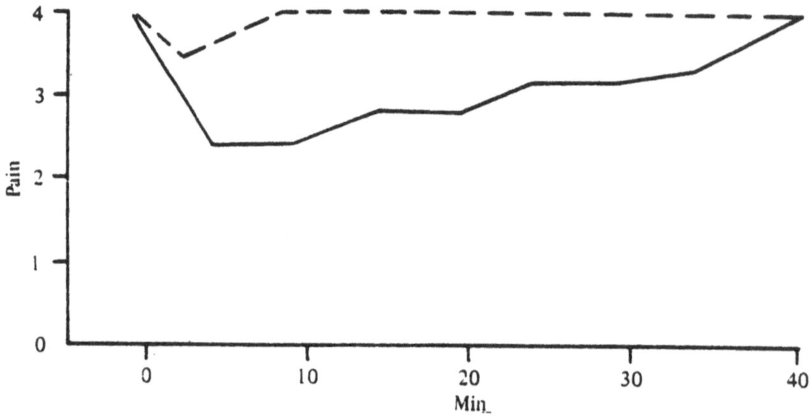

Fig. 59. Decrease, and persistence of decrease, in pain sensation (subjective pin-prick recording) in the knee region during acupuncture at three points on the lower leg (Yang-ling-chhüan, VF 34, Yin-ling-chhüan, LP 9, and Hsien-ku, V 43). The dotted line represents the effects when needles were implanted at random incorrect sites. Man & Baragar (1), Canadian subjects.

(1). They found that acupuncture[a] was significantly more effective than suggestion in raising overall body pain thresholds and tolerances, though in the latter case acupuncture off the tracts but in the same dermatomes was about as effective as classical acupuncture. Moreover, a significant disproportionate effect on the epigastrium predicted by the choice of classical acupuncture points was found for tolerances though not thresholds, so that the effect was morphinoid. They concluded that the Chinese traditions of a highly localised analgesic action remote from the point selected were verifiable.

There have also been pain threshold experiments in animals. Using a radiant heat dolorimeter with rabbits it has been found that a rise of 128% in pain threshold after acupuncture at the Tsu-san-li (V 36) point is quite constant and reproducible.[b] Similarly, pinching of the Achilles tendon with the fingers at the Khun-lun point (VU 60) will give rises of the order of 133%.

At an earlier point (p. 213) something was said of the possible role of the autonomic nervous system and the suprarenal cortex in acupuncture therapy. That it is not involved with acupuncture analgesia has been shown by Chiang Chen-Yü & Chu Tê-Hsing (*1*), who found that the pain threshold increases brought about by acupuncture in rabbits (150%) were not at all affected by prior total bilateral adenalectomy and cervical sympathectomy.

Large-scale statistical studies of pain relief with acupuncture are still not very numerous, but some interesting information is forthcoming from the Smythe Pain Clinic at the Toronto General Hospital.[c] Of cases with primarily functional disease 100% responded immediately, but after a week only 80% were responding and after a month only 40%. By contrast the figures for patients with organic disease were

[a] Bilaterally at Ho-ku and Tsu-san-li.
[b] Anon. (118).
[c] Our grateful thanks are due to Dr Raymond Evans for the information here given.

40%, 25% and 20% respectively. This means that in the first case the effects were well above the placebo base-line (p. 239 above), while in the second they were much nearer to it. The findings so far would thus bear out to some extent what was said at an earlier point about functional as opposed to organic conditions (p. 197). Another contribution[a] has reported on a series of male American veterans suffering from different types of chronic pain (post-laminectomy, causalgia, phantom limb pain, post-herpetic, osteo-arthritic, etc.). About 60% of the patients experienced at least 50% relief of their pain.[b] But a logical fallacy seems to have been present in the remark of the authors that they were 'surprised that the procedure was twice as effective as other placebo treatments'. If one finds in a given population a placebo effect of 30–35% this surely implies that something else (e.g. morphine and related narcotics) will work unfailingly for all or nearly all the members of the group. But in this case there was nothing possessing that character of overall effectivity to use as a comparison, since 'the patients had all failed to attain relief by conventional Western medical treatments'.[c] Consequently the term placebo is at least half out of order.

A certain linguistic uneasiness arises again in connection with a report on the evaluation of acupuncture analgesia by signal detection theory.[d] Here again there was a marked pain threshold increase. But at the same time the subjects' capacity for discrimination of very weak stimuli of lower or higher intensity remained unchanged. The conclusion was that the subjects simply raised their pain criterion in response to the expectation that acupuncture would work. Acupuncture in this case did not decrease discriminability though chemical analgesics do. Therefore the preponderant action would be (in our terms) efferent rather than afferent, events in the cortex or mid-brain being more important than those in the spinal cord segments registering inputs from the needles. According to Clark & Yang, the subjects 'experienced equal amounts of "physiological" pain in the arms, but were less likely to admit that a given sensory experience was painful when it occurred in the arm which had received the acupuncture treatment'. Consequently there was no 'true' analgesia.[e] But does this not depend on how we define analgesia? By all means let us do everything possible to differentiate between the efferent and the afferent components, but if a person reports freedom from pain, is it not rather gratuitous to insist that he is in fact really experiencing it but refusing to tell us?

All this raises interesting and unsolved questions in the 'psycho-physics' of SDT (sensory decision, or signal detection, theory). Critics of Clark & Yang[f] find much

[a] Beebe, Anderson & Perkins (1).

[b] See further J. Y. P. Chhen (1); Benzer *et al.* (1), Shifman (1), who also found a 60% satisfactory response in a series of 328 patients; Sato & Nakatani (1); Katz, Kao, Spiegel & Katz (1); Spoerel, Varkey & Liang (1). In a series of some 600 cases of chronic pain treated with acupuncture at Birmingham, Alabama, 62·4% obtained satisfactory relief; Gregory Chhen & Huang Yu-Chêng (1).

[c] See also the comments of Dr Mary Moore, in Jenerick (1), pp. 130–1.

[d] Clark & Yang (1).

[e] As is well known, frontal lobe damage causes a loss of the 'affective' component of pain. Is this not a form of analgesia?

[f] Such as Chapman (1); Chapman, Wilson & Gehrig (1, 2); Chapman, Gehrig & Wilson (2); Hayes, Bennett & Mayer (1); McBurney (1).

greater decreases in pain sensitivity than they did, but agree that acupuncture causes a positive increase in 'response bias', i.e. an increase in reluctance to report noxious stimuli as painful. This does not necessarily mean a volitional stoicism or cortical refusal to admit the perception of pain. Most people under certain conditions have experienced quite strong sensations not strictly pain, such as the tearing or wrenching effect when a tooth is being extracted under novocaine. Visceral traction in operations under acupuncture is apparently quite unpleasant, but not always, strictly speaking, pain. Why should one not count these 'peculiar feelings' of bearable quasi-pain as characteristic of this type of conscious behavioural analgesia?

In any case, direct afferent inhibition from the acupuncture needles has been demonstrated. At the National Institute of Physiology at Shanghai in 1973 the Norwegian group learnt that it had been shown by electro-physiological methods that pain impulses in single fibres in the dorso-lateral tracts could be inhibited by acupuncture. This worked from either limb but was particularly effective when the needling was done on the same limb as the painful stimulus. Now as these cats had high spinal transections it was evident that there could be no question of efferent inhibitory influences from the cortex or other brain or brain-stem centres.[a] This work was later published by Wu Chien-Phing *et al.* (1). The fibres were those of the spino-cervical tract in segments below L_4, electric shocks were used, and the inhibition, demonstrable oscillographically, was best if the same nerve-trunk was used both for the nociceptive and the acupuncture impulses. Wu Chien-Phing, like Melzack & Wall, regarded the probable gate as somewhere in the dorsal horn of the cord, and the most important thing was that descending efferent signals could be completely ruled out.

These results were in agreement with earlier experiments made by Wagman & Price (1) on decerebrate monkeys.[b] They found that spontaneous or evoked activity in spinal cord cells registering inputs from areas, even quite large areas, on a leg, can be inhibited by intense stimulation of the opposite leg. Moreover the latency in this effect was so extremely short that it could not have been mediated through more than a couple of segments; and once again the inhibition was afferent only, since it could not be due to any efferent impulses originating in the brain or brain-stem. A similar inhibition could be obtained by intense stimulation of the hands, and though here the inhibitory signals must have been descending, their speed was great, and they were certainly not emanating from any cerebral centres. Although the latency was so short, the inhibition would persist more than a second after the stimulation was ended, suggesting that the spinal gates would close rather faster than they would open.

Much other work supports the conception of an 'afferent barrage'. For example, Linzer & van Atta (1) found that stimulation of peripheral nociceptors by acupuncture in the cat affects only those thalamic neurons which respond differentially to pain stimuli.

This raises again the question of the location of the gates. So far we have been

[a] Kaada *et al.* (1), p. 425.
[b] Cf. Melzack (1), pp. 184–5.

thinking mostly of levels in the spinal cord, but Chang Hsiang-Thung (1), in a notable paper, brought forward electro-physiological evidence that they should rather be thought of in the lower parts of the fore-brain, especially the thalamus.[a] Here he identified in particular the nucleus parafascicularis[b] and the nucleus centralis lateralis. Cells in both of these fire in response to nocuous stimuli, rhythmically if a wound has been made; and their discharges are abolished by morphine. But they are abolished also by electro-acupuncture, and by pinching the Achilles tendon (cf. pp. 212, 230 above). Since any interference with the thalamus or the reticular formation produces hyperalgesia or analgesia, Chang believes that under ordinary conditions the thalamic pain centres are under continuous inhibitory control by incoming sensory impulses —a kind of normal beneficial jamming—and that if and when this fails, hyperalgesia may ensue, leading to spontaneous intractable central pain.[c] Experimentally pain signals persist after section of the dorsal cord columns, and they cannot be reproduced by stimulating cells in these columns above the cut.[d] Chang also believes that the excitation of a nerve entering a given spinal segment can inhibit pain from any part of the body, but if it belongs to the same or an adjacent spinal segment the inhibitory effect will be much greater. This agrees with a great volume of clinical experience in acupuncture analgesia.[e]

Location of the main gating mechanism in the brain stem is also supported by the remarkable work of Shen Ê, Tshai Thi-Tao & Lan Chhing (1). Viscero-somatic reflex discharges evoked by single-pulse stimuli of the splanchnic nerve in cats were recorded in the lower intercostal nerves. Electro-acupuncture at hind-limb points inhibited these signals. Now the acupuncture effect was diminished or abolished by complete spinal transection at cervical or upper thoracic levels, so inhibitory messages from somewhere were being cut off. But the same happened after bilateral lesions near the dorsal horns at upper thoracic levels, and also after bilateral section of the ventro-lateral funiculi similarly high up the cord.[f] On the other hand the cerebral cortex was not the source of the inhibition since decerebration at intercollicular level led to no reversal of the acupuncture effect. Consequently the mechanism must be located somewhere in the brain stem (the midbrain, pons or medulla oblongata).

This work has been followed up by Tu Huan-Chi & Chao Yen-Fang (1) using similar electro-physiological techniques. The inhibition of the viscero-somatic reflex

[a] Other papers bearing him out are Anon. (*135*) for the reticular formation in the mid-brain, and Anon. (*136*) for the thalamus (within the diencephalic part of the fore-brain). All used electro-physiological recording.

[b] Barr (1), pp. 171–2.

[c] Cf. Melzack (1), p. 166. Chang showed that certain thalamic neurons fire in a characteristic way, having a long latency, high discharge rate, prolonged after-discharge, lack of adaptability, and specific fatigue properties. Their activity can thus be recognised.

[d] McLeod *et al.* (1), pp. 121 ff., not easily impressed, were highly appreciative of the work of Chang Hsiang-Thung and Wu Chien-Phing.

[e] Summarised by Woodley (1).

[f] Chiang Chen-Yü, Liu Jen-I *et al.* (1) have also found that lesions in the ventral two-thirds of the lateral funiculus on the contra-lateral side completely abolish the analgesic effect of hindlimb acupuncture on radiant heat sensitivity of the rabbit nose in dolorimeter experiments. Thus the channels of conduction of the afferent inhibitory impulses in the spinal cord are becoming more and more clear. Cf. p. 233 above.

discharges was preserved intact after decerebration in cats, though the long-continuing after-inhibition was lost. On the other hand, transection at the level of the lower medulla or the cervical cord completely abolished the inhibitory effect of acupuncture; while median lesions in the medulla, including the nucleus raphe magnus, greatly decreased it. The long after-inhibition was naturally lost in both these conditions. However, ablation of the cerebellum did not affect either the inhibitory effect during acupuncture or the after-inhibition. Accordingly it would seem that the region of the raphe magnus in the medulla must be an essential link in the chain of causation of acupuncture analgesia, especially as regards the role of the supra-spinal structures in the efferent inhibition of viscero-somatic reflex activities such as are induced by painful traction of the visceral organs.

Again, it has been possible to show that the firing of pain-sensitive neurons in the spinal trigeminal nucleus in the medulla, caused by electrical stimuli to the inferior alveolar nerve or the dental pulp of cats, can be completely inhibited by electro-acupuncture at Chia-chhê (V 3), Ho-ku (IG 4), Tsu-san-li (V36) and Erh-shen-mên (on the auricula).[a] The higher the voltage used in the needling the longer the inhibition lasted (in milli-seconds). Since picrotoxin shortened this period while strychnine left it unchanged and sodium amytal prolonged it, the effect was considered to be mainly pre-synaptic.

On the other hand there are experiments on spinal reflexes which point to the substantia gelatinosa rather than the thalamus.[b] Hoffmann's reflex is known to be carried by large fast (Aα) fibres. Normally irregular, under spinal anaesthesia it is abolished entirely, but with acupuncture analgesia it is activated rather than suppressed; it becomes exaggerated and more frequent. So here it looks as if the large fibre signals are being reinforced by the acupuncture. Other experiments support this (Anon. *147*). The tibial nerve in man may be stimulated by a pulsating current passing between two acupuncture needles inserted in the popliteal fossa, and the current intensity may be chosen just strong enough to evoke the H-reflex in the calf muscles without the presence of the M-wave as shown oscillographically, thus demonstrating that only the large proprioceptive fibres are being excited. Then the pain threshold at six points on the legs, abdomen and thorax was tested by the potassium iontophoresis method. The tibial stimulation brought about rises of up to 150% of the normal control level, taking some twenty-five minutes to come on and rather less than twenty minutes to wear off. If the H-reflex was suppressed by applying an inflated cuff to the thigh, with consequent ischaemia, the analgesia disappeared too. 'Since the generalised analgesic effect', said the authors, writing from Hsü-yi Hospital in Chiangsu, 'produced by direct stimulation of the large afferent fibres closely resembles that obtained by acupuncture at various traditional acu-points, it seems reasonable to assume that the afferent impulses elicited by acupuncture are mainly transmitted by the large fast fibres of the peripheral nerves.'[c] Of course it has

[a] Anon. (152).
[b] Anon. (*137*).
[c] Again, it has been shown by Chan & Fêng (1) that stimulation at the locus Tsu-san-li (V 36) brings about specific inhibition of the cutaneous polysynaptic reflexes evoked by excitation of the suralis nerve.

long been evident, too, that acupuncture analgesia is effective on the head and the face for areas which are not supplied by any segmental spinal nerve.[a] One can only conclude, with the Norwegians, that the inhibitory effect of acupuncture on pain impulses can be recorded at several different levels of the neuraxis, spinal, mid-brain and thalamus.[b] And this is also, broadly speaking, the position of the Chinese neurophysiologists and anaesthesiologists themselves.[c]

Here may be the place to mention the suggestion of Melzack[d] that acupuncture at the periphery of the body need not necessarily be working upon the gates in an afferent direction from below. There could be a non-psychological, non-cortical efference if the deep receptors stimulated by the needles should have a direct line to the central biassing mechanism in the mid-brain. This would be a variety of hyper-stimulation analgesia, an experimental activation of central inhibition, but operating at a level lower than the cognitive and the cortical. The cells of the reticular formation are known to have large receptive fields, neuronically connected with many parts of the body,[e] and as already mentioned, electrical stimulation of the tegmental tract can make a whole half or quarter of the body analgesic (p. 242 above). This idea arose because the locations of acupuncture needles prescribed are sometimes rather puzzling from the dermatome point of view; but of course if there were direct access from the needle inputs to the mid-brain then this gate inhibition could be efferent too.[f] Might it not be that in some cases, where the effect can be readily understood in terms of the segmental distribution of nerves, that the action is wholly afferent, while in other cases some partially efferent mechanism of this kind comes into play?

(viii) *Neuro-chemical factors*

For some time it had been suspected, as we have seen (p. 242), that there might be a humoral[g] as well as a neural effect in acupuncture analgesia. Data which indeed seem to show this have been reported by Kung Chhi-Hua *et al.* (*1*), who carried out cross-circulation experiments on guinea-pigs using dolorimeter measurements and acupuncture at the point corresponding to Yin-mên (VU 51). One animal was needled, the other not. When the curves for the rise and fall of pain threshold over 90 minutes were compared it was found that the analgesia of the animal connected but not acupuncturised lay about half-way between the acupuncture one and the control. The conclusion could only be that some neuro-humour with analgesic properties was passing round in the blood-stream.[h]

[a] This was the point made by Man & Chen (1).

[b] Kaada *et al.* (1), p. 427. Bull (1) has even suggested a gate in the cortex itself. Continuous stimulation of certain receptors would 'lock on' to neurons there, as if the lines were 'busy', so that pain impulses could not be received.

[c] Anon. (*114*), Engl. tr., pp. 300ff. See also the interesting review of the possible physiological pathways by Wagman, Dong & McMillan (1). On the possible role of reflex actions see McDonald (1).

[d] (1), pp. 188–9.

[e] Rossi & Zanchetti (1).

[f] The views of Wall (2) would be compatible with this.

[g] *Thi i hsi thung*,[1] in Jen Khang-Thung's words.

[h] These results have been confirmed by Takeshige *et al.* (1); cf. Kaada (2), p. 738.

[1] 体液系統

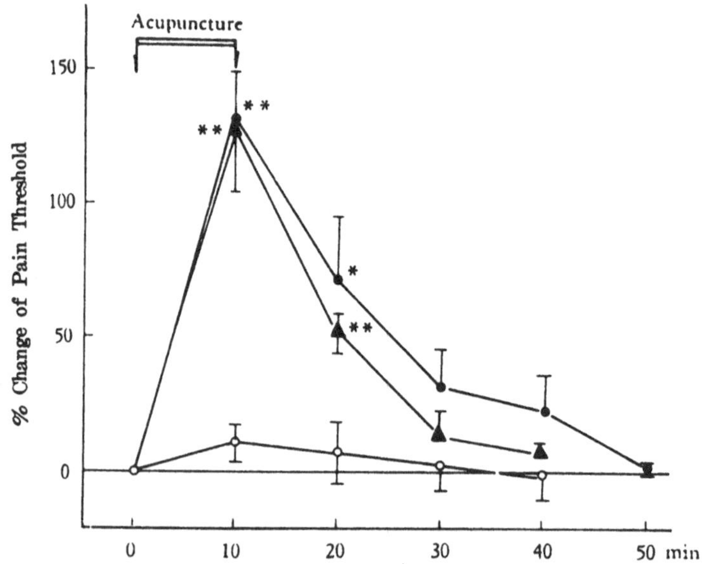

Fig. 60. Demonstrations of humoral transmission; the control experiment. Effect on pain threshold of acupuncture at Tsu-san-li (V 36) and of strong pressure at Khun-lun (VU 60) in rabbits; the former indicated by solid triangles, the latter by solid circles, controls by empty circles. Vertical bars represent ± standard error, single asterisks $P < 0{\cdot}05$ in statistical t test, double asterisks $P < 0{\cdot}01$ in the same. Anon. (118).

If this were so, it would be likely to be present in the cerebro-spinal fluid also, and this appears indeed to be the case according to other experiments.[a] The lateral brain ventricle of a rabbit under acupuncture analgesia was perfused with artificial CSF, and the perfusate injected into the brain of a receptor rabbit. In these circumstances the receptor animal showed dolorimetrically 82% of the effect observed in the donor (Figs. 60, 61). Therefore some analgesic substance was being produced in the brain and secreted into the CSF. The analgesic effect of acupuncture could be enhanced and prolonged by intravenous injection of reserpine (which blocks morphine analgesia, Fig. 62), but reduced to the original level by the intra-ventricular replacement of nor-adrenaline, dopamine (dihydroxy-phenyl-ethylamine) or serotonin (5-hydroxytryptamine, Fig. 63). So reserpine depletes the mono-amines of the brain. Conversely, after intra-ventricular atropine (which blocks the action of acetyl-choline in the brain) the analgesic effect of acupuncture was much weakened, though morphine analgesia competence was preserved. The general conclusion, apart from the clear demonstration of the neuro-humoral effect, was that acupuncture analgesia involves mechanisms slightly different from those of morphine analgesia. The former depends upon acetylcholine as a central neuro-transmitter, and it is rendered more effective by the depletion of the cerebral mono-amines;[b] the latter continues unchanged when the

[a] Anon. (118).

[b] This is of course the basis of the effectiveness of reserpine as a tranquillising agent. Conversely, the anti-depressants are inhibitors of the mono-amine oxidases, and so maintain or raise the concentration of the mono-amines in the brain (Burn (1), p. 69).

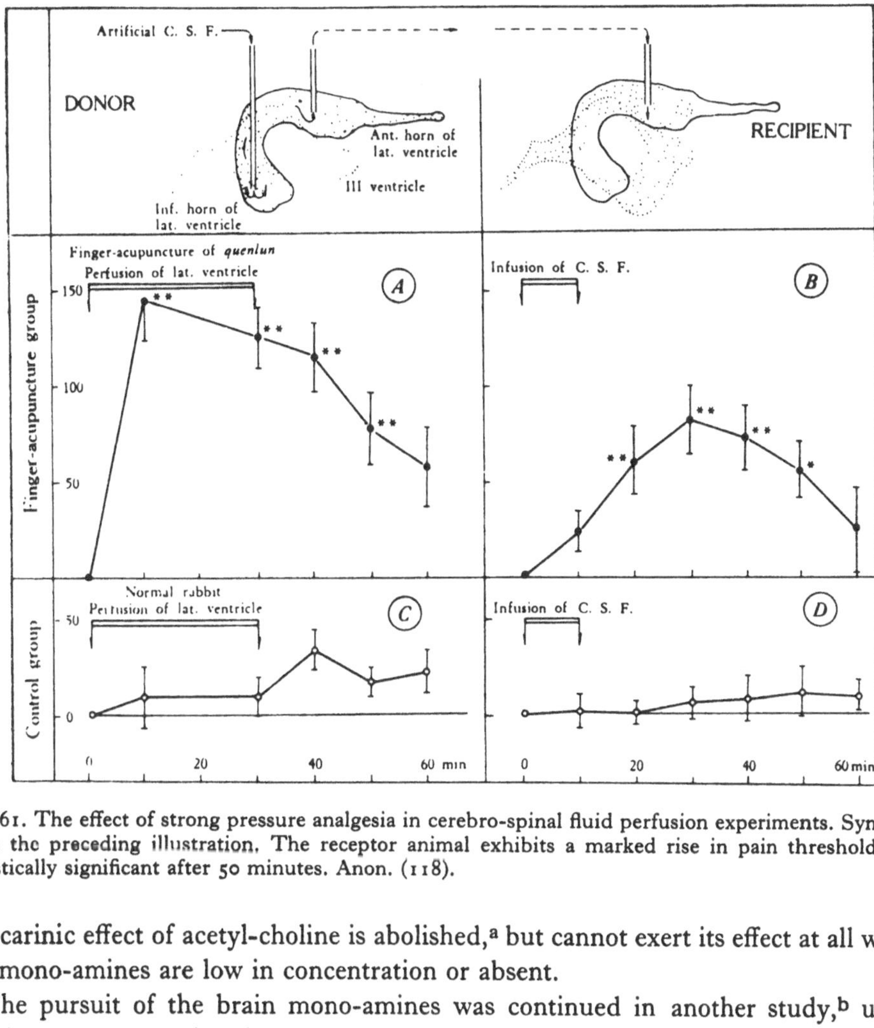

Fig. 61. The effect of strong pressure analgesia in cerebro-spinal fluid perfusion experiments. Symbols as in the preceding illustration. The receptor animal exhibits a marked rise in pain threshold still statistically significant after 50 minutes. Anon. (118).

muscarinic effect of acetyl-choline is abolished,[a] but cannot exert its effect at all when the mono-amines are low in concentration or absent.

The pursuit of the brain mono-amines was continued in another study,[b] using rabbits acupunctured at Fêng-lung (V 40) and Yang-fu (VF 38) on the hind legs. As a result of this the serotonin content of the medulla and thalamus rose, while glutamic acid in the thalamus fell; there was no change in either the nor-adrenaline or the γ-amino-butyric acid. Such effects could be interpreted as due to increased brain metabolism during a period of marked rise in pain threshold.[c] A further step was taken by Yi, Lu, Wu & Tsou (1), who measured the release of tritium-labelled serotonin into the CSF under various conditions. Pain thresholds in rabbits were raised by acupuncture at Tsu-san-li (V 36), and also (a good deal more) by morphine, but the former procedure resulted in a marked liberation of the labelled serotonin

[a] Muscarine is the classical parasympathetico-mimetic drug; cf. Burn (1), p. 4.
[b] Anon. (*144*).
[c] In other work, based on experimental laparotomy in rabbits, it has been claimed that nor-adrenaline and acetyl-choline, injected before acupuncture, enhance the analgesia produced (Anon. 149).

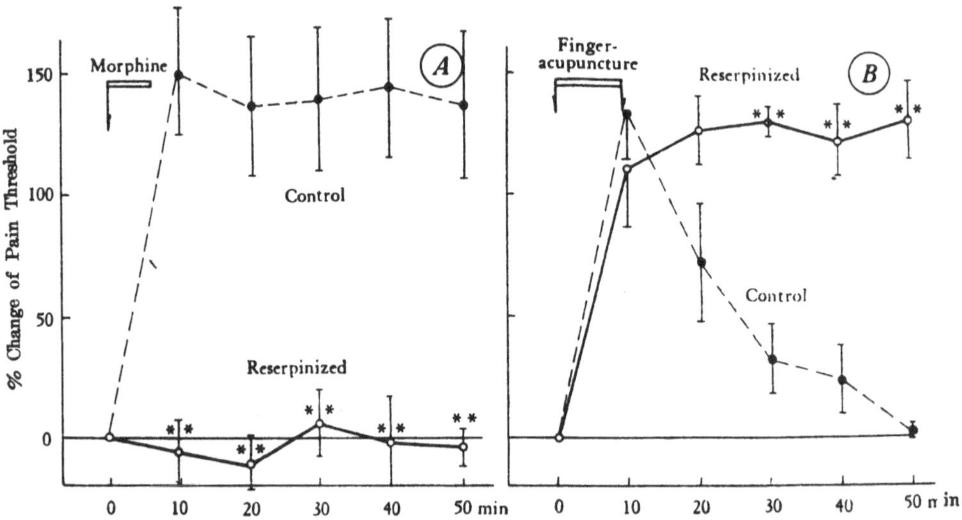

Fig. 62. The effects of reserpine on morphine and strong pressure analgesia in rabbits. The analgesic action of the acupuncture-surrogate is enhanced and prolonged by reserpine, but morphine analgesia completely blocked. Anon. (118).

to the perfusate, while the latter had no such effect. They concluded that acupuncture activates serotonergic neurons in the brain while morphine does not. Other researches had shown that inhibitors of serotonin synthesis attenuate the analgesic effect of electrical stimulation of the median raphe nuclei and neighbouring structures. But the exact relation between analgesia and serotonin activity, and the exact difference between acupuncture and morphine analgesia, still elude us.

All in all, the Norwegians may well have been right in their conclusion that while spinal inhibition may account for the segmental effect in acupuncture analgesia, the prolonged and general effect may perhaps best be explained by humoral factors. The total analgesic phenomenon may therefore be a synthesis of the actions of neural and humoral mechanisms.[a]

That the mono-amines in the brain (such as serotonin, nor-adrenaline and dopamine) are all involved in morphine analgesia is extremely likely,[b] but they seem not to be the immediate chemical substrate on which the alkaloid works.[c] Before the composition of this monograph began, and during the writing of it, a great deal of research was going on which demonstrated the existence of an 'opiate receptor' substance, possibly a membrane protein or polypeptide, in the corpus striatum and other parts of the brain.[d] Whether or not the neuro-anatomical sites of morphine action (especially

[a] Kaada *et al.* (1), p. 425.

[b] For example, the analgesic effect of morphine (and the enkephalins of which we shall be speaking in a moment) may be mediated by a descending serotonergic pathway originating in the raphe nuclei and inhibiting nociceptive transmission in the spinal cord; Deakin, Dickenson & Dostrovsky (1).

[c] Cf. Pert & Yaksh (1).

[d] Cf. Pert & Snyder (1); Kuhar, Pert & Snyder (1); Lowney, Shultz, Lovery & Goldstein (1).

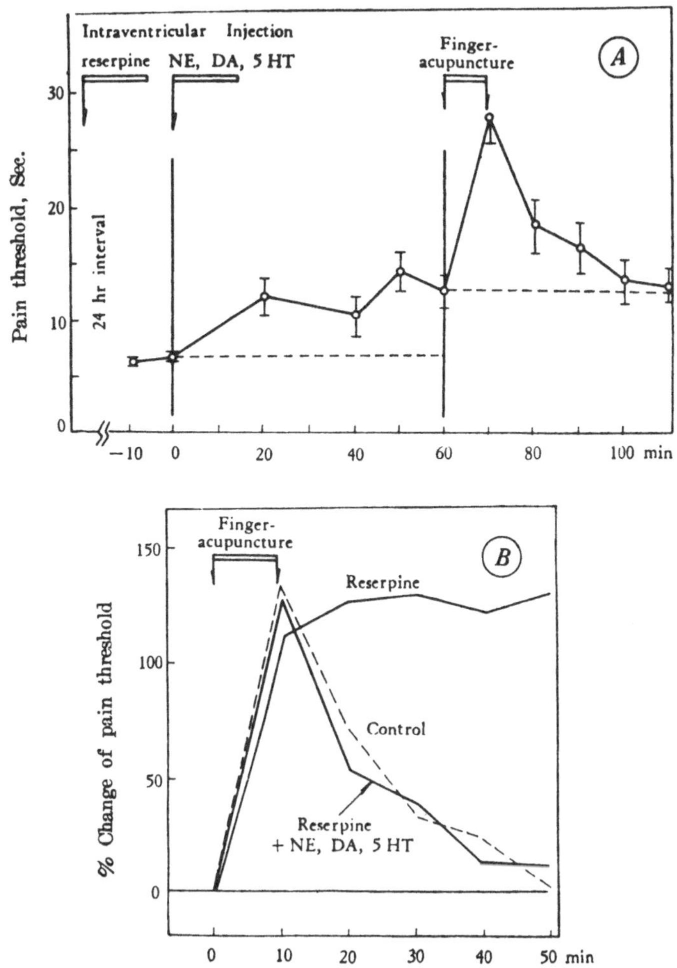

Fig. 63. The effect on acupuncture-surrogate analgesia of replacement of three cerebral mono-amines, nor-adrenalin (NE), dopamine (DA) and serotonin (5 HT), after reserpinisation the previous day. The mono-amines reversed the action of the reserpine, for the pressure analgesia showed no enhancement or prolongation. The reserpine effect is therefore probably due to a depletion of the brain's mono-amine content. Anon. (118).

in the peri-aqueductal grey matter)[a] can respond also directly to the afferent impulses of acupuncture analgesia is a difficult problem. More likely is an alternative hypothesis which will be mentioned below.

It was then ingeniously argued that Nature could hardly have provided this opiate receptor in the foreknowledge that mankind would discover the properties of the opium poppy. Search for a physiologically-produced and normally-occurring 'morphine-like factor' thus began. The phrase was that of Terenius (1), and he was in

[a] Pert & Yaksh (1, 2); Jacquet & Lajtha (1, 2).

fact one of the first to demonstrate its veritable existence. Later, a great breakthrough was made in 1975 with the isolation, identification and synthesis of two endogenous morphine analogues, the enkephalins, by Hughes, Smith, Kosterlitz *et al.* (1).[a] Both are labile polypeptides, but one, the more powerful, contains methionine, the other leucine. M-enkephalin is in some circumstances no less than twenty times as active as morphine, and three times as effective in dislodging the antagonist naloxone. The enkephalins are almost certainly neuro-transmitters, and their receptors are found in brain areas known to be involved in the physiology of pain, such as the reticular formation; they reduce the firing of neurons, whether spontaneous or evoked.[b] The fact that they escaped detection for so long is probably due to the great rapidity of their enzymic destruction under normal conditions. There is a cross-tolerance with morphine, i.e. increasing doses are needed to produce the same effect, and the natural and the introduced molecules can substitute for each other, so they must have the same receptors.[c]

More extraordinary still was the subsequent discovery that the sequence of amino-acids constituting the enkephalins was also present in the string of 91 amino-acids that forms the pituitary hormone β-lipotropin.[d] Fragments of this hormone can therefore act as enkephalins, but they do so even more strongly, for whereas the strongest enkephalin is, as we have seen, twenty times as effective as morphine, the strongest of the endorphins (as they are called) is fifty times as powerful in suppressing pain. This β-endorphin retains its activity to some extent when injected into the blood-stream, but it must normally work within the cerebrospinal fluid and the brain tissue.[e] A rich review of the opiate receptor problem and the opioid peptides is due to Snyder & Simantov (1).

The enkephalins and endorphins were then firmly incorporated into the story of acupuncture analgesia by the demonstration that naloxone inhibits this completely, just as it does morphine analgesia and the analgesia produced by m-enkephalin.[f] At the same time it has been shown that this antagonist does not inhibit hypno-anaesthesia at all[g]—a vindication of the conviction of so many observers that hypnosis and acupuncture work in quite different ways. So also removal of the pituitary (probable source of the endorphins) abolishes acupuncture analgesia.[h] Similarly, in

[a] Cf. Lewin (2); Büscher, Hill, Römer, Cardinaux *et al.* (1); Belluzzi, Grant, Garsky *et al.* (1).

[b] Cf. Bradley, Briggs, Gayton & Lambert (1); Gent & Wolstencroft (1).

[c] Waterfield, Hughes & Kosterlitz (1). These may be of more than one distinguishable type, as Terenius & Wahlström (2) found.

[d] Graf, Szekely, Ronai *et al.* (1); Lo, Tsêng, Wei & Li Cho-Hao (1); Terenius & Wahlström (1). Its function is not yet clearly understood, and it may be primarily a precursor of biologically active fragments.

[e] Tsêng Liang-Fu, Lo & Li Cho-Hao (1).

[f] Akil, Mayer & Liebeskind (1); Mayer (1); Mayer, Price & Raffii (1); Belluzzi, Grant, Garsky *et al.* (1); Pomeranz (1); McCarthy, Walker & Woodruff (1); Chapman & Benedetti (1). The depressive effect of enkephalin on single neurons and its abolition by naloxone is described by Frederickson & Norris (1). Pomeranz & Chiu (1) could demonstrate the complete inhibition of electro-acupuncture analgesia in mice by naloxone. In man the effect is much stronger when low frequencies (1 to 4 cycles/sec.) are used, than when the frequency is high (80 to 100 cycles/sec.), according to Dr H. Ågren (priv. comm., Oct. 1977).

[g] Goldstein & Hilgard (1).

[h] Pomeranz (1).

chronic facial pain and trigeminal neuralgia the endorphin content of the cerebro-spinal fluid is reduced,[a] but these conditions respond quite well to acupuncture and electro-acupuncture.[b] Once again, this analgesia is abolished by naloxone.[c] The role of the endogenous opiates in pain modulation is well brought out in the work of Madden *et al.* (1), who found that acute and inescapable stress in experimental animals caused a significant increase in the enkephalin–endorphin levels in the cerebro-spinal fluid with concurrent decrease in pain responsiveness. Repeated exposures reversed this and the opioid peptides followed suit. There are many grounds therefore for thinking that the enkephalins and endorphins go far to explaining the cross-circulation experiments described on p. 255 above.[d]

Early in 1979 the placebo effect itself was found to be explainable in terms of endogenous morphine analogues. Levine, Gordon & Fields (1) found that in post-operative dental pain the placebo response could be completely abolished by naloxone, showing that responders have the capacity to mobilise their own endorphins. This was a remarkable finding, since the placebo effect had been mysterious for so long. It also explained many old observations, such that with repeated use placebo becomes less effective, requiring an 'increase of dose' as time goes by (tolerance), or that sudden withdrawal may give an abstinence syndrome, or that placebo can partially reverse withdrawal symptoms in narcotic addicts, and so on. But of course it remains true that the placebo level in any population is an indispensable base-line in estimating the analgesic effects of such treatments as acupuncture.

All in all, the participation of a humoral component in the phenomena of acupuncture analgesia is now assured beyond doubt. The first suggestion that acupuncture analgesia might involve the naturally-occurring morphine-analogues seems to have been due to Pappenheimer, whose work on the sleep-inducing Factor-S in cerebro-spinal fluid has become so well known.[e] But many have recognised that the rather long latent period which occurs in acupuncture analgesia (up to half an hour), and the lengthy period of analgesia following the cessation of the peripheral stimulus (up to an hour), could be explained much more easily if chemical humoral factors were intervening rather than nervous conduction alone.[f] The enkephalin–endorphin system is not at all incompatible with the gating theories which we have described above (pp. 233, 252-3), for it could well be the opiate receptors which transmit efferent gate-closing impulses, not necessarily to spinal cord levels but perhaps to the mid-

[a] Terenius & Wahlström (1).

[b] Zaretsky, Lee & Rubin (1). Cf. Eriksson & Sjölund (1); Spoerel, Varkey & Liang (1). And evidence has now been brought forward by Sjölund, Terenius & Eriksson (1) that electro-acupuncture can raise the endorphin-content of the cerebro-spinal fluid, even as much as six times, in patients whom it relieves from chronic pain.

[c] Sjölund & Eriksson (1).

[d] As has been pointed out by Blakemore (1), p. 636.

[e] Pappenheimer, Koski, Fencl *et al.* (1). Cf. Blakemore (1), p. 638.

[f] This has been emphasised particularly well by Pomeranz (1); cf. Anon. (149). See also Eriksson & Sjölund (1). In 1974 the eminent Swedish neuro-physiologist, my old friend Yngve Zotterman, fractured the radius bone of his arm and had to have it in plaster for two months. Much pain was felt at times in the hand, but it could be abolished by vibratory stimulation through the plaster; moreover, the relief would persist for half an hour or more after the ending of the stimulus. This was puzzling for the neuro-physiologists at the time, but the discovery of the endorphins has made it quite comprehensible (private communication from Prof. Zotterman, Jan. 1977).

brain or medulla. The 'afferent barrage' would thus act primarily on the endorphin-producing cells, and these polypeptides would then send efferent signals to block the pain pathways that normally connect the pain nerve-endings with the cortex.[a]

Furthermore, neuro-transmitter peptides with powerful actions are not confined to the higher levels of the brain-stem. Forty-six years ago von Euler & Gaddum (1) discovered a hypotensive and oxytocic principle in brain and spinal cord, naming it Substance-P, and later it was found to be concentrated in the dorsal roots of cord segments much more than in the ventral roots. This led Lembeck (1) to suggest, a couple of decades later, that substance-P might be a neuro-transmitter of sensory and pain-conducting dorsal root fibres; but further progress hung fire until the isolation and identification of substance-P as an undeca-peptide by M. M. Chang and his collaborators in 1971.[b] There is indeed about a thousand times more of it in the dorso-lateral part of the dorsal horns than there is in the ventral or motor horns, and the experiments of Otsuka & Konishi (1, 2) now clearly indicate that it should be regarded as the excitatory transmitter of primary afferent sensory neurons (cf. Fig. 52).[c] The antagonist lioresal, for example, which blocks dorsal root transmission, also completely inhibits the effects of substance-P. Thus yet another peptide is involved in the transmission of pain impulses, and hence in the general system where acupuncture intervenes. The control of its release could constitute a further inhibitory or gating phenomenon.

(6) Influences on Other Cultures

(i) *Asian receptions*

Though originating in China, acupuncture and moxa cautery spread out in the course of time over the whole world; but it was natural that the peoples of the Chinese culture-area should have received these medical arts a long time before they were known in South or West Asia or Europe. Perhaps the first local culture in which they became implanted was that of Korea; indeed a Korean legend attributed the invention of the moxa and the stone needles (cf. p. 70 above) to Than chün,[1] the legendary first ruler of Korea.[d] But Chinese colonial prefectures like Lo-lang[2] existed in Korea in Han times,[e] so that in view of what we know about the state of Chinese medicine during those centuries (pp. 88, 106 above) it is more than probable that acupuncture was practised there, and it must have been so at least by the San Kuo period.[f] Among

[a] Cf. Deakin, Dickenson & Dostrovsky (1).

[b] Chang & Leeman (1); Chang, Leeman & Niall (1).

[c] Fluorescence-microscopy with antibodies to substance-P detects it in many places, but especially in the spinal ganglia and the substantia gelatinosa of the dorsal roots where the primary sensory neurons are; Hökfelt *et al.* (1). The mechanism of its release from synapses in the hypothalamus has been studied by Jessell, Iversen & Kanazawa (1). A large volume of research on this polypeptide transmitter is continuing.

[d] Miki Sakae (*1*), p. 384.

[e] *SCC*, Vol. 4, pt. 1, pp. 263–4, Vol. 4, pt. 2, p. 71, Vol. 4, pt. 3, pp. 25, 562. Cf. Vol. 3, pp. 682–3.

[f] The museum at Loyang in Honan possesses a fine stele dated +278 which describes the Imperial University of the Chin dynasty, and gives the names of a great many students, some of whom came 'from east of the sea' (presumably Korea and Liaoning), and others 'from west of the shifting sands'.

[1] 檀君 [2] 樂浪

our earliest firm dates is +514, in which year the Liang emperor Wu Ti[1] sent a number of physicians to Paekche to improve medical education, along with a doctor of literature, expert in interpreting the *Book of Odes*, to enlighten culture.[a] The physicians almost certainly took with them the *Chen Chiu Chia I Ching* of Huangfu Mi (cf. p. 119 above) which had been finished about +270, for this was used as a teaching text in Korea before the +7th century. Korea, unified under the dynasty of Silla forty years or so after the advent of the Thang, was now in possession of all the medical classics such as the *Shen Nung Pên Tshao Ching* (first of the pharmaceutical natural histories), the *Shang Han Lun* on fevers, and that great work of pathological aetiology produced in the Sui, the *Chu Ping Yuan Hou Lun* (+610). The Koreans also followed the Thang system in the ordering of their medical administration, with a Royal College of Medicine (I Hsüeh Yuan[2]) at the capital, having professors (I Po Shih[3]) in a number of specialities, as well as something approaching a State Medical Service.[b] This college seems to have been established at the beginning of the reign of Hyoso Wang[4] in +692, and one of the teachers was Professor of Acupuncture (Chen Po Shih[5]) using a *Chen Ching*[6] of some kind, and on anatomy and acu-tracts a *Ming Thang Ching*[7].[c] Throughout these centuries, too, there was a great export of Korean drugs to China.[d] Correspondingly, the Sung emperors twice presented texts of the *Thai-Phing Shêng Hui Fang* to Koryŏ (successor of Silla), in +988 and +1021.[e] In +1078, when a prince of Munjong's[8] court was ill, the Han-Lin Medical Academician Hsing Tshao[9] was sent from China by the Sung emperor to look after him, taking a hundred items of materia medica—and doubtless supplies of acupuncture needles. This kind of thing continued till the end of Northern Sung; for in +1103, again in response to an invitation, Sung Hui Tsung[10] despatched the medical official Mou Chieh[11] to teach at the Korean Medical College, and he was followed in +1118 by Yang Tsung-Li[12] and other Han-Lin Medical Academicians.[f] Records of the Koryŏ State medical examinations show that after +958 a *Chiu Ching*,[13] moxibustion manual, was studied as well as the *Chia I Ching* and *Chen Ching*.[g] One need hardly follow the medical relationships later than this time, for they never ceased, but it is interesting that after the +11th century, some version of a *Thung Jen Ching*[14] (Bronze Acupuncture Figure Manual) was in constant use in medical training.[h]

(Sinkiang). We have not come across any study of this monument, which we had the pleasure of seeing in 1958. The university in Chin times was located near the famous Pai-ma Ssu[15] temple about five miles east of the modern city, and consisted of more than 10,000 students and professors.

[a] Anon. (*131*), p. 168; Anon. (*83*), p. 48.
[b] See Lu Gwei-Djen & Needham (2).
[c] Miki Sakae (*1*), pp. 394–5; Li Yuan-Chi (*1*).
[d] Anon. (*83*), pp. 48 ff.
[e] Anon. (*83*), p. 78. The last two chapters of this are on acupuncture and moxa (cf. *SIC*, p. 926).
[f] *Ibid.*, pp. 78 ff.; Chhen Pang-Hsien (*1*), p. 419.
[g] It was about this date that Shen Hsiu[16] of Khaifêng was a favourite Royal Physician in Korea; cf. Wang Chi-Min (*2*).
[h] Miki Sakae, loc. cit. He gives a list of Chinese books on acupuncture and moxa in use in Korea in the Yi dynasty of Choson, after +1392, and also of the Korean books on these subjects then written. The greatest of all Korean medical treatises, the *Tongŭi Pogam*[17] of Hŏ Chun[18] (+1613), devotes its last chapters to acupuncture and moxibustion (pp. 754 ff.).

1 梁武帝 2 醫學院 3 醫博士 4 孝昭王 5 針博士 6 針經
7 明堂經 8 文宗 9 邢慥 10 宋徽宗 11 牟介 12 楊宗立
13 灸經 14 銅人經 15 白馬寺 16 愼修 17 東醫寶鑑 18 許浚

What song the sirens sang, or what medical arts Hsü Fu[1] (Jofuku) took with him from China to Japan in the time of Chhin Shih Huang Ti (−219),[a] might admit, as Sir Thomas Browne would have said, of a wide solution. But we are on firm ground when we come to the +6th century, for in +553, a little over a hundred years before Korea was unified under Silla, the kingdom of Paekche sent an I Po Shih[2] of noble rank, Wang Yurŭngt'a[3],[b] to re-organise medical education in Japan and propagate Chinese medicine there.[c] He was accompanied by two Masters of Drug Production, Pan Kyŏngnye[4][d] and Chŏng Yut'a,[5] but his teaching must clearly have included acupuncture and moxibustion, from all that we already know. This was the first link in a chain of medical missions from Korea and China which resulted finally in +702 in the establishment by the emperor Mommu of an Imperial Medical College at Nara with five faculties and regular monthly and annual examinations.[e] But before that time many other things had happened.

Indeed, ten years had not passed before another influx of Chinese medical influence occurred through the intermediation of a learned monk from Wu, Chih-Tshung[6] (Chisō). In +562 he travelled to Japan in the company of a general, Sadehiko, who had won a victory over some Koreans; and he took with him many books on pharmaceutical natural history (*yao tien*[7]), anatomy and acupuncture. The last is demonstrated by the presence of some version of[a] *Ming Thang Thu*[8] (cf. p. 100 above) among the 164 scrolls which were in the baggage of the monastic physician.[f] Most probably the *Chen Chiu Chia I Ching* was among them too.

Another famous scientific mission to Japan was that of the Korean monk Kwŏllŭk[9] (Kwanroku[4]) from Paekche, who in +602 introduced to the islanders the first of the learned calendrical systems, Genka-reki (i.e. the Yuan Chia Li of Ho Chhêng-Thien, worked out in +443). But Kwŏllŭk was also skilled in medicine, pharmacy and apotropaics, which he taught with much success, leaving behind eminent Japanese disciples such as Hinamitachi[10] (Yamashiro no Omi[10]).[g] Since the works of Huangfu Mi and Chhin Chhêng-Tsu were widely current at this time among acupuncture physicians (cf. pp. 119, 177), while those of Masters Tshao and Lei were celebrated for moxibustion (p. 176), it could hardly be believed that such specialities were unknown to Kwŏllŭk and his students. The activities of these Chinese and Korean

[a] Cf. *SCC*, Vol. 4, pt. 3, pp. 551 ff., Vol. 5, pt. 3, p. 17.

[b] Or Wangyu Rungtḥa. It is not at all clear how this name should be divided. His title was Naesu. Sŏng Wang[11] was reigning at the time (*Samguk Sagi*, ch. 26, pp. 6–7).

[c] Miki Sakae (*1*), p. 26; Lu Gwei-Djen & Needham (2); Kim Tujong (*1*), pp. 81, 89, 113, Engl. tr., p. 11; Tamura Sennosuke (*1*), p. 112.

[d] His given names are also read Yungphung.

[e] The beginnings of centralised official teaching in medicine go back to +493, when posts of Regius Professor and Regius Lecturer were established in the Imperial University at the capital of the Northern Wei (Lu Gwei-Djen & Needham, *ibid.*).

[f] Kim Dujong (*1*), p. 59; Chhen Pang-Hsien (*1*), pp. 415–16; Wang Chi-Min (*1*); Li Thao (*15*), p. 143; Anon. (*131*), p. 168; Li Yuan-Chi (*1*); Anon. (*83*), p. 49; Shirai Mitsutarō (1); Hara Shimetarō (*1*).

[g] Miki Sakae (*1*), p. 27; Shirai Mitsutarō (1).

[1] 徐福 [2] 醫博士 [3] 王有㥄陀 [4] 潘景豊 [5] 丁有陀
[6] 知聰 [7] 藥典 [8] 明堂圖 [9] 勸勒 [10] 日並立
[11] 聖王

monastic astronomers and physicians who offered the treasures of their learning to the Japanese during the +6th and +7th centuries are irresistibly reminiscent of the Jesuit missions from Europe to China a thousand years later. Both were scientific benefactions in the interests of a particular religion and a specific theology or philosophy—but the Chinese and Koreans were more successful in the latter part of their aim than were the Jesuits, for Buddhism took root in Japan as Christianity never did in China.

From the beginning of the +7th century, the Japanese themselves, greatly impressed and stimulated by the healing powers of mediaeval Chinese medicine, began to send out missions of students and physicians to learn in the great centres of the mainland. It makes one think of nothing so much as John Caius and William Harvey travelling to spend some years in Padua, but the storms in the China seas and the hardships of the journey were probably even more severe than conditions nine centuries later. Perhaps the first group was that headed by the pharmacist (*yakushi*[1]) Enichi,[2] and including a scholar of noble birth Yamato no Aya no fumi no Atahe;[3] they were sent out by the empress Suiko[4] in +608 and returned home in +623. Enichi may have gone to China again in his old age (+659) and some sources say that he was there three times.[a] At their first homecoming they brought many valuable books with them, especially the *Chu Ping Yuan Hou Lun* already mentioned.

Between +630 and +838 there were no less than thirteen official embassies from the Japanese court to the Chinese,[b] and it was customary for students in all kinds of disciplines, from engineering through philosophy to medicine, to accompany them, though often they stayed longer than the diplomatic staff. According to tradition, the student-priest Kiga Hotorike no Namba[5] learnt acupuncture in the Silla kingdom, and returning to the Japanese capital in +642 was promoted to a doctorate in the subject (Chen Po Shih[6]).[c] Another story is stranger; the *Nihon Shoki* tells how in +645 student-priests of Koguryŏ reported that their fellow-student the Japanese Kura-tsukuri no Tōkushi[7] had become a great master of acupuncture by sitting at the feet of a tiger of the woods, but had been poisoned there before he could return home.[d]

Fifty years later (as already mentioned) came the adoption in Japan of the Chinese State Medical Administration System, with an Imperial Medical College. Its course was seven years long, and acupuncture (with moxa) was one of the five faculties;[e] studies included not only the classic of classics, *Nei Ching*, *Su Wên*, but also a *Huang Ti Chen Ching* (cf. p. 88 above) as well as some *Ming Thang* (anatomical) text, and the *Chen Chiu Chia I Ching*.[f] Fifty years later again there appeared another great wave of influence of Chinese medicine, in the person of the High Monk Chien-Chen[8] (Kanshin, Ganjin[8]) and the library of books which he brought with him when he

[a] Chhen Pang-Hsien (*1*); Wang Chi-Min (*1*); Anon. (*83*), pp. 49 ff.
[b] Chou I-Liang (*2*).
[c] Miki Sakae (*1*), p. 384.
[d] Aston tr., vol. 2, p. 190.
[e] Chang Shih-Piao (*1*), ch. 4, p. 1.
[f] Anon. (*83*), p. 49; Wang Chi-Min (*1*), p. 13; Fujikawa (1), p. 4.

1 藥師 2 惠日 3 倭漢直福因 4 推古 5 紀河邊幾男磨
6 針博士 7 鞍作得志 8 鑑眞

came to Japan in +735.[a] This celebrated Buddhist cleric, whose lay family name was Shunyü[1],[b] born in +687 and trained at Yangchow, stayed in Japan the first time for thirteen years, participating in the Nara cultural Renaissance,[c] to which he brought much science and medicine as well as the lore of the Vinaya school.[d] He later returned there in +753 or the following year, and died in the neighbourhood of +762. At Chien-Chen's first coming he was accompanied by the Persian physician Li Mi-I[2],[e] but it seems generally agreed that the medical library came with him on his second visit, and that the last years of his life were particularly occupied with the teaching of medicine, in which acupuncture was certainly included; not only by himself but by many younger physicians who had accompanied him.[f] The 'Abbot who passed across the Seas' (Kuo Hai Ta-Shih[3]) was certainly an important influence in the dissemination of acupuncture and moxa.

It is hardly necessary to follow further developments since Chinese medicine was now firmly established in Japan (Fig. 64), all ready for the first observations of Westerners which we shall consider in a moment. A doctorate in acupuncture and moxa (*shinkyū hakushi*[4]) appears again in an edict of +1362.[g] From the +9th century onwards Chinese merchants habitually traded with Japan, either in their own ships or in those of Silla or Koryŏ, or in trading-vessels of Chinese type built at Nagasaki and other Japanese ports;[h] and large quantities of medicines and medical books were exported thither from China.[i] But they were not always very clearly understood, so the appearance of a Chinese physician, Chêng I-Yuan,[5] in the late +15th century at Nagasaki, where he settled, much improved Japanese medical learning and practice.[j] After +1640 others came, such as the Buddhist scholar-poet and physician Tai Man-Kung[6] (+1596 to +1672).[k] By the nineteenth century four principal schools of acupuncture had differentiated (e.g. the Daimyō-ryu,[7] the Yoshida-ryu,[8] etc.),[l] lasting down almost to our own time. And moxa had its schools too (e.g. the Gotō-ryu[9]).[m]

Naturally what happened to the north and east happened in the south also, and

[a] The chronology of Chien-Chen's life is still a little uncertain, and it is not agreed among specialists that he was in Japan twice. However we do have the names of the two student-priests who visited him in his temple at Yangchow and gave him the invitation—Yōei[10] and Fushō.[11]

[b] A strange coincidence that he was of the same clan as Shunyü I (cf. p. 106).

[c] During the Nara period there were four cultural and scientific missions accompanying Japanese embassies to China, in +717, +733, +752 and +777. It was members of the second and third of these who evoked Chien-Chen's visits to Japan. There were usually four ships in each expedition, and many were wrecked or blown in storms to Vietnam and other distant places.

[d] On the Vinaya masters (Ritsushi[12]) expert in the disciplines of Mahāyana monastic life, see Chou I-Liang (*2*). Chien-Chen's home was the Tōshodaiji[13] near Nara. There is a biography of him by Andō Kōsei (*1*). Cf. also *SCC*, Vol. 4, pt. 3, p. 130.

[e] *SCC*, Vol. 1, p. 188.

[f] See Anon. (*83*); Wang Chi-Min (*1*); Chhen Pang-Hsien (*1*).

[g] Chang Chün-I (*1*).

[h] See Ōba Osamu (*2*).

[i] A large number of titles are given in the study of Ōba Osamu (*1*).

[j] See Yeh Chü-Chhüan's editorial preface to the *Kharg-Phing Shang Han Lun.*

[k] There is much information about him in Chang Tzhu-Kung (*3*).

[l] See Homma Shōhaku (*1*); Nakayama Tadajiki (*1*), pp. 165ff.; Sung Ta-Jen (*3*), p. 11.

[m] Hara Shimetarō (*1*); Chang Shih-Piao (*1*), ch. 4.

1 淳于	2 李密醫	3 過海大師	4 針灸博士	5 鄭一元
6 戴曼公	7 大明流	8 吉田流	9 後滕流	10 榮叡
11 普照	12 律師	13 唐招提寺		

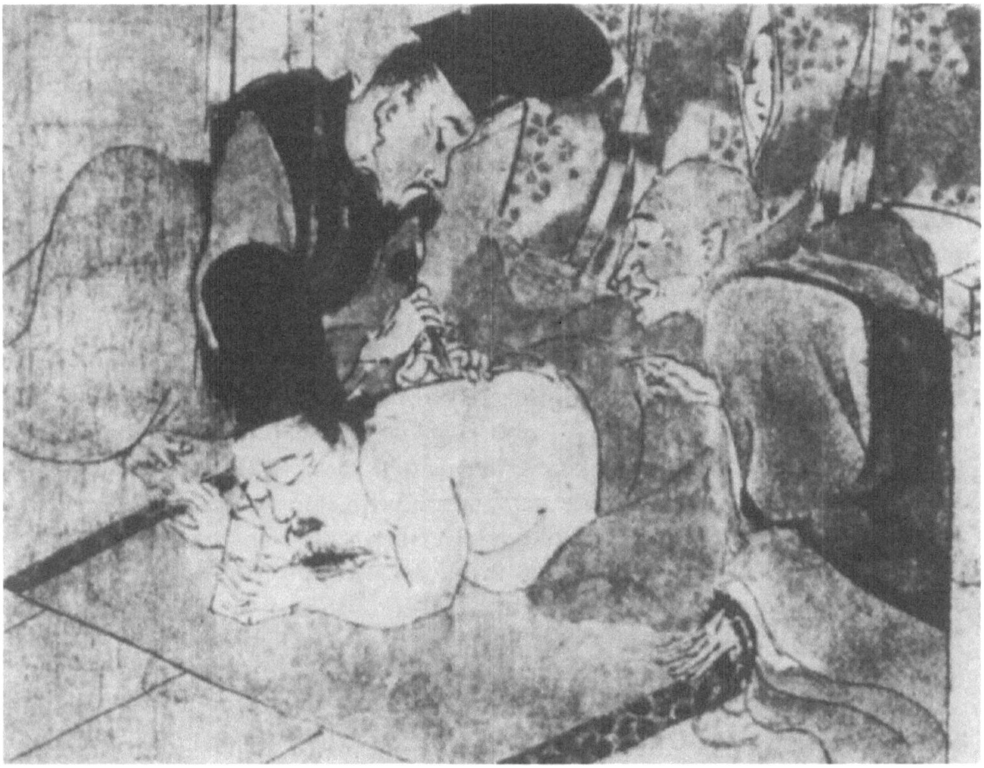

Fig. 64. Acupuncture in mediaeval Japan, a scene from the 'Scroll of Diseases' painted on paper by an unknown artist during the Kamakura period (+1193 to +1333). The physician is using the characteristic tube to locate the acu-point and insert the needle, while an old monk looks on with interest and a woman peeps through the curtains. Photo: Yamato Bunkakan, Nara.

places such as Yunnan and Annam received most of their medicine, including acupuncture, from the Chinese heartland. Vietnam was under such influence from the −2nd century onwards, and it lasted all through the Middle Ages.[a] The *Nan Chao Yeh Shih*[1] tells us that in +1103 Tuan Chêng-Shun,[2] the first king of the second Tali (Hou Li) dynasty of the Nan Chao kingdom in Yunnan, sent Kao Thai-Yün[3] to the Sung court to obtain canonical and other books; he got 69 of the former, with the significant addition of no less than 62 on medicine.[b] Or again, in +1340 a Chinese physician, Tsou Kêng,[4] successfully restored a Vietnamese crown prince from coma (cf. p. 80 above), and later became his Archiater Regius. He then cured him of impotence so that he was able to have three sons, and accomplished many other feats by the use of acupuncture.[c] But these are just pieces of evidence plucked at random for a case that needs no proving.

[a] We remember from *SCC*, Vol. 5, pt. 3, p. 75 the Chinese alchemical physician Tung Fêng,[5] who in +187 cured a Vietnamese king of some comatose condition. Cf. Chhen Tshun-Jen (*2*), p. 119.

[b] Ch. 21, tr. Sainson (1), p. 101.

[c] See Chhen Tshun-Jen (*5*). At this time, and henceforward, many medical students from Vietnam went to China for their training; cf. Wang Chi-Min (*1*).

[1] 南詔野史 [2] 段正淳 [3] 高泰運 [4] 鄒庚 [5] 董奉

All these regions bordered on the Indian culture-area, so it is natural to look for parallels in medical ideology there, even though acupuncture itself was never practised in the sub-continent of the Ayurveda. In the time of the *Samhitas*, about the beginning of the era, *praṇa* was quite as prominent as Greek *pneuma* or Chinese *chhi*,[a] but not much was said about the vessels in which it flowed. Only in late Tantrism was there elaborated a system of such channels (*vivaras*). Here six centres (*chakras* or *padmas*) of vital force were recognised, each the seat of a divinity; these were strung along the spinal column from the bottom to the top,[b] and connected by three main channels (*nādīs*), the left one (*idā*) corresponding to the moon (Yin) and the right one to the sun (Yang), while the central one combined both forces. Besides these three there were fourteen further principal *nādīs*, connecting in complicated ways the head or the abdomen with the ends of the upper and lower limbs; while beyond them again seven hundred major *nādīs* were recognised, and innumerable minor ones as well.[c] There was no clear circulation doctrine, however, as the *nādīs* radiated from the *chakras*. Since the main source for this pneumatic physiology dates only from +1577 (though perhaps embodying earlier materials), it may be reasonable to regard it as a somewhat garbled and theologised echo of the acu-tracts and *chhi* channels so ancient in Chinese medicine. Close relations between Tantrism and Taoism have long been suspected,[d] so the influence may well be as old as the Thang or Sung.[e]

The following centuries saw many out-going influences from China, but it is difficult to know how far Chinese medical techniques were adopted in the countries of the Nan Hai. During the first half of the +15th century the great fleets of Admiral Chêng Ho ranged far and wide,[f] and it must be relevant that some of them carried no less than 180 naval surgeons in their ships, so some medical transmissions may have occurred in Malaya, Indonesia, Thailand, even Ceylon. Similarly in the +16th century not only carpenters and other tradesmen, but also doctors, passed from China to take up residence in the Philippines.[g] But one can never underrate the extent to which Chinese medicine was ethnically bound, and it must have been practised in mixed communities decade after decade side by side with indigenous and Ayurvedic systems with only extremely little give and take between them. The strangest problem is why acupuncture and moxa never took root, so far as we know, among the Arabic cultures;[h] all the more so because the elixir idea did fully penetrate them,[i] and

[a] See Filliozat (1).

[b] We write thus because the system was central to Kundalīnī-yoga, the technique of psycho-physiological alchemy which involved the forced ascent of a beneficent spermatic influence from the reins to the cerebrum. This links with Chinese *nei tan* techniques, on which we discourse at length in *SCC*, Vol. 5, pt. 5.

[c] See Woodroffe (1), pp. 640ff., (2), pp. 129ff., 133.

[d] *SCC*, Vol. 2, pp. 425ff.

[e] A few modern Western acupuncturists have taken an interest in the Tantric *chakra* system, notably Finckh (1), who sought to analogise it with Jen Mo and Tu Mo.

[f] Cf. *SCC*, Vol. 4, pt. 3, pp. 487ff.

[g] Wang Chi-Min (*1*), p. 8.

[h] Something like moxa is traditional in Afghanistan, however, under the name of *dogh* (priv. comm. from Dr D. Blumhagen).

[i] This we showed fairly clearly in Vol. 5, pt. 4.

Avicenna's sphygmology undoubtedly drew much from earlier Chinese pulse-lore,[a] intimately bound up as that was with acupuncture and moxibustion.[b]

(ii) *Europe and the West*

The moment has now come for a brief survey of the passage of information about acupuncture and moxibustion to the Western parts of the Old World. It is a history of a garbling, for knowledge about ideas and practices came through in fragmentary and often partly incomprehensible form, recalling nothing so much as the converse transmission of Copernican heliocentrism in the opposite direction.[c] The sequence of events is very involved, and indeed as yet not fully cleared up; there are uncertainties of authorship, and some of the writings are now so rare that hardly any scholars have been able to examine and collate them all. One is struck by the very varying lapses of time between the original observations of Europeans in China and their publication in the West, as also by their extreme incompleteness, so that it would be fair to say that the full systematisation of the Chinese acu-tracts and acu-points was never appreciated by Westerners until our own time. This does not mean that acupuncture and moxa did not have waves of popularity in eighteenth- and nineteenth-century Europe, but with few if any exceptions, they were applied rather at random and without any of the codification which two and a half millennia of practice had given them in China. Some would say that this might well account for their relative ineffectiveness in Europe, and their failure to gain integration within modern Western medicine. Nevertheless the Western literature on acupuncture and moxibustion throughout these times is strangely voluminous, as we shall see.[d]

It was throughout the second half of the +17th century that information about acupuncture began to attract the attention of Europeans.[e] The very first writer, so

[a] See *SCC*, Vol. 6, pt. 3. His debt was recognised in the +17th century by Isaac Vossius (1), p. 70.

[b] The curious might also be inclined to ponder the question why the Chinese, alone of all ancient peoples, discovered and propagated acupuncture. For example, as is generally known, the clergy and laity of the Mesoamerican Indian cultures, especially the Aztec, had a masochistic passion for stabbing themselves with maguey spines, bone bodkins and obsidian spikes in penitential exercises. There is an interesting paper on this by Heyden (1). True, the object was to draw blood, but it seems quite strange that no one ever noticed or recorded, so far as we know, beneficial effects on other pains or ailments.

[c] See Sivin (11); Hsi Tsê-Tsung *et al.* (1).

[d] There are detailed accounts of it in Feucht (1, 2, 4). More brief surveys are those of Fransiszyn (1); Feucht (5). Much interest has been taken by Chinese writers in the transmission of acupuncture and moxibustion to Europe. There are papers by Sung-Ta Jen (3); Li Yuan-Chi (*1*) reprinted in Chhêng Tan-An *et al.* (*3*); Hsiao Yung-Thang (*1*); Manaka & Schmidt (*1*), Ch. tr., pp. 174ff.; Wang Chi-Min (*1*); Wang Chi-Min & Wu Lien-Tê (1), pp. 45ff. A valuable bibliography of the Western works, from +1656 onwards, has been issued in Shanghai by Wang Chi-Min & Fu Wei-Khang (*1*). Another bibliography and anthology of translations from them into Chinese is due to Thao I-Hsün & Ma Li-Jen (*1*).

[e] It has sometimes been said that there are mentions in Marco Polo or the +13th-century Franciscans, but if there were, Olschki (11) or Lach (5) would surely have found them, to say nothing of Yule (1, 2) and Cordier. Similarly, in spite of Craffe (1), we have found no evidence that Jerome Cardan (+1501 to +1576) or any other +16th-century physician knew or used acupuncture. The detailed biography of him by Henry Morley (2) has nothing to the point. Again, Huard & Huang Kuang-Ming (10), p. 130, aver that acupuncture was mentioned by Fernão Mendes Pinto (+1511 to +1583; cf. *SCC*, Vol. 4, pt. 3, pp. 535, 888). Pinto knocked about up and down the China seas from Goa to Ningpo and Nagasaki for twenty-five years or so from +1537 onwards; he was twice in China (apparently visiting Nanking and Peking) and four times in Japan, so he may well have seen something of

far as we can see, who spoke about acupuncture was the Dane Jacob de Bondt (+1598 to +1631) who in his capacity as surgeon-general for the Dutch East India Company at Batavia had come into contact with Chinese and Japanese physicians. His earlier book, *De Medicina Indorum* (+1642) has little or nothing on it,[a] but later this was reprinted in a larger work which also included a natural history of the animals and plants of the East. The last chapter of Bk. 5 of his *Historia Naturalis et Medica Indiae Orientalis* (+1658) is entitled: 'Certain miraculous works of Nature which future medical researchers must investigate further'. Here we can read the following passage:[b]

> The results (with acupuncture) in Japan which I will relate surpass even miracles.[α] For chronic pains of the head,[β] for obstructions of the liver and spleen, and also for pleurisy,[γ] they bore through[δ] (the flesh) with a stylus[ε] made of silver or bronze[ζ] and not much thicker than the strings of a lyre. The stylus[η] should be driven slowly and gently through the above-mentioned vitals so as to emerge from another part,[θ] as I myself have seen in Java.
>
> [α] Without undermining belief in their authenticity. [β] And moreover for acute ones, especially those arising from winds,[c] [γ] And for other ailments, as is here made clear, [δ] And they perforate, [ε] He should have said, with a needle, [ζ] More correctly, of gold, [η] Here the good author is quite in error, [θ] This last point is clearly untrue as one can gather from what I have said.[d]

The rather amusing comments are those of Willem ten Rhijne added when he quoted the passage in his own book on acupuncture published twenty-five years later.[e]

Thus the earliest observations by a European medical man must have been made about +1628, though they were not known in Europe until three more decades had passed. De Bondt must have written them down soon after the appearance in China of the book which represented the acme of the tradition, the *Chen Chiu Ta Chhêng* (cf. p. 159 above); but at that time European physicians were only on the periphery

Chinese medicine. His *Peregrinaçam*...(+1614), written from +1562 onwards, perhaps the first of all autobiographical novels, was built on essentially true materials, even though not all the experiences described were his own. He wrote it almost as a satire on the proceedings of the Europeans in Asia, giving warning that without a greater measure of friendship and morality in their dealings with other peoples, religions, and cultures, their empire-building would come to nothing. But neither in the French translation of B. Figuier (+1645) nor in the English of H. Cogan (+1653) can we find anywhere mention of acupuncture or moxa.

---

[a] But it is interesting as containing the first Western description of beriberi (p. 22*a*). De Bondt had the strange idea that dysentery was caused by drinking Chinese rice wine distilled with holothurians (*hai shen*[1]) as well as the cereal (pp. 16*b*, 24*a*, 36*b*).

[b] *Historia Animalium*, Bk. v, ch. 33, on p. 85; tr. Carrubba & Bowers (1), p. 394; Stiefvater (2), p. 43.

[c] Perhaps this was a piece of phraseology influenced by Chinese pneumatic theories in medicine.

[d] We are not so sure of this if one includes subcutaneous passages. Heroic variants were 'in the air' at the time (cf. p. 244). But possibly de Bondt had been confused by the practices of certain Taoist thaumaturgists who in ecstatic ceremonies pierce both cheeks through with a large bodkin, or hang weights from arm muscles so transfixed (photographs in Wang Chi-Min & Wu Lien-Tê (1), pl. 14, opp. p. 73). Apparently they suffer little pain, and the wounds bleed little; the effects could be due to pharmacological analgesia or, more likely, psychological exaltation (cf. p. 236 above). Piercing right through the arm, from Nei-kuan (HC 6) to Wai-kuan (SC 5) has also been found effective for analgesia in modern times, though not greatly used.

[e] See p. 271. The last seven words were omitted by ten Rhijne.

[1] 海參

of the culture-area, picking up strange ideas and clinical experiences from Japanese and other wanderers rather than being able to drink from the fountain-head in China itself.

Having just read Willem ten Rhijne's interjections on the text of Bontius it is fitting that we should look at his work next, even though, as we shall see, it is not exactly the next in chronological order. Still, it has justly been called 'the Western world's first detailed treatise on acupuncture', even though, again, it was not as detailed as all that. Ten Rhijne (+1647 to +1700) was also in the Dutch East India Company service, which he joined in +1673; six months later he was sent to Deshima[a] as resident physician, where for two years he had considerable opportunities for conferring with the physicians of Japan. The remaining twenty-four years of his life were spent in medical work in Java.[b] The title of his book is intriguing: *Dissertatio de Arthritide; Mantissa Schematica; De Acupunctura; et Orationes Tres: I. De Chymiae et Botaniae Antiquitate et Dignitate, II. De Physionomia, III. De Monstris*; and it appeared simultaneously in +1683 at London, The Hague and Leipzig.[c]

In the introduction to the part which concerns us, ten Rhijne wrote:

> Theory furnishes laws, and experience furnishes dexterity; the best practitioner is the one who, taught and trained with both theory and experience, is a master of his art. Cautery and acupuncture are the two primary operations among the Chinese and Japanese, who employ them to be free from every pain. If these two peoples (especially the Japanese) were to be deprived of these two techniques, their sick would be in a pitiful state without hope of cure or alleviation.[d] Both nations detest phlebotomy because, in their judgment, venesection draws forth both healthy and diseased blood, and thereby shortens life. They have accordingly attempted to rid unhealthy blood of impurities by moxibustion, and to expel from it the winds,[e] causes of all pain, by moxibustion and acupuncture. Although the Chinese physicians (who are the forerunners from whom Japanese physicians borrowed these systems of healing) are ignorant in anatomy, nonetheless they have perhaps devoted more effort over many centuries to learning and teaching with very great care the circulation of the blood, than have European physicians, either individually or as a group.[f] And they base the foundation of their entire medicine upon the rules of this circulation, as if these were oracular sayings from Apollo at Delphi.[g]

There follows a certain amount of historical information about persons and books, together with a few names of plant drugs, all of which are now quite difficult to identify because it is no small puzzle to find out the Chinese words which in the

[a] From +1641, when Japan was closed to all foreign contacts, the Dutch maintained a trading-station on this island in Nagasaki bay, and for almost two centuries it constituted the channel through which European science and medicine reached the Japanese. Ten Rhijne's work is an example of East Asian medicine passing in the opposite direction.

[b] His portrait is figured and described by Feucht (3). A brief account of his work appears in Feucht (5).

[c] A German translation was produced by Stiefvater (2) in 1955, but it omitted all the copious footnotes. The English translation of Carrubba & Bowers (1) twenty years later includes them.

[d] He probably knew that the pharmacy of the Chinese was relatively more advanced and important.

[e] Note again the emphasis on *fêng*[1] and *chhi*.[2]

[f] Cf. pp. 24 ff. above.

[g] Carrubba & Bowers tr., p. 375.

[1] 風 [2] 氣

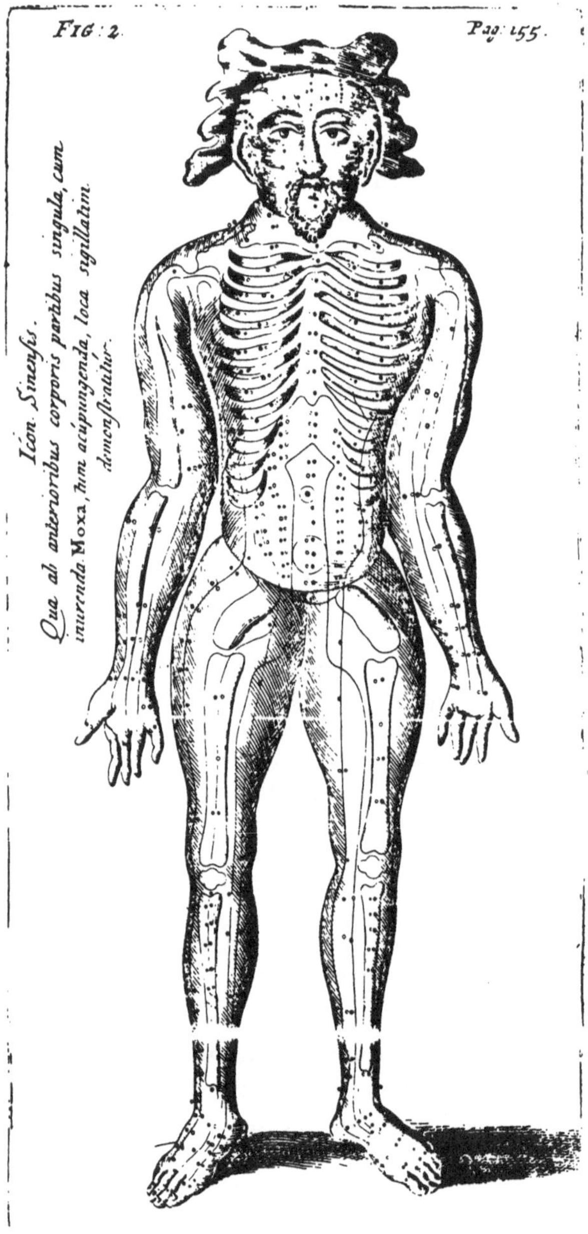

Fig. 65. The first illustration of acu-points in the Western world, a page from Willem ten Rhijne's book of + 1683. He took it from some Chinese work but had it redrawn in European style. The Latin caption says: 'A Chinese figure which shows the particular points on the anterior parts of the body for both moxibustion and acupuncture'. Reproduced by Carrubba & Bowers (1).

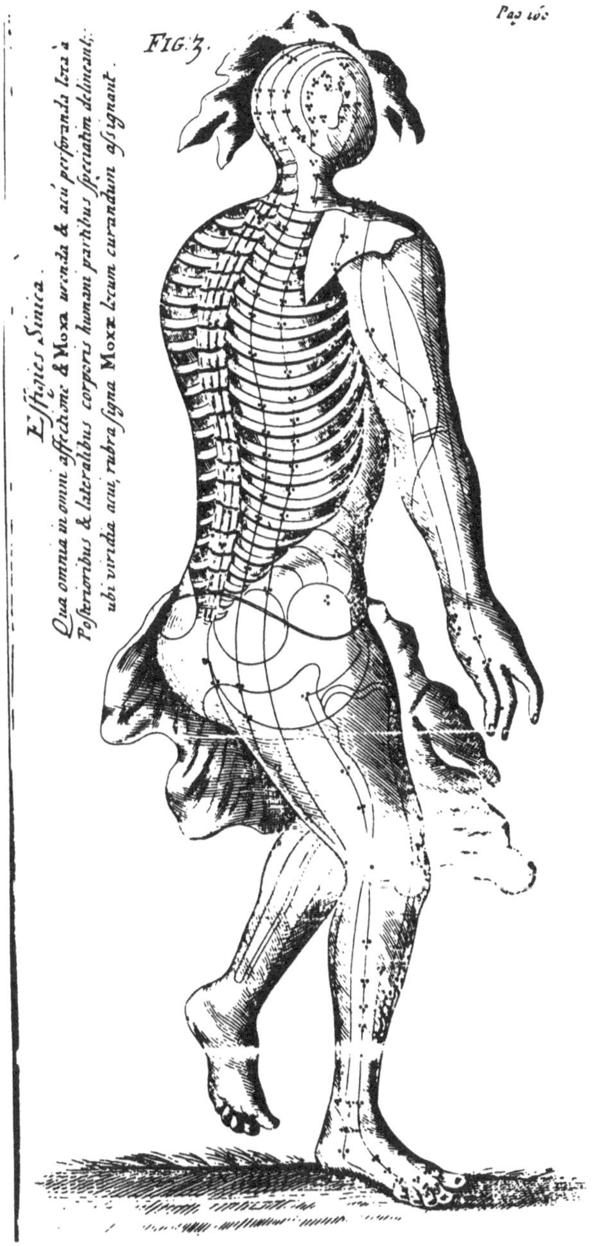

Fig. 66. Ten Rhijne's second figure, also Chinese, 'on which are clearly drawn all the locations on the posterior and lateral parts of the human body which should be burned with moxa and punctured with a needle in every condition. The green markings indicate the healing points for acupuncture, the red those for moxibustion.' The acu-tracts appear somewhat more clearly in this drawing than in the preceding one, for example, one can well make out the double course of VU lateral to the spinal column. It is curious that the European-style draughtsman put in flaps of resected skin, perhaps to make it more convincingly 'anatomical', though this was hardly necessary. We do not reproduce the colours which ten Rhijne intended.

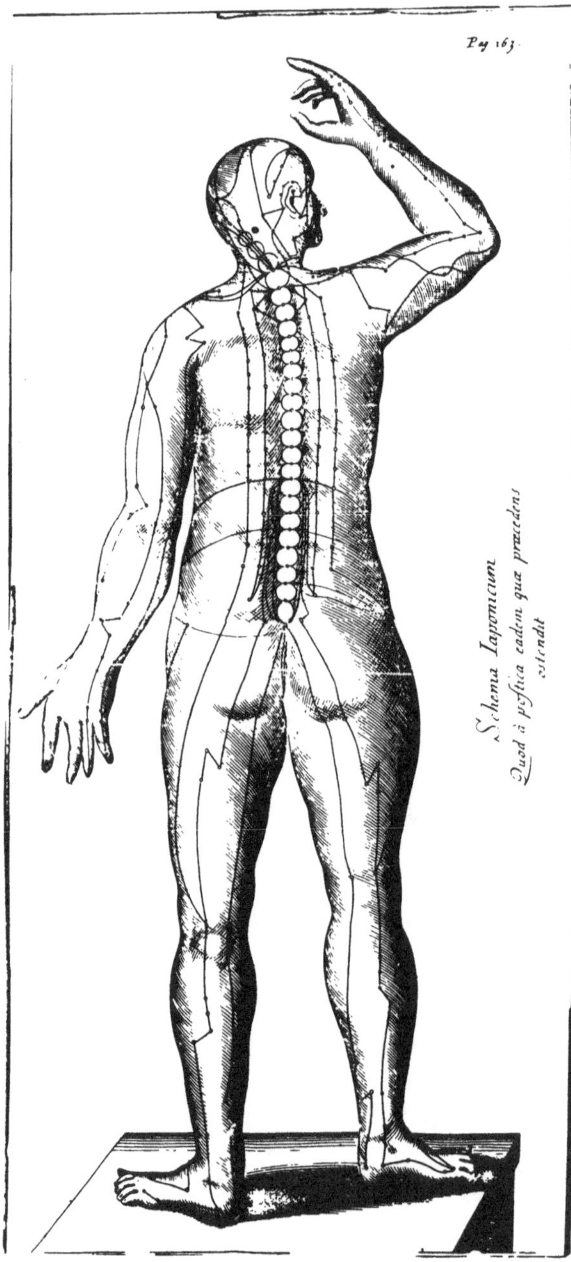

Fig. 67. Ten Rhijne's third picture, from a Japanese source, 'which shows, on the posterior of the body, the same items as the preceding diagram'. Here there are acu-tracts but no individual points, and an attempt has been made to correlate them with the vertebrae.

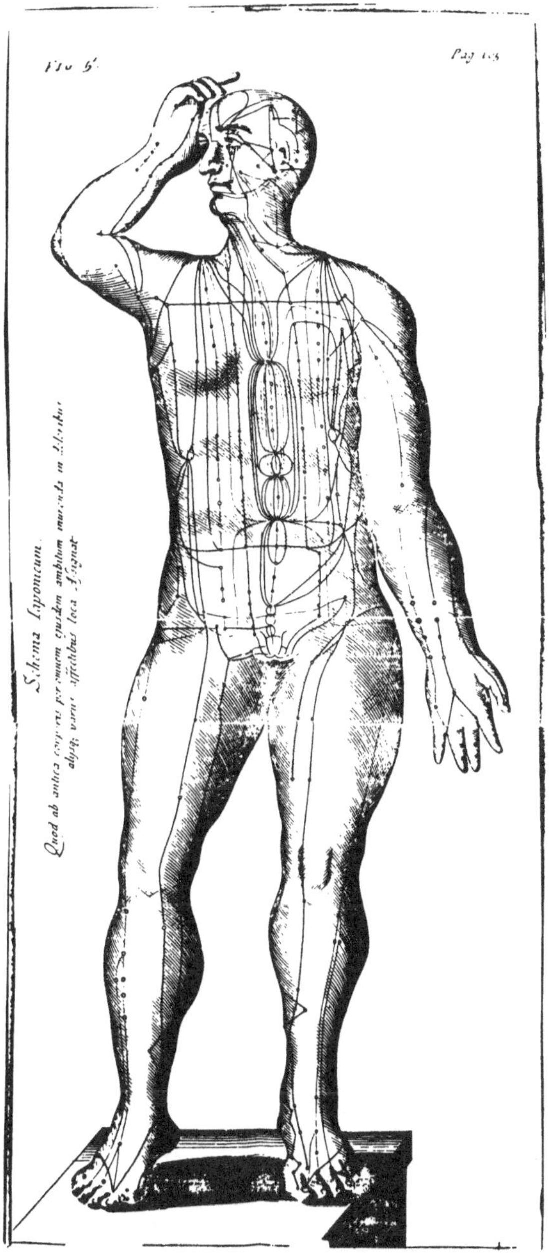

Fig. 68. In the fourth illustration, apparently from the same Japanese source, a number of acu-points are marked, though without names, and the tracts, especially on the trunk, seem rather more complicated than in the main tradition. The picture 'indicates the points, on the entire front of the body, which are to be burned for pains and various conditions'.

+17th century the Dutchman thought he heard the Japanese say. However, ten Rhijne went on to present four pictures, two Chinese and two Japanese(Figs. 65 to 68) which show the acu-tracts and the loci appropriate for acupuncture and for moxa cautery. He mentioned also the bronze acupuncture models, referring to Wang Wei-I (as 'Oyt', cf. p. 131 above);[a] a point which was taken up by his anonymous but prompt reviewer in the *Philosophical Transactions*, who wrote that 'the Chirurgions keep by them Images whereon all the places in the Body proper for the Needle are designed by Markes'.

Unfortunately, from this time onwards the whole study of acupuncture in the West was bedevilled by the confusion in ten Rhijne's mind between acu-tracts and blood-vessels; veins and arteries as he frequently called them. He rightly described fourteen; the twelve regular tracts (cf. p. 44 above) plus 'Nimiakph' (Jen Mo[1]) and 'Tokmiakph' (Tu Mo[2]). Besides these, he knew of two additional 'external veins, that is arteries' called 'Yn Kio' (Yin ching[3]) and 'Jo Kio' (Yang ching,[4] cf. Table 1). Other 'blood-vessels' were 'Kee miak' (*chhi mo*[5])[b] and 'Rak miak' (*lo mo*[6]), the former having a 'soul' (presumably a larger proportion of *chhi*[7]), the latter not.[c] And here came in a singular marriage very characteristic of the +17th century and later, the translation of Yang by the Galenic-Aristotelian 'innate heat' or *calidum innatum*, paralleling for Yin the 'radical' or 'primigenial, moisture', i.e. *humidum radicale*.[d] Naturally there were three types of each (Thai Yin, Yang Ming, etc.), and Willem ten Rhijne quite correctly associated them with the twelve regular *chhi* channels, the acu-tracts. For the rest, he said that the needles used were of gold or silver, and that they were sometimes applied heated as well as cold. To commend the needles to Westerners, he inserted a long paragraph describing their uses already customary in Greek and occidental surgery, and he ended by giving an interesting list of diseases in which acupuncture was successful, including an eye-witness account of a case of colic, *senki*,[e] suffered by a bodyguard of his own on one of the annual journeys to the capital.

In the year before the publication of ten Rhijne's book (i.e. +1682) there appeared at Frankfurt a work the true authorship of all of which is still not clear, Andreas

[a] Carrubba & Bowers tr., pp. 380, 396.

[b] Short for *chhi ching pa mo* (cf. p. 48), a common abbreviation.

[c] Ten Rhijne himself wrote *anima*, but glossed it as probably meaning vital spirits.

[d] These two concepts recur in all +17th-century medical and physiological writing, as in the works of William Harvey himself. They were prominent in the *Phil. Trans.* review, but they probably made European scholars feel that they understood the Chinese system more clearly than they really did. The correlations with Yang and Yin respectively run through most of the European accounts of Chinese medical philosophy; and *chhi*[7] itself was generally translated as 'vital spirits'.

[e] *Hsien-chhi*.[8] Colic, we write, but the matter is much more complicated, and needs further remark. *Hsien-chhi* is a group of syndromes in Chinese traditional medicine (and in the specific pathology and epidemiology of China and Japan) for which we have not been able to find any succinct equivalent in modern terminology. It can involve pains like acute colic but need not do so, the scrotum may be swollen or suppurating and painful as well as the lower abdomen, the pains and swellings may be accompanied by a gaseous inflation of the small intestine, and all these symptoms may be accompanied by anuria, dysuria, constipation or diarrhoea. See Anon. (*167*), pp. 379ff.; Chang Chün-I (*1*), p. 63. This description may be kept in mind when *hsien-chhi* is mentioned again in the following pages.

1 任脉 2 督脉 3 陰經 4 陽經 5 奇脉 6 絡脉
7 氣 8 疝氣

Cleyer's *Specimen Medicinae Sinicae, sive Opuscula Medica ad mentem Sinensium*... Cleyer was another surgeon-general at Batavia, a German, and he must have known ten Rhijne personally since he resided there between +1665 and +1697, though twice in Deshima and Japan in the eighties.[a] The *Specimen* is mainly on the Chinese doctrines of the pulse,[b] and Cleyer did not claim to be the author of it, only the editor, attributing several parts to the pen of an *eruditus Europaeus* living in Canton, most probably one of the Jesuits but not necessarily so. However the book opens with panegyric verses by Francis Bernard to the effect that 'what Greeks, Romans, Egyptians never knew you have now set forth, so let us bid farewell to urinoscopy, and you by the Pulse shall be the Mage of the Heart...' The Latin translations are supposedly from Wang Shu-Ho,[1] the writer of the *Mo Ching*[2] (Sphygmological Manual) of *c.* +300, but in fact they must be taken from some late medieval version of the *Mo Chüeh*[3] (Sphygmological Instructions) the oldest text of which, by Kao Yang-Shêng,[4] comes from about +940. Now although the discussion is primarily concerned with the numerous varieties of the pulse in health and disease, the correlations between the pulse and the acu-tracts were so close in traditional Chinese medicine that in fact there had to be much mention of the *viae* or 'ways' corresponding with the several viscera (Fig. 69). Indeed there is a special section *De viis*,[c] and elsewhere talk of the *duodecim vias* in connection with the speed of the circulation,[d] and in another place again, a sub-section *De octo viis extraordinariis* (the *chhi ching pa mo*[5]) from the *Nuý Kim̄* (*Nei Ching*[6]).[e] Unfortunately these are nowhere very clearly explained, either by Cleyer or the learned European in Canton, so that readers must have been a little mystified by the remarkable series of 30 plates which the book contains.[f] Apart from extras, these run systematically through the twelve regular tracts, each with an accompanying drawing of the relevant viscus, and the two median tracts Tu Mo and Jen Mo (Figs. 70, 71, 72). A comparison readily shows that these must have been taken from the *Lei Ching*[7] (The Classics Classified; a System of Medicine) written by Chang Chieh-Pin[8] in +1624.[g] The trouble was that the pictures were dubbed 'anatomical'

[a] They may not have been on very good terms, or else for some reason or other ten Rhijne disapproved of Cleyer's book, and succeeded in preventing its publication at Amsterdam; this was why it came out at Frankfurt. See Szczesniak (6), pp. 516–17, whose views on the whole controversy, however we cannot make our own.

[b] Fig. 8 shows the title-page of the MS. preserved in the Staatsbibliothek at Berlin. It was not reproduced in the printed version. Grmek (1), fig. 21. A complete list of the sub-titles in the *Specimen* is given by Szczesniak (6), pp. 508ff.

[c] First pagination, pp. 26–8.

[d] Second pagination, p. 15.

[e] *Ibid.*, pp. 98–9. They were all given their romanised names, from which it is easy to identify them (cf. Table 1).

[f] The originals of these are now in the Gabinetto delle Stampe dell'Accademia dei Lincei in Rome; see Vacca (11).

[g] Chinese books on acupuncture, moxa and pulse-lore given by Cleyer were in the Royal Library in Berlin in 1822, when they were catalogued by Klaproth (7), pp. viii, 153ff. If they are still there it should be possible to pin-point the exact editions used by Cleyer, perhaps also by Boym and the Anonymus (cf. p. 284 below). Actually, the question of the source of Cleyer's pictures is a little complicated. It would perhaps be better to say that as our comparisons show, the plates of the individual

1 王叔和 2 脈經 3 脈訣 4 高陽生 5 奇經八脉 6 內經
7 類經 8 張介賓

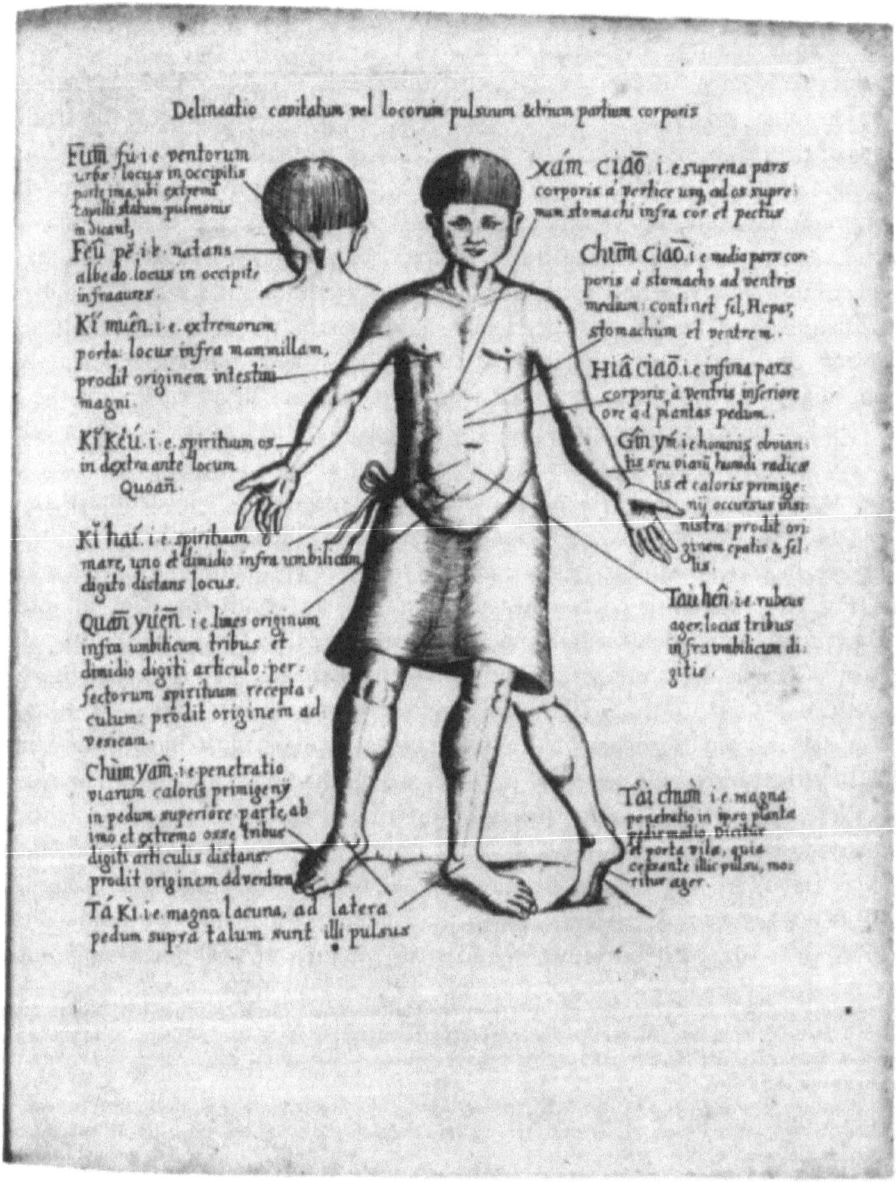

Fig. 69. An illustration from Andreas Cleyer's *Specimen Medicinae Sinicae* of +1682 (pl. 30). It is entitled 'A delineation of the pulses of the cavities or loci, and the three parts of the body'. It certainly bears witness to the close connection between sphygmology and acupuncture (cf. p. 26), but it may have been based on some misunderstandings. We know of no Chinese original for this picture. The three coctive regions (*shang chiao*, *chung chiao* and *hsia chiao*) are clearly to be made out, but most of the other markings are those of individual acu-points. Among those identifiable are the following:

taù hên	Tan-thien JM 4, 5, 6 (synonyms)
fum fú	Fêng-fu TM 15
feû pě	Fou-pai VF 16
kí muên	Chhi-mên H 14
kı haí	Chhi-hai JM 6
quañ yu'eñ	Kuan-yuan JM 4
chùm yam	Chhung-yang V 42
tá kì	Thai-chhi R 3

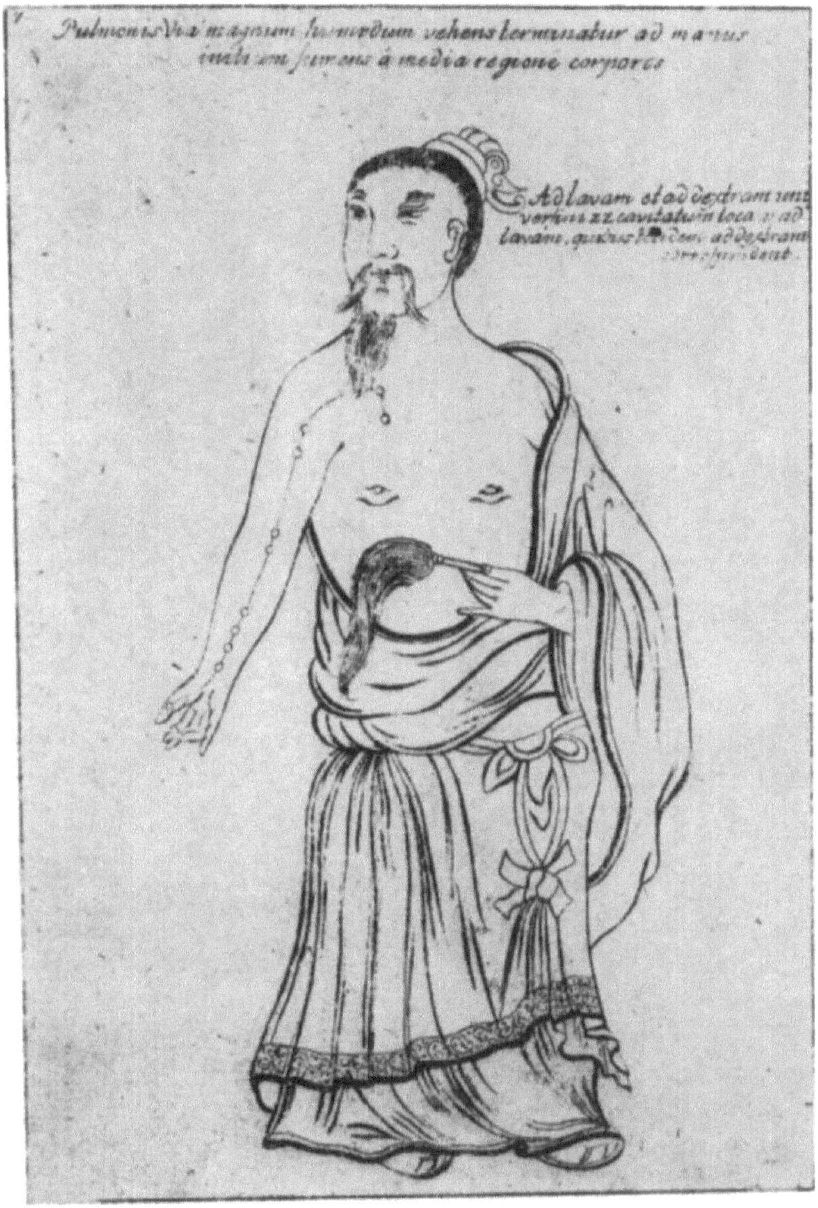

Fig. 70. One of Cleyer's plates of the acu-tracts in his *Specimen* . . . of + 1682; the cheirotelic pulmonic Thai-Yin tract (pl. 7). In the caption Thai-Yin appears as ***magnum humidum*** in accordance with European ideas of the 'primigenial moisture', and it is rightly stated that the tract starts on the thorax in front of the shoulder, and ends in the hand. The subsidiary caption adds that counting both sides there are 22 loci (acu-points), corresponding laterally to each other.

A comparison with Fig. 17 will show that the iconographic tradition used was assuredly that of the *Lei Ching* (+ 1624), but that the picture, apart from some occidentalisation by the copyist, is reversed as well as redrawn; this, no doubt, because of the copper plate process used.

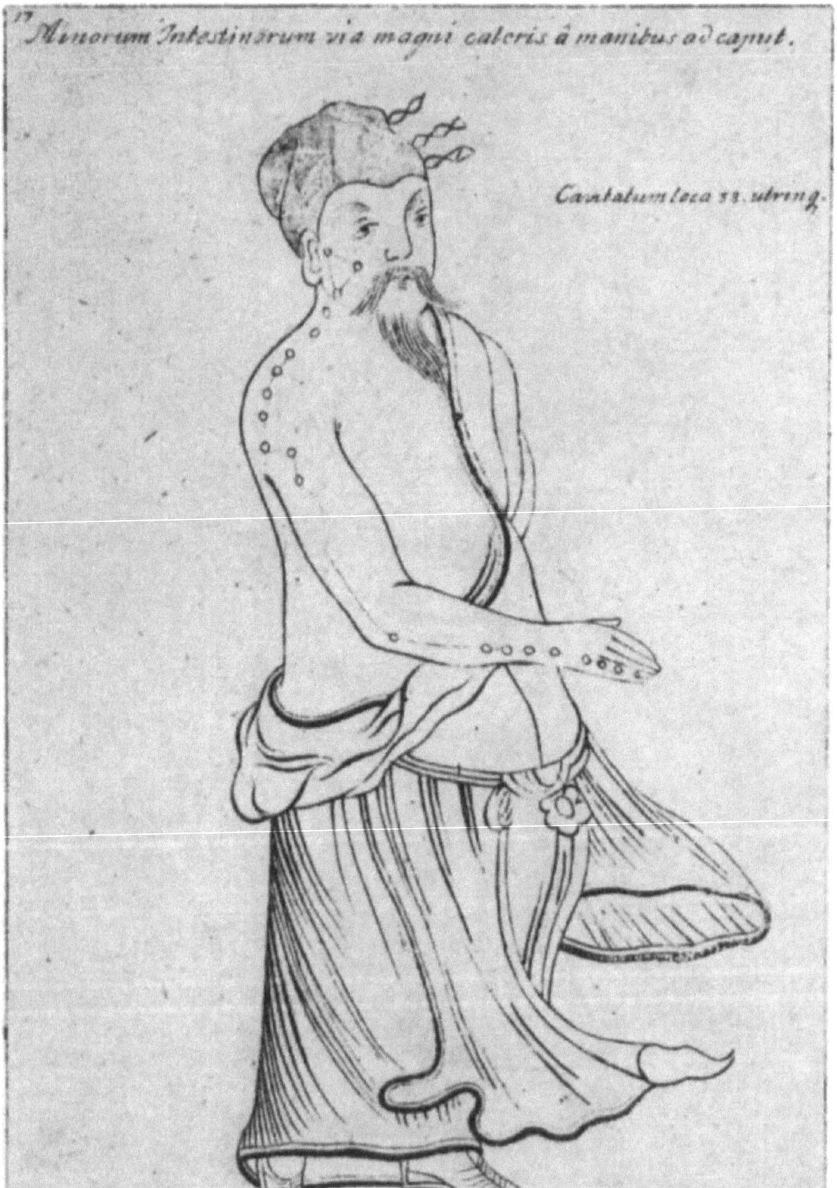
17
Minorum Intestinorum via magni caloris à manibus ad caput.
Cantatum loca 38. utrinq.

Fig. 71. Another of Cleyer's tract illustrations (pl. 17); the cheirogenic tenu-intestinal Thai-Yang tract. Running from the hand to the side of the head, it is copied with considerable faithfulness, as can be seen by comparison with any standard text, e.g. Anon. (135), p. 132. Thai-Yang appears as *magni caloris*, in harmony with the European conception of the 'innate, or radical, heat'. It is correctly added that bilaterally there are 38 acu-points.

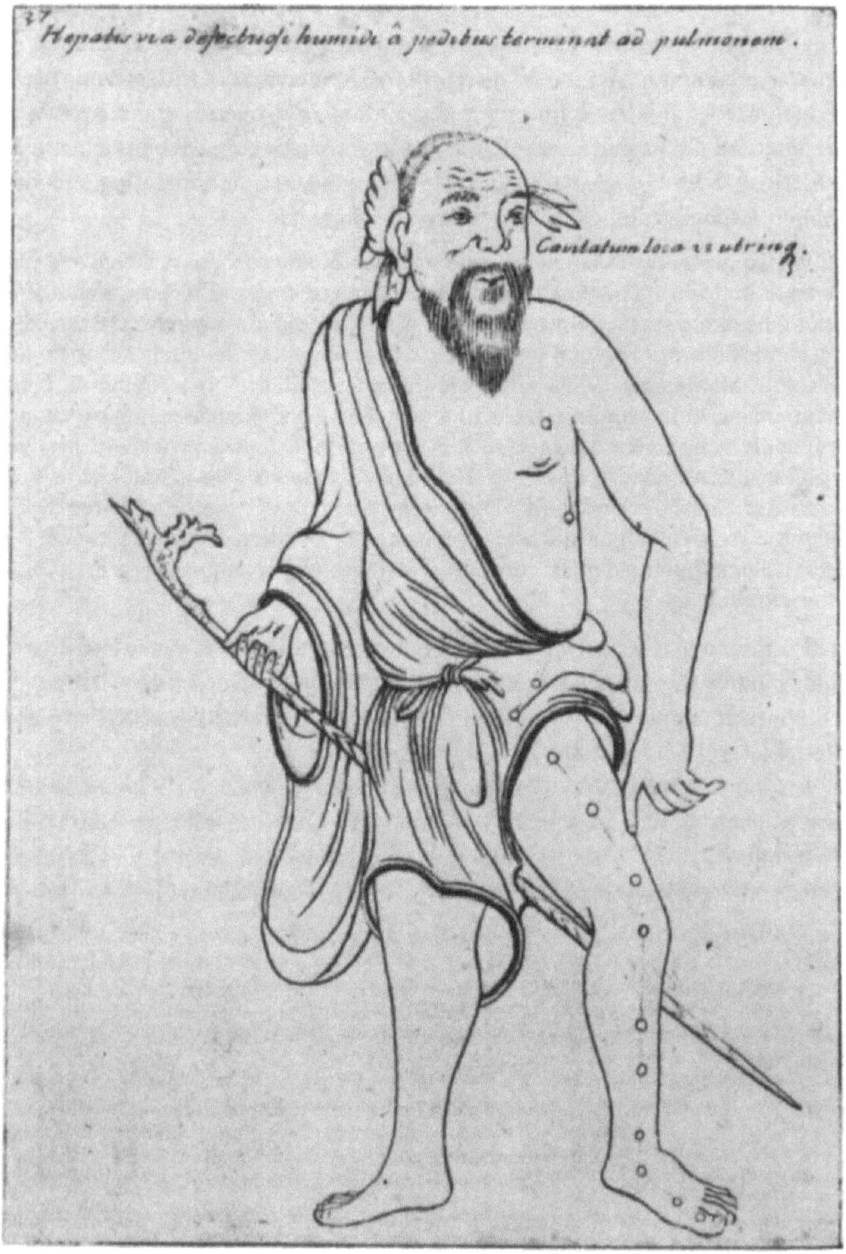

Fig. 72. A third example of Cleyer's tract plates (pl. 27); the podogenic hepatic Chüeh-Yin tract. The caption informs the reader rightly that this starts at the foot and terminates over the lungs, and it uses the quite reasonable expression *defectuosi humidi* for Chüeh-Yin. The number of 28 points bilaterally is also right. Once again the attitude of the figure, with its staff, is quite the same as that in the *Lei Ching*, but reversed as well as redrawn.

by Western writers, thereby challenging a pointless comparison with the drawings of Vesalian dissection,[a] and eliciting an amusing passage from William Wotton.

Wotton was a contender in the 'quarrel of the Ancients and Moderns' who paradoxically supported the latter by citing many Chinese discoveries and inventions but conversely attacked Chinese learning when it was supposed to have been more ancient than the Greek.[b] So here, in +1694, after giving an extract ridiculing the symbolic correlations in Chinese medical philosophy, he went on:[c]

> It would be tedious to dwell any longer upon such Notions as these, which every page of Cleyer's book is full of. The Anatomical Figures annexed to the Tracts, which also were sent out of China, are so very whimsical, that a Man would almost believe the whole to be a Banter, if these Theories were not agreeable to the occasional Hints that may be found in the Travels of the Missionaries. This, however, does no prejudice to their Simple Medicines,[d] which may, perhaps, be very admirable, and which a long Experience may have taught the Chineses to apply with great success; and it is possible that they may sometimes give not unhappy Guesses in ordinary Cases, by feeling their Patients Pulses: Still, this is little to Physic, as an Art; and however, the Chineses may be allowed to be excellent Empiricks, as many of the West-Indian Salvages are, yet it cannot be believed that they can be tolerable Philosophers; which, in an Enquiry into the Learning of any Nation, is the first Question that is to be considered.

And this at a time when blistering and phlebotomy, the four humours and elements, vegetable orthodoxy in pharmacy, with purges and glowing cauteries in therapy, were all part of unregenerate European medicine. Other contemporaries, less partisan, appreciated Cleyer's book better.

But he was not destined to enjoy for centuries in the Elysian Fields an untroubled recognition of merit; on the contrary, a sinological *cause célèbre* gathered about his name. First Bayer (2) in +1730 contended that Andreas Cleyer had appropriated the writings and translations of the Polish Jesuit, Michael Boym (Pu Mi-Ko[1]) and

acu-tracts in Cleyer were taken from a set in the same iconographic genre as those in the *Lei Ching*. Our copy of this is of +1749, but the best drawings of the kind are those of the Ssu Khu Chhüan Shu edition, *c.* +1780. A similar series, taken from some coloured MS. of Ming date, is reproduced by Chu Lien (*1*). The pictures occur from ch. 3, pp. 7*b* onwards in the Thu I[2] section (Appendix of Illustrations), which is absent from the modern facsimile edition, though this was taken from a Ming *pên*, perhaps the original of +1624.

The three plates of the acu-tracts as a whole, front (Chêng Jen Ming Thang Thu[3]), back (Fu Jen Ming Thang Thu[4]) and side (Tshê Jen Ming Thang Thu[5]), were taken, on the other hand, from Yang Chi-Chou's *Chen Chiu Ta Chhêng* of +1601 (p. 159 above). The various editions of this have the diagrams inserted as large folded sheets, and the double 'railway-line' convention in Cleyer is not found until the edition of +1680; that of +1665 has single lines. We reproduce the front view (Fig. 73).

[a] Anatomy in Europe, after all, had only just begun its great Renaissance rise from the condition it had been in during the late Middle Ages. A look at the *Fasciculus Medicinae* of Johannes de Ketham (+1491) shows that the drawings are similar to those of medieval China, indeed often not as good. Miyashita Saburo (1) even adduces evidence that Chinese anatomy, mediated through Persian and Arabic sources, stimulated or influenced the rise of the science in Europe. We shall, of course, discuss this question properly in Section 43 on anatomy. In the meantime there is the interesting paper by Rollins (1) on illustration in printed medical books.

[b] Cf. *SCC*, Vol 2, p. 297.

[c] (1), p. 164.

[d] Medicinal simples, of course.

[1] 卜彌格 [2] 圖翼 [3] 正人明堂圖 [4] 伏人明堂圖 [5] 側人明堂圖

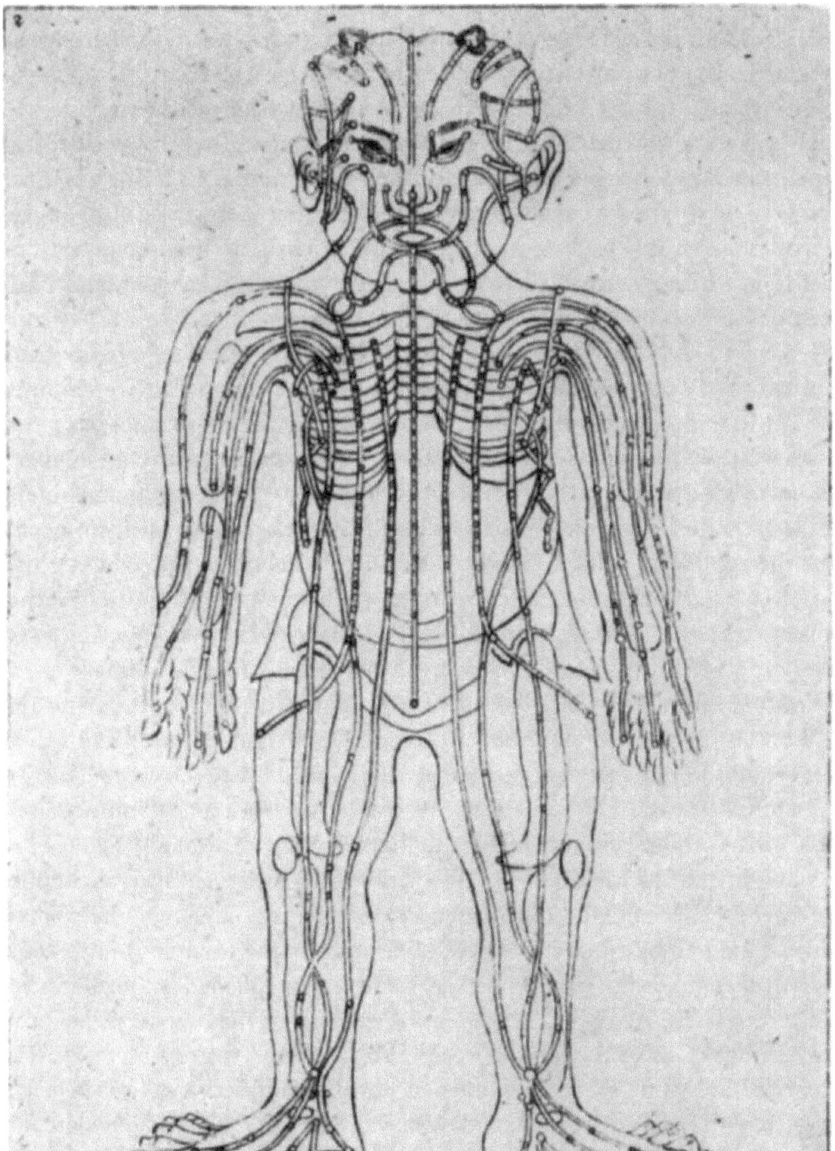

Fig. 73. One of Andreas Cleyer's illustrations of the system of acu-tracts as a whole, that for the front of the body (pl. 2). It must have been very up-to-date at the time, because the double 'railway-line' convention is not found until the +1680 edition of the *Chen Chiu Ta Chhêng*, first published in +1601. Many individual acu-points are marked along the lines, though not always very clearly.

published them under his own name;[a] and this accusation was followed by many later authors, notably Rémusat,[b] Chabrié[c] the biographer of Boym, Pfister, Cordier, Szczesniak (6) and even Vacca (11). It took Pelliot (50) with his usual sleuth-like penetration, to clarify the matter, and since then Grmek (1) and Kraft (1, 2) have added further evidence acquitting Cleyer of that charge. But who was Boym?

Michal Boym (or Dziurdzi-Boïm) was the son of an eminent physician of Lwów in Ruthenia, the family being patrician Hungarian in origin.[d] Entering the novitiate at Kraków in +1631 (the year that young de Bondt died) he arrived in Tongking in +1645 and worked there and in Hainan until +1649. In this latter year he was seconded to the Ming court in exile from the Manchus in Kuangtung and Kuangsi, leading members of which had then recently been converted to Christianity by Andreas Koffler (Chhü An-Tê[1]).[e] In +1650 Boym set off on an embassy from the Ming court to the Pope and the Doge of Venice which occupied the remaining nine years of his life and constitutes one of the most remarkable examples of devoted loyality an an utterly forlorn hope in all history. The missives taken and delivered by the Jesuit envoy were in vague and complimentary terms, requesting papal blessings, etc., but the intention must certainly have been to seek material aid from occidental powers for the expulsion of the Manchus and the restoration of the Ming – this hope proved of course perfectly vain. The Portuguese who had helped at first with small expeditionary forces now felt that the Chhing dynasty had come to stay, and therefore placed every obstacle in the path of Boym, who consequently had to make a difficult overland journey through Persia instead of taking ship from Goa. Arriving in Italy he found himself involved in all kinds of diplomatic intrigues, as well as in the Rites Controversy and the Jansenist attack against his order. Three whole years were spent in Rome before he at last got audience with the Pope, and then he immediately left again for China without once revisiting his homeland. He reached Siam in +1658 and Tongking in +1659, then fell ill and died on the Kuangsi border without even having succeeded in contacting the Ming pretender, Chu Yu-Lang,[2] by that time a refugee in Burma and destined to be executed at Kunming (Yunnan) in +1662.[f]

In spite of his extraordinary life Michael Boym accomplished important scientific work. His *Flora Sinensis* was published in Vienna in +1656 (though he probably never saw the book himself); the first description by any Westerner of plants of the Chinese culture-area, though dealing only with tropical and sub-tropical species, some more characteristic of Indo-China and Malaya. His catalogue of the latitudes of Chinese cities was used by other Jesuit geographers; and important maps made by Boym still exist at Paris and Rome, notably a series of the 18 provinces and their

[a] (1), vol. 1, p. 28.
[b] (11), vol. 1, p. 246, vol. 2, p. 363, (12), vol. 2, pp. 227–8.
[c] (1), pp. 235 ff., 264 ff.
[d] Cf. Pfister (1), no. 93. We have met him once before, in *SCC*, Vol. 3, pp. 444–5, and we shall often be with him again, as in the Section on botany in Vol. 6.
[e] *Op. cit.* no. 92.
[f] The most complete account of the epic of this embassy is that of Kleiser (1).

[1] 瞿安德　　[2] 朱由榔

mineral deposits. But above all he was interested in medicine, and so important for diagnosis was sphygmology in the Chinese medicine of the time that he too undertook a translation of some version of the *Mo Chüeh*. This appeared three years after Cleyer's book (i.e. +1686) under the title *Clavis Medica ad Chinarum Doctrinam de Pulsibus* ..., and the long Latin title goes on to mention as editors both Andreas Cleyer and Philippe Couplet (Po Ying-Li[1]),[a] the very Jesuit whom scholars had suspected of having conveyed Boym's writings improperly to Cleyer for his *Specimen*. But between these two works there is nothing in common but the subject, and the translations seem to be from different texts by different hands.[b] For our present purpose what is noteworthy is that Boym too tells his readers of the 12 regular acu-tracts (ch. 4, *Quae sit natura, quae sit temperamenta et qualitates viarum duodecim*...), as also of the circulations (ch. 13, *Circuitus ac motus sanguinis et spirituum*...) where he gives the quantitative measurements of distances, respiratory rates, etc. stemming originally from the *Nei Ching*. But though he provided several pictures of hands and wrists to illustrate pulse-taking,[c] he did not figure the acu-tracts themselves as Cleyer had done. In this case again Boym could never have seen his book, for he signed the preface of it at Ayutya in Siam in +1658, twenty-eight years before it appeared in print.[d] That was the same year in which de Bondt's book became available to Westerners, and Boym's own observations on the pulse and the acu-tracts were destined to reach them with almost as long a delay as his.

Now Boym, Cleyer and ten Rhijne had all been preceded in their dates of publication by an anonymous and now very rare book printed at Grenoble in +1671: 'Les Secrets de la Médecine des Chinois, consistant en la parfaite Connoissance du Pouls, envoyez de la Chine par un Francois, Homme de grand mérite'. This obscure French writer thus takes pride of place after de Bondt the Dane.[e] From internal evidence the writer must have been some French missionary resident at Canton between +1665 and +1668, and the work was based on a translation of the *Mo Chüeh* not at all the same as that contained in Boym's *Clavis Medica*. There is more similarity with the text contained in Cleyer's *Specimen*, and there seems every probability that the writer was none other than his *eruditus Europeaus* whose letters of +1669 and +1670 from Canton he printed. A number of Jesuits were held there for some years under house arrest at that time, and circumstantial evidence noted by Grmek points to either

[a] Cf. Pfister (1), no. 114.

[b] There may have been a little Boym material in the *Specimen*; if so, it would have been pt. 5, *Schemata ad meliorem praecedentium intelligentiam*. This contains a list of prescriptions, and then an account of 289 drugs, the entries being in most cases very brief. But the authorship of these is still not certain. See Pelliot (50), p. 149; Szczesniak (6), p. 511.

[c] Reproduced by Grmek (1), pp. 75, 77–8.

[d] A complete list of the sub-titles in the *Clavis* is given by Szczesniak (6), pp. 513ff.

[e] The book has been variously attributed to Louis Augustin Alemand (+1645 to +1728), or to an otherwise unknown writer named Alemand-Harvieu. The latter is an obvious confusion with the Jesuit Julien Hervieu (Ho Tshang-Pi[2]) who later on gave a partial translation of another version of the *Mo Chüeh* in du Halde (1), vol. 3, pp. 384–436 (+1735), Brookes tr., vol. 3, pp. 366ff. For Hervieu see Pfister (1), no. 259. The authorship of Michael Boym has also been conjectured, but Alemand was never in China and Boym was Polish, not French.

1 柏應理 2 赫蒼璧

Adrien Greslon, Humbert Augery, or Jacques le Favre[a] unless conceivably it was Philippe Couplet himself.[b] In any case, apart from references to the acu-tracts, the author had something to say about Japanese medicine, and mentioned that large needles of silver, slightly blunted at the end, were used, rolled between the fingers, to achieve effects in depth, though moxa cautery at acu-points was more common.[c] Such were the earliest European descriptions of the acupuncture and pulse-lore of China and Japan.

At this stage two passing quotations impose themselves. Isaac Vossius was, as we know,[d] a great admirer of Chinese discoveries and inventions, which he praised in his essay *De Artibus et Scientiis Sinarum*, part of the *Variarum Observationum Liber* (+1685). So here he said:

> Not less to be wondered at is that Surgery which they have cultivated in practice for so many centuries, especially in that perforation of all parts of the body which they do (with needles), even of the very brain itself, transfixed from one side of the head to the other with a metal bodkin a cubit in length or longer. Such things have often been seen by us (Europeans), either greatly mitigating or even totally removing by these means those pains to which the flesh is heir.[e]

This was rather too enthusiastic an echo of Bontius and ten Rhijne. More just and penetrating was the comment of Pierre Bayle on Boym's *Clavis*.[f]

> The Reverend Father expounds to us the Chinese system of medicine very clearly, and it is easy to see from what he says that the physicians of China are rather clever men. True, their theories and principles are not the clearest in the world, but if we had got hold of them under the reign of the Philosophy of Aristotle, we should have admired them much, and we should have found them at least as plausible and well based as our own. Unfortunately, they have reached us in Europe just at a time when the mechanick Principles invented, or revived, by our Modern Virtuosi have given us a great distaste for the 'faculties' (of Galen), and for the *calidum naturalis* and the *humidum radicale* too, the great foundations of the Medicine of the Chinese no less than of that of the Peripateticks.

Truly, as Grmek says, a passage of astonishing perspicacity, far exceeding the gibes of Wotton, and completely conscious of the difference between the 'new, or experimental, science', modern science, as opposed to all the preparative science of the ancient and medieval worlds.

Cleyer's book had a great influence in England a little later when it was abridged and paraphrased as part of Sir John Floyer's 'Physician's Pulse-Watch; or, an Essay to explain the Old Art of Feeling the Pulse, and to Improve it by the help of a Pulse-Watch'; the two volumes of this came out in +1707 and +1710. Floyer was a

[a] Of these the most likely was perhaps Greslon (Nieh Chung-Chhien[1]). Cf. Pfister (1), nos. 104, 101, 102 respectively.
[b] Grmek (1), p. 63.
[c] Cf. Craffe (1).
[d] Pp. 36, 37 above; cf. *SCC*, Vol 4, pt. 3, pp. 417, 666 and Vol. 5, pt. 4.
[e] (1), p. 76.
[f] In the 'Nouvelles de la République des Lettres', 1686, p. 1013.
[1] 聶仲遷

Lichfield man, and an eminent, if slightly eccentric, doctor.[a] While at Oxford between +1664 and +1680 he must certainly have known Thomas Hyde, Bodley's Librarian, who afterwards brought over from France Shen Fu-Tsung,[1] the companion of Philippe Couplet, to catalogue the Chinese books.[b] Perhaps the keynote of Floyer's work was struck in his second volume where he entitled part I 'an Essay to make a new Sphygmologia, by accommodating the Chinese and European Observations about the Pulse' into one system. His chief originality lay in his use of a new kind of stop-watch which ran for exactly sixty seconds,[c] and his studies of pulse-rate in many different diseases opened a completely new chapter for the Western world.

Here once again, sphygmology was so much tied up with the acu-tracts that they could not fail to come in, yet they were never in any real way explained. 'They make 12 Ways' wrote Floyer, following Cleyer, 'of the Primigenial Heat [Yang] and of the *humidum radicale* [Yin], six upwards and six downwards...'[d] Elsewhere he mentioned *via cordis*,[e] *via stomachae*,[f] 'the Way of the lungs',[g] and 'the eight extraordinary Ways' muttering, as it were, 'all these must be some description of the arteries, veins and nerves'.[h] He seems to have known extremely little of acupuncture itself, and not much more of moxa, for he believed that pharmacy was the predominating cure in China for the diseases which the pulse-taking had diagnosed. Westerners were indeed at this time seeing through a glass darkly.[i]

They must have obtained a rather clearer idea of what acupuncture was like in practice from the writings of Engelbert Kaempfer (+1651 to +1716). This admirable German naturalist, bold and adventurous in early life, qualified medically in Sweden, then went with a Swedish embassy to Persia, where he stayed more than four years. Voyaging onward through India and Ceylon, he took service with the Dutch East India Company and so found himself (+1690 to +1692) yet another of the Deshima physicians, whence he made the journey to Yedo, returning to Europe in the following year.[j] From his inaugural dissertation at Leiden in +1694, giving a 'decade of exotic

[a] +1649 to +1734. Szczesniak (11), in a biographical study, makes him out a credulous, superstitious figure, comical in the eyes of his contemporaries; but this, we think, is going much too far. He was certainly interested in balneology, advocating cold baths, and he thought that physicians should follow the Chinese system of being their own apothecaries, and dispensing as well as prescribing.

[b] Cf. *SCC*, Vol. 1, p. 38.

[c] Cf. the small 'stop-watch steelyard clepsydras' for short-time intervals used in China since the +5th century; Vol 3, pp. 316ff., 326–7. We mentioned the timing of eclipses, and races in sport, but it may well be that medical uses for heart-rate and respiration-rate will be found in due course in the relevant literature. Yet another use was the timing of meditation and respiratory exercises in Taoist physiological alchemy (Vol. 5, pt. 5).

[d] (1), vol. 1, p. 354. Cf. our terms cheirotelic and cheirogenic, podotelic and podogenic explained on p. 42 above.

[e] *Op. cit.*, p. 377. It was connected, he thought, with a 'choleric cachochymia' or morbid state of the humours.

[f] *Op. cit.*, p. 389.

[g] P. 387.

[h] P. 384.

[i] Yet Floyer, though unknowingly, was not entirely wrong, for just at this time acupuncture was passing through one of its periodical eclipses in China. Hsü Ling-Thai, writing about +1770, described this well in his *I Shu Chhüan Chi*, ch. 1, pt. 2, (pp. 96ff.).

[j] For his biography see Bowers (3).

[1] 沈福宗

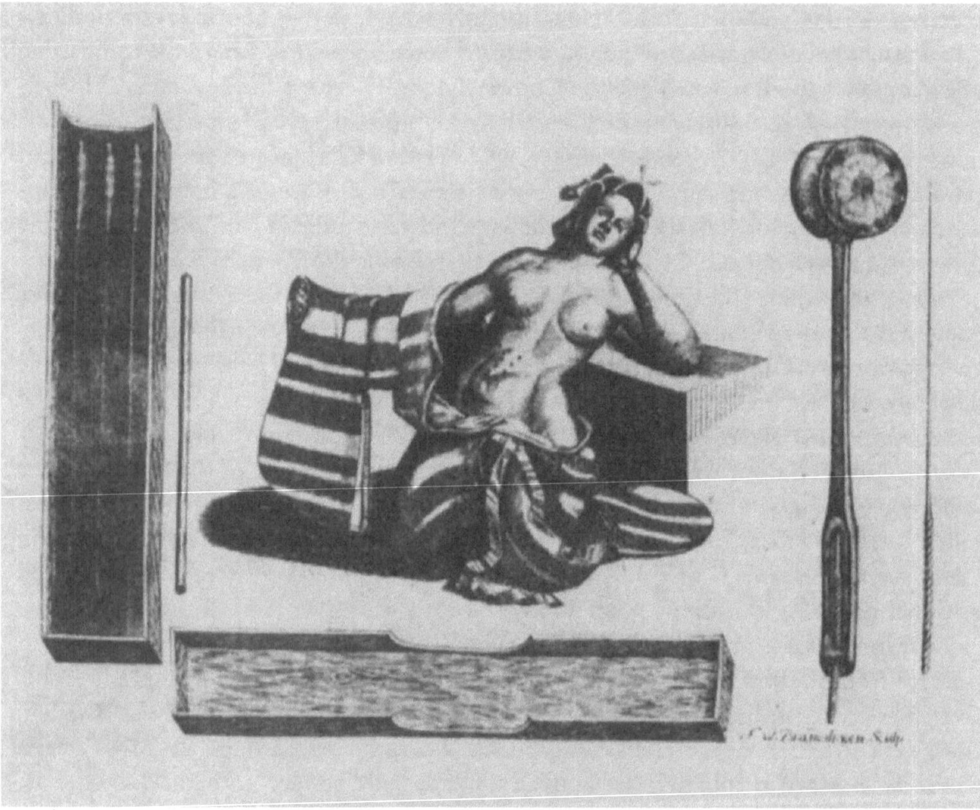

Fig. 74. An illustration from Engelbert Kaempfer's *Amoenitatum Exoticarum* . . . of 1712. A Japanese girl with uncovered torso is demonstrating the acu-points which were used in the cure of *senki* (*shan chhi*), a kind of diarrhoea with colicky cramps. Below and on the left is the box of acupuncture needles and the little brass tube used by the Japanese physicians to guide the needle as they inserted it; on the right is the samll hammer made of leather-covered horn and weighted with lead which they used to strike the head of the needle at some loci (cf. Fig. 64). Needles were stored in the handle of the hammer. See the translation of Kaempfer's Latin description by Bowers & Carrubba (2).

observations',[a] and from the re-written versions of it which he included in his famous *Amoenitatum Exoticarum Politico-Physico-Medicarum Fasciculi V*...(+1712) we have two excellent descriptions of acupuncture and moxa as he saw them among the Japanese. Unfortunately for the former he dealt only with one illness, the *senki*[1] or diarrhoea with colic-like cramp pains which he found very common in that country.[b]

[a] There is a translation by Bowers & Carrubba (1). Kaempfer's thesis contained the first descriptions of maduromycosis (pseudactinomycosis), filariasis and dracunculosis, a great contribution in the history of parasitology, even though he had no idea of the real aetiological agents involved in the first two.

[b] *Curatio Colicae per Acupuncturam, Japonibus usitata.* The version in the *Amoenitatum* has been translated by Bowers & Carrubba (2). It is interesting that the rather dramatic results in colicky diarrhoea should have loomed so large in the minds of these first transmitters, as in the case of ten Rhijne (p. 276 above).

[1] 疝氣

Fig. 74 from his book shows an afflicted woman with the loci on the abdominal wall where acupuncture was performed.[a] Kaempfer's account was quite detailed; he spoke of needles of silver or gold, and the twisting of them when in place by the operator, also the use of slim tubes of brass either because the needles were so fine or to prevent the needle being driven in too far when tapped on the head, as it often was, by a delicate little hammer. The depth of penetration was never more than an inch and usually but half that. He also mentioned the time during which the needles should remain implanted, and added that moxibustion was also employed at the same loci. 'Generally, after the three rows of punctures had been made according to the instructions of an expert and to the proper depth, the colic pains ceased immediately as if by magic.' Kaempfer was precise about the names of the acu-points. The highest row, he said, was called 'Sjoquan', the second 'Tsjuquan' and the third one, just above the umbilicus, 'Gecquan'.[b] From the picture it is quite clear that the centre line of three points was along Jen Mo (JM 10, 12, 13),[c] and perhaps it is no coincidence that the lowest one of these is Hsia-kuan.[1] For the two side lines one cannot be so certain; they may have been V 22, 23, 24,[d] or, nearer in, R 17 and 18, the last of which again, perhaps significantly, is Shih-kuan[2].[e] Perfect identification is thus difficult, but any reader of Kaempfer would have got quite a good idea of the technique, even though it was confined to just one particular malady.[f] On the other hand he had nothing to say about the acu-tract system which had been so puzzling to the sphygmologists.

On the moxa front, Kaempfer's account was again the clearest of any of the seventeenth-century reports.[g] He knew that the 'tinder' was made from the dried leaves of a species of mugwort (*Artemisia*),[h] and in the light of his wide experience he considered it the best cautery material of any part of Asia. He described the cones, and

[a] P. 583. It seems that Kaempfer had been through it himself. His only misunderstanding was that he thought the acupuncture needles released gases from distended parts.

[b] Presumably Shang-kuan, Chung-kuan and Hsia-kuan.

[c] See Anon. (*107*), p. 97, Anon. (135), p. 199. JM 9 and 11 are also recommended for similar conditions in modern books.

[d] Anon. (*107*), p. 229, Anon. (135), p. 107.

[e] Anon. (*107*), p. 161, Anon. (135), p. 155. Anon. (*123*), p. 233, suggests R 19, higher up, as well. In *CCTC*, ch. 9, (p. 289.1) we note an interesting technique for finding lateral points desired – a reed is cut to the length of the patient's mouth from commissure to commissure, then suspended from the umbilicus so as to form an equilateral triangle, its two ends indicating the points where moxa is to be applied. Such points, obviously below, not above, the navel, would have come somewhere between R 14 and V 27 on each side, no doubt as *chhi hsüeh* (cf. p. 52). *CCTC*, ch. 6, (p. 184. 2) also advised VU 18, on the back. Points still in use today for different kinds of *hsien chhi* are given in Chang Chün-I (*1*), ch. 6, p. 63.

[f] Kaempfer's description of the geometrical arrays of acu-points used in Japan was echoed in the middle of the following century by van Meerdervoort (1), who wrote an interesting account of his medical practice there and that of the Japanese traditional physicians; cf. Wittermans & Bowers tr., p. 98.

[g] His *Moxa, praestantissima Cauteriorum materia, Sinensibus Japonibusque multum usitata*, as it appeared in the +1694 dissertation, has been translated by Bowers & Carrubba (1). In the *Amoenitatum* it occurs on pp. 589 ff. much enlarged.

[h] Cf. *SCC*, Vol. 1, pp. 163–4, Fig. 29; Vol. 3, p. 678.

[1] 下脘 [2] 石關

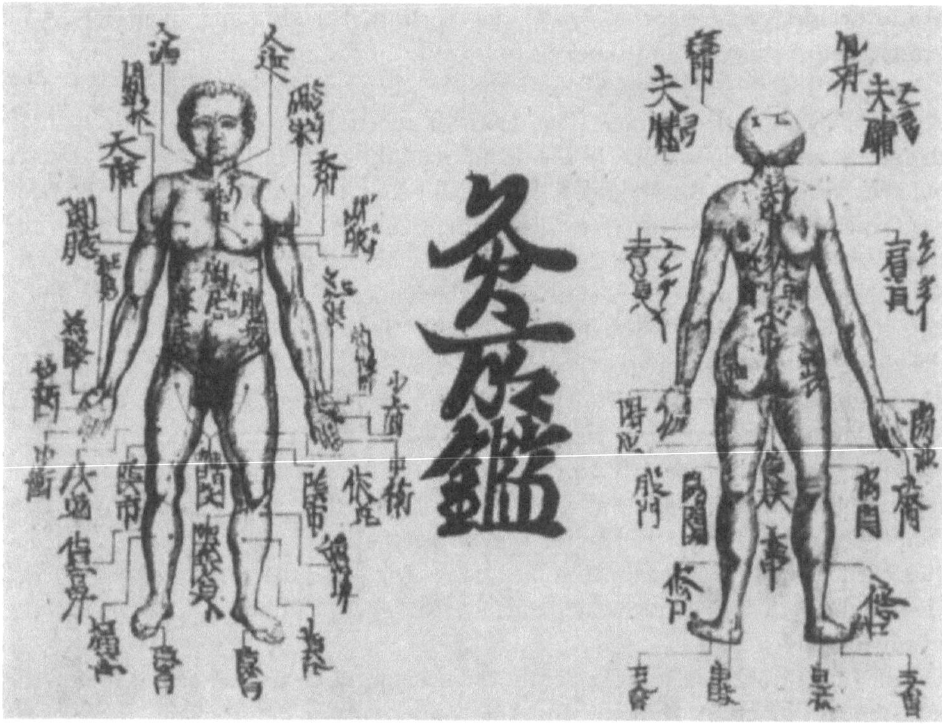

Fig. 75. Kaempfer's plate depicting the most important points where moxa was applied (1712). The title in the middle reads *Chiu So Chien*, Mirror of the Loci for Moxibustion. Since the plate must have been cut by someone who knew no Chinese or Japanese, the characters are recognisable only with great difficulty. However, if the drawings are compared with those in Figs. 39 and 40, a few correspondences can be made out, e.g. Yang-chhih (SC 4) at the back of the wrist, and Yin-ling-chhüan (LP 9) at the side of the knee. Unlike the preceding illustration, Kaempfer appended to this one a table of explanations extending to more than four pages (see text).

their close relation to temple incense, the constituents of which he studied,[a] going on to say:

The burning is not frightening in any respect. Although the appearance of the element does not particularly invite the eye, the smell of both the sticks and the small cones is most pleasant to the nose. Nor is the pain burdensome, except for the first three cones which the Japanese call *kawa kiri*,[1] that is, 'cutters of the skin'. . . The place subjected to the tinder harmonises with the affected part, though there may very often be no known anatomical connection, unless it were the common flux and fasciae of the body as a whole. Considering the places cauterised, you would think the unexpected successes illusory. For example: to facilitate birth, the tip of the small toe on the left foot; to prevent conception or to promote sterility, the navel; to relieve toothache, the adducting muscle of the thumb on the same side as the aching tooth.[b] The rest I pass over. The results do not allow us to accuse all of

[a] Cf. *SCC*, Vol. 5, pt. 2, pp. 134 ff.

[b] A clear reference to Ho-ku,[2] well-known today for its analgesic action (IG 4).

[1] 皮切 [2] 合谷

them of deception, yet sound reasoning does not permit us to testify in defence of all of them...

And to make this the more clear, Kaempfer appended an illustration (Fig. 75) with a caption headed *Kju sju Kagami*,[a] i.e. *Urendorum locorum Speculum* (Mirror of Moxibustion Loci), showing about sixty acu-points most commonly used.[b] The plate was cut by some European who did not know Chinese or Japanese, so the characters are recognisable only with difficulty. But Kaempfer added fourteen maxims indicating the treatment of a variety of affections, with ten more that deal with the conditions under which moxa should be done, and finally two on contraception and infertility.[c] Rather outstanding is his realisation that neither moxa nor acupuncture was done primarily *in loco dolenti*, a point which later Western acupuncturists would have done well to ponder; and his perplexity (knowing little of referred pain or viscero-cutaneous reflexes) about what the connections could be.

At this juncture we have to retrace oursteps a little because moxa had in fact been known in Europe at least twenty years earlier than Kaempfer's dissertation.[d] The word itself has given rise to confusion, for some have been inclined to believe that it was really Portuguese, *moxa* or *mogusa* meaning a wick or slow-match, like *mèche*

[a] I.e. *Chiu so chien.*[1]

[b] A slightly different form of this picture appeared again in Kaempfer's 'Geschichte und Beschreibung von Japan' (+1777). This has been reproduced by Veith (5), who also gives an English translation of large parts of chs. 3 and 4 of his Appendix on acupuncture and moxa. Here the material on *senki* is repeated.

[c] Kaempfer did not give clear directions about these save that for contraception moxa should be burnt at or near the umbilicus, while women wishing for children should take it on each side of the 21st vertebra (i.e. the second lumbar). Exact instructions are easy to find, however, in the old Chinese literature.

Thus contraceptive action was believed to occur with moxibustion at Shih-mên[2] (JM 5, syn. Tan-thien,[3] Ming-mên[4]) two inches below the navel; *CCTC*, ch. 7, (p. 215.2). But moxa at a point 1 in. above the ankle inside the right foot, and on the hand (IG 4), was also prescribed, as in *CCTC*, ch. 8, (p. 263.2). The ankle position was certainly one of those *ching wai chhi hsüeh*,[5] or acu-points away from any tract; and so was another named Chhi-mên,[6] recommended for the same purpose in *CCYF*, ch. 2, (p. 19.1) – this was 3 in. on each side of Kuan-yuan[7] (JM 4), again on the lower abdomen. On *chhi hsüeh* in general see Chhêng Tan-An (*1*), pp. 195 ff.; it has been usual to number 132 of them, but that was before the most recent developments regarding the ears and hands. Almost three-quarters of these *chhi hsüeh* were used for moxibustion only, not acupuncture. Anon. (135) selects 36 as the most important for description. It gives no name to the ankle point mentioned above, but calls the points lateral to Kuan-yuan Wei-pao[8] rather than Chhi-mên,[6] and numbers them as Chhi (Extra) 15.

As for the promotion of fertility, there were acu-points on the back, just as Kaempfer said, notably Shen-shu[9] (VU 23) and Shang-liao[10] (VU 31), the former corresponding pretty closely with his anatomical indication. See on them *CCTC*, ch. 6, (pp. 185.1, 186.1). But there were also points to be cauterised on the inner surface of the foot, e.g. R 2, cf. *CCYF*, ch. 2, (p. 19.1); and LP 5, cf. *CCTC*, ch. 8, (p. 263.1). And curiously enough there were also points on the abdomen, e.g. Kuan-yuan[11] itself (JM 4), Chung-chi[12] (JM 3), Tzu-kung[13] (Chhi or Extra 7 or 16, see Anon. (*107*), p. 238, Anon. (135), pp. 208–9) and Tzu-hu[14] (Chhi or Extra, see Anon. (*123*), p. 256). This we can see from an interesting picture in the *Chen Chiu Chhüan Shu*[15] (Complete Treatise on Acupuncture and Moxibustion) by Chhen Yen[16] (+1591), ch. 2, p. 93*a* of the +1601 ed. (facsim., p. 263) entitled Fu-jen Thai Lêng Wu Yün,[17] 'Women with wombs too cold to bear children', i.e. with insufficient Yang.

[d] There are special papers on its history in the West by von Reichert (1) and Feucht (2), supplemented by (1).

1 灸所鑑 2 石門 3 丹田 4 命門 5 經外奇穴 6 氣門
7 關元 8 維胞 9 腎兪 10 上髎 11 關元 12 中極
13 子宮 14 子戶 15 針灸全書 16 陳言 17 婦人胎冷無孕

in French or *myxa* in Spanish, this last the same as in classical Latin. It would thus have become current after the first Portuguese contacts in the +16th century. But this supposition is probably gratuitous since Japanese origins lie ready to hand – *mogusa*[1] (*jan tshao*,[1] herb for burning)[a] and *momigusa*[2] (*jou tshao*,[2] herb dried to soft tinder).[b] *Mogusa* was more properly pronounced *moe-gusa*,[1] hence perhaps the '*moje kousa*' of Hübotter (7).[c] Japanese lexicographers give as alternatives for *mogusa*, first *yomogi*[3] (*ai*,[3] *Artemisia* spp.), or *gaiyo*[4] (*ai yeh*,[4] *Artemisia* leaves), or *sashimogusa*[5] (*ai tshao*,[5] *Artemisia* herb). This last word occurs in a love-poem by Fujiwara Sanekata,[6] who compares his passionate feelings to the burning pain caused by the *sashimogusa* of Ibuki.[d] Since this poem occurs in the imperial collection entitled *Goshūiwakashū*,[7] which was compiled in +1086, it seems rather superfluous to appeal to words in the Romance languages.[e]

However this may be, its first appearance in a Western printed book was in +1674, when Hermann Buschof produced his 'Het Podagra...' on gout and arthritic conditions.[f] But he never saw it, as he died that year. Buschof was a learned Dutch Reformed minister friendly with ten Rhijne in Batavia, and himself deeply grateful for the good results which moxa cautery had brought in his own case, applied by a Chinese or Indonesian woman doctor. There followed many publications—Geilfuss in +1676, Gehema in +1682, Valentini in +1686, but of them all the 'Verhandeling van het Podagra...' of Stephen Blankaart (+1684) was perhaps the most influential.[g] It included a previously unpublished letter or memorandum of ten Rhijne: 'On the Chinese and Japanese Way of curing all kinds of Diseases completely and with certainty by burning with Moxa and implanting golden Needles.'[h] This phase of literature elucidated gradually the true nature of the moxa material used in East Asia, and sought to substitute for it all kinds of organic substances such as cotton, cobwebs, the pith of the elder or the bulrush, stalks of wild crowfoot, and so on.[i]

The time was marked by two other events of interest – the experiences of Sir William Temple (+1628 to +1699) and the eminent clinician Thomas Sydenham

[a] A synonym was *jukugai*[8] (*shu ai*,[8] hot *Artemisia*).

[b] The leaves were dried and rubbed, whereupon the body crumbles to dust leaving the white hairs on the under surface; these, matted together and mixed with a combustible vehicle, form the moxa.

[c] Not meaning, as he seems to have thought, 'burning the skin'.

[d] Ibuki in Shige is famous to this day for its *mogusa*.

[e] Of course this might have been another case of a reaction which we meet with elsewhere (*SCC*, Vol. 5, pt. 4, p. 474), where early travellers have remarked, thinking of some word already known to them but without any real linguistic connection, 'how strange, that's just what we say'.

[f] An English translation appeared two years later; Brockbank (1), p. 126 reproduces its frontispiece. A German translation of part of Buschof's lively dialogue text is given by Feucht (2). Parts were also included in the article of Elsholz (1) in +1676: 'Von den chinesischen Moxa, ein Mittel wider das Zipperlein'.

[g] German translation, +1692.

[h] Pp. 318ff.

[i] The nature of the original was confirmed in a letter from Andreas Cleyer in +1679. If the substitutes were not as efficacious as they might have been, the reason might lie in an actual absorption of some active principle from the *Artemisia* during its burning, surmised more recently by some (cf. p. 171). Among incidental mentions at this time there was a brief discussion of moxa in Jean Crasset's history of the Church in Japan (+1689).

1 燃草 2 揉草 3 艾 4 艾葉 5 艾草 6 滕原實方
7 後拾遺和歌集 8 熟艾

(+1624 to +1689). Temple, the eminent diplomat, and literary protagonist in the 'quarrel of the Ancients and Moderns', was suddenly attacked by extremely painful gout[a] during an international conference at Nijmegen in +1677. For this, moxibustion was so successful that he devoted an enthusiastic essay to 'the Cure of the Gout by Moxa' in the first part of his *Miscellanea* (+1693).[b] Ten years earlier Sydenham, too, had written upon gout, taking a less favourable view of moxa, however;[c] but what is more interesting, he pronounced himself 'against acupuncture (though a famous remedy) in dropsy'. This must mean that by the last two decades of the +17th century acupuncture (of a sort) as well as moxibustion was already practised fairly widely in Western Europe.

Neither took root, however. Less than a dozen years after Kaempfer and Floyer acupuncture and moxibustion were both treated of in the surgical textbooks of Heister (+1718)[d] and Junker (+1722)[e] but without any enthusiasm, as remedies which had gone out of fashion. Partly also there was a vigorous reaction from the partisans of cauterisation with red-hot irons, a barbarous procedure which lasted to a surprisingly late time. But if clinical usage declined, theoretical interest continued. In +1755 Gerhard van Swieten wrote a singularly prophetic passage:[f]

> The acupuncture of the Japanese and the cautery of various parts of the body with (Chinese) moxa seem to stimulate the nerves and thereby to alleviate pains and cramps in quite different parts of the body in a most wonderful way. It would be an extraordinarily useful enterprise if someone would take the trouble to note and investigate the marvellous communion which the nerves have with one another, and at what points certain nerves lie which when stimulated can calm the pain at distant sites. The physicians of Asia, who knew no (modern) anatomy, have by long practical experience identified such points.

And towards the end of the century Rougemont firmly classified acupuncture and moxibustion among the agents of counter-irritation.[g]

In the meantime further information and stimuli kept on coming from the East. Dujardin & Peyrilhe, in their history of surgery, published in +1774, thought fit to devote a special section to 'La Chirrugie des Chinois et des Japonais', where they reproduced ten Rhijne's four illustrations as plates.[h] In the following year a Chinese

[a] Acute paroxysmal arthritis, as we should today call it; cf. Cecil & Loeb (1), pp. 605ff. The role of purine metabolism and uric acid is still unclear, but some analgesic is unquestionably necessary.

[b] Pt. I, pp. 185ff. He returned to the subject in Pt. III, p. 189. See also his letters edited by Jonathan Swift. A similar experience befell Purmann in +1692, (1), pp. 306–7.

[c] Works, vol. 2, pp. 156–7; on dropsy, p. 181. One must remember that the acute attacks of gout are spaced out with complete remissions, but that does not mean that the analgesic action of acupuncture and moxibustion could not reduce the duration of the paroxysmal phases. To what extent they could cure radically what is probably a metabolic disease is another matter (cf. p. 197 above).

[d] (1), pt. 2, sect. 1, ch. 18

[e] (1), p. 624.

[f] (1), sect. 650.

[g] (1), sect. 159. A considerable number of writers were quite sagacious on this score, including P. F. von Siebold (+1796 to 1866) a famous naturalist and traveller in East Asia, who published a study of Japanese acupuncture in 1832 (1). Cf. Busk (1), p. 308, who in 1841 added a reference to Titsingh's book and 'doll'.

[h] (1), vol. 1, pp. 88ff. for moxa, pp. 95ff. for acupuncture. An edited reproduction of this section has been published by Khoubesserian (2).

merchant, Whan A-Tong,[a] appeared in London, and demonstrated to the curious a nude model figure with the acu-tracts and loci marked upon it; this was probably the first time that a *thung jen*[1] had been seen in the West. In +1787 the great physiological anatomist Vicq-d'Azyr wrote a short treatise on acupuncture, rather favourable in tone.[b] Then after the great naturalist C. P. Thunberg returned from his travels in East Asia in +1779, he had a good deal to say about the two techniques.[c] Of acupuncture he remarked that the places for implantation are most carefully selected by the operators, who have 'printed tables' of them, and that 'the needles are very fine, nearly as thin as the hairs of one's head', and twirled by the acupuncturists. As for moxa, it was used by everyone, 'as often as phlebotomy in Europe'; indeed he was convinced that it was 'of use in mo t disorders, but especially in the Pleurisy, Toothache, etc. and it proves of the greatest service in Gout and Rheumatisms'. After his return to Sweden Thunberg succeeded Linnaeus, and it is interesting to read the inaugural dissertation on moxibustion by young Hallman (1) benignly presided over by Thunberg at Uppsala in +1788.

(iii) *The nineteenth century and after*

The nineteenth century opened with the coming of another acupuncture statuette to Europe, among the possessions of Isaac Titsingh. Titsingh was a surgeon by training who had joined the Dutch East India Company in +1768 and become the head of the Deshima station from +1779 onwards; then unexpectedly in +1794 he found himself Ambassador to Peking, the last of the old series of Dutch embassies.[d] After the mission was completed he returned to Europe and spent the last few years of his life, till 1812, in arranging his collections, afterwards dispersed.[e] His acupuncture figure, called a '*tsoë bosi*',[f] became renowned, and we have a description of it in the catalogue of his treasures:

Japanese Acupuncture and Moxa

One very large folio notebook with twenty drawings, and a painted doll on which are indicated by means of points, lines and characters, the spots at which it is proper, and safe, to practise these two therapeutic methods. The doll was a gift from the Imperial Physician of highest rank. This little human image, about 30 in. high, is made from cardboard (or papier-maché) and painted flesh colour, with the ribs, the vertebral column, the muscles and the principal sinuosities of the body well brought out. The characters and numbers marked on it refer to a Japanese book of particulars in sexto-decimo, in which there are

[a] We do not know the characters, nor any further details, because the information depends upon Pelletan (2), so rare as to be unavailable for consultation in England. See Feucht (4*b*).

[b] *Oeuvres*, vol. 5, pp. 133 ff. He agreed with Rougemont about counter-irritation.

[c] (1), vol. 3, pp. 74, 226, vol. 4, pp. 73, 75.

[d] On this see Duyvendak (12).

[e] One of the best biographies of him is in Boxer (5). A catalogue of his library was published by de Landresse (1); on acupuncture see vol. 2, p. 38.

[f] Conjecturally *tsu hōshi*[2] or *tsū hōshi*.[3] The second word, Buddhist abbot, is quite reasonable, because the figure had a hairless head as if shaven, but the first is guesswork. There are many contemporary mentions and descriptions of it, e.g. Heyfelder (1); Anon. (140). Some thought that the figure was of metal, with pinholes, and paper glued all over it. Cf. Feucht (1), pp. 30, 36, 41.

[1] 銅人 [2] 通法師 [3] 痛法師

engravings and descriptions, and in which one can find, according to the number indicated, the name and nature of the part, the diseases to which it is subject, the manner in which it ought when necessary to be needled, and the number of times that this should be done, together with the remedies which ought (also) to be applied to it.

An ebony case containing various needles, and tinder prepared for moxa, belong with this item.[a]

Titsingh translated a tractate on acupuncture, entitled by Rémusat *Tchin Kieou Ki Pi Tchhao*[b] and said to have been written by a Japanese physician of Kimura in +1780. Titsingh was no great sinologist, but his manuscripts came before long to the knowledge of Sarlandière in Paris, and helped to stimulate a new wave of acupuncture practice.[c]

From 1800 onwards, during the first half of the century indeed, there was great activity in the use of acupuncture and moxibustion clinically. Yet in spite of the '*tsoë bosi*' figures and all the other information which had come through, albeit imperfectly, no attention whatever was paid to the acu-tract system of China, nor to the close connection between needling and pulse-diagnosis. Basically it was the *ah shih hsüeh* (cf. p. 127) all over again, acupuncture *in loco dolenti*.[d] Still, enough was obtained in good results to sustain the practice for many years. In France the first book (1816) was that of Berlioz (1), the father of the composer; he described many interesting cases, including 'nervous fever' in a girl resulting from fright,[e] and whooping-cough in countryfolk, but as might be expected, the best successes were in muscle and joint stiffness after falls, and many rheumatic and arthritic states, often with dramatic effectiveness.[f] Then came Sarlandière (1) in 1825 (already mentioned, p. 188), the first to apply electric currents to the implanted needles.[g] He reported curative successes in many respiratory affections including asthma, various forms of paralysis, migraines and of course the rheumatisms. Similar results were published from another Paris hospital at just the same time by Cloquet & Dantu (1), the experiences of Cloquet's clinic being reported *in extenso* by his disciple Dantu (1, 2). Here the emphasis was very much on analgesic effects, including the relief of facial neuralgia and other forms of intractable pain as well as the usual treatment of sciatica, arthritis etc. These clinicians would sometimes leave the needles in place for as long as eight

[a] Titsingh (1), p. xviii; (2), p. 315.

[b] Conceivably *Chen Chiu Chi Pi Chhao*,[1] but we have not been able to identify it in any catalogue, and we cannot interpret Rémusat's romanisation of the names of the author or his teacher; Rémusat (12), vol. 1, pp. 270, 374. The latter reference is in an interesting essay in which Rémusat (14) sketched the Western knowledge of acupuncture down to 1825. The former (15) is on Titsingh. De Landresse, *loc. cit.* made it a Chinese physician, Yuan Thai-Chung, writing at Fukushima.

[c] Apparently Julius Klaproth was instrumental in this transmission.

[d] This was not invariably true, for occasionally remote sites were used. For example, in the seventies, Dumontpallier applied acupuncture needles not where the pain was, but at the same place on the opposite side of the body (Anon. 144). But there was no Chinese theory behind this.

[e] Today this case history reads like conversion hysteria. On Berlioz cf. Craffe (1). He seems to have started experimenting with acupuncture at least as early as 1809.

[f] Following upon some controversies in which Berlioz was involved, a number of pathologists carried out animal experiments to determine the degree of danger inherent in acupuncture; cf. Feucht (4a). On the whole the judgments were favourable.

[g] Cf. Vergier (1).

[1] 針灸極秘鈔

hours, but again described many cases of dramatic cessation of pain within seconds of implantation. This brings us to 1828, and in the following year there appeared Honoré de Balzac's 'Physiologie du Mariage'. In the course of this witty book, which in many ways anticipated the enlightened sexology of the present day, Balzac, perhaps with tongue in cheek, gives much ironical and sage advice to husbands concerning the advances of the dreaded 'célibataires'. So in a chapter on strategies of distraction we suddenly find him saying:

> After all, in medicine when an inflammation breaks out at some capital point in the organism, they carry out a little counter-revolution at some other point by means of moxas, scarifications, acupuncture needles, etc. Or again, you can apply a moxa to your wife, or implant in her mind some deeply pricking needle which will assure a diversion in your favour.[a]

And he goes on to tell how a certain gentleman, conscious of the imminent acceptance by his wife of a lover, told her that half their fortune was lost and that they would have to retire to the country, where in due course by means of building a Gothic wing on to the château, arranging new lakes and fountains in the park, and a hundred other occupations – conjugal moxas, Balzac calls them – the danger was finally overpast. All this is simply to show that in 1829 acupuncture and moxibustion were a matter of course in polite European society, and readily available for metaphorical use.

All the principal European countries participated in this fashion. The first Italian book was that of Bozetti (1) in 1820, the most famous that of Carraro (1) in 1825, and perhaps the most curious and interesting writings those of da Camin (1, 2) in the thirties.[b] Da Camin followed Sarlandière in applying electric currents, for which he used Leyden jars. In general at this time nearly everyone, following the lead given by van Swieten long before, thought that the effects of acupuncture were mediated through the nervous system, but also that they were in some sense or other 'galvanic' or electrical.[c] Much rather primitive experimental work was devoted to investigating this, with some on animals, but the far more sophisticated ideas and instrumentation of our own time had to come into being before much progress could be expected in the understanding of the rationale of acupuncture and moxibustion in terms of modern physiology and pathology.

Acupuncture also made a new start at the beginning of the nineteenth century in Germany. In 1806 the playwright August von Kotzebue published in his magazine *The Candid Observer* (*Funny and Serious*) a letter, ostensibly from his son who was travelling in the Far East, which gave a rather satirical picture of acupuncture as seen in Japan.[d] This stimulated a long paper from an anonymous physician urging that it

[a] (1), p. 181. 'Les voyages en Italie, en Suisse, en Grèce, les maladies subites qui exigent les eaux, et les eaux les plus éloignées, sont d'assez bons moxas...'

[b] The centre of interest in Italy was in the lands of the Venetian Republic. There is a paper by Premuda (1) on the Italian clinicians interested in acupuncture at this time.

[c] So, for example, Pelletan (1) commenting on Berlioz; Pouillet (1); Rémusat (14) also accepted this. See Feucht (1), p. 32.

[d] Feucht (1), p. 29, (4*c*), p. 164. The reply contains the first mention in the West of the *wu hu hsüeh fa*[1] (cf. p. 178). On this see Hsieh Li-Hêng (*2*), p. 390.

[1] 五虎穴法

should be taken more seriously, if with due scepticism, and describing similar eye-witness experiences there of an open-minded Erlangen professor, J. P. J. Rudolf (+1729 to +1797). Rudolf had made a collection in +1770 of acupuncture needles and other things pertaining to Japanese medicine, together with books and drawings, but unfortunately these were dispersed and the notes never published. Clinical acupuncture was rather slow in developing in Germany, and at first physicians there were interested in it partly in connection with arousal from coma and partly for the prevention of premature burial. While in France it was quickly adopted in hospital clinics (as by Cloquet and Sarlandière) in Germany it was tried mostly by private practitioners. The earliest records date from about 1822,[a] and in the following year J. M. L. Farina (the son of the famous eau-de-cologne distiller) described a striking cure of facial neuralgia. By 1828 there were important papers by Bernstein (1) and Lohmayer (1), reporting good results in rheumatism, while Woost (1) in 1826 surveyed the whole scene in East and West in his dissertation *Quaedam de Acupunctura Orientalium...*[b] In Vienna many veterinary surgeons took it up. But by the time of Dieffenbach (1845) it was no longer attracting much interest.[c]

In England there was a very similar wave of activity during the first half of the century. Acupuncture was sufficiently well known for a country general practitioner like Coley (1, 2) to write about it in 1802, having performed paracentesis on an infant with tympanites.[d] He had the *senki*[1] of ten Rhijne and Kaempfer very much in mind, and acupunctured such patients at the loci that Kaempfer had described, as nearly as he could. But the first great protagonist was J. M. Churchill (1, 2), who published two books on it in 1821 and 1828. The first was entitled: 'A Treatise on Acupuncturation; being a Description of a Surgical Operation originally peculiar to the Japanese and Chinese, and by them denominated Zin-King,[e] now introduced into European Practice, with Directions for its Performance, and Cases illustrating its Success.'[f] The second book added many case-histories. Most of Churchill's achievements were with what he called 'local diseases of the muscular and fibrous structures of the body', i.e. rheumatic conditions, sciatica, back-pain, muscle strains, trismus, often traumatic in origin (e.g. after falls); but he also had some good results in dropsical states, oedema, anasarca, etc. (cf. Fig. 76). He clearly observed the *tê chhi*[2] effect, the immediate numbness or heaviness, though not knowing about this from Chinese writings, and the speed of its onset inspired him to write:

> It has long been supposed that the nerves are the media by which a fluid, analogous to the galvanic, is circulated or conveyed to the remotest parts of our structure...and as the effects

[a] Feucht (1), pp. 34, 41.
[b] Feucht (1), p. 38. Sweden contributed an interesting Uppsala thesis by Landgren (1) in 1829.
[c] (1), art. Akupunktur.
[d] See Haller (1) and Anon. (141), who both give good accounts of the development of the practice of acupuncture in England.
[e] *Chen Ching*?[3]
[f] The book was translated into German in 1824 and French in 1825 so that it had considerable influence on the continent. Among several recent writers interested in Churchill, Lippert & Lippert (1) are to be mentioned.

[1] 疝氣 [2] 得氣 [3] 針經

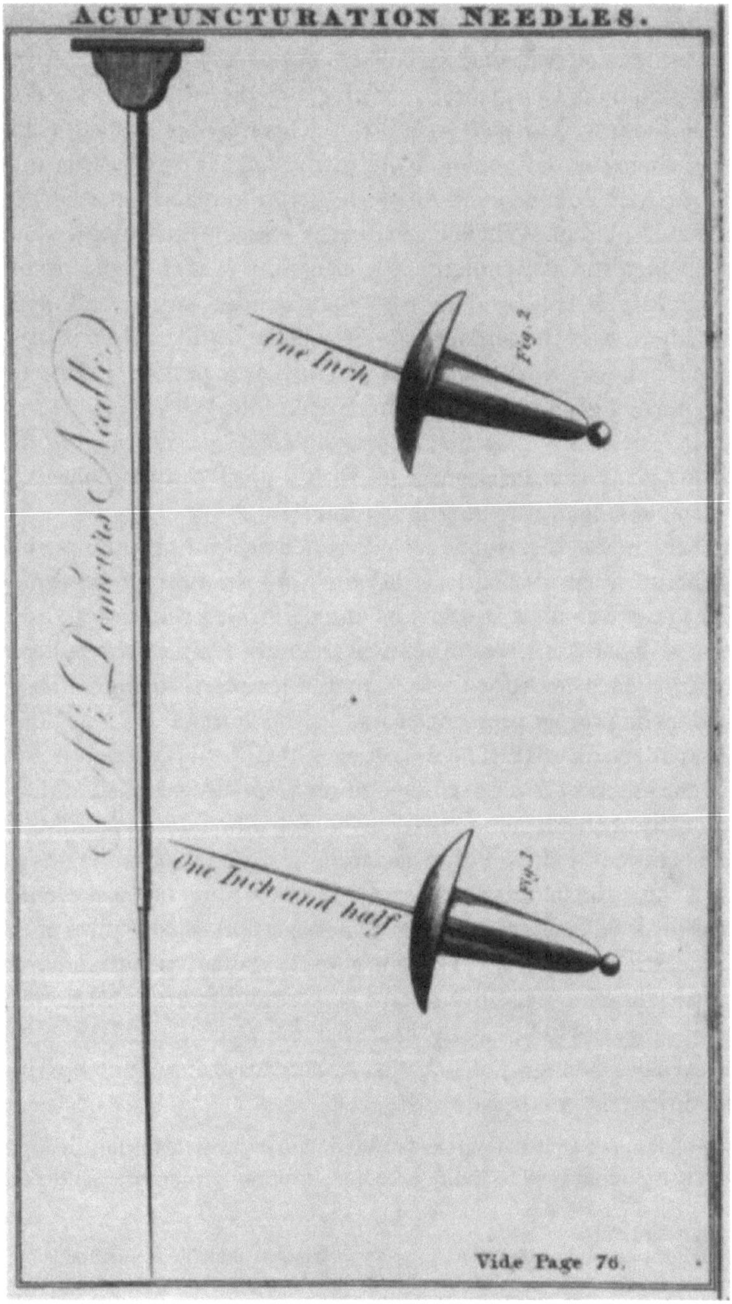

Fig. 76. Needles described in J. M. Churchill's 'Treatise on Acupuncturation . . .' of 1821.

of acupuncture are so instantaneous, it is very natural to infer that they proceed from, or are affected by, some principle like to, or connected with, the electric, pervading the animal machine.[a]

One wonders what exactly had brought acupuncture to England at the turn of the century, for Churchill had had his predecessors; he speaks of the practice of Dr Edward Jukes, whose patient, a Mr Scott of Westminster, had been probably the first to be treated successfully with acupuncture in this country. Though Churchill's enthusiasm did not quickly spread, interest grew, and Wansborough (1) described wittily a case of lumbago in which the pain had been driven by the needles from one part of the body to another, and finally relieved altogether. Later John Elliotson (+1791 to 1868), whom we have already encountered in connection with the history of hypnotism (p. 237), supported the use of acupuncture too. During the forties the Leeds Infirmary became a great centre of the technique, mainly for the treatment of chronic rheumatism and similar diseases, rivalling the fame of the Paris hospitals in this direction. From these European centres the art had already spread to North America, as is evidenced by the reports of Morand (1) and Bache (1), both of 1825.[b]

Subsequent developments were rather bizarre. In the middle of the century very little acupuncture was being done, though it could still find an entry in surgical treatises such as that of Billroth (1863); and what there was of it became attached to one of the major concerns of the medical charlatans of the time, 'spermatorrhoea'. The sexual fears of Victorian males were exacerbated by decade-long campaigns against masturbation and 'nocturnal pollutions', for the cure of which needles were inserted in the perineal region about half-way between the scrotal bursae and the anus.[c] Impotence and urethral irritation[d] were also greatly feared, hence acupuncture in the perineal and especially prostatic regions. The irrational fear of seminal loss went back, no doubt, to ancient Western medical ideas analogous to the doctrine of 'catarrh',[e] for just as the brain made phlegm so also the semen was a *cerebri stillicidium* dangerous to lose.[f] But here too there was a strangely Chinese echo. In the centuries-old tradition of physiological alchemy[g] we found the *idée fixe* that the conservation of semen was one of the most important aids to the attainment of material immortality —and not only its conservation but its actual engineered return upwards to nourish the brain. And it seems an almost more than extraordinary coincidence that the region between the scrotum and the anus was precisely where the Taoist adepts applied the pressure that re-routed the semen at the moment of ejaculation into the bladder and not the exterior.[h] It would be a fascinating achievement to trace out the path of transmission of ideas from the medieval Taoists to the prudish and superstitious Victorian doctors; in itself a truly incongruous juxtaposition.

[a] (1), p. 5.
[b] Cf. Cassedy (1).
[c] See Deslandes (1); Lallemand (1), pp. 392ff.; Anon. (143).
[d] A condition of infection terminated by a mere change in the urinary pH, as we know today.
[e] See Pagel (10), pp. 165ff.
[f] On the 'white' and the 'red' see Needham (2), p. 60.
[g] See *SCC*, Vol. 5, pt. 5.
[h] The acu-point is JM 1, clearly shown in Mann (3) and all the usual atlases.

In Germany a different aberration developed and flourished for a time. A mechanic from Edinich, Charles Baunscheidt, invented in the forties a 'resuscitator' (*Lebenswecker*) which consisted of 30 or more gold-plated needles fixed in a holder and driven into the skin of the patient at the release of a spring. The peculiarity of the method was that an *Oleum Baunscheidtii*, containing cyanide, croton oil and other irritants, was then painted over the place, resulting in an exanthematous eruption. The whole process, claimed as a panacea by Baunscheidt and his supporters, was thus but another form of counter-irritation by blistering, but it became fashionable among German-Americans and for a time gained much popularity in the United States.[a] The spring mechanism was evidently derived from similar arrangements in the 'scarifiers' used for bleeding, but the arrangement of needles is reminiscent of the multiple-needle techniques used in China,[b] so here again it would be interesting to trace possible Chinese influences on Baunscheidtism. The method was used as late as 1900 in America, but in Europe it had sunk without trace at a much earlier time.

In the preceding paragraphs we have neglected moxibustion, but it followed the fortunes of acupuncture with no less than 19 theses on the subject before 1850, after which it was almost lost to sight.[c] One of the best of these was the *De Usu Moxae* of Avery (1) defended at Edinburgh in 1821; and in the following year there appeared the English translation of the book of D. J. Larrey (1), the distinguished French army surgeon, who was a great believer in it. Asthma, tuberculosis, rheumatism, gout and paralysis were the sort of affections it was used for, but Larrey burnt cotton cylinders, and others the pith of sunflower stalks.[d] There was at this time a great dispute with men like Valentin (1) who in 1815 upheld cautery with red-hot irons, giving descriptions quite hair-raising to read today, especially in cases of hysteria and other nervous and mental diseases. In Dublin William Wallace (1827) employed the very Chinese technique of burning moxa on the ends of implanted needles, though paying little attention to classical acu-points;[e] he had some striking successes with facial neuralgia and the usual rheumatoid group. He often took the moxa off before it actually burnt the skin; if eschars formed he washed them with silver nitrate or copper sulphate and kept them covered with plaster. Sarlandière emphasised that *Artemisia* should be used, but as it was difficult to obtain in Europe the practice in general almost died out during the second half of the century.

Finally in the last decades of the last century the Western world gradually began to take acupuncture seriously again, and its study rose in a crescendo to the many investigations of the present time. One important event was the publication of Dabry de Thiersant's book on Chinese medicine (1) in 1863, where he gave a translation of

[a] Cf. the full description, with illustrations, in Haller (1).

[b] Cf. pp. 130, 164 above.

[c] The general pattern of interest in acupuncture and moxa during the first half of the century, followed by eclipse during the second half, presents itself in Russia too. The writings of Tsarukowsky in and around 1828 were a landmark, but subsequently the techniques were forgotten until under quite new political circumstances interest re-awakened and an official mission went to China to study them in 1956 led by Tikojinskaia. See Vogralik (2) with Chinese translation in Anon. (*108*), and Li Yuan-Chi (*1*), reprinted in Chhêng Tan-An *et al.* (*3*).

[d] Cf. Brockbank (1), pp. 127–8.

[e] (1), p. 71.

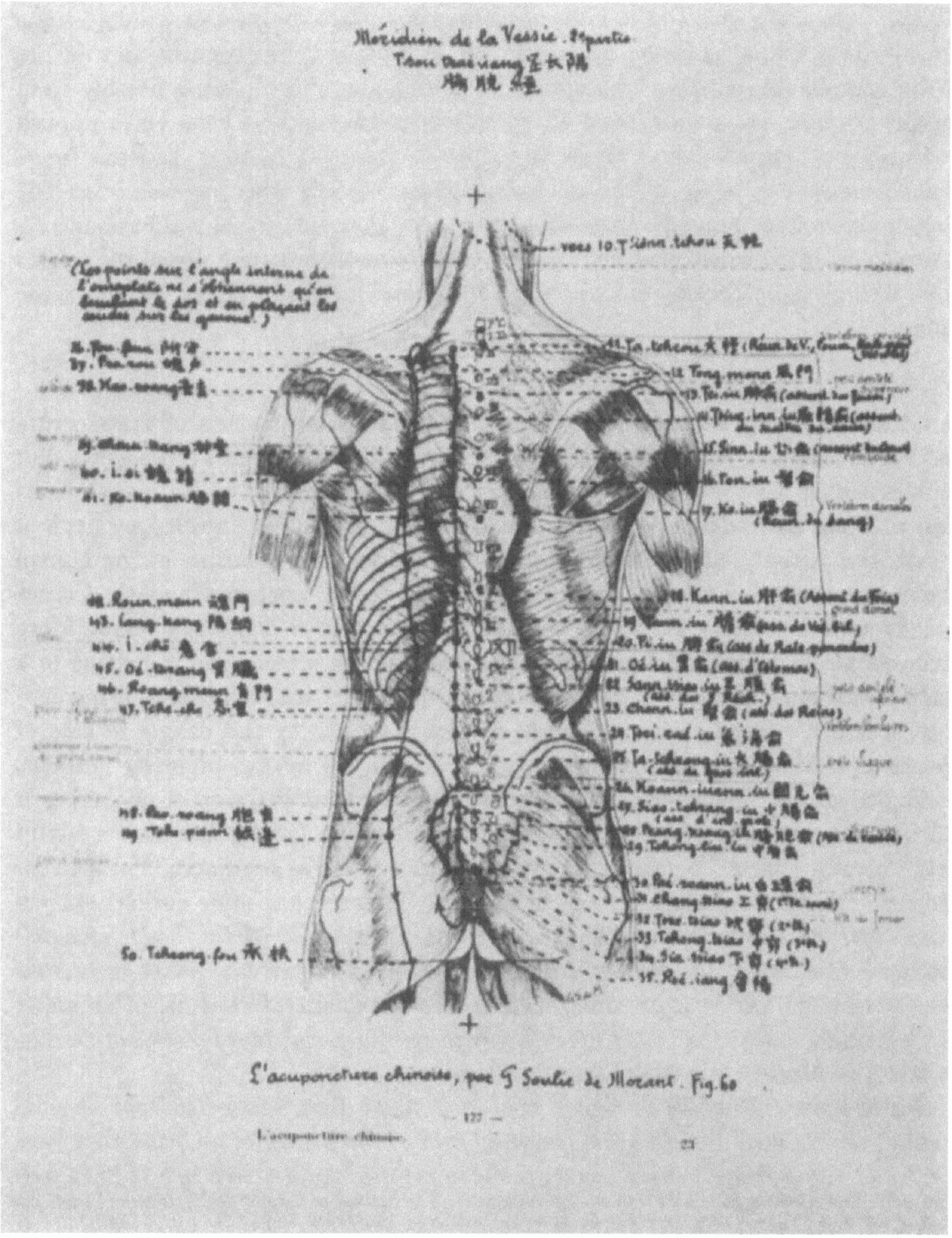

selected passages from the *Chen Chiu Ta Chhêng* (cf. p. 159). It was slow to make any impression, however, and presumably a more important factor was the great increase of contacts between Europeans and people of East Asia brought about by modern means of transport and communication, an increase which certainly involved medical men as well as others. The wheel has now come full circle, and we may recall what was said at the beginning of this monograph (p. 11) about the multiple streams of clinical experience which have influenced Western practitioners and writers—some directly from China, as in the case of Soulié de Morant in the twenties and thirties of the present century (Fig. 77), others from Vietnam, and of course notably from Japan.[a] Societies grew up in most of the European countries and started to publish bulletins and journals – the French in 1950, the Germans in 1951, and the International Society in 1954. In the celebrated phrase, this is where we came in. The development of acupuncture analgesia about 1960, alongside the age-old therapeutic system, placed the whole problem upon an entirely new basis, and alerted the worlds of physiology and pathology to something of profound interest. The rest belongs to the future.

(7) The Lore of Vital Spots

In all the foregoing discussions of therapy and analgesia by means of acupuncture and moxibustion we have been dealing with manifestations of man's compassion. But an outstanding feature of these two techniques, so characteristic of traditional medicine in China and Japan, was that they involved a large body of knowledge (much of which was certainly not illusory) about precise points on the surface of the human body, just as capable of cartography as the stars in the macrocosm above. Consequently such knowledge could also be used in the service of man's aggression. Were there points of particular danger in the anatomy which would give advantage to a warrior who knew them, even in unarmed combat? There are such points, as medico-legal specialists very well know,[b] spots of special sensitivity and danger in case of violent assault, where trauma, contusion or shock will be exceptionally perilous, leading to internal injury or death, sometimes with no external sign of wounding at all. Chinese expressions for these danger-points are either *to ming tien mo*,[1] 'a fateful spot', or *tien hsüeh*,[2] 'a vital acu-point', the latter clearly associating this present chapter with the acupuncture story as a whole. Japanese has some curious expressions, perhaps euphemisms, such as *atemi*[3] (confrontation of the body), *kyūsho*[4] (instant-effect places) and *kinsho*[5] (forbidden places). This last expression again links us with acupuncture, for at an earlier stage we had to explain the existence of a number of 'forbidden acu-points' (*chin hsüeh*[6]), where needling and moxa were not recommended, or allowed only under specific conditions (p. 68).

It is necessary therefore to take a brief look at the East Asian traditions of close combat, the 'martial arts' (*wu shu*,[7] *bujutsu*,[7] or *wu i shu*[8]).[c] In recent years they have

[a] A book such as that of T. Nakayama (1), published in Paris, may be recalled here. In China there has been great interest in the European developments. The school of Soulié de Morant has been described by Yeh Ching-Chhiu (*1*), and other work in France has been studied by Liu Yung-Shun (*2*). Modern Western opinions have been collected by Hsiao Yung-Thang (*1*), and many original papers both in Russian and other Western languages have been assembled and translated into Chinese (Anon. *108*).

[b] We are particularly grateful to Dr J. M. Cameron and Dr Bernard Sims of the London Hospital Department of Forensic Medicine for discussions on these and other questions.

[c] It is distinctly difficult to ascertain hard historical facts frcm the abundant literature on these subjects, most of it being quasi-esoteric and unscholarly. The absence of informative sinological references in the book of Huard & Huang Kuang-Ming (7) is particularly tantalising. See however Huang Wên-Shan (1), pp. 34ff.

[1] 奪命點脈 [2] 點穴 [3] 當身 [4] 急所 [5] 禁所 [6] 禁穴
[7] 武術 [8] 武藝術

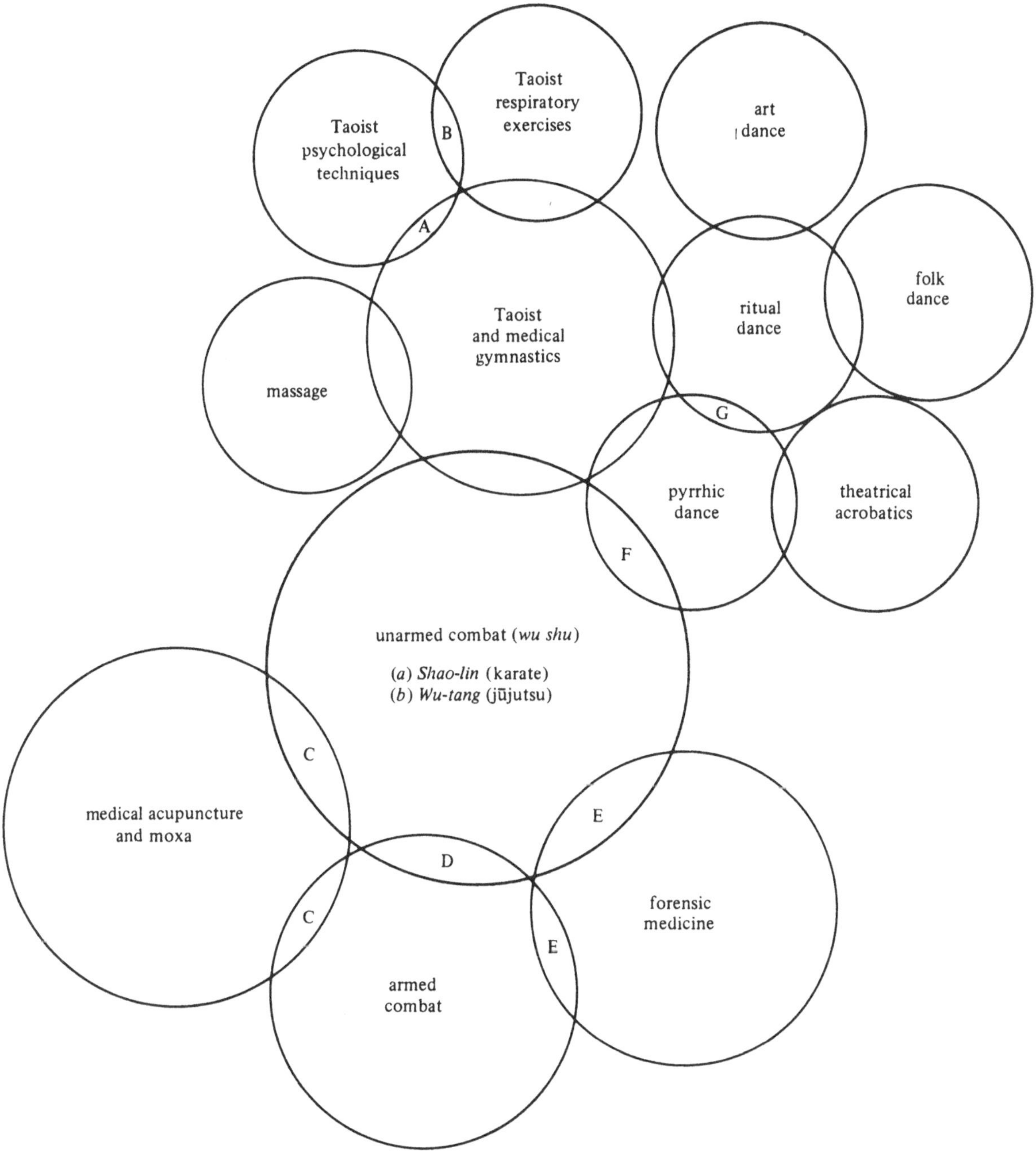

A āsana, quasi-yogistic positions
B anoxaemic states
C vital spots or danger points
D spike-and-chain, thrown darts, etc.
E practice of coroners
F *Thai-chi chhüan*
G Confucian temple dances

Fig. 78. Chart to show the relationships between the many Chinese psycho-somatic practices; see text.

become extremely well known and popular throughout the world under the name of *kung fu*[1],[a] but this term, 'attainment', applied primarily to the various kinds of bodily training or callisthenics which formed part of the Taoist armamentarium of techniques for longevity and material immortality. No more need be said about these in this context, for we describe them in detail elsewhere.[b] Yet it is useful to think of the martial arts as component elements of a wide range of psycho-somatic practices (Fig. 78), ranging from the psychological techniques of meditation through the respiratory exercises (*nei kung*[2]) and massage (*an mo*[3]) to physio-therapeutic gymnastics (*tao yin*[4])[c] and so to unarmed combat (*chhüan po*[5]).[d] This again shades off into armed combat on one side and to the pyrrhic dance on the other, while that again has relations with the ritual dance and beyond it to art or entertainment dance forms, with folk dances and theatrical acrobatics as close neighbours. Concentrating our attention on unarmed combat for the present purpose, one has to distinguish first between boxing and wrestling, i.e. between those forms in which hitting or striking happens and those in which gripping and overthrowing the adversary are more important. The natural use of the closed fist is called *chhüan fa*[6] (*kempō*[6]), but in some forms of combat the hand is kept open and used like a knife; this is known as *khai shou*[7] (*kaishu*[7]). Let us consider in turn the traditions of Shao-lin boxing, *karate*, *jūdō*, *sumō*, *Thai-chi chhüan*, the use of the spike-and-chain, and the throw of sharp darts, proceeding no further in the direction of arms.

It may not have been quite the beginning of the affair, but for our present purpose it is sufficient to start from an ancient Chinese sport known as *chio ti*[8,9,10], 'butting with horns', in which two combatants without weapons fought with one another, each wearing an ox skin with horns on the head.[e] This martial art, also called *hsiang phu*,[11] 'mutual assault',[f] was in vogue at least as early as the −3rd century, when it was a favourite spectacle of the second Chhin emperor.[g] A celebrated tournament of it was organised at the court of Han Wu Ti in −108,[h] and it was still widely practised in the +10th century, so that it overlapped for a long time with the boxing tradition emanating from the Shao-lin temple in Honan. To this day, the art of wrestling in Japan is named *sumō*, an expression which in Chinese characters is written in just the same way, *chio ti*,[8] or *chio li*,[12] or *hsiang phu*.[11] When Buddhist sūtras translated in the Liu Chhao period speak of unarmed combats with bare hands and feet they use the

[a] In 1974 a Hongkong bookshop published a catalogue or bibliography of books and tractates on the martial arts then in print. The total number of these was 225, including 36 on Thai-chi chhüan, 19 on Shao-lin, 13 on *jūdō*, and 18 on *karate*. Such is the current state of the Chinese literature alone.

[b] *SCC*, Vol. 5, pt. 5.

[c] Cf. Anon. (75), pp. 4ff.

[d] Lit. 'fisting and gripping'.

[e] See the account of Giles (5), pp. 132ff., which follows *TSCC*, *I shu tien*, ch. 810, *tsa lu*, pp 3*a*ff.

[f] The second word would imply hitting or striking, but it must be remembered that a common modern expression for wrestling is *phu chiao*.[13] Alternatively there is *shuai chio*[14] and *kuan chiao shu*.[15]

[g] According to Chu Hui's[16] *Shih Yuan*.[17]

[h] *CHS*, ch. 6, p. 24*a*, *b*.

1 功夫	2 內功	3 按摩	4 導引	5 拳博	6 拳法
7 開手	8 角觝	9 角牴	10 角抵	11 相撲	12 角力
13 撲交	14 摔角	15 躀跤術	16 朱繪	17 事原	

expression *hsiang chha hsiang phu*,[1] evidently closely related. Now Shao-lin Ssu[2] is a famous Buddhist temple on the slopes of Sung Shan[3] north-west of Têng-fêng[4] and not far from Loyang, and if the date of foundation in +494 is right it must indeed have been in the lifetime of Ta-Mo,[5] that egregious Chhan[6] (Zen) monk and patriarch, i.e. Bodhidharma (Phu-Thi-Ta-Mo[7]), who has always been associated with its semi-legendary origins.[a] According to tradition, it was he who embarked upon techniques of unarmed combat as part of the physical education which the monks had to go through, and at some early time the exercises crystallised into 18 distinct movements, the *Shih-pa Lo-han shou*[8].[b] At later dates, these were increased, first to 72, then finally systematised at 173.[c] The general chronology thus indicates that rather continuous traditions have come down from Chou and Chhin times, though possible influences from India remain an open question.[d] Yet the literature is sparse and the traditions overwhelmingly oral, presumably because in the ever-prevailing Confucian ethos military affairs were always regarded as vastly inferior in value and prestige to civilian preoccupations. If a scholar learnt boxing or wrestling it was not a thing that he would be inclined to talk about in polite company, though it might serve him well in occasional passages with brigands, or for the improvement of his own health.[e] Nor would he want to write much about it. We know the titles of some books and tractates of very uncertain date, often attributed to Ta-Mo but very likely as late as the +16th century — the *Hsi Sui Ching*[9] (Manual of the Purification of the Marrow) is probably lost, but the *I Chin Ching*[10] (Manual of Exercising the Muscles and Tendons) survives.[f] Chang Khung-Chao's[11] plainly named *Chhüan Ching*[12] (Manual of Boxing) was in all likelihood a product of the +18th century, but there must have been several more of the same name in earlier times, for Chhi Chi-Kuang,[13] the great general, devoted ch. 14 of his *Chi Hsiao Hsin Shu*[14] to boxing exercises, entitling it Chhüan Ching Chieh Yao Phien,[15] 'Basic Essentials of Training from the Boxing Manuals'; this was in +1575.

With Thai-chi chhüan,[16] 'Supreme-Pole' callisthenic boxing,[g] we come to a quite different tradition which verges on that of the dance. Today it is known all over the world, and has been extremely prevalent in contemporary China, being considered

[a] Cf. Pelliot (3), pp. 248 ff., 252 ff.; Mullikin & Hotchkis (1), p. 38.

[b] Smith (1), pp. 16 ff.

[c] A succinct account of Shao-lin boxing is given by Smith (1). Cf. Haines (1).

[d] There was a lore of vital spots or danger-points (*marmas*), some fatal, in ancient India, as we can see from the *Suśruta Saṃhitā*, one of the two greatest Ayurvedic classics. The present redaction of this is placed between the +2nd and +4th centuries (Renou & Filliozat (1), vol. 2, p. 147; Bose, Sen & Subbarayappa (1), p. 223). The 107 *marmas* were thought of as junction-points between blood-vessels, ligaments, muscles, bones and joints; and there is a considerable overlap with the danger-points described in Japanese treatises on unarmed combat (pp. 312 below). See the Bhishagratna ed., vol. 2, pp. 173 ff. and pls. 1, 2.

[e] One could hardly omit a reference here to the 'Boxer Rebellion' of 1900, 'the Uprising of the Righteous and Harmonious Fists' (I Ho Chhüan[17]), on which see Purcell (4). Characteristically it was peasant and popular, not upper-class.

[f] This work verges on the field of pure gymnastics, in which context we consider it in *SCC*, Vol. 5, pt. 5.

[g] We cannot embark here on the explanation of this name, but must refer only to Vol. 2, pp. 460 ff.

[1] 相叉相撲 [2] 少林寺 [3] 嵩山 [4] 登封 [5] 達摩 [6] 禪
[7] 菩提達磨 [8] 十八羅漢手 [9] 洗髓經 [10] 易筋經 [11] 張孔昭 [12] 拳經
[13] 戚繼光 [14] 紀效新書 [15] 拳經捷要篇 [16] 太極拳 [17] 義和拳

especially good for the elderly. During the Thang and Sung periods unarmed combat skills were polarised into two schools, the nine Northern or 'exoteric' traditions (*wai chia*[1]) called the Shao-lin Phai[2] (though Shao-lin chhüan[3] was only one of them), contrasting with six Southern or 'esoteric' traditions (*nei chia*[4]) called the Wu-tang Phai[5] (of which Thai-chi chhüan was one).[a] This was because of another mountain temple complex, on Wu-tang Shan,[6] a peak of the range of the same name on the south slopes of the Han River and about twice as far north-west of Hsiangyang[7] as Sung Shan was east of Loyang. Since this was over the border into Hupei it was necessarily called southern, and in so far as the Shao-lin traditions were Buddhist in origin, those of Wu-tang were Taoist. The *nei chia* techniques, it has been said, were 'inspired by Taoist conceptions of yielding, and defeating the enemy less by force than by a knowledge of his weak spots'.[b] In the present context this is truly significant. The Taoist background also brings out the traditional associations of that religion with the sciences, both in their compassionate and their aggressive applications, here acupuncture on the one hand and a knowledge of the danger-points on the other. The patron saint of the Wu-tang Phai was Chang San-Fêng,[8] a rather shadowy Taoist alchemist who must have lived between +1368 and +1424; he acquired such a reputation for longevity techniques, including gymnastics, sexology and aurifaction, that he was sought for (unsuccessfully) by one emperor after another.[c] But no evidence for his connection with the Wu-tang Phai is available before the time of the unarmed-combat master Chang Sung-Chhi[9] (*fl.* +1522 to +1566).[d] The scarcity of documentation makes the study of all these traditions difficult, and modern accounts of them are very confused.[e]

Although it would no doubt be a gross simplification one could perhaps say that *karate*[10] was what the Japanese developed from the Northern Shao-lin school,[f] and *jūjutsu*[11] (or *jūdō*[12])[g] was what they made of the Southern Wu-tang school. Although the former has in recent times been written *khung shou*,[13] 'empty-hand fighting', its proper orthography was always *Thang shou*,[14] 'Thang, or Chinese, hand-work'.[h] Although the latter involved no hitting or kicking, it is capable of inflicting grave damage or death on an opponent, aided by the considerable knowledge of anatomy which goes along with it, and its emphasis upon 'weakness' at the same time manifests

[a] See Huang Wên-Shan (1), pp. 37ff.; Tsêng Chao-Jan (*1*).

[b] Seidel (1), p. 505.

[c] Cf. *SCC*, Vol. 5, pt. 3, p. 209, and Vol. 5, pt. 5, *passim*. The biography by Seidel (1) is of much value.

[d] *Ibid.*, p. 504.

[e] This does not mean that specific further research could not piece a good deal together. For example there is a document written by Huang Pai-Chia[15] (the son of the famous scholar Huang Tsung-Hsi[16]) towards the end of the +17th century, entitled *Nei Chia Chhüan Fa*[17] (The Techniques of the Esoteric, i.e. the Southern, School of Unarmed Combat).

[f] A clear and practical account of *karate*, well illustrated, is given by Nakayama Masatoshi & Draeger (1).

[g] Often written wrongly *jiu-jitsu*.

[h] Cf. Haines (1).

[1] 外家 [2] 少林派 [3] 少林拳 [4] 內家 [5] 武當派 [6] 武當山
[7] 襄陽 [8] 張三峯 [9] 張松溪 [10] 唐手 [11] 柔術 [12] 柔道
[13] 空手 [14] 唐手 [15] 黃百家 [16] 黃宗羲 [17] 內家拳法

its Taoist origins. In the transmission of Shao-lin and karate techniques to Japan, the Liu-Chhiu[1] island kingdom[a] seems to have played a particularly important role, especially Okinawa.[2] Chinese *chhüan fa*[3] may have come there, it is thought, as early as the Thang period, and it was certainly cultivated by the Okinawans when Liu-Chhiu became a tributary State of China in +1372. Apparently they had embassies all over south-east Asia at that time, hence numerous contacts with Indonesian and Malayan boxing–wrestling–dance techniques which we cannot explore further here.[b] Then when the Satsuma clan annexed Liu-Chhiu (Ryūkyū) to Japan in +1609 the way was open for the further development, so well known, in that country. But the details of the whole story are obscure.[c] Certain it is that direct Chinese influence was active in Japan in the late Ming and early Chhing, as witness the potter Chhen Yuan-Pin[4] (+1587 to +1671) who lived in Nagasaki and spread widely the knowledge of the Shao-lin and Wu-tang schools, especially the latter.[d]

It only remains to touch upon a couple of other martial arts which trend upon the domain of weapons, and again, both developed highly in Japan. In the *manriki-gusari*[5] art, of which there are said to be 20 schools,[e] a man attacks his opponent or defends himself, by the aid of a steel chain connecting two spikes or handles. Chinese origins for this are very probable because we can find illustrations and descriptions of two similar implements, almost flails, in the *Wu Ching Tsung Yao*[6] of +1044, the *thieh mao*[7] and the *theih lien chia phêng*[8].[f] Here again the knowledge of the anatomical danger-points is very much to the fore.[9] Pain, unconsciousness and death can be brought about by their use. The other art is that of thrown spikes, *shuriken*,[9] small sharp darts which could be concealed in the sleeves of a man's dress; this most probably derives from a similar technique practised in medieval China, that of the *fei tao*[10] 'flying knives'. Naturally with perfected accurate aim great damage could be done at the 'vital spots'.[h]

Our own starting-point here was the oldest extant book on forensic medicine in any civilisation, the *Hsi Yuan Lu*[11] (Records of the Washing Away of Unjust Imputations), written by Sung Tzhu[12] in +1247 under the Southern Sung.[i] Born in +1186 in Fukien, Sung became a student of Wu Chih,[13] who had himself studied under the great Neo-Confucian philospher Chu Hsi[14],[j] and he was also helped by the eminent

[a] Cf. *SCC*, Vol. 4, pt. 3, *passim*.

[b] Cf. Haines (1); Huard & Huang Kuang-Ming (7), p. 285.

[c] It is not only that secondary sources in Western languages like the foregoing are unsatisfactory, those in Chinese are vague and contradictory as well.

[d] Haines (1), p. 92; Huang Wên-Shan (1), p. 38.

[e] See the account of Gruzanski (1).

[f] *Chhien chi*, ch. 10, p. 22*a*, *b*, ch. 13, p. 14*a*, *b*.

[g] As many as 47 are recognised, 28 on the front of the body and 19 on the back. See further regarding numbers on p. 313 below.

[h] This also is described by Gruzanski, *op. cit.*

[i] There are translations, old but still useful, into Dutch by de Grijs (1) and into English by Giles (7).

[j] Cf. *SCC*, Vol. 2, pp. 455 ff.

1 琉球 2 冲繩島 3 拳法 4 陳元斌 5 萬力鎖
6 武經總要 7 鐵猫 8 鉄鏈夾捧 9 手裡劍 10 飛刀 11 洗寃錄
12 宋慈 13 吳稚 14 朱熹

scholar Chen Tê-Hsiu.[1] He took his degree in +1217, but he was 41 before he succeeded in obtaining an official post. Eventually he was gazetted to Gan-hsien (Chiangsi) and then to Chhang-ting (Fukien), but became most famous for his work as a judge in Canton. Sung Tzhu's book, remarkably rational and scientific for its time, contains many things of interest which we shall discuss in the appropriate place;[a] what is important here is that it shows a deep knowledge of the danger-points significant in unarmed combat.

The *Hsi Yuan Lu*, early though it was in comparison with the rest of the world, was not the first text of the kind in Chinese culture, as bibliographical records show. Working backwards, there had been the *I Yü Chi*[2] (Records of Doubtful Criminal Cases), written in the Wu Tai period (+10th century) by a father and son, Ho Ning[3] and Ho Mêng.[4] Earlier still, in the +6th century, *c.* +565, there had been the *Ming Yuan Shih Lu*[5] (True Records of the Clarification of Wrongs), written by Hsü Chih-Tshai.[6] Both these works have long been lost, but if indeed the origins of Shao-lin pugilism go back to the +5th century, it is certainly to be assumed that Ho Ning and Hsü Chih-Tshai wrote of the injuries which trained men could inflict upon others even without weapons. Indeed one can carry the tradition back to the Han, for the *Li Chi*[7] (Record of Rites) contains some details about the juridical examination of corpses resulting from violent actions and in connection with subsequent legal procedures.[b] This would have been about contemporary with the *chio ti*[8] combats (p. 304 above), which themselves must have led now and then to fatal results.

After Sung Tzhu's time the literature continued to grow. Before the Renaissance in Europe which brought Western forensic medicine into being there were several more Chinese treatises, for instance the anonymous *Phing Yuan Lu*[9] (Pacification of those Unjustly Accused) before the end of the Sung, and Wang Yü's[10] *Wu Yuan Lu*[11] (Nullification of False Accusations) in the Yuan (early +14th century). There was thus a great Chinese tradition of forensic medicine many centuries before the beginning of the +17th, when in +1602 Fortunato Fedeli published his epoch-making *De Relationibus Medicorum*. Towards the middle of that century the great work of Paolo Zacchia, *Quaestiones Medico-Legales* (+1635), took the subject within the realm of modern science.

In the *Hsi Yuan Lu* it is easy to find the information about the vital spots or danger-points, for it occurs with two diagrams (Figs. 79, 80) in the third section of the first chapter.[c] Points of particular danger on which a person's fate depends (*chih ming chih chhu*[12]) are enumerated as 16 on the front of the body (*shih*[13]), or 22 if all the bilateral ones are counted; with 6 on the back, or 10 if all the bilaterals count – making 32 in all. The connection with acupuncture arises because one notices that while most of the danger-points are given in essentially anatomical terms, some are fixed more

[a] Sect. 44 in Vol. 6.
[b] Yüeh Ling; ch. 6, p. 73*a*, tr. Legge (7), vol. 1, p. 275. On the whole genre see Jen An (*1*).
[c] Ch. 1, p. 12*a*ff., diagrams on p. 15*a*, *b*.

[1] 眞德秀 [2] 疑獄集 [3] 和凝 [4] 和㠓 [5] 明寃實錄
[6] 徐之才 [7] 禮記 [8] 角牴 [9] 平寃錄 [10] 王與 [11] 無寃錄
[12] 致命之處 [13] 屍

歌訣
仰面傷痕十六方。
頂心左右顖門當。
額角額顱頭看畢，
耳竅咽喉并太陽，
兩乳胸膛心肚腹，
臍同肚脇更須詳。
腎囊有子看雙獨，
婦女陰門恐暗傷。

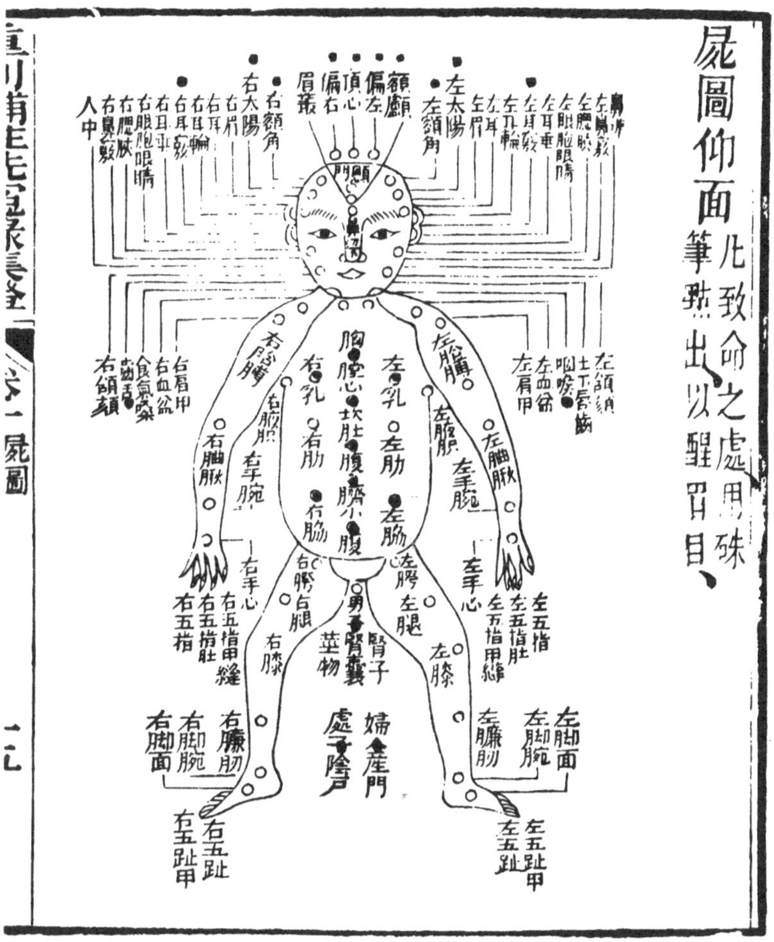

Fig. 79. Vital spots, or danger-points where any trauma is liable to be mortal, shown in the *Hsi Yuan Lu* of + 1247, the oldest extant book on forensic medicine in any civilisation. Front of the body. The sub-caption recommends the book's owner to mark them in with a red pen. The commentary above is a mnemonic verse.

歌訣

合面傷痕亦有六。
腦後耳根宜日囑。
脊背脊膂穴須詳
後脇腰眼相連屬（致命此）
肩甲血盆腋肢傷
兩邊筋骨死亦速
除此皆非致命痕
二十二傷可更僕

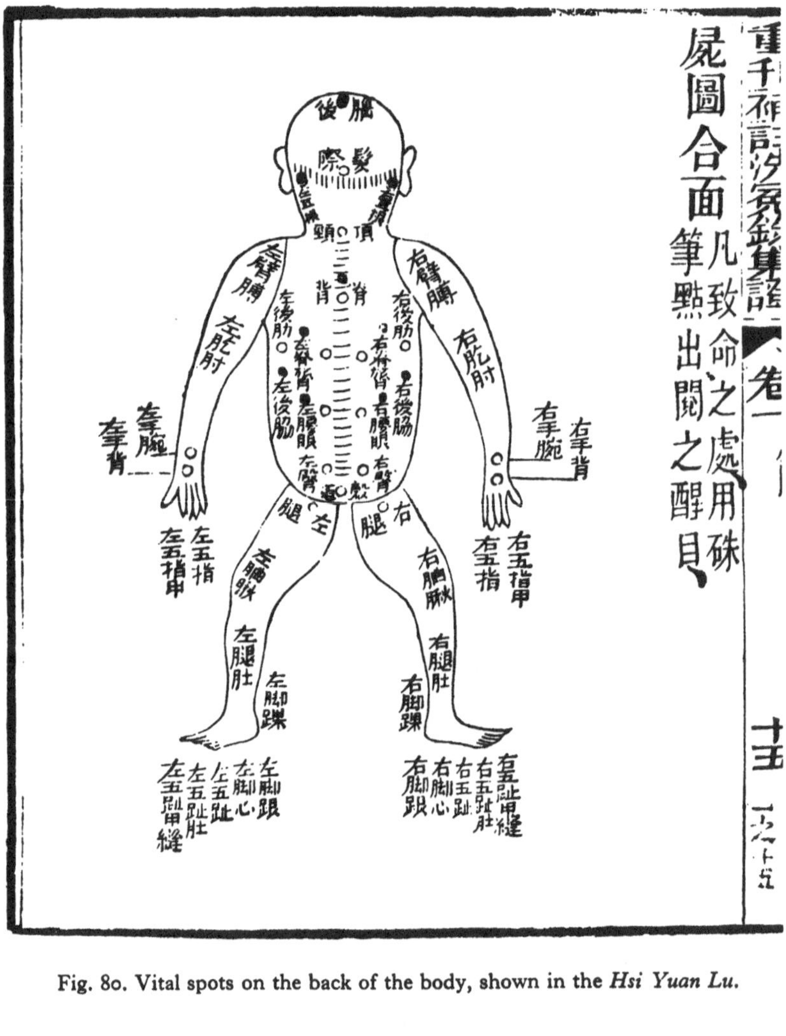

Fig. 80. Vital spots on the back of the body, shown in the *Hsi Yuan Lu*.

precisely by acu-point names. Thus *hsing mên*[1] refers to the anterior fontanelle, one of those gaps between the bones of the skull never completely obliterated by their natural suturing in adult life, and *hsin khan*,[2] the 'heart-pit', means the indentation at the sternal notch on the breast. But Thai-yang hsüeh[3] is an acu-point on the temple on each side, not one of those on the regular or auxiliary tracts but a special and isolated one.[a] So also Yao-yen hsüeh[4] is another isolated acu-point low down on the back in the lumbar region on each side not far from the lateral border of the sacro-spinalis muscle.[b] It was this which alerted us to the fact that some of the vital spots or danger-points discovered by the specialists in unarmed combat, and consequently reflected in the medico-legal literature, were indeed defined as sites familiar already to the practitioners of acupuncture and moxibustion.

If then we look at a few of the danger-points identified by Sung Tzhu, and compare them with information current in modern forensic medicine,[c] we immediately begin to see what was the meaning of the discoveries of the Buddhist and Taoist combat schools. Half a dozen will be more than enough to make the point.

(1) The fontanelles of the skull. Concussive vibration would cause bleeding in the brain tissue, and subarachnoid haemorrhages; there could also be fractures of the skull bones. The Ta-hsing-mên[5] of Japanese charts[d] would be equivalent to Pai-hui[6] (TM 19);[e] and the Hsiao-hsing-mên[7] would be either Hsing-hui[8] (TM 21) or Shang-hsing[9] (TM 22). These are all mid-line points, but there would be others on the sides of the head.[f]

(2) Occipital and cervical regions. Trauma at the base of the skull or near the nape of the neck can lead to fracture of the odontoid process of the second (Axis) cervical vertebra, or the transverse process of the first (Atlas) cervical vertebra, accompanied by injury to the vertebral artery and hence severe subarachnoidal haemorrhages.[g] This is one of the circumstances where no external signs of the damage may be visible after death. Japanese charts[h] indicate Ya-mên[10] (TM 14), but VF 20 (Fêng-chhih[11]) and VU 10 (Thien-chu[12]) higher up and at the sides occipitally would also be dangerous.

(3) Behind the ear. Here again haemorrhages in the brain tissue and between its membranes (dura mater and pia mater) will result. Japanese charts[i] indicate Wan-ku[13] (VF 17).

(4) Above the sternum, at the throat. A blow in the Adam's apple region may lead to vertical fracture of the thyroid cartilage accompanied by haemorrhages from the carotid artery and the carotid sinus (the dilatation at the point where it divides into the external and

[a] Chhi (Extra) 2; see Anon. (*107*), p. 236, (*123*), p. 122; Anon. (135), p. 205.
[b] Chhi (Extra) 5; see Anon. (*107*), pp. 237–8.
[c] Cf. the treatise of Camps & Cameron (1).
[d] Fujita *et al.* (1), p. 63. We shall have more to say about this interesting work on p. 312 below.
[e] This is a locus of much importance; cf. pp. 81ff. above.
[f] Cf. Adams (1), pp. 19ff. This is a valuable and unusual contribution on the medical significance of *karate* blows.
[g] Cameron & Mant (1); cf. Adams (1), pp. 54ff.
[h] Fujita *et al.* (1), p. 35, but very clear also in the charts on pp. 16, 24, etc. P. 35 is a Shao-lin ssu (Shorinji) diagram.
[i] Fujita *et al.* (1), p. 38, but very clear also in that on p. 23.

1 顖門 2 心坎 3 太陽穴 4 腰眼穴 5 大顖門 6 百會
7 小顖門 8 顖會 9 上星 10 瘂門 11 風池 12 天柱
13 完骨

the internal branches); there may also be sudden vagal inhibition with consequent cardiac arrest.[a] Sung Tzhu contented himself with the broad description *yen hou*[1] (the throat), but the Japanese charts indicate Lien-chhüan[2] (JM23).[b]

(5) The sternal notch, or 'pit of the stomach'. The most likely effect would be the sudden heart stoppage formerly called vagal inhibition, but there could also be damage to a number of important structures just below the diaphragm in this epigastric region. The coeliac (or 'solar') plexus, largest of the sympathetic plexuses, lies about the level of the 1st lumbar vertebra, and there could be damage to the liver and haemorrhage from the coeliac artery.[c] Japanese charts indicate Shan-chung[3] (JM17).[d]

(6) Perineal region and scrotum (*yin nang*[4]). Apart from the pain caused, pubic fractures would be expected, damage to the whole pelvic girdle, and testicular haemorrhages.[e] Chhang-chhiang[5] (TM1) was doubtless one of the targets, half way between coccyx and anus, a site named *kuei wei*[6] (*kamebi*[6]) by some of the Japanese schools.[f]

Thus Sung Tzhu must have realised, and all his predecessors and successors too, without knowing anything of the detail of modern anatomy, that the aggression of one unarmed man upon another could be productive of the most fatal consequences, especially if one of the two was trained in the techniques of the *chhüan fa*[7] schools of martial art while the other was not.

Sung Tzhu was the great representative of the learning needful for coroners,[g] but over against it stood the developing knowledge of the military trainers, so often lamentable when it got into the hands of those who would use it for evil purposes. As in other instances it reached special perfection in Japan, hence the interesting book of Fujita Saiko, Plée & Devêvre (1) on the *atemi*,[8] *shi-ketsu*[9] and *katsu-ketsu*[10] (life and death points) of the body. Here we may find the vital spots recognised by twenty-one of the principal schools (*ryu*[11]) of *karate*, and when these are averaged the result (28·6) comes out remarkably close to the 32 described in Sung Tzhu's book (Table 24).

It is interesting that the *sumō* term is *kinketsu*[12] (*chin hsüeh*[12]), exactly as in acupuncture, while the Shorinji experts use *tenketsu*[13] (*tien hsüeh*[13]) exactly as in modern Chinese (p. 302), and the spike-and-chain practitioners *kyūsho*.[14h] But in spite of these implicit references to acu-points the great majority of the names for the vital spots are fancy ones, differing according to the traditions of the different schools. Nevertheless, one can identify quite a number of acu-point terms in the Japanese charts.[i] Chiu-wei[15]

[a] Camps & Hunt (1); Adams (1), pp. 47ff.; Smith (1), p. 59.
[b] Fujita *et al.* (1), p. 34.
[c] Adams (1), pp. 62ff.; Smith (1), p. 60.
[d] Fujita *et al.* (1), p. 36.
[e] Adams (1), pp. 92ff., who visualises also rupture of the bladder and crushing of the testes. Cf. Smith (1), p. 61.
[f] Fujita *et al.* (1), p. 23.
[g] Indeed his book has often been given the translated title 'Handbook for Coroners', banal compared with the original.
[h] Gruzanski (1), pp. 77ff.
[i] Cf. Fujita *et al.* (1), pp. 34, 38, two summarising charts (Figs. 81, 82.).

1 咽喉 2 廉泉 3 膻中 4 陰囊 5 長强 6 龜尾
7 拳法 8 當身 9 死穴 10 活穴 11 流 12 禁穴
13 點穴 14 急所 15 鳩尾

Table 24. *Vital points recognised by coroners and combat masters*

	points on the front of the body	points on the back of the body	total
Hsi Yuan Lu (Sung Tzhu)	16	6	22
if bilaterals included	22	10	32
Shao-lin Ssu (Shorinji) boxing	24	12	36
Points from a +13th-century Japanese military treatise (the 'Buyo Chronicle'; Fujita *et al.* (1), p. 36)	22	—	22
Japanese *karate* schools; Fujita *et al.* (1)	17	8	25
The *sumō* wrestling tradition (Fujita *et al.* (1), p. 37)	13	—	13
The *manriki-gusari* and *shuriken* traditions (Gruzanski, 1)	28	19	47

(JM 15), below the sternal notch, occurs often, as does Chang-mên[1] (H 13) in the lumbar region at the back close to the free end of the 11th rib, and Shui-fên[2] (JM 9) just above the umbilicus. There is also Yin-thang[3] on the forehead centrally between the eyes.[a] Shao-lin (Shorinji) boxing has much to say of Thai-yang[4] on the temples, just as Sung Tzhu did (p. 311), dangerous because of possible skull fractures and haemorrhage from the middle meningeal artery.[b] It also emphasises Jen-chung[5] (syn. Shui-kou[6]) on the philtrum (TM 25) because of the serious sequelae of maxillary fractures.[c] In the *sumō* tradition Chiu-wei appears again, as also Tan-thien[7] (syn. Shih-mên[8]) on the lower abdomen (JM 5).[d]

The work of Fujita Saiko and his collaborators says nothing about the *jūjutsu*[9] schools, presumably because where direct blows were impermissible and everything was accomplished by falls and throws a knowledge of danger-spots would be unnecessary. But nevertheless it could surely happen that an opponent might be made to fall heavily against the ground or some hard object precisely at one of the danger-spots. Hence Fujita's account may be supplemented by a discussion in the book of Hashimoto Masae, which compares the vital spots (*kyūsho*[10]) recognised in *aikidō*[11] with

[a] A Chhi (Extra) point 1, see Anon. (*107*), pp. 234–5; Anon. (135), pp. 204, 206. It occurs in Fujita *et al.* (1), p. 18; and Adams (1), pp. 34ff. expounds the dangers of fractures of the nasal bones and the orbital sockets.

[b] Cf. Adams (1), pp. 27ff. Fujita *et al.* (1), p. 62, give a detailed comparison between vital spots in the facial region and acu-points there.

[c] Adams (1), pp. 39ff.

[d] Cf. pp. 50, 56 above.

1 章門 2 水分 3 印堂 4 太陽 5 人中 6 水溝
7 丹田 8 石門 9 柔術 10 急所 11 合氣道

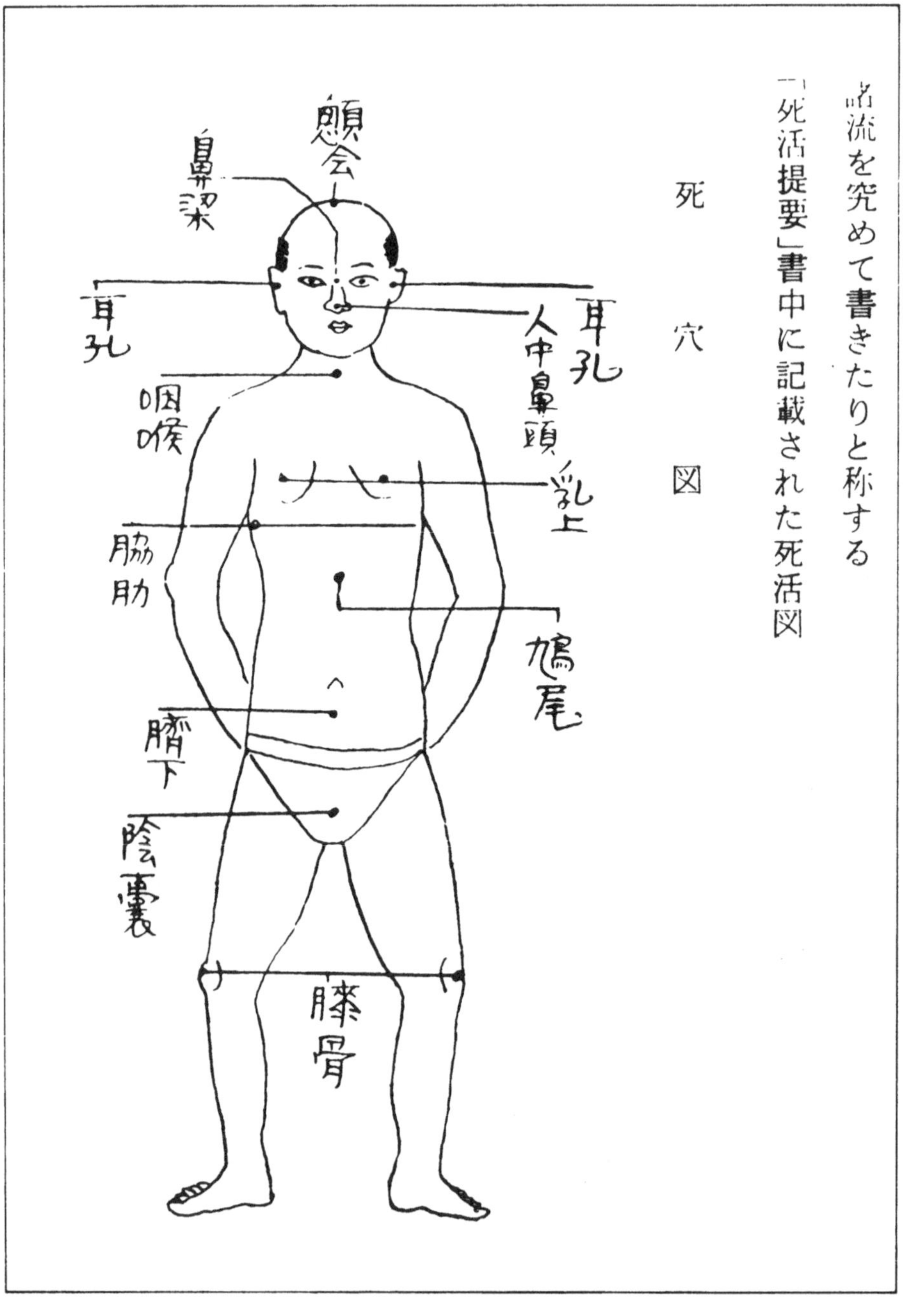

Fig. 81. Vital spots on the front of the body, as recognised by the principal schools of Japanese *karate* (Fujita *et al.* (1), p. 34). They are called *atemi* (*tang shen*), 'body-withstanders', *shiketsu* (*ssu hsüeh*), 'death loci', or *katsu-ketsu* (*huo hsüeh*), 'life loci'. This drawing and the following one may be compared with Figs. 79 and 80.

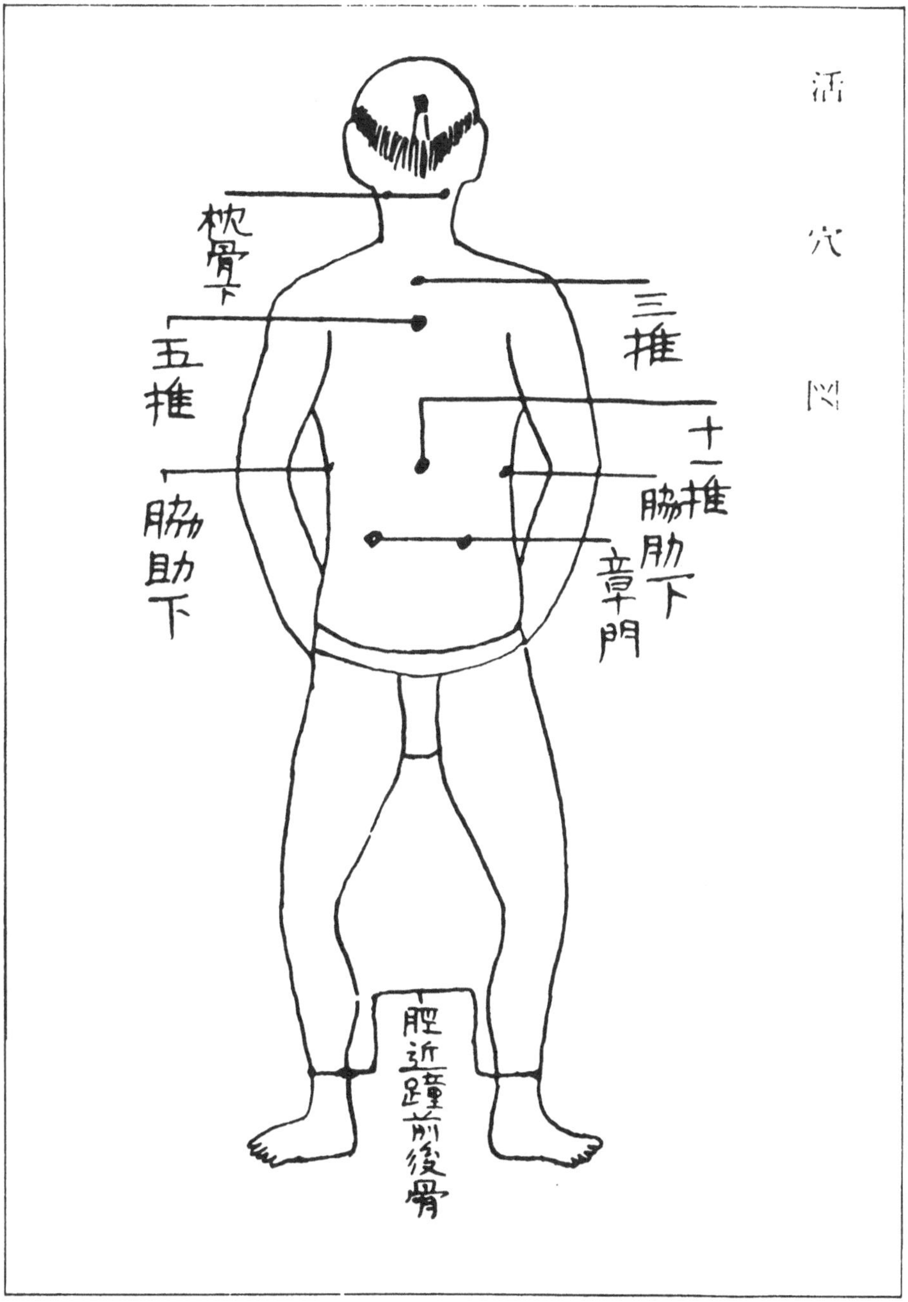

Fig. 82. Vital spots on the back of the body, as recognised in Japanese *karate*.

acu-points.[a] *Aikidō* is a relatively recent development of *jūjutsu* based on leverage holds and throws,[b] yet it identifies 22 danger-points on the front of the body and 3 on the back, making 25 in all. These figures invite comparison with those in Table 24. Correspondingly Hashimoto tabulates the acu-points concerned,[c] making the figures 24, 3 and 27 respectively. Some have not yet been mentioned, but loci such as Pai-hui, Shan-chung, Chhang-chhiang, Chiu-wei and Chang-mên are all familiar to us from the preceding pages. Finally, she emphasises not only the possibility of cardiac arrest, but the sudden inhibition of respiratory movements when certain of these points are heavily struck, with the possibility of suffocation.[d]

How did these danger-points compare with the 'forbidden' points (*chin hsüeh*[1]) of the acupuncturists themselves? Something has already been said of these (p. 68 above), and one would expect a certain correlation, though of course the dangers guarded against were not necessarily the same; the physicians would have been worrying about bleeding, fainting, piercing large nerve-trunks, and other unwanted eventualities, while the physical training specialists would have had quite other ideas in mind. Here one can turn to an ancient and very authoritative source, the +3rd-century *Chen Chiu Chia I Ching* of Huangfu Mi (p. 119 above), which gives a list of forbidden points, both for acupuncture and moxa.[e] Of these 12, five have already been encountered among the danger-points in unarmed combat. Chiu-wei (JM 15) and Ya-mên (TM 14) are typical loci, but others of interest are Shen-thing[2] (TM 23) near the fontanelles or sutures of the skull, Lu-hsi[3] (SC 19) just behind the ear, and Jen-ying[4] (V 7) near the Adam's apple over the sternomastoid muscle on each side. Ju-chung[5] (V 17), at the nipple, has always been contra-indicated, and there are two occipital acu-points banned by the doctors yet encouraged by the fighters—Nao-hu[6] (TM 16) and Fêng-fu[7] (TM 15). All in all, there is some correspondence between the medical and the military preoccupations, but not beyond a limited extent, since the nature of their objectives was so divergent.

As a pendant to this account of 'vital spots' it may be worth while to look briefly at a famous, though often forgotten, series of points on the body of an animal—the *nila* or 'nerve-centres' on the surface of elephants which the groom or *mahout* prods with his goad[f] in order to control their movements.[g] Since some of these can

[a] (*1*), pp. 33–4.

[b] Cf. Haines (1), p. 151; Huang Wên-Shan (1), p. 37. *Ho chhi*, the 'uniting of the *chhi*', is a phrase which has had a legion of technical meanings through the centuries. Its use here is not as attractive as that of the early Taoists, cf. *SCC*, Vol. 2, p. 150.

[c] She calls them *tsubo*,[8] apparently a usage among Japanese acupuncturists for the more official *kōketsu*.[9]

[d] It should be added that all the authoritative books and manuals of unarmed combat nowadays, whether in Chinese, Japanese or Western languages, give details of measures of resuscitation in case of such accidents.

[e] *CIC*, ch. 5, (p. 111). A modern list, in the form of a mnemonic rhyme, can be found in Anon. (*91*), p. 362.

[f] The *henduva* or *amkussa* has a head like a boat-hook with two iron spikes of equal length, one being flattened into a spatula-like blade and curved backwards.

[g] The relevance of this to acupuncture was perhaps first pointed out by Mann (1), 1st ed., pp. 34ff.

1 禁穴 2 神庭 3 顱息 4 人迎 5 乳中 6 腦戶
7 風府 8 壺 9 孔穴

cause the death of the beast if pricked sufficiently deeply, and for other reasons obvious enough, the lore of the *nila* has been for centuries kept professionally secret, but Deraniyagala (1) has succeeded in giving a remarkable account of it,[a] partly from the direct information of *mahouts* and traditional elephant veterinarians, and partly from Indian and Sinhalese MSS.[b] On the body of the Asian *Elephas maximus*, one of the only two surviving species, there are some 90 points at which pricking will bring about all kinds of results, many no doubt due to reflex action. They may be tabulated as follows:

control as such	7
control,	
of trunk movement	3
of trumpeting	2
of head, neck, shoulders and fore-limbs, with offering of seat for mounting	14
of hind legs	4
to kneel	4
to lie down	1
to go forward	11
to stop, or slow	13
to turn round	5
to go backward	1
rouse, or excite	7
frighten[c]	6
benumb[d]	1
lethal, to kill the animal[e]	14

Further physiological research on the sensitive points of the elephant would be likely to bring results of much interest.[f] And we see that in this case again, there are certain points of particular danger, where an injury even no more than a deep prick can cause irreparable fatal damage.

(8) Conclusions

In the foregoing pages we have attempted to describe the nature of acupuncture and moxibusion, to sketch their history, to elucidate the physiological basis of their actions in therapy and analgesia, and to show how the knowledge of them gradually spread

[a] (1), pp. 9, 68 ff., 140 ff.

[b] For example, the *Hasti Lakshana Vidyāva*, the *Mahāgaja Lakshana Sangarahava*, etc. The dates of these are very hard to determine. Deraniyagala, *op. cit.*, pp. 130 ff.

[c] Three of these are on the head, and three on the back in the posterior midline.

[d] The possibility of an analgesia here is interesting (cf. pp. 231 ff. above). The point lies at the back of the neck in the midline (on TM, as one might say).

[e] Plus three more points if the *amkussa* is thrust sufficiently deep. Two inches is enough at most of them (Deraniyagala (1), p. 68).

[f] The thought even arises that the relation of the *nila* with acupuncture might be closer than a mere parallelism, for the Chinese elephant (*E. maximus rubridens*) survived wild down to the beginning of the nineteenth century. In the days of Huangfu Mi and Wênjen Chhi-Nien it must have been quite common, at least in the south and south-east. Cf. Deraniyagala, *op. cit.*, pp. 124–5; Laufer (43); Chang Hung-Chao (5).

all over the world. The reader may have been surprised to find how great a medical literature concerning them grew up in China through the centuries. In the course of our survey we have come across many matters of absorbing interest; for example (*a*) the convictions of Chinese scholars and physicians about the circulation of *chhi* and blood in the body, estimating a rate of flow only sixty times slower than that which modern physiology since Harvey has recognised; (*b*) the discovery of viscero-somatic reflexes, and the connections of many parts of the body's surface with events occurring in the internal organs; (*c*) the appreciation of diurnal (circadian) and longer biological rhythms in man, and the development of an abstruse calculus on the basis of this to determine when acupuncture and moxibustion should best be performed; (*d*) the development of a modular system for locating acu-points in human bodies of different sizes and proportions.

There have been a number of misunderstandings in the West about acupuncture and moxibustion. They have nothing to do with parapsychology, occult influences or 'psychic powers', and consequently do not deserve the praises of those who believe in such things. They do not depend entirely on suggestion, nor on hypnotic phenomena at all, and they are not contradictory of modern scientific medicine; consequently they do not deserve the *odium theologicum* of the medical profession in the West. Acupuncture (with moxa) is simply a system of medical treatment which was already two thousand years old when modern science was born, and which had developed in a civilisation quite different from that of Europe. Today the explanations of its actions are being sought in terms of modern physiology and pathology; great advances have been made in this direction though the end is not yet in sight. It looks as though the physiology and biochemistry of the central and autonomic nervous systems will be the leading elements in our understanding, but many other systems, endocrinological and immunological, are also sure to be involved. Another problem of great interest is the exact nature of the acu-points in terms of histology and bio-physics. Since modern science did not spontaneously grow up in Chinese culture, acupuncture and moxa are traditionally based upon a theoretical system essentially medieval in character, though very sophisticated and subtle, indeed full of valuable insights and salutary lessons for modern scientific medicine. Again the exact re-interpretation and re-formulation of these theories, if such a thing is possible, will be a difficult matter for the future. However, we think it likely that in the oecumenical medicine of the coming years there will be a definite place for acupuncture both in therapy and analgesia – exactly how far this will be so it is too early as yet to say.

BIBLIOGRAPHIES

A CHINESE AND JAPANESE BOOKS BEFORE +1800

B CHINESE AND JAPANESE BOOKS AND JOURNAL ARTICLES SINCE +1800

C BOOKS AND JOURNAL ARTICLES IN WESTERN LANGUAGES

In Bibliographies A and B there are two modifications of the Roman alphabetical sequence: transliterated *Chh-* comes after all other entries under *Ch-*, and transliterated *Hs-* comes after all other entries under *H-*. Thus *Chhen* comes after *Chung* and *Hsi* comes after *Huai*. This system applies only to the first words of the titles. Moreover, where *Chh-* and *Hs-* occur in words used in Bibliography C, i.e. in a Western language context, the normal sequence of the Roman alphabet is observed.

When obsolete or unusual romanisations of Chinese words occur in entries in Bibliography C, they are followed, wherever possible, by the romanisations adopted as standard in the present work. If inserted in the title, these are enclosed in square brackets; if they follow it, in round brackets. When Chinese words or phrases occur romanised according to the Wade–Giles system or related systems, they are assimilated to the system here adopted (cf. Vol. 1, p. 26) without indication of any change. Additional notes are added in round brackets. The reference numbers do not necessarily begin with (1), nor are they necessarily consecutive, because only those references required for this volume of the series are given.

Korean and Vietnamese books and papers are included in Bibliographies A and B. As explained in Vol. 1, pp. 21 ff., reference numbers in italics imply that the work is in one or other of the East Asian languages.

ABBREVIATIONS

See also p. XV

A/AIHS	*Archives Internationales d'Histoire des Sciences* (continuation of *Archeion*)
AAND	*al-Andelus*
AEPP	*Archiv. f. exp. Pathol. u. Pharmakol.*
AETR	*Acupuncture and Electro-therapeutics Research*
AFDGP	*Archiv. f. d. gesamte Physiol.* (Pflügers)
AGM	*Archiv. f. d. Gesch. d. Medizin* (Sudhoff's) contd as *AGMN*
AGMN	*Archiv. f. d. Gesch. d. Medizin u. d. Naturwissenschaften* (Sudhoff's)
AHJ	*American Heart Journal*
AHOR	*Antiquarian Horology*
AHRA	*Agric. History Research Annual* (*Nung Shih Yen-Chiu Chi-Khan*, formerly *Nung Yeh I-Chhan Yen-Chiu Chi-Khan*)
AIB	*Archives Italiennes de Biol.*
AIM	*Archives of Internal Medicine*
AJAP	*Amer. Journ. Acupuncture*
AJCM	*Amer. Journ. Chinese Medicine.*
AJCM/CM	*Comparative Medicine East and West*
AJM	*Asian Journ. Med.*
AJPSY	*Amer. Journ. Psychiatry*
AJPY	*Amer. Journ. Physics*
AMH	*Annals of Medical History*
AMNH/AP	*Anthropological Papers of the American Museum of Natural History* (New York)
AMSD	*Acta Medica Scandinavica*
ANAESTH	*Anaesthesiology*
ANAL	*Anaesthesia and Analgesia*
ANATR	*Anatomical Record*
ANEURP	*Archives of Neurol. & Psychiatr.*
ANS	*Annals of Science*
ANSURG	*Annals of Surgery*
ANT	*Antaios* (Stuttgart)
AOL	*Acta Oto-Laryngologica*
APRT	*Advances in Pain Research and Therapy*
APSD	*Acta Physiologica Scandinavica*
ARO	*Archiv Orientalni* (Prague)
ARSI	*Annual Reports of the Smithsonian Institution*
AS/CJA	*Chinese Journal of Archaeology, Academia Sinica*
ASKL	*Asklepios*
ASURG	*Annals of Surgery*
ATOM	*Atomes* (Paris)
AX	*Ambix*
BCGS	*Bull. Chinese Geological Soc.*
BIHM	*Bulletin of the (Johns Hopkins) Institute of the History of Medicine*
BINAH	*Boletin de los Instituticiones Nacionales de Antropologia y Historia* (Mexico)
BIOM	*Biometrika*
BJA	*British Journ. Anaesthesia*
BJAU	*British Journ. Audiology*
BJPM	*British Journ. Physical Medicine*
BMFEA	*Bulletin of the Museum of Far Eastern Antiquities* (Stockholm)
BMB	*British Mecical Bulletin*
BMJ	*British Medical Journal*
BNYAM	*Bulletin of the New York Academy of Medicine*
BR	*Biological Reviews*
BRN	*Brain*
BRNR	*Brain Research*
BSAC	*Bulletin de la Société d'Acupuncture*
BSEIC	*Bulletin de la Société des Études Indochinoises*
BSRCA	*Bulletin of the Society for Research in [the History of] Chinese Architecture*
CCHY	*Chen Chiu Huo Yeh Tshan-Khao Tzu-Liao* (*Materials for the Study of Acupuncture*, i.e. collections of photocopied papers selected and bound in a series of volumes)
CCL	*Chê Chiang Lu* (Biographies of Chinese Engineers, Architects, Technologists and Master-Craftsmen, by Chu Chhi-Chhien and collaborators, q.v. [a series, not a journal])
CHIH	*Chao-Hsien I Hsüeh* (*Korean Medicine*)
CIBA/MZ	*Ciba Zeitschfift* (Medical History)
CIBA/R	*Revue Ciba* (Medical History)
CIBA/S	*Ciba Symposia*
CITC	*Chung I Tsa Chih* (*Journal of Traditional Chinese Medicine*)
CLIME	*Clinical Medicine*
CLS	*Clinical Science*
CR/MSU	*Centennial Review of Arts and Science* (Michigan State University)
CMAJ	*Canadian Medical Association Journal*
CMJ	*Chinese Medical Journal*
CMJ/C	*Chinese Medical Journal* (Chinese edition)
CNOW	*China Now* (Society for Anglo-Chinese Understanding, London)

CONCM	*Concomis Médical*
CR	*China Review* (Hong Kong and Shanghai)
CRAS	*Comptes Rendus de l'Académie des Sciences* (Paris)
CREC	*China Reconstructs*
CRIT	*Critère* (Ahuntsic College Review, Montreal, Que.)
CSHSQB	*Cold Spring Harbour Symposia on Quantitative Biology*
CUL	Cambridge University Library
CUTHR	*Current Therapeutic Research*
DAAM	*Deutsches Ärzteblatt Ärztliche Mitteilungen.*
DAGM	*Deutsches Archiv f.d. Geschichte d. Medizin und medizinischen Geographie*
DHEW	Department of Health, Education and Welfare (USA)
DNM	*Tzu-Jan Pien-Chêng Fa Tsa Chih* (*Dialectics of Nature Magazine*)
DRS	*Drugs and Society*
DZA	*Deutsche Zeitschrift für Akupunktur*
EAPPA	*Ergebrisse d. allg. Pathologie u. Pathol. Anat. i. Mensch u. Tiere.*
EARLC	*Early China*
EB	*Encyclopaedia Britannica*
EHOR	*Eastern Horizon* (Hong Kong)
EJPH	*European Journ. Pharmacol.*
END	*Endeavour*
ERJB	*Eranos Jahrbuch*
ERYB	*Eranos Yearbook*
EXN	*Experimental Neurology*
GMI	*Gazzetta Medica Italiana*
HAM	*Hamdard, Voice of Eastern Medicine* (Karachi)
HC	*Hung Chhi Tsa Chih* (*Red Banner Miscellany*)
HEJ	*Health Education Journal*
HEM	*Hemisphere*
HIP	*Hippokrates*
HJAS	*Harvard Journal of Asiatic Studies*
HMSO	Her Majesty's Stationery Office
HOFR	*l' Homéopathie Française*
HOSC	*History of Science* (annual)
HSCIY	*Hsin Chung I Yao* (*New China's Medicine and Pharmacy*)
IEEET/BME	*Transactions of the Institute of Electrical and Electronics Engineers* (NY); *Bio-medical Engineering*
IMPAC	*Impact of Science on Society* (UNESCO)
ISIS	*Isis*
ISTC	*I Shih Tsa Chih* (*Chinese Journal of the History of Medicine*)
JADA	*Journ. Amer. Dental Assoc.*
JAMA	*Journ. Amer. Med. Assoc.*
JAOA	*Journ. Amer. Osteopath. Assoc.*
JAOS	*Journal of the American Oriental Society*
JBC	*Journ. Biological Chemistry*
JCI	*Journ. Clinical Investigation*
JCN	*Journ. Compar. Neurology*
JCPP	*Journ. Compar. and Physiological Psychol.*
JEB	*Journ. Expl Biol.*
JEZ	*Journal of Experimental Zoology*
JGER	*Journ. Gerontology*
JHMAS	*Journal of the History of Medicine and Allied Sciences*
JKAMS	*Journ. Dem. Peop. Rep. Korea Acad. Medical Sciences*
JMJ	*Japanese Medical Journal* (contd. as *Jap. Journ. Med. Sci & Biol.*)
JMPC	*Jen Min Pao Chien* (*Journ. Pub. Health*)
JMSMA	*Journ. Mississippi State Med. Assoc.*
JNC	*Journ. Neurochem.*
JNMD	*Journ. Nervous & Mental Diseases*
JNNSP	*Journ. Neurol., Neurosurgery & Psychiatr.*
JNP	*Journ. Neurophysiol.*
JNS	*Journ. Neurosurgery*
JNT	*Journ. Neurotransmission*
JOFOM	*Journ. Forensic Medicine*
JOGBC	*Journ. Obstet. & Gyn. Brit. Commonwealth* (formerly *Empire*)
JOP	*Journal of Physiology*
JPHK	*Journ. f. prakt. Heilkunde* (Hufeland & Osmann's)
JPOS	*Journal of the Peking Oriental Society*
JPS	*Journ. Psychol.*
JRAS	*Journal of the Royal Asiatic Society*
JRSA	*Journal of the Royal Society of Arts*
JSIS	*Journ. Social Issues*
JSPC	*Journ. Social Psychol.*
JWCBRS	*Journal of the West China Border Research Society*
JWCI	*Journal of the Warburg and Courtauld Institutes*
KHSC	*Kho Hsüeh Shih Chi-Khan* (*Ch. Journ. Hist. of Sci.*)
KHTP	*Kho Hsüeh Thung Pao* (*Science Correspondent*)
KKTH	*Khao Ku Thung Hsün* (*Archaeological Correspondent*) (cont. as *Khao Ku*)
KM	*Die Katholischen Missionen*
KNU/BIOOS	*Bull. Institute of Oriental and Occidental Studies, Kansai University*

KSCI	*Chiangsu Chung I* (*Chiangsu Provincial Journal of Traditional Chinese Medicine*)
KTD	*Korea Today*
LBM	*La Biologie Médicale* (Paris)
LD	*London Doctor*
LI	*Listener* (BBC)
LMR	*London Medical Record*
LS	*Life Sciences*
LT	*Lancet*
LTD	*Läkartidningen* (Stockholm)
M	*Mind*
MBG	*Mitt. d. Batavisch Genotschap.*
MBH	*Medical Bookman & Historian*
MCB	*Mélanges Chinois et Bouddhiques*
MCHR	*Medical Chronicle*
MDGHK	*Magazin f.d. ges. Heilkunde* (Rust's)
MDGNVO	*Mitteilungen d. deutsch. Gesellschaft f. Natur- u. Volkskunde Ostasiens*
MDT	*Medical Times* (USA)
MH	*Medical History*
MHJO	*Medizin-Historisches Journal* (Hildesheim)
MIGN	*Migraine News*
MIMS	*Monthly Index of Medical Specialities*
MINM	*Minnesota Medicine*
MIT	Massachusetts Institute of Technology
MMEDA	*Modern Medicine in Asia*
MMW	*Munchener Medizinische Wochenschrift*
MPJ	*Medical & Physical Journal*
MS	*Monumenta Serica*
MSL	*Medicine, Science and the Law*
N	*Nature*
NAMSJ	*North American Medical and Surgical Journal*
NCNA	*New China News Agency Bulletin*
NGNHK	*Notizen aus dem Gebiete der Natur- und Heikunde* (Froriep's)
NIH	National Institutes of Health (Bethesda, Md.)
NM	*Nordisk Medicin* (Stockholm)
NMJC	*National Medical Journal of China*
NN	*Nation*
NRIAC	*Nouv. Revue Internat. d'Acupuncture*
NRNAW	*News Reports of the Nat. Acad. Sciences, Washington*
NS	*New Scientist*
NSRPB	*Neuro-sciences Research Progress Bulletin*
NSW	*Newsweek*
NTIM	*Nursing Times*
NYSJM	*New York State Journ. Med.*
OARZ	*Österreichische Ärztezeitung*
OLN	*Osler Library Newsletter* (McGill Univ. Montreal)
OSIS	*Osiris*
PAIN	*Pain*
PAPS	*Proc. Amer. Philos. Soc.*
PC	*People's China*
PGMED	*Post-Graduate Medicine*
PHREV	*Pharmacological Reviews*
PNASW	*Proc. Nat. Acad. Sci. Washington.*
PRACT	*Practitioner*
PRSM	*Proceedings of the Royal Society of Medicine*
PSEBM	*Proc. Soc. Exp. Biol. & Med.*
PSM	*Psychosomatic Medicine*
PTRS	*Philosophical Transactions of the Royal Society*
QJEP	*Quartery Journal of Experimental Physiology*
QSGNM	*Quellen u. Studien z. Gesch. d. Naturwiss. u. d. Medizin* (continuation of *Archiv f. Gesch. d. Math., d. Naturwiss. u. d. Technik, AGMNT*, formerly *Archiv f. d. Gesch. d. Naturwiss. u. d. Technik, AGNT*)
RAC	*Revue d' Acupuncture*
RAI/OP	*Occasional Papers of the Royal Anthropological Institute*
RAL/MSF	*Rendiconti d. Accademia* (*reale*, now *nazionale*) *dei Lincei* (*Cl. Sci. Moral. Stor. e Filol.*)
RBS	*Revue Bibliographique de Sinologie*
RGE	*Review of Gastro-enterology.*
RHSID	*Revue d'Histoire de la Sidérurgie* (Nancy)
RIAC	*Revue Internat. d'Acupuncture* (contd. as *NRIAC*)
RKANF	*Der Römischen Kaiserlichen Akamedie der Naturforscher auserlesene medizinisch, chirurgisch, anatomisch, chemisch und botanische Abhandlungen* (Deutsche Ausgabe) Nürnberg
RTS	*Religious Tract Society*
S	*Sinologica* (Basel)
SAM	*Scientific American*
SBE	*Sacred Books of the East* Series
SC	*Science*
SCISA	*Scientia Sinica* (Peking)
SGO	*Surgery, Gynaecology and Obstetrics*
SHIY	*Shanghai Chung I Yao Tsa Chih* (*Shanghai Journ. Traditional Chinese Medicine and Pharmacy*)
SPECT	*Spectator*
SSEB	*Symposia of the Society of Experimental Biology*

SSM	*Social Science and Medicine*
TCPP	*Transactions and Studies of the College of Physicians of Philadelphia*
TCULT	*Technology and Culture*
TH	*Thien Hsia Monthly* (Shanghai)
TM	*Terrestrial Magnetism and Atmospheric Electricity* (continued as *Journal of Geophysical Research*)
TNLF	*Tidsskrift Norske Laegeforening*
TNS	*Transactions of the Newcomen Society*
TP	*T'oung Tao* (*Archives concernant l'Histoire, les Langues, la Géographie, l'Ethnographie et les Arts de l'Asie Orientale*, Leiden)
TRNS	*Trends in Neuro-Sciences*
VS	*Variétés Sinologiques*
WI	*Wine Industry*
WKW	*Wienen Klinische Wochenschrift*
WWTK	*Wên Wu* (formerly *Wên Wu Tshan Khao Tzu Liao, Reference Materials for History and Archaeology*)
ZDMG	*Zeitschrift d. deutsch. morgenlöndischen Gesellschaft*
ZGEM	*Zeitschrift f. d. gesamte Experimentelle Medizin*
ZGNP	*Zeitschrift f. d. gesamte Neurologie u. Psychiatrie*
ZKM	*Zeitschr. f. Klinische Medizin*
ZVHFF	*Zeitschr. f. Vitamin-, Hormon- und Ferment-forschung*

A. CHINESE AND JAPANESE BOOKS BEFORE +1800

Each entry gives particulars in the following order:

(*a*) title, alphabetically arranged, with characters;
(*b*) alternative title, if any;
(*c*) translation of title;
(*d*) cross-reference to closely related book, if any;
(*e*) dynasty;
(*f*) date as accurate as possible;
(*g*) name of author or editor, with characters;
(*h*) title of other book, if the text of the work now exists only incorporated therein; or, in special cases, references to sinological studies of it;
(*i*) references to translations, if any, given by the name of the translator in Bibliography C;
(*j*) notice of any index or concordance to the book if such a work exists;
(*k*) reference to the number of the book in the *Tao Tsang* catalogue of Wieger (6), if applicable;
(*l*) reference to the number of the book in the *San Tsang* (Tripiṭaka) catalogues of Nanjio (1) and Takakusu & Watanabe, if applicable.

Words which assist in the translation of titles are added in round brackets.

Alternative titles or explanatory additions to the titles are added in square brackets.

It will be remembered (p. 305 above) that in Chinese indexes words beginning *Chh-* are all listed together after *Ch-*, and *Hs-* after *H-*, but that this applies to initial words of titles only.

Where there are any differences between the entries in these bibliographies and those in Vols. 1–4, the information here given is to be taken as more correct.

An interim list of references to the editions used in the present work, and to the *tshung-shu* collections in which books are available, has been given in Vol. 4, pt. 3, pp. 913 ff., and is available as a separate brochure.

Abbreviations

C/Han	Former Han.
E/Wei	Eastern Wei.
H/Han	Later Han.
H/Shu	Later Shu (Wu Tai).
H/Thang	Later Thang (Wu Tai).
H/Chin	Later Chin (Wu Tai).
S/Han	Southern Han (Wu Tai).
S/Phing	Southern Phing (Wu Tai).
J/Chin	Jurchen Chin.
L/Sung	Liu Sung.
N/Chou	Northern Chou.
N/Chhi	Northern Chhi.
N/Sung	Northern Sung (before the removal of the capital to Hangchow).
N/Wei	Northern Wei.
S/Chhi	Southern Chhi.
S/Sung	Southern Sung (after the removal of the capital to Hangchow).
W/Wei	Western Wei.

Chan Kuo Tshê 戰國策.
Records of the Warring States.
Chhin.
Writer unknown.

Chang Shih Lei Ching
See *Lei Ching*

Chen Chhüan Chen Ching 甄權鍼經
Chen Chhüan's Manual of Acupuncture.
Sui or Thang *c.* +610/+620.
Chen Chhüan 甄權
Now available only in quotations, e.g. in (*Thung Jen*) *Chen Chiu Ching*.
Cf. Chang Tsan-Chhen (*5*).

Chen Ching Chieh Yao 鍼經節要.
Summary of the Important Points in the Acupuncture Classics.
Ascr. +3rd.
Attrib. Huangfu Mi 皇甫謐.
First pr. Yuan, +1315.
Ed. Tu Ssu-Ching 杜思敬.
In *Chi Shêng Pa Sui*, no. 1.

Chen Ching Chih Nan 鍼經指南.
A Rutter (Set of Compass-Bearings) for the Acupuncture Manuals [mnemonic rhymes].
J/Chin or Yuan, +1241.
Tou Han-Chhing (b) 竇漢卿.
Includes *Piao Yu Fu*, *Ting Pa Hsüeh Chih Nan*, and *Hsieh Chê Kung Thu*.

Chen Ching Tsê Ying Chi 鍼經摘英集.
A Collection of Gems culled from the Acupuncture Classics.
Yuan, before +1315.
Writer unknown, perhaps Tu Ssu-Ching 杜思敬.
In *Chi Shêng Pa Sui*, no. 3.

Chen Chiu Chhüan Shu 針灸全書.
Complete Treatise on Acupuncture and Moxibustion.
Ming, +1591.
Chhen Yen 陳言, based on the teachings and private treatise of Yang Ching-Chai [= Chi-Chou] 楊敬齋 [繼州].
Cf. Hsieh Li-Hêng (*1*), p. 32*b*, and the postface by Fan Hsing-Chun.

Chen Chiu Chia I Ching 針灸甲乙經
Treatise on Acupuncture and Moxibustion.
S/Kuo & Chin, finished some time between +256 and his death in +282.
Huangfu Mi 皇甫謐.

Chen Chiu Chieh Yao 鍼灸節要.
Important Essentials of Acupuncture and Moxibustion.
Ming, +1536 or +1537.
Kao Wu 高武.
ICK, p. 345.

Chen Chiu Chü Ying 鍼灸聚英.
A Collection of Gems in Acupuncture and Moxibustion.
Ming +1529, first pr. +1537. First pr. Japan, +1546.
Kao Wu 高武.
Kho-Hsüeh Chi-Shu, Shanghai, 1963.
Based on a Japanese edition of +1645 with some corrections.
Cf. Anon. (*83*), p. 103.

Chen Chiu Chü Ying Fa Hui
See *Chen Chiu Chü Ying*
Chen Chiu Su Nan Yao Chih
See *Chen Chiu Chieh Yao*
Chen Chiu Ta Chhêng 針灸大成 (alternative titles: *Chen Chiu Ta Chhüan* 全, *Chen Chiu Chi Chhêng* 集).
Principles of Acupuncture and Moxibustion.
An enlargement of the *Wei Shêng Chen Chiu Hsüan Chi Pi Yao.*
Ming, pref. +1601.
Yang Chi-Chou 楊繼州.
Cf. Anon (*83*), p. 104; *ICK*, pp. 351–2; Li Thao (*10*), p.58.
Chen Chiu Tsê Jih Pien (*Chi*) 鍼灸擇日編(集).
On the Choice of Days (and Times) for Acupuncture and Moxibustion.
Ming, +1447.
Chhüan Hsün-I 全循義 & Chin I-Sun 金義孫 with a preface by Chin Li-Mêng 金禮蒙.
Bound with *Pei Chi Chiu Fa*, q.v.
Preserved only in Japan till repr. in 1890.
Chen Chiu Tzu Shêng Ching 鍼灸資生經.
Manual of Acupuncture and Moxibustion Profitable for the Restoration of Health.
Sung +1220, repr. +1231, +1236.
Wang Chih-Chung 王執中.
ICK, pp. 327 ff.
Chen Chiu Wên Tui 鍼灸問對
Questions and Answers about Acupuncture and Moxibustion.
Ming, +1532.
Wang Chi 汪機.
ICK, pp. 344–5.
Chêng Lei Pên Tshao
See *Chhung-Hsiu Chêng-Ho Ching-Shih Chêng Lei Pei Yung Pên Tshao.*
Chi Hsiao Hsin Shu 紀效新書.
A New Treatise on Military and Naval Efficiency.
Ming, *c.* +1575.
Chhi Chi-Kuang 戚繼光.
Chi Shêng Pa Sui (*Fang*) 濟生拔粹(方).
Selected Materials for the Preservation of Health (a collectaneum of nineteen medical books).
Yuan, +1315.
Tu Ssu-Ching (ed.) 杜思敬.
Chieh-Ku Yün-Chhi Chen Fa 潔古雲岐鍼法.
Acupuncture Methods of (Chang) Chieh-Ku and Yün Chhi (Tzu, Chang Pi, his son).
J/Chin and Yuan, *c.* +1235.
Chang Chieh-Ku [Yuan-Su] 張潔古 and Chang Pi 張璧.
In *Chi Shêng Pa Sui*, no. 2.
Chin Kuei Yao Lüeh (*Fang Lun*) 金匱要略(方論) (originally part of *Sheng Han Tsa Ping Lun*).
Systematic Treasury of Medicine (lit.: Main Principles of the (Prescriptions in the) Golden Medicine-Chest).
H/Han, orig. *c.* +200, revised *c.* +300.
Chang Chung-Ching 張仲景, revised and edited by Wang Shu-Ho (Chin) 王叔和.
Chin Lan Hsün Ching Chhü Hsüeh Thu Chieh 金蘭循經取穴圖解.
The Golden Orchid; an Illustrated Study of Finding the Acu-points according to the Tracts.
Yuan, +1303.
Hu-Thai-Pi-Lieh 忽泰必烈 (Hu Kung-Thai) 忽公泰
ICK, pp. 334–5.
Ching-Yo Chhüan Shu 景岳全書.
A Comprehensive Collection of the Medical Writings of (Chang) Ching-Yo [i.e. Chang Chieh-Pin, d. +1640].
Ming, +1624 (prefaces of +1503 and +1711).
Chang Chieh-Pin 張介賓.
Kho-Hsüeh Chi-Shu, Shanghai, no date.
Chiu Lao Fa 灸勞法.
Moxibustion Method for Tuberculosis.
See *Ku Chêng Ping Chiu Fang.*
Chou Hou Pei Chi Fang 肘後備急方.
(= *Chou Hou Tsu Chiu Fang*
= *Chou Hou Pai I Fang*
= *Ko Hsien Ong Chou Hou Pei Chi Fang*)
Handbook of Medicines for Emergencies.
Chin, *c.* +340.
Ko Hung 葛洪.
Chou Li 周禮.
Record of the Institutions (lit. Rites) of (the) Chou (Dynasty) [descriptions of all government official posts and their duties].
C/Han, perhaps containing some material from late Chou.
Compilers unknown.
Tr. E. Biot (1).
Chu Chieh Shang Han Lun 註解傷寒論.
Annotations on the *Treatise on Febrile Diseases.*
Sung, +1144.
Original text by Chang Chung-Ching 張仲景 (H/Han).
Chhêng Wu-Chi 成無巳.
Chu Ping Yuan Hou Lun 諸病源候論.
(= *Chhao Shih Chu Ping Yuan Hou* (*Tsung*) *Lun*).
Treatise on Diseases and their Aetiology [systematic pathology].
Sui, *c.* +607.
Chhao Yuan-Fang 巢元方.
Chuang Tzu 莊子.
(= *Nan Hua Chen Ching.*)
The Book of Master Chuang.
Chou, *c.* −290.
Chuang Chou 莊周.
Tr. Legge (5); Fêng Yu-Lan (5); Lin Yü-Thang (1).
Yin-Tê Index no. (suppl.) 20.

Chhao Shih Chu Ping Yuan Hou Tsung Lun
See *Chu Ping Yuan Hou Lun*
Chhi Hsüan Tzu Yuan Ho Chi Yung Ching 啓玄子元和紀用經.
Manual of (Medical) Dealings in the Yuan-Ho reign-period (+806 to +820), by the Revealing-of-Mysteries Master.
Thang, +889.
Hsü Chi 許寂.
Cf. Fan Hsing-Chun (9).
Chhi Lüeh 七略.
The Seven Summaries [bibliography].
C/Han, −6.
Liu Hsiang 劉向, completed by his son Liu Hsin 劉歆.
Now extant only as incorporated into the *Chhien Han Shu* bibliography (*I wên chih*).
Chhi Tung Yeh Yü 齊東野語.
Rustic Talks in Eastern Chhi.
Sung, *c.* +1290.
Chou Mi 周密.
Chhien Chin I Fang 千金翼方.
Supplement to the *Thousand Golden Remedies* [i.e. Revised Prescriptions saving lives, worth a Thousand Ounces of Gold].
Thang, between +660 and +680.
Sun Ssu-Mo 孫思邈.
Chhien Chin Yao Fang 千金要方.
A Thousand Golden Remedies [i.e. Essential Prescriptions saving lives, worth a Thousand Ounces of Gold].
Thang, between +650 and +659.
Sun Ssu-Mo 孫思邈.
Chhien Fu Lun 潛夫論.
Comments of a Hermit Scholar.
H/Han, *c.* +150.
Wang Fu 王符.
Chhing I Lu 清異錄.
Exhilarating Talks on Strange Things.
Wu Tai and Sung, *c.* +965.
Thao Ku 陶穀.
Chhüan Ching 拳經.
Manual of Boxing.
Chhing, +18th.
Chang Khung-Chao 張孔昭.
Chhuan Chung Lu
Essays on the Orthodox Doctrines (of Chinese Traditional Medicine).
Part of Chang Chieh-Pin's *Ching-Yo Chhüan Shu*, q.v.
Chhung-Hsiu Chêng-Ho Ching-Shih Chêng Lei Pei-Yung Pên Tshao 重修政和經史證類備用本草.
New Revision of the Pharmacopoeia of the Chêng-Ho reign-period; the Classified and Consolidated Armamentarium. (A Combination of the *Chêng-Ho...Cheng Lei...Pên Tshao* with the *Pên Tshao Yen I*).
Yuan +1249; reprinted many times afterwards, esp. in the Ming +1468, and at least seven Ming editions, the last in +1624 or +1625.
Thang Shen-Wei 唐慎微.
Khou Tsung-Shih 寇宗奭.
pr. (or ed.) Chang Tshun-Hui 張存惠.
Goshūiwakashū 後拾遺和歌集.
Japan, compiled +1086.
(Fourth Imperial) Anthology of Japanese Poetry.
Huai Nan Tzu 淮南子.
(= *Huai Nan Hung Lieh Chieh.*)
The Book of (the Prince of) Huai-Nan [compendium of natural philosophy].
C/Han, *c.* −120.
Written by the group of scholars gathered by Liu An (prince of Huai-Nan) 劉安.
Partial trs. Morgan (1), Erkes (1), Hughes (1), Chatley (1), Wieger (2).
Chung-Fa Index, no. 5.
TT/1170.
Huang Ti Chen Chiu Hsia-Ma Chi (*or Thu, or Ching*) 黃帝鍼灸蝦蟆忌（圖,經）
The Yellow Emperor's (Illustrated Manual of the) Preferential and Forbidden Days for Acupuncture and Moxibustion according to the Lunar Cycle (lit. the Yellow Emperor's Toad Manual).
Sui or pre-Sui, perhaps Liang.
Writer unknown.
Cf. *Ming Thang Hsia-Ma Thu.* A *Hsia-Ma Ching* is extant in Japan.
ICK, p. 305; *SIC*, p. 246; Hsieh Li-Hêng (*1*), p. 11*b*.
Much quoted in ch. 2 of *I Hsin Fang* (+984), (pp. 69 ff.).
Huang Ti Nei Ching, Ling Shu 黃帝內經靈樞.
The Yellow Emperor's Manual of Corporeal (Medicine); the Vital Axis [medical physiology and anatomy].
Probably C/Han, *c.* −1st century.
Writers unknown.
Edited Thang, +762, by Wang Ping 王冰.
Analysis by Huang Wên (1).
Tr. Chamfrault & Ung Kang-Sam (1).
Commentaries by Ma Shih 馬蒔 (Ming) and Chang Chih-Tshung 張志聰 (Chhing) in *TSCC*, *I shu tien*, chs. 67 to 88.
Huang Ti Nei Ching, Ling Shu, Pai Hua Chieh
See Chhen Pi-Liu & Chêng Cho-Jen (*1*).
Huang Ti Nei Ching Ming Thang (*Chu*) 黃帝內經明堂（注）.
A Description of the Microcosm (i.e. the Human Body) [visceral anatomy and acupuncture according to the tracts] (to accompany the) Yellow Emperor's Manual of Corporeal (Medicine).
Sui, *c.* +610.
Writer unknown.
Contemporary commentary by Yang Shang-Shan 楊上善.
Only one chapter preserved in Japan.
ICK, pp. 306, 313–14; *SIC*, pp. 257–8; Anon (*90*), p. 4.

Huang Ti Nei Ching, Su Wên 黃帝內經素問.
The Yellow Emperor's Manual of Corporeal (Medicine); Questions (and Answers) about Living Matter [clinical medicine]. (Cf. *Pu Chu Huang Ti Nei Ching, Su Wên.*)
Chou, remodelled in Chhin and Han, reaching final form *c.* −2nd century.
Writers unknown.
Ed. & comm., Thang (+762), Wang Ping 王冰; Sung (*c.* +1050), Lin I 林億.
Partial trs. Hübotter (1), chs. 4, 5, 10, 11, 21; Veith (1); complete, Chamfrault & Ung Kang-Sam (1).
See Wang & Wu (1), pp. 28 ff.; Huang Wên (1).

Huang Ti Nei Ching Su Wên, Pai Hua Chieh.
See Chou Fêng-Wu, Wang Wan-Chieh & Hsü Kuo-Chhien (*1*).

Huang Ti Nei Ching, Thai Su 黃帝內經太素.
The Yellow Emperor's Manual of Corporeal (Medicine); the Great Innocence [i.e. the *Yellow Emperor's Manual of Corporeal (Medicine); Questions (and Answers) about Living Matter; and the Vital Axis;* arranged in their original form].
Chou, Chhin & Han, essentially in present form by −1st century, commented upon in Sui, +605 to +618.
Ed. and comm. Yang Shang-Shan 楊上善.
Identifications of chapters and component passages with the corresponding texts in the *Questions (and Answers) about Living Matter;* and the *Vital Axis*; in Wang Ping's recension, and in the *Chen Chiu Chia I Ching* (Treatise on Acupuncture and Moxibustion) of Huangfu Mi; by Hsiao Yen-Phing 蕭延平 (1924).

Hsi Fang Tzu Ming Thang Chiu Ching
西方子明堂灸經.
Moxibustion Manual for the Microcosm (i.e. the Human Body), by the Western-Direction Master [based on the *Thung Jen Shu Hsüeh Chen Chiu Thu Ching* of Wang Wei-I].
Sung, *c.* +1050.
Hsi Fang Tzu (personal name not known) 西方子.
ICK, p. 320.

Hsi Yuan Lu 洗寃錄.
Records of the Washing Away of Unjust Imputations [treatise on forensic medicine].
Sung, +1247.
Sung Tzhu 宋慈.
Partial tr., H. A. Giles (7).

Hsia-Ma Ching 蝦蟆經.
See *Huang Ti Chen Chiu Hsia Ma Chi.*

Hsieh Chê Kung Thu 叶蟄宮圖
A Chart for the (Diseases of the) Wintry North [lit. the Realm of Universal Hibernation; cf. Hsieh Li-Hêng (*2*), vol. 1, p. 718].
J/Chin or Yuan, *c.* +1240.
Tou Han-Chhing (b) 竇漢卿.
Part of *Chen Ching Chih Nan*, q.v.

Hsin Khan Pu Chu Thung Jen Shu Hsüeh Chen Chiu Thu Ching 新刊補註銅人腧穴鍼灸圖經.
See *Thung Jen Shu Hsüeh Chen Chiu Thu Ching.*
A 1909 reprint of the J/Chin Ta-Ting r.p. issue (thus between +1161 and +1189) with additional comments.

Hsü Shih Chen Chiu Ta Chhüan
徐氏鍼灸大全.
Master Hsü's Compendium of Acupunture and Moxibustion.
Ming, +1439.
Hsü Fêng, 徐鳳.
Cf. Li Thao (*10*), p. 58; *ICK*, p. 351.

Hsü Tzu Chih Thung Chhien Chhang Phien
續資治通鑑長編.
Continuation of the *Comprehensive Mirror (of History) for Aid in Government* [+960 to +1126].
Sung, +1183.
Li Tao 李燾.

Hsüan Chu Mi Yü 玄珠密語
[= *Su Wên Liu Chhi Hsüan Chu Mi Yü*].
Confidential Sayings of the Mysterious-Pearl (Master). [Taoist medical theory dealing especially with *wu-yün liu-chhi*].
Ascr. Thang, +7th or +8th. Actually written at some time in the +10th to +12th centuries.
Attrib. Wang Ping 王冰.
Real writer unknown.
SKCS/TMTY, ch. 100, p. 22*b*; *ICK*, pp. 1390–3; *SIC*, pp. 49 ff.

Hsün Ching Khao Hsüeh Pien 循經考穴編.
An Investigation of the Acu-points along the Tracts.
Ming, not before +1575.
Prob. Yen Chen-Shih 嚴振識.
MS. ed. with postface by Fan Hsing-Chun 范行準, 2 vols., Chhun-lien, Shanghai, 1955.

Hsün Tzu 荀子.
The Book of Master Hsün.
Chou, *c.* −240.
Hsün Chhing 荀卿.
Tr. Dubs (7).

I Chin Ching 易筋經.
Manual of Exercising the Muscles and Tendons [Buddhist].
Ascr. N/Wei.
Chhing, perhaps +17th.
Attrib. Ta-Mo (Bodhidharma) 達摩.
Author unknown.
Reproduced in Wang Tsu-Yuan (*1*).

I Hsin Fang (Ishinhō) 醫心方.
The Heart of Medicine [partly a collection of ancient Chinese and Japanese books].
Japan, +982 (not printed till 1854).
Tamba no Yasuyori 丹波康賴.

I Hsüeh Ju Mên 醫學入門.
Janua Medicinae [a general system of medicine].
Ming, +1575.
Li Chhan 李梴.

I Shu Chhüan Chi 醫書全集.
Collection of Medical Writings (by Hsü Ling-Thai).
Chhing, *c.* +1770.
Hsü Ling-Thai 徐靈胎.

I Shuo 醫說.
Discourses on Medicine (and its History).
Sung, *c.* +1189.
Chang Kao 張杲.

Ishinhō
See *I Hsin Fang*.

Kao-Huang Chiu Fa 膏肓灸法.
On Moxibustion at the Kao-huang acupoint [VU 38].
Sung, +1128.
Chuang Cho 莊綽.
ICK, p. 326.

Khang-Phing Shang Han Lun 康平傷寒論.
The Khang-Phing (Kōhei) text of the *Treatise on Febrile Diseases*.
H/Han, +205.
Chang Chung-Ching 張仲景.
This text, edited in Japan in +1060, is the only pre-Sung text which clearly distinguishes the original book from its commentaries.
Ed. Yeh Chü-Chhüan 葉橘泉.
Chhien Chhing Thang Shu Chü, Shanghai, 1947, repr. 1954.

Ko Hsien Ong Chou Hou Pei Chi Fang
See *Chou Hou Pei Chi Fang*

Ku Chêng Ping Chiu Fang 骨蒸病灸方.
[= *Chiu Lao Fa.*]
Moxibustion for Tuberculosis-like Diseases.
Thang, *c.* +670.
Tshui Chih-Thi 崔知悌.
SIC, p. 250; *ICK*, p. 316.

Kuan Tzu 管子.
The Book of Master Kuan.
Chou and C/Han. Perhaps mainly compiled in the Chi-Hsia Academy (late −4th century) in part from older materials.
Attrib. Kuan Chung 管仲.
Partial trs. Haloun (2, 5); Than Po-Fu *et al.* (1).

Kuang Ya 廣雅.
Enlargement of the *Erh Ya*; *Literary Expositor* [dictionary].
San Kuo (Wei), +230.
Chang I 張揖.

Lei Ching 類經.
The Classics Classified; a System of Medicine.
Ming, +1624.
Chang Chieh-Pin 張介賓.

Lei Kung Phao Chih Lun 雷公炮炙論.
The Venerable Master Lei's Treatise on the Decoction and Preparation (of Drugs).
L/Sung, *c.* +470.
Lei Hsiao 雷斅.
Preserved only in quotations in *Chêng Lei Pên Tshao* and elsewhere, and reconstituted by Chang Chi 張驥; see Lung Po-Chien (*1*), p. 116.

Lei Shuo 類說.
A Classified Commonplace-Book [a great florilegium of excerpts from Sung and pre-Sung books, many of which are otherwise lost].
Sung, +1136.
Ed. Tsêng Tshao 曾慥.

Li Chi 禮記.
(= *Hsiao Tai Li Chi*).
Record of Rites [compiled by Tai the Younger] (cf. *Ta Tai Li Chi*).
Ascr. C/Han, *c.* −70 to −50, but really H/Han, between +80 and +105, though the earliest pieces included may date from the time of the *Analects* (*c.* −465 to −450).
Attrib. ed. Tai Shêng 戴聖.
Actual ed. Tshao Pao 曹褒.
Trs. Legge (7); Couvreur (3); R. Wilhelm (6).
Yin-Tê Index, no. 27.

Li Tai Ming I Mêng Chhiu 歷代名醫蒙求.
Brief Lives of the Famous Physicians of all Ages.
Sung, +1220.
Chou Shou-Chung 周守忠.
SIC, p. 507.

Lieh Tzu 列子.
[= *Chhung Hsü Chen Ching*]
The Book of Master Lieh.
Chou and C/Han, −5th to −1st centuries. Ancient fragments of miscellaneous origin finally cemented together with much new material about +380.
Attrib. *Lieh Yü-Khou* 列禦寇.
Tr. R. Wilhelm (4); L. Giles (4), Weizer (7); Graham (6).
TT/663.

Liu Chu Chih Wei Fu 流注指微賦.
Ode on the Minutiae of the Circulations (of the Chhi).
J/Chin or Yuan, *c.* +1235.
Ho Jo-Yü 何若愚 but by Kao Wu attrib. Tou Kuei-Fang 竇桂芳.
A small tractate preserved in *Chen Chiu Chü Ying*, ch. 4A, (p. 229).
SIC, pp. 297–8.

Lü Shih Chhun Chhiu 呂氏春秋.
Master Lü's Spring and Autumn Annals [compendium of natural philosophy].
Chou (Chhin), −239.
Written by the group of scholars gathered by Lü Pu-Wei 呂不韋.
Tr. R. Wilhelm (3).
Chung-Fu Index, no. 2.

Mêng Chhi Pi Than 夢溪筆談.
Dream Pool Essays.
Sung, +1086; last supplement dated +1091.
Shen Kua 沈括.
Ed. Hu Tao-Ching (*1*); cf. Holzman (1).
Mêng Tzu 孟子.
The Book of Master Mêng (Mencius).
Chou, *c.* −290.
Mêng Kho 孟軻.
Tr. Legge (3); Lyall (1).
Yin-Tê Index, no. (suppl.) 17.
Ming Huang Tsa Lu 明皇雜錄.
Miscellaneous Records of the Brightness of the Imperial Court (of Thang Hsüan Tsung).
Thang, +855.
Chêng Chhu-Hui 鄭處誨.
Ming I Pieh Lu 名醫別錄.
Informal (or Additional) Records of Famous Physicians (on Materia Medica).
Ascr. Liang, *c.* +510.
Attrib. Thao Hung-Ching 陶弘景.
Now extant only in quotations in the pharmaceutical natural histories, and a reconstitution by Huang Yü (*1*).
This work was a disentanglement, made by other hands between +523 and +618 or +656, of the contributions of Li Tang-Chih (*c.* +225) and Wu Phu (*c.* +235) and the commentaries of Thao Hung-Ching (+492) from the text of the *Shen Nung Pên Tshao Ching* itself. In other words it was the non-*Pên-Ching* part of the *Pên Tshao Ching Chi Chu* (q.v.). It may or may not have included some or all of Thao Hung-Ching's commentaries.
Ming Thang Chen Chiu Thu 明堂鍼灸圖.
Charts of the Microcosm (i.e. the Human Body) for Acupuncture and Moxibustion.
Date uncertain, ascr. H/Han, perhaps even Sung.
Attrib. Huang Ti.
Possible writer Yang Chieh (Sung) 楊介.
Now extant only in quotations.
SIC, pp. 265–6.
Ming Thang Chiu Ching 明堂灸經.
Manual of Moxa for all Parts of the Body.
Thang, +7th (possibly pre-Thang).
Writer unknown.
Included, at least partially, in *Thai-Phing Shêng Hui Fang*, q.v.
Ming Thang Chiu Ching 明堂灸經.
See *Hsi Fang Tzu Ming Thang Chiu Ching*.
Ming Thang Hsia-Ma Thu 明堂蝦蟆圖.
Illustrated Toad Manual for the Microcosm (i.e. the Human Body), [preferential and forbidden days for acupuncture according to the lunar cycle].
Sui or pre-Sui, perhaps Liang.
Writer unknown.
Cf. *Huang Ti Chen Chiu Hsia-Ma Chi*.
ICK, p. 313; *SIC*, p. 248; Hsieh Li-Hêng (*1*), p. 11*b*.
Ming Thang Jen Hsing Thu 明堂人形圖.
Charts of the Human Form Divine (with Explanations), [anatomy and acupuncture].
Sui, *c.* +610.
Chen Chhüan 甄權.
Preserved only in quotations, chiefly in the works of Sun Ssu-Mo.
SIC, p. 255.
Ming Thang Khung Hsüeh Chen Chiu Chih Yao 明堂孔穴鍼灸治要.
Essentials of Therapy of the Microcosm (i.e. the Human Body) by the Application of Acupuncture and Moxa at the Acu-points.
Prob. H/Han, +1st or +2nd.
Writer unknown.
Extant now only in quotations, as in Huangfu Mi's *Chia I Ching* (+282).
SIC, p. 245.
Ming Thang Khung Hsüeh Thu 明堂孔穴圖.
Charts of the Acu-points on the Human Body (lit. the Microcosm).
Liang or pre-Liang.
Writer unknown.
Still extant in Sui and Thang, now known only in rare quotations.
SIC, p. 253.
Ming Thang Ta Tao Lu 明堂大道錄.
A Broad Outline of the Microcosm [human anatomy in relation to acupuncture].
Chhing.
Hui Tung 惠棟.
Mo Ching 脈經.
The Pulse Manual; or, Manual of Sphygmology.
Chin, *c.* +300.
Wang Shu-Ho 王叔和.
Ed. Lin I (+1068) 林億.
Mo Chüeh 脈訣.
Sphygmological Instructions.
Wu Tai, *c.* +907 to +960.
Kao Yang-Shêng 高陽生.

Nan Chao Yeh Shih 南詔野史.
History of the Nan Chao Dynasty (Yünnan).
Ming, +1550 (enlarged in +1775 by Hu Wei 胡蔚).
Yang Shen 楊愼.
Tr. Sainson (1).
Nan Ching 難經.
Manual of (Explanations concerning Eighty-one) Difficult (Passages in the *Yellow Emperor's Manual of Corporeal Medicine*).
C/Han, *c.* −1st, or H/Han, +1st.
Attrib. Chhin Yüeh Jen 秦越人, but author not identical with Pien Chhio.
Nan Ching Pên I 難經本義.
The Original Ideas of the *Manual of Difficult Passages* (commentary on the text).
Yuan, +1361.
Hua Shou 滑壽.

Nan Hua Chen Ching
See *Chuang Tzu*
Nei Chia Chhüan Fa 內家拳法.
Techniques of the Esoteric (Southern, or Wu-tang Shan) School (of Unarmed Combat).
Chhing, *c.* +1690.
Huang Pai-Chia 黃百家.
Nei Ching 內經.
See *Huang Ti Nei Ching, Su Wên* and *Huang Ti Nei Ching, Ling Shu.*
Nei Ching, Thai Su 內經太素.
See *Huang Ti Nei Ching, Thai Su.*
Nei Ching Yün Chhi Yao Chih Lun
內經運氣 旨論.
A Discussion of the Most Important Points about the Permutations of the (Five Elements and the Six) Chhi in the (*Yellow Emperor's*) *Manual of Corporeal* (*Medicine*).
Sung, *c.* +1180.
Liu Wan-Su 劉完素.
ICK, pp. 1395 ff.
Nihongi 日本記.
(= *Nihon-shoki*)
Chronicles of Japan [from the earliest times to +696].
Japan (Nara), +720.
Toneri-shinnō (prince) 舍人親王, Ōno Yasumaro 大安萬呂, Ki no Kiyobito *et al.*
Tr. Aston (1). Cf. Anon (103), pp. 1 ff.
Nihon-shoki 日本書記.
See *Nihongi.*

Pa-shih-i Nan Ching 八十一難經.
See *Nan Chhing.*
Pai Chêng Fu 百症賦.
Mnemonic Ode on the Hundred Syndromes.
Ming, +1529.
Kao Wu 高武.
Incorporated in *Chen Chiu Chü Ying*, q.v. (ch. 4A, p. 241).
Pei Chi Chhien Chin Yao Fang.
The Thousand Golden Remedies for Use in Emergencies.
See *Chhien Chin Yao Fang*, of which it is the full title.
Pei Chi Chiu Fa 備急灸法.
Methods of Moxibustion for Use in Emergencies.
Sung, +1226, with pref. of +1245.
Wênjen Chhi-Nien 聞人耆年.
ICK, p. 329, *SIC*, p. 294.
Based on two earlier books written between +1100 and +1126 by Chang Huan 張渙.
Bound with *Chen Chiu Tsê Jih Pien* q.v.
Preserved only in Japan till repr. in 1890.
Pên Tshao Ching Chi Chu 本草經集注.
Collected Commentaries on the *Classical Pharmacopoeia* (*of the Heavenly Husbandman*).
S/Chhi, +492.
Thao Hung-Ching 陶弘景.
Now extant only in fragmentary form as a Tunhuang or Turfan MS, apart from the many quotations in the pharmaceutical natural histories under Thao Hung-Ching's name.
Pên Tshao Hui Pien 本草會編.
The Congregation of the Pharmaceutical Naturalists; Correlated Notes on Materia Medica.
Ming, *c.* +1540.
Wang Chi 汪機.
Pên Tshao Kang Mu 本草綱目.
The Great Pharmacopoeia; or, The Pandects of Natural History (Mineralogy, Metallurgy, Botany, Zoology, etc.) Arrayed in their Headings and Subheadings.
Ming, +1596.
Li Shih-Chen 李時珍.
Paraphrased and abridged tr. Read & collaborators (2–7) and Read & Pak (1) with indexes. Tabulation of plants in Read (1) (with Liu Ju-Chhiang). Cf. Swingle (7).
Phao Chih Lun.
See *Lei Kung Phao Chih Lun.*
Phu Chi Fang 普濟方.
Practical Prescriptions for Everyman.
Ming, *c.* +1418.
Chu Hsiao (Chou Ting Wang) 朱橚（周定王）.
ISK, p. 914.
Piao Yu Fu 標幽賦.
Mnemomic Ode Explaining the Obscurities (in the Theory and Practice of Acupuncture).
J/Chin or Yuan, *c.* +1235.
Tou Han-Chhing (b) 竇漢卿.
Part of *Chen Ching Chih Nan*, q.v.
Pien Chhio Shen Ying Chen Chiu Yü Lung Ching
扁鵲神應鍼灸玉龍經.
Jade Dragon Manual of Acupuncture and Moxibustion according to the Marvellously Successful Principles of Pien Chhio [Yü Lung here refers to an exquisitely carved dragon of jade found in +542 (*Yu-Yang Tsa Tsu*, ch. 10, p. 3*a*), and symbolises rarity and intricacy.]
Yuan, +1329.
Wang Kuo-Jui 王國瑞.
Cf. Chhen Pi-Liu & Chêng Cho-Jen (2), p. 85; *ICK*, p. 336.
Pu Chu Huang Ti Nei Ching Su Wên
補註黃帝內經素問.
Commentaries on the *Yellow Emperor's Manual of Corporeal* (*Medicine*); *Questions* (*and Answers*) *about Living Matter.*
Thang, +762.
Wang Ping 王冰.
Re-edited in Sung, *c.* +1050.
Lin I *et al.* 林億

Samguk Sagi 三國史記.
History of the Three Kingdoms (of Korea) [Silla (Hsin-Lo), Kokuryo (Kao-Chü-Li) and Pakche (Pai-Chhi), −57 to +936].
Korea, +1145 (imperially commissioned by King Injong) reprd. +1394, +1512.
Kim Pusik 金富軾.
San Fu Huang Thu 三輔黃圖.
Illustrated Description of the Three Cities of the Metropolitan Area (Chhang-an (mod. Sian), Fêng-i and Fu-fêng).
Chin, original text late +3rd century or perhaps H/Han; present version stabilised, including much older material, between +757 and +907.
Attrib. Miao Chhang-Yen 苗昌言.
Cf. des Rotours (1), p. lxxxvi.
San Kuo Chih 三國志.
History of the Three Kingdoms [+220 to +280].
Chin, *c.* +290.
Chhen Shou 陳壽.
Yin-Tê Index, no. 33.
For translations of passages see the index of Frankel (1).
Shan Hai Ching 山海經.
Classic of the Mountains and Rivers.
Chou and C/Han.
Writers unknown.
Partial tr. de Rosny (1).
Chung-Fa Index no. 9.
Shang Han Lun 傷寒論.
(Originally part of *Shang Han Tsa Ping Lun*.)
Treatise on Febrile Diseases.
H/Han, *c.* +200.
Chang Chung-Ching 張仲景.
Shen Nung Pên Tshao Ching 神農本草經.
Classical Pharmacopoeia of the Heavenly Husbandman.
C/Han, based on Chou and Chhin material, but not reaching final form before the +2nd century.
Writers unknown.
Lost as a separate work, but the basis of all subsequent compendia of pharmaceutical natural history, in which it is constantly quoted.
Reconstituted and annotated by many scholars; see Lung Po-Chien (*1*), pp. 2 ff., 12 ff.
Best reconstructions by Mori Tateyuki (1845) 森立之, Liu Fu (1942) 劉復.
Shen Ying Chen Ching Yao Chüeh 神應鍼經要訣.
Confidential Essentials of a Manual of Marvellously Effective Acupuncture.
Sung, *c.* +1034.
Hsü Hsi 許希.
SIC, p. 283.
Shen Ying Ching 神應經.
Manual of Marvellously Successful (Acupuncture and Moxibustion).
Ming, +1425.
Chhen Hui 陳會 & Liu Chin 劉瑾.
With a preface by Ning Hsien Wang 寧獻王.
ICK, pp. 341–2.
Shêng Chi Tsung Lu 聖濟總錄.
Imperial Medical Encyclopaedia (lit. General Treatise (on Medical Care) Commissioned by the Majestic Beneficence) [issued by authority].
Sung, *c.* +1111 to +1118. Repr. Yuan, +1300.
Ed. by twelve physicians, headed by Shen Fu 申甫.
SIC, pp. 1002 ff.
Shih Chi 史記.
Historical Records [or perhaps better: Memoirs of the Historiographer (-Royal); down to −99].
C/Han, *c.* −90 [first pr. *c.* +1000].
Ssuma Chhien 司馬遷, and his father Ssuma Than 司馬談.
Cf. Burton Watson (2).
Partial trs. Chavannes (1); Burton Watson (1); Pfizmaier (13–36); Hirth (2); Wu Khang (1); Swann (1), etc.
Yin-Tê Index, no. 40.
Shih Ching 詩經.
Book of Odes [ancient folksongs].
Chou, −9th to −5th centuries.
Writers and compilers unknown.
The definitive redaction was that of Mao Hêng 毛亨, *c.* −160.
Tr. Legge (1, 8); Waley (1); Karlgren (14).
Shih I Chi 拾遺記.
Memoirs on Neglected Matters.
Chin, *c.* +370.
Wang Chia 王嘉.
Cf. Eichhorn (5).
Shih-ssu Ching Fa Hui 十四經發揮.
An Elucidation of the Fourteen Acu-Tracts [the Twelve Regular Tracts plus Tu-Mo and Jen-Mo].
Yuan, +1341.
Hua Shou 滑壽.
ICK, pp. 336 ff.
Shih Wu Chi Yuan 事物紀原.
Records of the Origins of Affairs and Things.
Sung, *c.* +1085.
Kao Chhêng 高承.
Shih Yuan 事原.
On the Origins of Things.
Sung.
Chu Hui 朱繪
Shu Ching 書經.
Historical Classic [or, Book of Documents].
The 29 'Chin Wên' chapters mainly Chou (a few pieces possibly Shang); the 21 'Ku Wên' chapters a 'forgery' by Mei Tsê 梅賾, *c.* +320, using fragments of genuine antiquity. Of the former, 13 are considered to go back to the −10th century, 10 to the −8th, and 6 not before

Shu Ching (cont.)
the −5th. Some scholars accept only 16 or 17 as pre-Confucian.
Writers unknown.
See Wu Shih-Chhang (1); Creel (4).
Tr. Medhurst (1); Legge (1, 10); Karlgren (12).

Shuo Yuan 說苑
Garden of Discourses.
Han, *c.* −20.
Liu Hsiang 劉向.

Ssu Khu Chhüan Shu Tsung Mu Thi Yao 四庫全書總目提要.
Analytical Catalogue of the *Complete Library of the Four Categories* (made by imperial order).
Chhing, +1782.
Ed. Chi Yün 紀昀.
Indexed by Yang Chia-Lo; Yü & Gillis.
Yin-Tê Index, no. 7.

Su Wên Hsüan Chi Yuan Ping Shih 素問玄機原病式.
The Pattern of the Causation of Disease according to the Mysterious Mechanism (of the Cyclical Periods of the Chhi) in Accordance with the *Questions (and Answers) about Living Matter*.
Sung, *c.* +1180.
Liu Wan-Su 劉完素.
ICK, pp. 830 ff.

Su Wên Ju Shih Yün Chhi Lun Ao 素問入式運氣論奧.
A Discussion of the Mysterious Pattern of the Cyclical Changes of the (Five Elements and the Six) Chhi in the *Questions (and Answers) about Living Matter* [the earliest medical book on this subject].
Sung, +1099.
Liu Wên-Shu 劉溫舒.
ICK, p. 1394.

Su Wên Liu Chhi Hsüan Chu Mi Yü
See *Hsüan Chu Mi Yü*.

Sung Chhao Lei Yuan 宋朝類苑.
Garden of History and Bibliography of the Sung Dynasty.
Sung, *c.* +1120.
Chiang Shao-Yü 江少虞.

Tao Tsang 道藏.
The Taoist Patrology [containing 1464 Taoist works].
All periods, but first collected in the Thang about +730, then again about +870 and definitively in +1019. First printed in the Sung (+1111 to +1117). Also printed in J/Chin (+1168 to +1191), Yuan (+1244), and Ming (+1445, +1598 and +1607).
Writers numerous.
Indexes by Wieger (6), on which see Pelliot's review (58); and Ong Tu-Chien (Yin-Tê Index, no. 25).

Thai Phing Ching 太平經.
(= *Thai Phing Chhing Ling Shu*.)
Canon of the Great Peace (and Equality).
Ascr. H/Han, *c.* +150 (first mentioned +166) but with later additions and interpolations.
Part attrib. Yü Chi 于吉.
Perhaps based on the 'apocryphal classic' *Thien Kuan Li Pao Yuan Thai Phing Ching* (*c.* −25) of Kan Chung-Kho 甘忠可.
TT/1087; reconstructed edn. Wang Ming, ed. (Chung-hua, Peking, 1960).
Cf. Yü Ying-Shih (2), p. 84; Kaltenmark (7).
According to Hsiung Tê-Chi (*1*) the parts which consist of dialogue between a Heavenly Teacher and a disciple correspond with what the *Pao Phu Tzu* bibliography lists as *Thai Phing Ching* and were composed by Hsiang Khai 襄楷.
The other parts would be mainly fragments of the Chia I Ching 甲乙經, also mentioned in *Pao Phu Tzu*, and due to Yü Chi and his disciple Kung Chhung 宮崇 between +125 and +145.

Thai Phing Chhing Ling Shu 太平淸領書.
Received Book of the Great Peace and Purity.
Now synonymous with *Thai Phing Ching*, q.v. But originally this was the title of a second text dating from *c.* −140, parts of which are now incorporated in what remains of the *Thai Phing Ching*. It has recipes for longevity in which acupuncture and sphygmology figure prominently.
Cf. Kaltenmark (7).

Thai Phing Hui Min Ho Chi Chü Fang 太平惠民和劑局方.
Standard Formularies of the (Government) Great Peace People's Welfare Pharmacies [based on the *Ho Chi Chü Fang*, etc.].
Sung, +1151.
Ed. Chhen Chhêng 陳承, Phei Tsung-Yuan 裴宗元 & Chhen Shih-Wên 陳師文.
Cf. Li Thao (1, 6); *SIC*, p. 973.

Thai-Phing Kuang Chi 太平廣記.
Copious Records collected in the Thai-Phing reign-period [anecdotes, stories, mirabilia and memorabilia].
Sung, +978.
Ed. Li Fang 李昉.

Thai-Phing Shêng Hui Fang 太平聖惠方.
Prescriptions Collected by Imperial Solicitude in the Thai-Phing reign-period.
Sung, commissioned, +982; completed +992.
Ed. Wang Huai-Yin *et al.* 王懷隱.
SIC, p. 921

Thai Phing Tung Chi Ching 太平洞極經.
Canon of the Uttermost Penetration of the Mystery of the Great Peace (and Equality), [apotropaic medicine, absolution of sins, techniques of acupuncture and sphygmology].
Ascr. between Han and Sui (+1st to +6th centuries).
Writer unknown.
Partly incorporated in *Thai Phing Ching*, q.v.
Cf. Kaltenmark (7).

Thai-Phing Yü Lan 太平御覽.
Thai-Phing reign-period Imperial Encyclopaedia (lit. the Imperial Speculum of the Thai-Phing reign-period, i.e. the Emperor's Daily Readings).
Sung, +983.
Ed. Li Fang 李昉.
Some chs. tr. Pfizmaier (84–106).
Yin-Tê Index no. 23.

Thien Kung Khai Wu 天工開物.
The Exploitation of the Works of Nature.
Ming, +1637.
Sung Ying-Hsing 宋應星.

(*Thung Jen*) *Chen Chiu Ching* 銅人鍼灸經.
Manual of Acupunture and Moxibustion (for Use with the Bronze Figure). This final phrase is an erroneous later addition.
Thang (between *Chen Chhüan Chen Ching*, *c.* +620, and *Thai-Phing Shêng Hui Fang* *c.* +990).
Writer unknown.
See also *Thung Jen Shu Hsüeh Chen Chiu Thu Ching*, and on the differentiation of the two books, Chang Tsan-Chhen (5).
ICK, p. 319, uses the title *Wang Ming Shih Chen Ching* (Anonymous Acupuncture Manual).

Thung Jen Shu Hsüeh Chen Chiu Thu Ching 銅人腧穴鍼灸圖經.
Illustrated Manual explaining Acupuncture and Moxibustion with the aid of the Bronze Figure and its Acu-points.
Sung, +1026 or +1027.
Wang Wei-I 王惟一.
SIC, pp. 266 ff. Cf. Chang Tsan-Chhen (5).
See also *Hsin Khan Pu Chu Thung Jen*...

Ting Pa Hsüeh Chih Nan 定八穴指南.
A South-Pointer (Compass) for Finding the Eight (Assembly) Acu-Points.
J/Chin or Yuan, *c.* +1240.
Tou Han-Chhing (b) 竇漢卿.
Part of *Chen Ching Chih Nan*, q.v.

Tongŭi Pogam.
See *Tung I Pao Chien*.

Tou Thai-Shih Hsien-Sêng Liu Chu Fu 竇太師先生流注賦.
Master Doctor Tou (Han-Chhing's) Ode on the Circulations of the Chhi (in connection with acupuncture).
J/Chin or Yuan, *c.* +1235.
Tou Han-Chhing (b) 竇漢卿.
In *Chi Shêng Pa Sui*, no. 2*a*.

Tso Chuan 左傳.
Master Tsochhiu's Tradition (or Enlargement) of the *Chhun Chhiu* (*Spring and Autumn Annals*) [dealing with the period −722 to −453].
Late Chou, compiled from ancient written and oral traditions of several States between −430 and −250, but with additions and changes by Confucian scholars of the Chhin and Han, especially in Hsin. Greatest of the three commentaries on the *Chhun Chhiu*, the others being the *Kungyang Chuan* and the *Kuliang Chuan*, but unlike them, probably originally itself an independent book of history.
Attrib. Tsochhiu Ming 左邱明.
See Karlgren (8); Maspero (1); Chhi Ssu-Ho (1); Wu Khang (1); Wu Shih-Chhang (1); van der Loon (1); Eberhard, Müller & Henseling (1).
Tr. Couvreur (1); Legge (11); Pfizmaier (1–12).
Index by Fraser & Lockhart (1).

Tung I Pao Chien 東醫寶鑑.
Precious Mirror of Eastern Medicine [system of medicine].
Korea, commissioned in +1596, presented +1610, printed +1613.
Hŏ Chun 許浚.

Tung Thien Chen Chiu Ching 洞天鍼灸經.
Penetrating Elucidation of Acupuncture and Moxibustion.
Sung, *c.* +1080.
Liu Yuan-Pin 劉元賓.
Now extant only in quotations.
ICK p. 325

Tung-Pho Chih Lin 東坡志林.
Journal and Miscellany of (Su) Tung-Pho [compiled while in exile in Hainan].
Sung, +1097 to +1101.
Su Tung-Pho 蘇東坡.

Tzu Shêng Ching 資生經.
See *Chen Chiu Tzu Shêng Ching*.

Tzu Wu Ching 子午經.
Noon and Midnight Manual [i.e. Acupuncture according to the Diurnal Rhythm in the Circulation of the Chhi].
Ascr. Chou, but not noted in any bibliography earlier than the *Chün Chai Tu Shu Hou Chih* of Chhao Kung-Wu, +1151.
Prob. Thang or Sung.
Attrib. Pien Chhio 扁鵲. Actual writer unknown.
SIC, p. 285; *ICK*, p. 306; *Shih Shan Thang Tshang Shu Mu Lu*, ch. 2, p. 41*b*.

Tzu Wu Liu Chu 子午流注.
On Diurnal Rhythms in the Circulation (of the Chhi), [lit.: Noon and Midnight Differences in the Flowing (of the Chhi)].
Yuan or J/Chin, *c.* +1240.
Tou Han-Chhing (b) 竇漢卿.

Tzu Wu Liu Chu Cho Jih An Shih Ting Hsüeh Ko 子午流注逐日按時定穴歌.
Mnemonic Rhyme to aid in the Selection of Acu-points according to the Diurnal Cycle, the Day of the Month and the Season of the Year.
Ascr. Chin & L/Sung, *c.* +419. More probably Wu Tai, *c.* +930, acc. to Chhêng Tan-An, Chhen Pi-Liu & Hsü Hsi-Nien (*1*).
Attrib. Hsü Wên-Po 徐文伯.
A small tractate preserved in *Chen Chiu Chü Ying*, ch. 4B (p. 263).

Wai Thai Pi Yao (Fang) 外臺秘要(方).
Important (Medical) Formulae and Prescriptions now revealed by the Governor of a Distant Province.
Thang, +752.
Wang Thao 王燾.
On the title see des Rotours (1), pp. 294, 721. Wang Thao had had access to the books in the Imperial Library as an Academician before his posting to the provinces as a high official.

Wei Shêng Chen Chiu Hsüan Chi Pi Yao 衛生鍼灸玄機秘要.
Confidential Principles of the Mysterious Mechanisms (of the Human Body involved in) Acupuncture and Moxibustion for the Preservation of Health.
Title of the first form of Yang Chi-Chen's *Chen Chiu Ta Chhêng* (q.v.); it was mainly on the practice and traditions of his own family but later he enlarged it by taking account of the whole of the earlier literature.
Usually attributed under his other name; Yang Chi-Shih 楊濟時.

Wu Ching Tsung Yao 武經總要.
Collection of the Most Important Military Techniques [compiled by Imperial Order].
Sung, +1040 (+1044).
Ed. Tsêng Kung-Liang 曾公亮.

Wu Li Lun 物理論.
Discourse on the Principles of Things [astronomical].
San Kuo, end +3rd century.
Yang Chhüan 楊泉.

Wu Yuan Lu 無冤錄.
The Cancelling of Wrongs (i.e. False Charges) [treatise on forensic medicine].
Yuan, +1308.
Wang Yü 王與.

Wu Yüeh Chhun Chhiu 吳越春秋.
Spring and Autumn Annals of the States of Wu and Yüeh.
H/Han.
Chao Yeh 趙曄.

Yen Thieh Lun 鹽鐵論.
Discourses on Salt and Iron [record of the debate of −81 on State control of commerce and industry].
C/Han, *c.* −80 to −60.
Huan Khuan 桓寬.
Partial tr. Gale (1); Gale, Boodberg & Lin (1).

Yen Tshê Tsa Chen Chiu Ching 偃側雜鍼灸經.
Manual of Acupuncture and Moxibustion Loci seen on the Recumbent Figure Laterally.
L/Sung, *c.* +460.
Chhin Chhêng-Tsu 秦承祖.
The charts are all lost, and only a few fragments of the text remain.
SIC, p. 229.

Yü Hai 玉海.
Ocean of Jade [encyclopaedia].
Sung, +1267 (first pr. Yuan, +1351).
Wang Ying-Lin 王應麟.
Cf. des Rotours (2), p. 96.

Yu-Yang Tsa Tsu 酉陽雜俎.
Miscellany of the Yu-yang Mountain (Cave) [in S.E. Szechuan].
Thang, +863.
Tuan Chhêng-Shih 段成式.
See des Rotours (1), p. civ.

Yüeh Ling 月令
Monthly Ordinances (of the Chou Dynasty).
Chou, between −7th and −3rd centuries.
Writers unknown.
Incorporated in the *Hsiao Tai Li Chi* and the *Lü Shih Chhun Chhiu* q.v.
Tr. Legge (7), R. Wilhelm (3).

B. CHINESE AND JAPANESE BOOKS AND JOURNAL ARTICLES SINCE +1800

Andō Kōsei (*1*) 安藤更生.
Kanshin 鑑眞.
Life of Chien-Chen (+688 to +763), [outstanding Buddhist missionary to Japan, skilled also in medicine and architecture].
Bijutsu Shuppansha, Tokyo 1958, repr. 1963.
Abstr. *RBS*, 1964, **4**, no. 889.

Anon (*23*).
Chêngchow Erh-Li-Kang 鄭州二里岡.
Report on the Erh-Li-Kang (Tombs) at Chêngchow.
Academia Sinica, Peking, 1959.

Anon. (*27*).
Shang-Tshun-Ling Kuo Kuo Mu Ti 上村嶺虢國墓地.
The Cemetery (and Princely Tombs) of the State of (Northern) Kuo at Shang-tshun-ling (near Shen-hsien in the San-mên Gorge Dam Area of the Yellow River).
Institute of Archaeology, Academia Sinica, Peking, 1959 (Yellow River Excavations Report, no. 3).

Anon. (*75*).
'*Chin Kuei*' *Chiao Hsüeh Tshan Khao Tzu Liao* 金匱教學參考資料.
Materials for the Study of the Medical System of the *Chin Kuei Yao Lüeh* (Systematic Treasury of Medicine, +3rd century, by Chang Chung-Ching).
Kho-Hsüeh Chi-Shu, Shanghai, 1961.
(Nanking College of Traditional Medicine.)

Anon. (*76*) (ed.).
'*Ku Chin Thu Shu Chi Chhêng*' *I Pu Chhüan Lu* (*I Ching Chu Shih*) 古今圖書集成醫部全錄(醫經註釋).
A Rearrangement of the Medical Section of the Great Encyclopaedia (*Thu Shu Chi Chhêng*, +1726); Commentaries and Explanations on the Medical Classics [gives together the commentaries of Wang Ping, Ma Shih and Chang Chih-Tshung on the *Nei Ching*, *Su Wên*].
Jen-Min Wei-Shêng, Peking, 1959.

Anon. (*80*).
'*Nan Ching*' *I Shih* 難經譯釋.
Modern Interpretations of the *Manual of Difficult Passages*.
Kho Hsüeh Chi-Shu, Shanghai, 1964.

Anon. (*81*).
'*Nei Ching*' *Chiang I* 內經講義.
Lecture Notes on the *Manual of Corporeal* (*Medicine*).
Kho-Hsüeh Chi-Shu, Shanghai, 1964.
(Peking College of Traditional Medicine.)

Anon. (*83*).
Chung-Kuo I Hsüeh Shih Chiang I 中國醫學史講義.
Lecture Notes on the History of Chinese Medicine.
Kho-Hsüeh Chi-Shu, Shanghai, 1964.
(Peking College of Traditional Medicine.)

Anon. (*90*).
Chen Chiu Hsüeh Chiang I 鍼灸學講義.
Lecture Notes on Acupuncture and Moxibustion.
Kho-Hsüeh Chi-Shu, Shanghai, 1963.
(Shanghai College of Traditional Medicine.)

Anon. (*91*).
Chen Chiu Hsüeh Chiang I 針灸學講義.
Lecture Notes on Acupuncture and Moxibustion.
Kho-Hsüeh Chi-Shu, Shanghai, 1964.
(Nanking College of Traditional Medicine.)

Anon. (*98*).
Chung I Ko Chia Hsüeh Shuo Chiang I 中醫各家學說講義.
Lecture Notes on the Different Schools of Chinese Medicine.
Jen-Min Wei-Shêng, Peking, 1961.
Revised and enlarged edition, Kho-Hsüeh Chi-Shu, Shanghai, 1964.
(Peking College of Traditional Medicine.)

Anon. (*106*).
Wên-Hua Ta Ko-Ming Chhi Chien Chhu Thu Wên Wu 文化大革命期間出土文物.
Cultural Relics Unearthed during the period of the Great Cultural Revolution (1965–71). Vol. 1 [album].
Wên Wu, Peking, 1972.

Anon. (*107*).
Chung-Kuo Chen Chiu Hsüeh Kai Yao 中國針灸學概要.
Concise Treatise on Acupuncture and Moxibustion.
Ta Kuang, Hongkong, 1970.

Anon. (*108*) (ed.).
Chen Chiu Chuan Chi 針灸專輯.
Special Studies on Acupuncture and Moxa [translations of papers in Western languages into Chinese, issued by the Shanghai Committee for Research in Medical and Pharmaceutical Science].
Kho-Hsüeh Chi-Shu, Shanghai, 1962.

Anon. (*109*).
Chung-Kuo Kao Têng Chih-Wu Thu Chien 中國高等植物圖鑑.

Anon. (*109*) (*cont.*)
Iconographia Cormophytorum Sinicorum (Flora of Chinese Higher Plants).
Kho-Hsüeh, Peking, 1972– (for Nat. Inst. of Botany), Vols. 1 and 2, 1972, Vol. 3, 1974, Vol. 4, 1975, Vol. 5, 1976.

Anon. (*110*).
Chhang Yung Chung Tshao Yao Thu Phu 常用中草葯圖譜.
Illustrated Handbook of the Most Commonly Used Chinese Plant Materia Medica (prepared by the Chinese Academy of Medicine and the Chekiang Provincial College of Traditional Medicine).
With index of Latin binomials as well as Chinese names.
Jen-Min Wei-Shêng, Peking, 1970.

Anon. (*114*).
Chen Tzhu Ma Tsui 針刺麻醉.
Acupuncture Analgesia.
Shanghai Jen-Min, Shanghai, 1972.
Engl. translation: 'Acupuncture Anaesthesia', U.S. Government Printing Office, Washington, D.C., 1975 (DHEW Publication NIH/75–784; Fogarty International Centre China Health Studies, no. 11). Preface by M. D. Leavitt. Bibliographical specification of original used not provided, translator or translators anonymous, no Chinese characters for technical terms, no index.

Anon. (*119*).
Erh Chen Liao Fa 耳針療法.
The Therapeutic use of the Acu-Points on the External Ear.
Kho-Hsüeh, Peking, 1971.

Anon. (*120*).
Chung-I Chien I Chiao Tshai 中醫簡易教材.
Elementary Handbook of Chinese Medicine.
Tientsin Jen-Min, Tientsin, 1971.

Anon. (*121*).
Chen Chiu Ching Hsüeh Mo-Hsing 針灸經穴模型.
(Booklet accompanying) Model of the Human Body showing the Acupunture Points and the Courses of the Meridians [Tracts].
Contains romanised acu-point names and definitions of anatomical positions in English, as well as Chinese.
China Nat. Machinery Import and Export Corp. Tientsin, 1972.

Anon. (*122*).
Chen Chiu Lin Chhuang Chhü Hsüeh Thu Chieh 針灸臨床取穴圖解.
Illustrated Explanation of the Selection of Acu-points for Clinical Acupuncture and Moxibustion.
Peking Inst. Trad. Chinese Med., 1958
Reprinted by Commercial Press, Hongkong, 1972.

Anon. (*123*).
Chen Chiu Hsüeh 針灸學.
Treatise on Acupuncture and Moxibustion.
Updated edition of an earlier publication in 4 small parts under the same title.
Jen-Min Wei-Shêng, Peking, 1974.

Anon. (*124*).
Tshung Sian Nan-Chiao Chhu-Thu ti I-Yao Wên Wu Khan Thang-Tai I-Yao ti Fa Chan 從西安南郊出土的醫藥文物看唐代醫藥的發展.
The Development of Pharmaceutical Chemistry in the Thang Period as seen from the specimens of (inorganic) drugs recovered from the Hoard in the Southern Suburbs of Sian [the silver boxes with the labelled chemicals, *c.* +756].
WWTK, 1972, no. 6, 52.

Anon. (*128*).
Chen-Tzhu Jen Thi Mou Hsieh Hsüeh-Wei tui Phi-Fu Thung Yü ti Ying-Hsiang 針刺人体某些穴位對皮膚痛閾的影响.
The Effect of Acupuncture on the Pain Threshold of Human Skin.
CMJ/C, 1973, no. 3, 151 (Eng. summ., p. 35).
(Acupuncture Analgesia Research Group, Peking Med. Coll.)

Anon. (*129*).
Tsai Chen-Tzhu Ma-Tsui hsia Wei-shen-mo Nêng Khai Tao? 在針刺麻醉下爲什麼能開刀?
How is it that Surgical Operations can be performed under Analgesia induced by Acupuncture?
HC, 1971, no. 9, 713 (59). With two articles following on pp. 724 (70) and 729 (75).
Repr., with a fourth article, in Anon. (*130*)
Eng. tr. in *AJCM*, 1973, **1** (no. 1), 159 (slightly abridged).

Anon. (*130*).
Chen-Tzhu Ma-Tsui Yuan-Li Than Thao 針刺麻醉原理探討.
An Investigation of the Nature of Acupuncture Analgesia.
Jen-Min, Peking, 1972.
Eng. tr. in *AJCM*, 1973, **1** (no. 1), 159 (slightly abridged).

Anon. (*131*).
Chen-Tzhu Ma-Tsui Li-Lun Yuan-Li Thao Lun Chi 針刺麻醉理論原理討論集.
A Collection of Papers on the Nature of Acupuncture Analgesia.
Jen-Min, Shanghai, 1972.

Anon. (*132*).
I-chhien-san-pai-pa Li Hsiao Erh Shou-Shu Ying-Yung Chen-Tzhu Ma-Tsui ti Thi

Anon. (*132*) (*cont.*)
Hui 1308例小兒手術應用針刺痲醉的体會.
Acupuncture Analgesia in Paediatric Surgery; a Report of 1308 Cases (from the Peking Children's Hospital).
CMJ/C, 1973, no. 2, 91 (Engl. summ., p. 23).

Anon. (*133*).
Hsiu-Kho, Wei Chung Ping Yuan Shou Shu Shih Ying-Yung Chen-Tzhu Ma-Tsui ti Chhu-Pu Kuan Chha 休克危重病員手術時應用針刺痲醉的初步觀察.
Acupuncture Analgesia for Operations in Shock and Critical Cases.
CMJ/C, 1973, no. 2, 95 (Eng. summ., p. 24).

Anon. (*134*).
Chen-Tzhu Ma-Tsui Shih Hsing Phi Chhieh Chhu Shu San-pai-ling-wu Li ti Thi-Hui 針刺痲醉施行脾切除術305例的体會.
Acupuncture Analgesia in Splenectomy; a Report of 305 cases (from the Chhangshan County Hospital, Chekiang).
CMJ/C, 1973, no. 2, 90 (Eng. summ., p. 22).

Anon. (*135*).
Chung Nao Wang Chuang Chieh-Kou tsai Chen-Tzhu Ma-Tsui chung ti Tso Yung 中腦網狀結構在針刺痲醉中的作用
The Role of the Reticular Formation of the Midbrain in Acupuncture Analgesia.
CMJ/C, 1973, no. 3, 136 (Engl. summ., p. 32).

Anon. (*136*).
Thu Chhiu Nao Chung-Yang Wai Tshê Ho tui Shang-Hai Hsing Tzhu Chi ti Tien Fan Ying Chi chhi I Chih 兔丘腦中央外側核對傷害性刺激的電反應及其抑制.
The Electrical Response in the Nucleus Centralis Lateralis of the Thalamus to Nocuous Stimulation, and its Inhibition by Acupuncture, in the Rabbit.
CMJ/C, 1973, no. 3, 131 (Eng. summ., p. 31).

Anon. (*137*).
Chen-Tzhu Ma-Tsui hsia Chi Sui Shen-Ching Fan-Shê ti Tien Shêng-Li-Hsüeh Yen-Chiu 針刺痲醉下脊髓神經反射的電生理學研究.
An Electro-physiological Study of Spinal Reflexes under Acupuncture Analgesia (from Hsü-yi County Hospital Research Unit).
CMJ/C, 1973, no. 3, 139 (Eng. summ., p. 33).

Anon. (*138*).
Chen-Tzhu Ma-Tsui tsai Shen-Ching Wai-Kho Shou-Shu ti Ying-Yung 針刺痲醉在神經外科手術的應用.
Acupuncture Analgesia in Neuro-surgery (482 craniotomies at the Hsüan-Wu Hospital, Peking).
CMJ/C, 1973, no. 2, 67 (Eng. summ., p. 15).

Anon. (*139*).
Chen-Tzhu Chhüan-Liao Hsüeh tui Lu Nao Shou-Shu Chen Thung Hsiao-Kuo ti Kuan Chha 針刺顴髎穴對顱腦手術鎮痛效果的觀察.
Observations on the Analgesic Effect of Acupuncture at the Chhüan-Liao Point in Neuro-surgery; Report of 619 Cases (from the Shanghai First Medical College).
CMJ/C, 1973, no. 2, 71 (Eng. summ., p. 16).

Anon. (*140*).
Chen-Tzhu Ma-Tsui Chia-Chuang-Hsien Chhieh Chhu Shou-Shu ti Hsiao-Kuo Fên-Hsi 針刺痲醉甲狀腺切除手術的效果分析.
Acupuncture Analgesia in Thyroidectomy (700 cases from the Shanghai First People's Hospital).
CMJ/C, 1973, no. 2, 74 (Eng. summ., p. 17).

Anon. (*141*).
Chen-Tzhu Ma-Tsui Ying-Yung Yü Fei Chhieh-Chhu Shu ti Lin Chhuang Tsung Chieh 針刺痲醉應用于肺切除術的臨床總結.
Pulmonary Resections under Acupuncture Analgesia (611 Cases from the Shanghai First Tuberculosis Hospital).
CMJ/C, 1973, no. 2, 80 (Eng. summ., p. 19).

Anon. (*142*).
Chen-Tzhu Ma-Tsui Shih Hsing Khai Hsiung Shou-Shu Pa-pai-shih-pa Li Lin Chhuang Fên-Hsi 針刺痲醉施行開胸手術818例臨床分析.
Acupuncture Analgesia in Thoracic Surgery, a Clinical Analysis of 818 Cases (from the Peking Thoracic Coordinating Group).
CMJ/C, 1973, no. 2, 85 (Eng. summ., p. 20).

Anon. (*143*).
Chen-Tzhu Jen Chung Kou tui Mao Shih Hsüeh Hsing Hsiu Kho ti Ying-Hsiang 針刺人中溝對猫失血性休克的影响.
The Effect of Acupuncture of the Philtrum in Cats on Haemorrhagic Shock and its relation to Shock in Man.
CMJ/C, 1973, no. 2, 98 (Eng. summ., p. 25).

Anon. (*144*).
Chen-Tzhu Chen Thung yü Nao nei Shen-Ching Chieh-Chih ti Kuan-Hsi 針刺鎮痛與腦內神經介質的關係.
The Relation between Acupuncture Analgesia and Neuro-transmitter Substances in Rabbit Brain.
CMJ/C, 1973, no. 8, 478 (Eng. summ., p. 105).

Anon. (*145*)
'Tê Chhi' Shih Chen-Tzhu Pu Wei ti Chi Tien Huo Tung 得氣時針刺部位的肌電活動.
Electromyographic Activity produced locally in Acupuncture Manipulation.
CMJ/C, 1973, no. 9, 532 (Eng. summ., p. 118).

Anon. (*146*).
Mou Hsieh Shen-Ching Hsi Thung Chi-Ping tui Chen-Tzhu 'Tê Chhi' Ying-Hsiang ti Chhu Pu Kuan Chha 某些神經系統疾病對針刺[得氣]影响的初步觀察.
Acupuncture Sensation and the Electromyogram of the Needled Point in Patients with Diseases of the Nervous System.
CMJ/C, 1973, no. 10, 619 (Eng. summ., p. 137).

Anon. (*147*).
Chen Tzhu Chen Thung Wai Chou Chhuan Ju Thu Ching ti Chin-i-Pu Than Thao 針刺鎮痛外周傳入途徑的進一步探討.
The Peripheral Afferent Pathway in Acupuncture Analgesia.
CMJ/C, 1974, **54** (no. 6), 360, with Engl. abstr., p. 102.

Anon. (*148*).
Chung-I Hsüeh Shu Lun Wên Hsüan Chi 中醫學術論文選集.
Selected Papers on Traditional Chinese Medicine.
Academy and Hospital of Traditional Medicine, Peking, 1965.

Anon. (*149*).
Chen Chiu Wên Hsien So Yin 1959–1965 針灸文獻索引.
A Bibliography of Papers on Acupuncture and Moxibustion.
History of Medicine Museum, Shanghai, 1969.

Anon. (*160*).
Shou I Chen Chiu Chi-Shu Chih Shih Kua Thu 獸醫針灸技術知識挂圖.
Wall Chart of Veterinary Acupuncture and Moxibustion (prepared by the Chiangsi Provincial Veterinary Research Institute).
Hsin-Hua, Shanghai, 1970.

Anon. (*161*).
Chen Chiu Ko Kho Chih Liao Fa 針灸各科治療法.
Clinical Applications of Acupuncture and Moxibustion in the Various Types of Diseases [a handbook of the Shanghai College of Traditional Medicine].
Shanghai, 1968, reprinted 1974, and Hsüeh Lin Shu Chü (Academy Press), Hongkong, 1969.

Anon. (*162*).
Chen Chiu Ching-Lo Hsüeh 針灸經絡學.
The study of the Tract-and-channel System in Acupuncture and Moxibustion, [a handbook of the Shanghai College of Traditional Medicine].
Shanghai, 1969, reprinted, Shao-Hua Wên-Hua-Shê, Hongkong, n.d.

Anon. (*163*).
Tien-Chen Chih Liao Fêng Shih Hsing Kuan-Chieh-Yen 307 Li Liao Hsiao Chhu Pu Kuan Chha 電針治療風濕性關節炎307例療效初步觀察.
A Preliminary Study of 307 cases of Arthritis due to exposure to cold and damp treated by Electro-acupuncture (from the Dept. of Internal Medicine, Shensi Provincial Neurological Hospital).
SHIY, 1959, no. 12, 20.

Anon. (*164*).
Erh Chen 耳針.
Auricular Acupuncture.
Jen-Min, Shanghai, 1972.

Anon. (*165*).
Chen Chiu Erh Chen Liao Fa 針灸耳針療法.
Therapeutic Auricular Acupuncture (by the Shanghai Auriculo-Acupuncture Committee).
Wan-Yeh, Hongkong, n.d. (*c.* 1974).

Anon. (*166*).
Chung Tshao Yao Yu Hsiao Chhêng-Fên ti Yen-Chiu 中草葯有效成分的研究.
A Study of the Chemical Constituents of Chinese Drug-Plants (Vol. 1).
Jen-Min, Peking, 1972.

Anon. (*167*).
Chung I Ming Tzhu Shu Yü Hsüan Shih 中醫名詞术語選釋.
Glossary of Selected Technical Terms in Traditional Chinese Medicine (compiled by the Kuangtung College of Traditional Medicine and the National Academy of Traditional Medicine, Peking).
Jen-Min Wei-Shêng, Peking, 1972.

Anon. (*169*).
Lung Ya Ping ti Chih Liao 聾啞病的治療.
The Therapy of Deaf-Mutism.
Jen-Min Wei-Shêng, Peking, 1971.

Anon. (*170*).
Chen Chiu Chih Liao Chi Hsing Lan-Wei-Yen Liao Hsiao Chi Chhi Tso Yung Chi Chih ti Chhu Pu Than Thao 針灸治療急性闌尾炎療效及其作用機制的初步探討.
A Preliminary Discussion of the Treatment of Acute Appendicitis with Acupuncture; its Effectiveness and Possible Mechanism (from the Appendicitis Group of the Acupuncture Research Unit of the Shanghai Municipality).
SHIY, 1959, no. 10, 18.

Anon. (*171*).
Tien-Chen Liao Fa tsai Shou-I Lin Chhuang shang ti Ying-Yung 電針療法在獸醫臨床上的應用.

Anon. (*171*) (*cont.*)
Practical Clinical Applications of the Therapeutic Methods of Electro-Acupuncture in Veterinary Medicine.
Hopei Jen-Min, Shih-chia-chuang, 1973.

Anon. (*172*).
Chhih-Chiao I-Shêng Shou-Tshê 赤脚醫生手册.
Medical Manual for 'Barefoot Doctors'.
Hunan Jen-Min, Chhangsha, 1971.
Engl. translation: 'A Barefoot Doctor's Manual', Bethesda, Maryland, 1975. (DHEW Publication no. NIH/75-695).

Anon. (*173*).
Mei-Hua-Chen Liao Fa 梅花針療法.
Acupuncture Therapy with the 'Plum-Blossom' Multiple-Needle Device (five needles).
Jen-Min Wei-Shêng, Peking, 1973.

Anon. (*174*).
Tshang-Shu Ai-Yeh-Hsiang Yü Fang Kan-Mao chi Khung Chhi Hsiao Tu Hsiao-Kuo ti Kuan Chha 蒼朮艾葉香預防感冒及空氣消毒效果的觀察.
An Investigation of the Response of Patients with Influenza, Chronic Bronchitis and other Infections of the Respiratory Tract to Fumigation with an Incense composed of *Artemisia* leaves and *Atractylis ovata*.
CMJ/C, 1975, **55** (no. 9), 624.

Anon. (*175*).
Chen-Tzhu Ma-Tsui Wei Ta Pu Chhieh Chhu Shu 800 Li Lin Chhuang Kuan Chha 針刺麻醉胃大部切除術800例臨牀觀察.
A Report on the Clinical Observation of 800 Cases of Gastric and Duodenal Ulcer involving partial Resections of the Stomach and Duodenum under Acupuncture Analgesia.
CMJ/C, 1975, **55** (no. 10), 703.
(Committee of Acupuncture Anaesthesia of the Shu-Kuang Hospital of the Shanghai College of Traditional Medicine.)

Anon. (*194*).
Yung-Chhang Yuan-Yang-Chhih Hsin Shih Chhi Shih-Tai Mu Ti ti Fa Chüeh 永昌鴛鴦池新石器時代墓地的發掘.
Excavation of a Neolithic Tomb at Yuan-yang-chhih in Yung-chhang District (Kansu province).
KKTH, 1974, **5**, 299.

Anon. (*195*).
Anyang Yin Hsü Wu-hao Mu ti Fa Chüeh 安陽殷墟五號墓的發掘
Excavation of Tomb no. 5 at Yin Hsü, Anyang (richest and best preserved of all the Royal Tombs of the Shang).
The tomb was that of Fu Hao (Pu Hsin), a consort of the King Wu Ting
AS/CJA 1977 (no. 2), no. 47, 57; Engl. summ. 97.

Anon. (*196*)
Ma-wang-tui Po Shu Ssu Chung Ku I-Hsüeh I Shu Chien Chieh 馬王堆帛書四種古醫學佚書簡介
A Brief Study of Four Lost Ancient Medical Texts contained in the Silk Manuscripts recovered from Tomb (no. 3) at Ma-wang-tui (by the History of Medicine Research Group of the Academy of Traditional-Chinese Medicine). Date of Burial, −168.
WWTK 1975 (no. 6), no. 229, 16.

Anon. (*197*)
Ma-wang-tui Han Mu Chhu Thu I Shu Shih Wên (pt. 1) 馬王堆漢墓出土醫書釋文
A Transcription of Some of the Medical Texts (contained in the Silk Manuscripts) unearthed at the Han Tomb (no. 3), at Ma-wang-tui (−168).
WWTK 1975 (no. 6), no. 229, 1.

Anon. (*198*)
Ma-wang-tui San Hao Mu Po Hua Tao-Yin Thu ti Chhu Pu Yen-Chiu 馬王堆三號墓帛畫導引圖的初步研究
Preliminary Investigations of the Text and Paintings of (Medical) Gymnastics, etc. contained in the Silk Manuscripts recovered from Tomb no. 3 at Ma-wang-tui (−168)—with drawings.
WWTK 1975, (no. 6), no. 229, 6.

Anon. (*199*)
Ma-wang-tui Han Mu Chhu Thu I Shu Shih Wên (pt. 2) 馬王堆漢墓出土醫書釋文
A Transcription of a Medical Text (the 'Book of Fifty-two Diseases') unearthed (as a Silk Manuscript) at the Han Tomb (no. 3) at Ma-wang-tui (−168).
WWTK 1975, (no. 9), no. 232, 35.

Anon. (*200*)
Chen Chiu (*shih hsing pên*) 針灸（試行本）
Acupuncture and Moxibustion (a trial manual prepared by the Health Department of Hopei Province).
Jen-Min Wei-Shêng, Peking, 1970. Tr. Silverstein, Chang I-Lo & Macon (1).

Anon. (*201*)
Chiang Hu I Shu Pi Chhuan 江湖醫術祕傳
Confidentially Handed-down Therapeutic Traditions of the Hedge-Doctors of the Countryside.
Li-Li, Hongkong, n.d. (*c.* 1958).

Chang Chün-I (*1*) 張俊義.
Chen Chiu Hsüeh chih Li-Shih 針灸學之歷史.
A History of Acupuncture.
Tung-Fang Chen Chiu Shu Chü, Shanghai, 1937.

Chang Hsin-Chhêng (*1*) 張心澂.
Wei Shu Thung Khao 僞書通考.
A General Study of Books of Uncertain Date and Authorship.
2 vols., Shanghai, 1939, revised ed. 1955.

Chang Hsüan (*1*) 張瑄.
Chung Wên Chhang Yung San Chhien Tzu Hsing I Shih 中文常用三千字形義釋
Etymologies of Three Thousand Chinese Characters in Common Use.
Hongkong Univ. Press, 1968.

Chang Shih-Piao (*1*) 張世鑣.
Wên Chiu Hsüeh Chiang I 溫灸學講義.
Lectures on Moxibustion Heat-Treatment.
Tung-Fang I-Hsüeh Shu Chü, Shanghai, 1928; 6th repr. 1943.

Chang Tsan-Chhen (*1*) 張贊臣.
Chung-Kuo Li-Tai I-Hsüeh Shih Lüeh 中國歷代醫學史略.
A Brief History of Chinese Medicine.
Chhing Chhien Thang Shu Chü, Shanghai, 1st ed., 1933; 2nd ed. 1954.

Chang Tsan-Chhen (*5*) 張贊臣.
'Thung Jen Shu Hsüeh Chen Chiu Thu Ching' Ho 'Thung Jen Chen Chiu Ching' ti I Thung 「銅人腧穴鍼灸圖經」和「銅人鍼灸經」的異同.
On the Similarities and Differences between Two books with the Title *Manual of...Acupuncture and Moxibustion...for Use with the Bronze Figure*.
ISTC, 1954, **6** (no. 2), 104.

Chang Tzhu-Kung (*3*) 章次公.
Man-Kung Shih Chi Khao 曼公事跡考.
A Study of (Tai) Man-Kung (Late Ming physician in Japan).
ISTC, 1951, **3** (no. 1), 35.

Chao Yü-Chhing 趙玉青 & Khung Shu-Chên 孔淑貞 (*1*).
Chung-Kuo ti I Shêng Pien Chhio – Chhin Yüeh-Jen 中國的醫聖扁鵲–秦越人.
China's Medical Sage Pien Chhio – Chhin Yüeh-Jen.
ISTC, 1954, **6** (no. 3), p. 135.

Chiang Chen-Yü 江振裕 & Chu Tê-Hsing 朱德行 (*1*).
Chhieh-Chhu Thu Shuang Tshê Shen Shang Hsien, ho Ching Chiao-Kan Shen-Ching Hou ti Chen-Tzhu Chen Thung Hsiao Ying 切除兎双側腎上腺和頸交感神經後的針刺鎭痛效應.
Acupuncture Analgesia following Bilateral Adrenalectomy and Cervical Sympathectomy in Rabbits.
CMJ/C, 1974, **54** (no. 5), 303, with Engl. abstr. p. 82.

Chou Fêng-Wu 周鳳梧, Wang Wan-Chieh 王萬杰 & Hsü Kuo-Chhien 徐國仟 (*1*).
Huang Ti Nei Ching, Su Wên, Pai Hua Chieh 黃帝內經素問白話解.
The *Yellow Emperor's Manual of Corporeal (Medicine); Questions (and Answers) about living Matter*, expressed in Modern Colloquial Language.
Jen-Min Wei-Shêng, Peking, 1958.

Chou I-Liang (*2*) 周一良.
Chien-Chen ti Tung Tu yü Chung Jih Wên Hua Chiao-Liu 鑑眞的東渡與中日文化交流.
The Mission of Chien-Chen (Kanshin) to Japan (+735 to +748) and Cultural Exchanges between China and Japan.
WWTK, 1963 (no. 9), 1.

Chu Chhi-Chhien 朱啓鈐 & Liu Tun-Chên 劉敦楨 (*1, 2*).
Chê Chiang Lu [parts 8 and 9] 哲匠錄.
Biographies of [Chinese] Engineers, Architects, Technologists and Master-Craftsmen (continued).
BSRCA, 1935, **6** (no. 2), 114 [CCL (8)]; 1936, **6** (no. 3), 148 [CCL (9)].

Chu Hsiao-Nan (*1*) 朱小南.
Ching-Lo Hsüeh Shuo ho Fu Kho 經絡學說和婦科.
The Acupuncture Tracts in relation to Gynaecology.
SHIY, 1959, no. 6, 285.

Chu Lien (*1*) 朱璉.
Hsin Chen Chiu Hsüeh 新針灸學.
A New Treatise on Acupuncture and Moxibustion.
Jen-Min Wei-Shêng, Peking, 1954.

Chu Lung-Yü (*1*) 朱龍玉.
Tien Chen Liao Fa 電針療法.
The Techniques of Electro-acupuncture Therapy.
Shensi Jen-Min, Sian, 1957.

Chu Yen (*1*) 朱顏.
Chung-Kuo Ku-Tai I-Hsüeh ti Chhêng Chiu 中國古代醫學的成就.
Achievements of Ancient Chinese Medicine.
Kho-Hsüeh Phu-Chi, Peking, 1955, 1957.

Chung I-Yen (*1*) 鍾依研.
Hsi Han Liu Shêng Mu Chhu Thu ti I-Liao Chhi Chü 西漢劉勝墓出土的醫療器具.
Medical Instruments and Objects unearthed from the Western (Former) Han Tomb of Liu Shêng (Prince of Chungshan, −113).
KKTH, 1972, no. 3, 49.

Chung I-Yen (*1*) & Ling Hsiang 鍾依研 凌襄
Wo Kuo Hsien I Fa-Hsien-ti Tsui Ku I Fang—Po Shu 'Wu-Shih-erh Ping Fang' 我國現已發現的最古醫方，帛書「五十二病方」
The Oldest Chinese Work on Therapeutics, the 'Book of Fifty-two Diseases' now discovered as a Silk Manuscript (in Tomb no. 3 at Ma-wang-tui, dating from −168).
WWTK 1975 (no. 9), no. 232, 49.

Chhen Chih (*1*) 陳直.
Hsi Yin Mu Chien chung Fa-Hsien ti Ku-Tai I-Hsüeh Shih-Liao 璽印木簡中發現的古代醫學史料.
Ancient Chinese Medicine as recorded in Seals and on Wooden Tablets.
KHSC, 1958, **1**, 68; *ISTC*, 1958, no. 2, 139.

Chhen Kho-Chhin (*1*) 陳克勤.
Tien Chen ho Chen-Tzhu-Chi Ying-Hsiang hsia Mien I Fan-Ying ti Fa Shêng 電針和針刺激影响下免疫反應的發生.
The Effect of Acupuncture and Electro-Acupuncture on the Production of Antibodies and Immunity Reactions.
NMJC, 1958, **44** (no. 12), 1173 (Engl. summ., p. 66).

Chhen Pang-Hsien (*1*) 陳邦賢.
Chung-Kuo I-Hsüeh Shih 中國醫學史.
History of Chinese Medicine.
Com. Press, Shanghai, 1937, 1957.

Chhen Pi-Liu (*1*) 陳璧琉.
Nan Ching, Pai Hua Chieh 難經白話解.
The *Manual of Difficult Passages* expressed in Modern Colloquial Language.
Jen-Min Wei-Shêng, Peking, 1963.

Chhen Pi-Liu 陳璧琉 & Chêng Cho-Jen 鄭卓人 (*1*).
(*Huang Ti Nei Ching*) *Ling Shu Ching, Pai Hua Chieh* 靈書經白話解.
The *Yellow Emperor's Manual of Corporeal* (*Medicine*); *the Vital Axis* expressed in Modern Colloquial Language.
Jen-Min Wei-Shêng, Peking, 1963.

Chhen Pi-Liu 陳璧琉 & Chêng Cho-Jen 鄭卓人 (*2*).
Chen Chiu Ko Fu Hsüan Chieh 鍼灸歌賦選解.
Interpretations of Selected Mnemonic Verses and Chants in Acupuncture and Moxibustion.
Jen-Min Wei-Shêng, Peking, 1960.

Chhen Tshun-Jen (*1*) *et al.* 陳存仁.
Chung-Kuo Yao-Hsüeh Ta Tzhu Tien 中國藥學大辭典.
Encyclopaedia of Chinese Materia Medica.
In 2 vols. with a supplementary volume of illustrations.
Shih-Chieh, Shanghai, 1935.

Chhen Tshun-Jen (*2*) 陳存仁.
Chung-Kuo I-Hsüeh Shih Thu Chien 中國醫學史圖鑑.
A Pictorial History of Chinese Medical Science.
With an extensive summary and copious captions in English.
Shanghai Printing Co., Hongkong, 1968.

Chhen Tshun-Jen (*3*) 陳存仁.
Ou-Chou Yen-Chiu Ching Hsüeh (*Kuo Chi Pien Hao*) *Chieh Shao* 歐洲研究經穴（國際編號）介紹.
Introduction to the European Researches towards an International Standard Nomenclature for the Acupuncture Tracts and Points.
ISTC, 1955, **7** (no. 2), 86.

Chhen Tshun-Jen (*4*) 陳存仁.
Jih-Pên So Tshang Thung Jen ti Khao-Chha 日本所藏銅人的考察.
On the Bronze Acupuncture Figures conserved in Japan.
ISTC, 1954, **6** (no. 4), 233.

Chhen Tshun-Jen (*5*). 陳存仁
Chung-Kuo I-Hsüeh Chhuan Ju Yüeh-Nan Shih Shih ho Yüeh-Nan I-Hsüeh Chu Tso 中國醫學傳入越南史事和越南醫學著作.
On the Transmission of Chinese Medicine to Vietnam, and on Vietnamese Medical Books and Authors.
ISTC, 1957, **8** (no. 3), 193.

Chhêng Tan-An (*1*) 承澹盦(淡安).
Chung-Kuo Chen Chiu Hsüeh 中國針灸學.
Chinese Acupuncture and Moxibustion.
Jen-Min Wei-Shêng, Peking, 1956.

Chhêng Tan-An (*2*) 承澹盦.
Tsêng Ting Chung-Kuo Chen Chiu Chih Liao Hsüeh 增訂中國針灸治療學.
Acupuncture and Moxibustion Therapy in China; a Revised Treatise.
Chhien Ching Thang Shu Chü, Shanghai, 1931, 1932, 1933, 1934.

Chhêng Tan-An (*3*) (ed.) 承澹盦.
Hsien-Tai Chen Chiu Tzu-Liao Hsüan-Chi 現代針灸資料選集.
Collected Papers on Acupuncture (and Moxa) in Modern Medical Practice.
Jen-Min Wei-Shêng, Peking, 1956.

Chhêng Tan-An 承澹盦(淡安), Chhen Pi-Liu 陳璧琉 & Hsü Hsi-Nien 徐惜年 (*1*).
Tzu Wu Liu Chu Chen Fa 子午流注針法.
The Time Cycle Method of Acupuncture; or, The Diurnal Rhythm in the Circulation of the Chhi, and its significance for Acupuncture.
Jen-Min, Chiangsu, 1958.

Fan Hsing-Chun (*1*) 范行準.
Chung-Kuo Yü Fang I-Hsüeh Ssu-Hsiang Shih 中國預防醫學思想史.
History of the Conceptions of Hygiene and Preventive Medicine in China.
Jen-Min Wei-Shêng, Peking, 1953, 1954.

Fan Hsing-Chun (*9*) 范行準.
Wu Yün Liu Chhi Shuo ti Lai Yuan 五運六氣說的來源.
On the Origins of the Doctrine of the Five Cycles and the Six Chhi.
ISTC, 1951, **3** (no. 1), 3.
Cf. Wang Shih-Fu (*1*).

Fan Hsing-Chun (*12*) 范行準.
'*Huang Ti Chung Nan Ching Chu*', '*Yü Kuei Chen Ching*' *Tso-chê Lü Kuang ti Nien-Tai Wên Thi* [黃帝衆難經註, 玉匱鍼經]作者呂廣的年代問題.
On the Date of Lü Kuang, the writer of the commentary on the *Huang Ti Nan Ching* and of the *Yü Kuei Chen Ching* (Liang, mid. +6th century).
SHIY, 1957, no. 10, p. 32 (p. 464).

Fang Yu-An (*1*) 方幼倉.
Chen-Tzhu Chih Liao Lung-Ya Chêng 100 Li Lin Chhuang Tsung Chieh 針刺治療聾啞症 100 例臨床總結.
Summary Clinical Report on 100 Cases of Deaf-Mutism Treated with Acupuncture.
SHIY, 1959, no. 10, 46.

Fang Yün-Phêng (*1*) 方云鵬.
Chen-Tzhu Hou, Chhu Hsien Thê I ti Phi Chen, Chêng Ming Ching Lo ti Tshun Tsai 針刺后出現特異的皮疹，証明經絡的存在.
A Demonstration of the Reality of the Acu-Tract System by Observations of Red Spots on the Skin following Acupuncture.
SHIY, 1959, no. 12, 42.

Fujita Rokurō (*1*) 藤田六朗.
Gogyō Junkan 五行循環.
The Circulation of the Five Elements (*Works of Fujita Rokurō*, vol. 4).
Ido no Nippon-shu, Yokosuka, 1972.

Hao Chin-Khai (*1*) 郝金凱.
Chen Chiu Ching Wai Chhi Hsüeh Thu Phu 針灸經外奇穴圖譜.
Illustrated Account of the Auxiliary Acu-points (i.e. those not on any Acu-tract).
Shensi Hsin-Hua, Sian, 1974

Hara Shimetarō (*1*) 原志免太郎.
Chiu Fa I-Hsüeh Yen-Chiu 灸法醫學研究.
Medical Researches on Moxibustion.
Tr. by Chou Tzu-Hsü 周子敍 from the Japanese *Kyūhō Igaku Kenkyū* (1925).
Chung-Hua, Shanghai, 1933.

Hashimoto Masae (*1*) 橋本昌枝.
Atsukunai Okyū Nyūmon あつくないお.灸入門.
An Introduction to (Acupuncture and) Moxibustion without Cautery.
Tokyo, 1964.

Ho Ai-Hua (*1*) 何愛華.
Phing Lung Po-Chien ti 'Huang Ti Nei Ching ti Chu Tso Shih-Tai' 評龍伯堅的[黃帝內經的著作時代].
A Critique of Lung Po-Chien's paper on the Dates of Composition of the *Yellow Emperor's Manual of Corporeal* (*Medicine*).
ISTC, 1958, **9** (no. 4), 62.

Homma Shōhaku (*1*) 李間祥白.
Ching-Lo Chih Liao Chiang Hua 經絡治療講話.
Dialogues on Therapy by the Ching-Lo Network.
Tr. Chiu Chih 九芝.
Chiangsu Jen-Min, Nanking, 1957.

Huang Chu-Chai *et al.* (*1*) 黃竹齋.
Chen Chiu Chih Liao Tso-Ku-Shen-Ching Thung I-pai Li Pao-Kao 針灸治療坐骨神經痛一百例報告.
Sciatica treated by Acupuncture; Report of 100 Cases.
NMJC, 1958, **44** (no. 10), 968.

Huang Hsien-Ming *et al.* (*1*) 黃羨明等.
Erh Chen Chih Liao 800 Li Fên Hsi Pao-Kao 耳針治療 800 例分析告報.
A Report of 800 Cases Treated with Auricular Acupuncture Therapeutically.
SHIY, 1959, no. 4, 27.

Hsiao Han (*1*) 曉菡.
Chhangsha Ma-Wang-tui Han Mu Po Shu Kai Shu 長沙馬王堆漢墓帛書概述.
Brief Notes on the Silk Manuscripts of Ancient Books found in the Han Tomb (no. 3) at Ma-wang tui near Chhangsha (−168).
WWTK, 1974, (no. 9), no. 220, 40.

Hsiao Yung-Thang (*1*) 蕭詠唐.
Shih-Chieh I-Hsüeh Chia tui Chung-Kuo Chen Chiu Liao-Fa chih Thui Chhung 世界醫學家對中國針灸療法之推崇.
On the International Spread of the Chinese Therapy of Acupuncture and Moxibustion.
Shih-Yung, Hongkong, 1962.

Hsieh Li-Hêng (*1*) 謝利恆.
Chung-Kuo I-Hsüeh Yuan Liu Lun 中國醫學源流論.
A Discourse on the Historical Development of Chinese Medicine.
Chhêng Chai I Shih, Shanghai, 1935.

Hsieh Li-Hêng (*2*) 謝利恆.
Chung-Kuo I-Hsüeh Ta Tzhu Tien 中國醫學大辭典.
Encyclopaedia of the Chinese Medical Sciences.
Shang Wu (Com. Press), 1921 (1st ed.); reprinted 1954.

Hsü Hsün-Chan 許訓湛 & Chhen Ta-Chang 陳大章 (*1*).
Têng-Hsien Tshai-Sê Hua Hsiang Chuan Mu 鄧縣彩色畫象磚墓.
The Tomb of the Painted Brick Reliefs at Têng-hsien (Honan), [+5th century, N/Wei].
Wên-Wu, Peking, 1958.

Hsü Jung-Chai (*1*) 徐榮齋.
Lüeh Than Chhêng Wu-Chi 'Chu Chieh Shang Han Lun' ti Nei Jung ho So Fu Thu Chieh Wên-Thi 略談成無已[註解傷寒論]的內容和所附圖解問題.
A Brief Discussion of the Problem of the Content of the [Yün Chhi Hsüeh] Diagrams and Explanations added to the *Shang Han Lun* by Chhêng Wu-Chi [+1144].
SHIY, 1958, no. 3, 6.

Jen An (*1*) 靱庵.
Chung-Kuo Ku-Tai I-Hsüeh Chia 中國古代醫學家.
Chinese Physicians of Ancient Times.
Shanghai Shu Chü, Hongkong, 1963.

Jen Khang-Thung (*1*) 任康桐
Chen-Tzhu Ma-Tsui Chung ti Pien Chêng Fa 針刺痲醉中的辯証法.
A Dialectical Study of the Evidence on the Rationale of Acupuncture Analgesia.
DNM, 1974, no. 1, 62.

Jen Ying-Chhiu (*1*) 任應秋.
Thung Su Chung-Kuo I-Hsüeh Shih Hua 通俗中國醫學史話.
Popular Talks on the History of Chinese Medicine.
Jen-Min, Chungking, 1957.

Jen Ying-Chhiu (*3*) 任應秋.
Wu Yün Liu Chhi 五運六氣.
The Five Cycles and the Six Chhi.
Kho-Hsüeh Chi-Shu, Shanghai, 1959.

Kan Tsu-Wang (*1*) 干祖望.
Tou Han-Chhing Khao 竇漢卿考.
A study of Tou Han-Chhing (b), [eminent physician, fl. +1210, d. +1280].
HSCIY, 1955, no. 6, 220.
Abstr. in *ISTC*, 1955, **7** (no. 3), 175.

Khung Chhing-Lai *et al.* (*1*) 孔慶萊 (13 collaborators).
Chih-Wu-Hsüeh Ta Tzhu Tien 植物學大辭典.
General Dictionary of Chinese Flora.
Com. Press, Shanghai and Hongkong, 1918; repr. 1933 and often subsequently.

Kim Bonghan (*1*) 金鳳漢.
Kuan-Yü Ching-Lo Shih Chih ti Yen-Chiu; Lun Wên Chai Yao 關于經絡實質的研究;論文摘要.
Researches on the Material Basis for the System of Tracts and Branches (in Acupuncture Theory); Essential Findings taken from the Full Report.
In Anon. (*108*), pp. 55 ff.
Trans. from the full publication in Korean, *CHIH*, 1962, no. 1, 5.

Kim Tujong (*1*) 金斗鐘.
Hanguk Ŭihak Sa 韓國醫學史(上中世編).
A History of Medicine in Ancient and Mediaeval Korea.
Chŏngsŭm Sa, Seoul, 1955.
With mimeographed summary in English.

Kung Chhi-Hua 龔啓華, Sun Ai-Chên 孫愛貞, Tshao Chi-Jen 曹及人, Chang Yu-Liang 張友良 & Fan Li 范黎 (*1*)
Ta Pai Shu Chen-Tzhu Chen Thung Hsiao Ying Chung Thi I Yin Su Kuan Chha 大白鼠針刺鎭痛效應中体液因素觀察.
An Investigation of the Transmission of Analgesic Neuro-humours in Cross-circulation Experiments on Rats after Acupuncture.
KHTP, 1973, **18** (no. 4), 187.
Eng. tr. by E. Mei & J. J. Kao (ascribing the paper to 'C. H. Lung' *et al.*) in *AJCM*, 1974, **2** (no. 2), 203.

Kung Shun (*1*) 龔純.
Wo Kuo Wei Ta ti Kho-Hsüeh Chia Hua Tho 我國偉大的科學家華佗.
Hua Tho (*c.* +145 to +208); a Great Chinese Scientist.
ISTC, 1955, **7** (no. 1), 24.

Li Ching-Wei (*2*) 李經緯.
Chen Chiu Fa Chan Chien Shih 針灸發展簡史.
A Brief History of the Development of Acupuncture and Moxibustion.
CITC, 1959, no. 7, 69 (501).

Li Thao (*2*) (ed.) 李濤.
Chung I ti Chih Shih 中醫的智識.
Introduction to [Traditional] Chinese Medicine.
Hsüeh-Wên Shu-Tien, Hongkong, 1956.

Li Thao (*4*) 李濤.
Sui Thang Shih-Tai (+589/+907) Wo Kuo I-Hsüeh ti Chhêng Chiu 隋唐時代(589–907)我國醫學的成就.
Achievements of Chinese Medicine in the Sui and Thang Periods.
ISTC, 1953, **5** (no. 1), 14.

Li Thao (*6*) 李濤.
Chin Yuan Shih-Tai ti I-Hsüeh 金元時代的醫學.
Medicine in the (Jurchen) Chin, and the Yuan, Periods [+1115 to +1234 and +1280 to +1368].
ISTC, 1954, **6** (no. 2), 88.

Li Thao (*10*) 李濤.
Ming-Tai I-Hsüeh (+1369/+1644) ti Chhêng Chiu 明代醫學(1369–1644)的成就.
Achievements of Medicine in the Ming Period.
ISTC, 1957, **8** (no. 1), 43.

Li Thao (*12*) 李濤.
Pei Sung Shih-Tai ti I-Hsüeh 北宋時代的醫學.
Medicine in the Northern Sung Period [+960 to +1126].
ISTC, 1953, **5** (no. 4), 212.

Li Thao (*13*) 李濤.
Chung-Kuo ti-i-pu I Shu 'Nei Ching Su Wên' Chien Chieh 中國第一部醫書內經素問簡介.
A Brief Introduction to China's First Medical Work, the (*Yellow Emperor's*) *Manual of Corporeal* (*Medicine*); *the Pure Questions* (*and Answers*).
ISTC, 1954, **6** (no. 4), 236.

Li Thao (*14*) 李濤.
Chung-Kuo tui-yü Chin-Tai Chi Chung Chi Chhu I-Hsüeh ti Kung-Hsien 中國對於近代幾種基礎醫學的貢獻.
Chinese Contributions to some of the Fundamental Principles of Modern Medicine.
ISTC, 1955, **7** (no. 2), 110.

Li Thao (*15*) 李濤.
I-Hsüeh Shih Kang 醫學史綱.
A Brief Conspectus of the History of Medicine (in China).
Shanghai and Peking, 1940.

Li Yuan-Chi (*1*) 李元吉.
Chung-Kuo Chen Chiu Hsüeh Yuan Liu Chi Lüeh 中國針灸學源流紀略.
Notes on the Development of Acupuncture and Moxibustion in China.
ISTC, 1955, **7** (no. 4), 263.
Repr. in Chhêng Tan-An (*3*), p. 1.

Li Yuan-Chi (*2*) 李元吉.
Thang-Tai Chen Chiu Hsüeh ti Fa Chan ho Chhêng Chiu 唐代針灸學的發展和成就.
The Development and Achievements of Acupuncture and Moxibustion during the Thang Period [+618 to +906].
KSCI, 1963, no. 10.

Liang Chhi-Chhao (*6*) 梁啓超.
Ku Shu Chen Wei chi chhi Nien-Tai 古書眞僞及其年代.
On the Authenticity of Ancient Books and their Probable Datings.
Lectures recorded by Chou Chuan-Ju 周傳儒, Yao Ming-Ta 姚名達 & Wu Chhi-Chhang 吳其昌.
Chung-Hua, Peking, 1955, repr. 1957.

Liu Tun-Yuan (*1*) 劉敦愿.
Han Hua Hsiang Shih shang ti Chen Chiu Thu 漢畫象石上的針灸圖.
Acupuncture and Moxibustion in Stone Reliefs of the Han Period.
WWTK, 1972 (no. 6), no. 193, 47.

Liu Yung-Shun (*2*) 劉永純.
Chung-Kuo 'Chin Chen Chih Liao Fa' tsai Fa-Kuo Chih Kai Khuang 中國[金針治療法]在法國之概況.
Chinese 'Gold Needle Acupunture Therapy' in France.
CMJ/C, 1949, **35** (no. 11/12), 455; repr. *CCHY*, 1973, no. 426.

Lung Po-Chien (*2*) 龍伯堅.
'Huang Ti Nei Ching' ti Chu Tso Shih-Tai 黃帝內經的著作時代.
On the Dates of Composition of the *Yellow Emperor's Manual of Corporeal (Medicine)*.
ISTC, 1957, **8** (no. 2), 106.
Cf. Ho Ai-Hua (*1*).

Ma Chi-Hsing (*4*) 馬繼興.
Thang Jen Hsieh Hui Chiu Fa Thu Tshan Chüan Khao 唐人寫繪灸法圖殘卷考.
A Study of a Fragmentary Paper MS. Hand-scroll of the Thang Period on Moxibustion (and Acupuncture) with Illustrations (S 6168 and S 6262 in the British Museum Stein Collection).
WWTK, 1964 (no. 6), no. 164, 14.
Abstr. *RBS*, 1973, **10**, no. 899.

Ma Chi-Hsing (*5*) 馬繼興
Chieh-Fang Hou Chhu Thu Wên-Wu tsai I-Hsüeh Shih shang-ti Kho-Hsüeh Chia-Chih 解放後出土文物在醫學史上的科學價值
On the Archaeological Finds made since the Cultural Revolution important and valuable for the History of the Medical Sciences.
WWTK 1978 (no. 1), no. 260, 56.

Ma Khan-Wên (*1*) 馬堪溫.
Nei-Chhiu Hsien Shen-Thou Tshun Pien Chhio Miao Tiao Chha Chi 內丘縣神頭村扁鵲廟調查記.
A Report on the Votive Temple of Pien Chhio at Shen-thou Tshun in Nei-chhiu Hsien (S.W. Hopei).
ISTC, 1955, **7** (no. 2), p. 100.

Manaka Yoshio 間中喜雄 & Schmidt, H. 許米特 (*1*).
Chen Shu ti Chin-Tai Yen-Chiu 針術的近代研究.
A Modern Study of Acupuncture.
Tr. from the Japanese: *Ika no Tame no Shinjutsu Nyūmon Kōza*, Yokosuka, 1954, by Hsiao Yu-Shan 蕭友山 & Chhien Tao-Sun 錢稻孫.
Jen-Min Wei-Shêng, Peking, 1958.

Mêng Ching-Pi (*1*) 孟競璧.
Chen Chiu Liao Fa Ting Hsüeh Tan Wei 鍼灸療法定穴單位.
On the Determination of the Exact Points for Acupuncture and Moxibustion in Therapy.
JMPC, 1959, no. 11, 1022.

Miki Sakae (*1*) 三木榮.
Chōsen Igakushi oyobi Shippeishi 朝鮮醫學史及疾病史.
A History of Korean Medicine and of Diseases in Korea.
Sakai, Osaka, 1962.

Nagahiro Toshio (*3*) 長廣敏雄.
Kandai Oso no Kenkyū 漢代畫象の研究.
Studies on the Art of the Han Period.
Chuo-Koron Bijutsu, Tokyo, 1965.

Nakayama Tadajiki (*1*) 中山忠直.
Kampō Igaku Kenkyū 漢方醫學研究.
Researches on (the History of) Chinese Medicine in Japan.
Tokyo, 1931.

Ōba Osamu (*1*) 大庭脩.
Edo Jidai ni okeru; Tōsen Jidosho no Kenkyū 江戸時代における；唐船持渡書の研究.
Researches on the Importation of Books to Japan on Chinese Trading-Ships during the Yedo Period.
Institute of Oriental & Occidental Studies, Kansai University, 1967.

Ōba Osamu (*2*) 大庭脩.
Hirado Matsuura Shiryō Hakubutsukan Zō 'Tōsen no Zu' ni tsuite; Edo Jidai ni Kikō Shita Chūgoku Shōsen no Shiryō
平戸松浦史料博物館藏[唐船之圖]について;江戸時代に來航した中國商船の資料.
On the Scroll of Chinese Ships in the Possession of the Matsuura Museum (at Hirado near Nagasaki); Materials for the Study of Chinese Trading-Ships and Japan in the Yedo Period.
KNU/BIOOS, 1972, no. 5, 13.

Phêng Ching-Shan (*1*) 彭靜山.
Chien I Chen Chiu Liao Fa
簡易針灸療法.
Simplified Therapy of Acupuncture and Moxibustion.
Chhien Chhing Thang Shu Chü, Shanghai, 1954, 1955.

Sugihara Noriyuki (*1*) 杉原德行.
Chung-I-Hsüeh Chi Chhu Chien Shih
中醫學基礎簡釋.
A Simple Exposition of the Fundamental Theories of Chinese Medicine.
Tr. Pai Yang 白羊.
Jen-Min Wei-Shêng, Peking, 1957, repr. 1958.

Sun Chin-Chhing (*1*) 孫錦淸.
Ching-Lo Hsüeh Shuo tsai Chen Chiu Liao Fa shang ti Ying-Yung Chia-Chih
經絡學說在針灸療法上的應用價值.
The Value and Application of the Theory of the Ching-Lo (Tract) System for the Therapeutic Practice of Acupuncture and Moxibustion.
SHIY, 1959, no. 4, 151.

Sung Ta-Jen (*3*) 宋大仁.
Chen Chiu ti Fa Chan ho tsai Shih-Chieh Ko Kuo Yen-Chiu ti Hsien Chuang
鍼灸的發展和在世界各國硏究的現狀.
On the Development of Acupuncture and Moxibustion, with some Account of their Use in various Countries of the World at the Present Day.
ISTC, 1954, **6** (no. 1), 9.

Sung Ta-Jen (*5*) 宋大仁.
Pao Ku; Chin-Tai Chiu Fa Chuan Kho Nü I-Shih 鮑姑;晉代灸法專科女醫師.
A Woman Medical Specialist in Moxibustion and Cautery – Pao Ku (wife of Ko Hung).
ISTC, 1958, **9** (no. 4), 283.

Taki Mototane (*1*) 多紀元胤.
I Chi Khao (*Iseki-kō*) 醫籍考.
Comprehensive Annotated Bibliography of Chinese Medical Literature (Lost or Still Existing).
C. 1825, pr. 1831, repr. Tokyo, 1933, and Chinese-Western Medical Research Society, Shanghai, 1936 with introd. by Wang Chi-Min.

Tamura Sennosuke (*1*) 田村專之助.
Tōyōjin no Kagaku to Gijutsu 東洋人の科學與技術.
(Essays on the History of) Science and Technology among East Asian Peoples [mainly astronomical and meteorological, with much on Korea as well as China and Japan].
Awaji Shobō Shinsha, Tokyo, 1958.
RBS abstr., 1964, **4**, no. 936.

Thang Lan (*3*) 唐蘭
Ma-wang-tui Po Shu 'chhio ku shih chhi' Phien Khao 馬王堆帛書「却谷食氣」篇考
A Study of the Tractate on 'Abstaining from Cereals and Imbibing the chhi' in the Silk Manuscripts recovered from Tomb (No. 3) at Ma-wang-tui (–168).
WWTK, 1975 (no. 6), no. 229, 14.

Thao I-Hsün 陶義訓 & Ma Li-Jen 馬立人 (*1*) (ed. & tr.).
Chen Chiu Liao Fa Kuo Wai Wên Hsien Chi Chin 針灸療法國外文獻集錦.
An Anthology and Bibliography of Western Works on Acupuncture Therapy.
Wei-Shêng, Shanghai, 1956.

Tsêng Chao-Jan (*1*) 曾昭然.
Thai-Chi Chhüan Chhüan Shu 太極拳全書.
A Complete Study of Thai-chi Boxing [Callisthenics].
Hongkong, 1964.

Tsou Chieh-Chêng (*1*) 鄒介正.
Thang Tai ti Chen Lao Shu 唐代的針烙術.
The Technique of Acupuncture and Cautery [in Veterinary Practice] during the Thang period.
AHRA 1960, *2*, 151.

Tung Chhêng-Thung 董承統 & Li Yün-Shan 李蘊山 (*1*).
Chen Chiu Liao Fa tui Chung-Shu-Shen-Ching Hsi Thung Chi Nêng ti Ying-Hsiang – Chung Tzhu Chi ho Chhing Tzhu Chi Shih Chung-Shu-Shen-Ching ti Chi Nêng Pien-Hua 針灸療法對中樞神經系統機能的影响—重刺激和輕刺激時中樞神經的機能變化.
The Influence of Various Intensities of Acupuncture Stimulation on the Functional State of the Central Nervous System.
NMJC, 1958, **44** (no. 5), 461.
Engl. summ., p. 31.

Wang Chi-Min (*1*) 王吉民.
Tsu Kuo I Yao Wên-Hua Liu Chhuan Hai-Wai Khao 祖國醫藥文化流傳海外考.
On the Transmission of Chinese Medical Culture beyond the Seas.
ISTC, 1957, **8** (no. 1), 8.

Wang Chi-Min (*2*) 王吉民.
Li Shih-Chen Wên-Hsien Chan-Lan Hui Thê-Khan 李時珍文獻展覽會特刊.
Catalogue of the Exhibition on the Contributions of Li Shih-Chen.
Museum of the History of Medicine, Shanghai, 1954.

Wang Chi-Min 王吉民 & Fu Wei-Khang 傅維康 (*1*).
Chung-Kuo I-Hsüeh Wai Wên Chu Shu Shu Mu 中國醫學外文著述書目.
Catalogue of Publications on Chinese Medicine in Foreign Languages, 1656 to 1962.
Museum of the History of Medicine, Shanghai Academy of Chinese Medicine, Shanghai, 1963.

Wang Jen-Chün (*1*) 王仁俊.
Ko Chih Ku Wei 格致古微.
Scientific Traces in Olden Times.
1896.

Wang Kuang-Chhien (*1*) 王光前.
Wu Mei Wan ho Huang Po Mu Hsiang Wan Chih Man Hsing Chün Li ti 55 Li Liao Hsiao Kuan Chha 烏梅丸和黃伯木香丸治慢性菌痢的55例療效觀察.
Observations on 55 cases of Chronic Bacterial Dysentery Treated with Wu-mei-wan and Huang-po-mu-hsiang wan.
SHIY, 1959, no. 8, 18, 29.

Wang Shih-Fu (*1*) 王士福.
Wu Yün Liu Chhi Shuo Chhi Yuan ti Shang Thao 五運六氣說起源的商討.
A Discussion of the Origin of the Theory of the Five Cycles and the Six Chhi.
ISTC, 1958, **9** (no. 2), 127.
Cf. Fan Hsing-Chun (*9*).

Wang Yu-Chung 王有忠 & Chang Ping-Yüeh 章秉鉞 (*1*).
(Chien-Ming) Chung-Hsi Hui Tshan I-Hsüeh Thu Shuo (簡明)中西滙參醫學圖說.
Illustrated Explanations of the Differences and Similarities between Chinese (-traditional) and (modern-) Western Medicine [the first book to superimpose the system of acupuncture tracts on modern anatomical diagrams].
Shanghai, 1906.

Wei Pao-Ling 魏保齡 & Chang Hsi-Hsien 張希賢 (*1*).
Chen-Tzhu tui Kou Hsin-Tsang Tung Tso Tien-Liu ti Ying-Hsiang 針刺對狗心臟動作電流的影响.
The Effect of Acupuncture on Cardiac Action in the Dog.
NMJC, 1958, **44** (no. 4), 343.
Engl. summ., p. 23.

Wên Yu (*1*) 聞宥.
Szechuan Han-Tai Hua Hsiang Hsüan Chi 四川漢代畫象選集.
A Collection of the Han Reliefs of Szechuan (album).
Chhün-Lien, Shanghai, 1955.

Wu I-Chhing (*1*) 吳藝卿.
Chhi-Hsing-Chen Liao Fa 七星針療法.
Acupuncture Therapy with the 'Seven Stars' Multiple-Needle Device (seven needles).
Jen-Min Wei-Shêng, Peking, 1960, 1963.

Wu I-Chhing (*2*) 吳藝卿.
Wo tui Chen Chiu ti Jen-Shih ho Thi-Hui 我對針灸的認識和體會.
On the Reactions to Acupuncture experienced by Patients, and their Meaning.
CITC, 1957, no. 3, 119.
Repr. in Chhêng Tan-An (*3*), p. 29.

Yang Tho (*1*) 洋佗.
Hsing Lin Kuang Chi 杏林廣記.
Far-ranging Records from the Apricot Garden [one hundred essays on the history of medicine].
Com. Press, Hongkong, 1973.

Yeh Ching-Chhiu (*1*) 葉勁秋.
Chen Chiu Shu Yao 鍼灸術要.
Essentials of Acupuncture and Moxibustion.
Chung-Hua Shu Chü, Shanghai, 1955.

Yeh Hsiao-Lin (*1*) 葉肖麟.
Erh Chen Liao Fa Chieh Shao 耳針療法介紹
Important Developments in Auriculo-Acupuncture [contains a Chinese translation of the first three German papers of Nogier (1) in *DZA*].
SHIY, 1958, Acupuncture Special No., 45.

Yü Kho (*1*) 于柯.
Sung 'Hsin Chu Thung Jen Shu Hsüeh Chen Chiu Thu Ching' Tshan-Shih ti Fa-Hsien 宋新鑄銅人腧穴鍼灸圖經殘石的發現.
Discovery of damaged Stone Tablets on which were inscribed the text of (Wang Wei-I's) *Illustrated Manual explaining Acupuncture and Moxibustion with the aid of the Bronze Figure and its Acu-points* (probably between +1027 and +1030).
KKTH, 1972 (no. 6) no. 123, 18.

Yü Yün-Hsiu (*1*) 余雲岫.
Ku-Tai Chi Ping Ming Hou Su I 古代疾病名候疏義.
Explanations of the Nomenclature of Diseases in Ancient Times.
Jen-Min Wei-Shêng, Shanghai, 1953.
Rev. Nguyen Tran-Huan, *RHS*, 1956, **9**, 275.

C BOOKS AND JOURNAL ARTICLES IN WESTERN LANGUAGES

ACKERKNECHT, E. H. (1). '"Mesmerism" in Primitive Societies.' *CIBA/S*, 1948, **9** (no. 11), 826.

ADAMS, BRIAN (1). *The Medical Implications of Karate Blows*. Barnes, Cranbury, N.J. and Yoseloff, London, 1969.

AGADJANIAN, N. (1). 'Hypothèse Nouvelle sur le Mode d'Action de l'Acupuncture.' *BSAC*, 1952, no. 6, 13.

ÅGREN, H. (1) (tr.). *Handbook of Acupuncture and Moxibustion Therapy* (from the Shanghai Acupuncture and Moxibustion Research Laboratory). Com. Press, Hongkong, 1971.

AKIL, H. & MAYER, D. J. (1). 'Antagonism of Stimulation-produced Analgesia by p-CPA, a Serotonin Synthesis Inhibitor.' *BRNR*, 1972, **44**, 692.

AKIL, H., MAYER, D. J. & LIEBESKIND, J. C. (1). 'Antagonism of Stimulation-produced Analgesia by Naloxone, a Narcotic Antagonist.' *SC*, 1976, **191**, 961.

ALBERTI, J. (1). 'Guérison Extraordinaire d'un Bébé de Six Mois, qui présentait une séquelle d'hémorrhagie cérébro-méningée néo-natale, grâce à l'Acupuncture, excluant ainsi toute suggestion en raison de l'âge de l'enfant.' *RIAC*, 1959, **12**, (no. 2) no. 48, 61.

ANDERSEN, P. (1). 'Inhibitory Reflexes elicited from the Trigeminal and Olfactory Nerves in Rabbits.' *APSD*, 1954, **30**, 137.

ANDERSSON, S. A., ERICSON, T. & HOLMGREN, E. (1). 'Electro-acupuncture; Effect on Pain Threshold measured by Electrical Stimulation of Teeth.' *BRNR*, 1973, **63**, 393.

ANDERSSON, S. A., ERICSON, T., HOLMGREN, E. & LINDQVIST, G. (1). 'Electro-acupuncture and Pain Threshold.' *LT*, 1973, pt. 2, 564, 915; *BRNR*, 1973, **63**, 393.

ANDERSSON, S. A. & HOLMGREN, E. (1). 'On Acupuncture Analgesia and the Mechanism of Pain.' *AJCM*, 1975, **3**, 311.

ANON. (80). *Chinese Therapeutical Methods of Acupuncture and Moxibustion*. Foreign Languages Press, Peking, 1962. (An authoritative statement prepared by the National Academy and Research Institute of Traditional Chinese Medicine in Peking.)

ANON. (103). *Introduction to Classical Japanese Literature*. Kokusai Bunka Shinkokai (Soc. for Internat. Cultural Relations). Tokyo, 1948.

ANON. (118). 'The Role of some Neuro-transmitters of the Brain in Finger-Acupuncture Anaesthesia.' *SCISA*, 1974, **17** (no. 1), 112.

ANON. (119). 'Recent Achievements in the Promotion of Traditional Chinese Medicine.' *CMJ*, 1959, **78** (no. 2), 103.

ANON. (120). 'Acupuncture and Moxibustion in Treatment of Bacillary Dysentery; Clinical Observations on 63 Cases.' *CMJ*, 1959, **78** (no. 2), 106. French tr. *BSAC*, 1959, no. 34, 30.

ANON. (121). 'China discovers Acupuncture Anaesthesia.' *CREC*, 1971, **20** (no. 10), 2.

ANON. (122). 'The Patient Sat Up and Drank.' *CREC*, 1972, **21** (no. 9), 30.

ANON. (123). 'Acupuncture Anaesthesia for Open-Heart Surgery.' *CREC*, 1974, **23** (no. 10), 26.

ANON. (124). 'Acupuncture and Traditional Drugs in the Treatment of Appendicitis; an Analysis of Forty-nine Cases.' *CMJ*, 1959, **79**, 72. Abstr. in Mann (5), pp. 110 ff. Abridged French tr., *BSAC*, 1959, no. 34, 39.

ANON. (125). 'The Traditional Chinese Medical Treatment of Appendicitis; some preliminary observations.' *CMJ*, 1959, **79**, 77.

ANON. (126). 'Acupuncture in the Treatment of Acute Appendicitis; Report of 116 Cases.' *CMJ*, 1960, **80** (no. 2), 103. German. tr. by G. Bachmann, *DZA*, 1960, **9** (no. 4), 73.

ANON. (127). *Exploring the Secrets of Treating Deaf-Mutes*. Foreign Languages Press, Peking, 1972. French tr. 'Franchir le Seuil du Mutisme', Peking, 1973.

ANON. (128). 'A Preliminary Study of the Mechanism of Acupuncture Anaesthesia' (Report from the Peking Acupuncture Anaesthesia Coordinating Group). *SCISA*, 1973, **16** (no. 3), 447.

ANON. (129). 'Otolaryngology in China since Liberation.' *CMJ*, 1959, **79** (no. 5), 423.

ANON. (130). 'Acupuncture in the Treatment of Deaf-Mutism.' *CMJ*, 1959, **78** (no. 1), 12. German tr. by J. Karoff, *DZA*, 1960, **9** (no. 6), 140. French abstr. in *BSAC*, 1959, no. 33, 37.

ANON. (131). 'Acupuncture in the Treatment of Schistosomiasis; Clinical Observations on 54 Cases' (from the Chekiang Institute of Traditional Chinese Medicine). *CMJ*, 1959, **78** (no. 1), 15. French abstr. in *BSAC*, 1959, no. 33, 38. Abridged French tr., *BSAC*, 1959, no. 34, 45.

ANON. (134). 'Acupuncture Anaesthesia; an Anaesthetic Method combining Traditional Chinese and [Modern] Western Medicine.' *CMJ*, 1975 (N.S.), **1** (no. 1), 13.

ANON. (135). *An Outline of Chinese Acupuncture.* (Compiled by the Chinese Academy of Traditional Medicine.) Foreign Languages Press, Peking, 1975.

ANON. (136). 'Intracardiac Operations [Open Heart Surgery] with Extra-corporeal Circulation under Acupuncture Anaesthesia.' *SCISA*, 1975, **18**, 271. More extensive material presented in Chinese from the same and similar hospital teams: *CMJ/C*, 1974, **54** (no. 8), 453, 460, 464; with English abstrs. 134, 135, 136.

ANON. (137). 'A Clinical Analysis of 1474 Operations under Acupuncture Analgesia among Children.' *CMJ*, 1975 (N.S.), **1** (no. 5), 369.

ANON. (138). *Acupuncture Anaesthesia.* (Translation of Anon. (*114*), *Chen-Tzhu Ma-Tsui.*) U.S. Government Printing Office, Washington, D.C. 1975. (DHEW Publication NIH/75-784; Fogarty International Centre China Health Studies, no. 11.) Preface by M. D. Leavitt. Bibliographical specification of original used not provided, translator or translators anonymous, no Chinese characters for technical terms, no index.

ANON. (139). *A Bibliography of Chinese Sources on Medicine and Public Health in the People's Republic of China, 1960 to 1970.* (Translation of Anon. (*149*)?) U.S. Government Printing Office, Washington, D.C., 1973. (DHEW Publication NIH/73-439, Fogarty International Centre China Health Studies.) Prefaces by M. D. Leavitt & M. M. Cummings. Bibliographical specification of original not provided, no Chinese characters for names or titles given.

ANON. (140). 'Ansicht und Verfahren der Chinesen und Japanesen in Bezug auf Acupunctur und Moxa.' *NGNHK*, 1826, **13**, 169.

ANON. (141). 'When Acupuncture Came to Britain.' *BMJ*, 1973, no. 5894, 687.

ANON. (142). *Les Secrets de la Médecine des Chinois, consistant en la parfaite Connoissance du Pouls, envoyez de la Chine par un François, homme de grand mérite.* Charrys, Grenoble, 1671. Variously attributed to Louis Augustin Alemand (+1645 to +1728) or to an otherwise unknown writer named Alemand-Harvieu, or to Michael Boym the Jesuit missionary in China. But the former was never in China and the latter was Polish, not French.

From internal evidence the writer must have been some French missionary resident at Canton between +1665 and +1668, and the work is based on a translation of some late mediaeval version of the *Mo Chüeh* (Sphygmological Instructions), not at all the same as that contained in Michael Boym's *Clavis Medica ad Chinarum Doctrinam de Pulsibus* (Frankfurt, +1686). There is more similarity with the text contained in Andreas Cleyer's *Specimen Medicinae Sinicae* (Frankfurt, +1682). The *eruditus Eurcpaeus* to whom he refers may well be the translator at Canton. Circumstantial evidence points to either Adrien Greslon, Humbert Augery or Jacques le Favre, possibly even Philippe Couplet, but identification is not yet possible (cf. Grmek (1), p. 63).

The book was republished as an appendix to M. Baudier's *L'Histoire de la Cour du Roy de la Chine*, Champ, Grenoble, 1699. Italian tr. *Secreti Svelati della Medicina de Chinesi Cioè della Cognitione de Polsi...* by F. d'Amphous. Vigone, Milan, 1676.

ANON. (143). *Reproductive Disorders, Spermatorrhagia, Exhausted Brain, etc.; by a Court Physician.* London, 1876.

ANON. (144). 'Dumontpallier on the Cure of Pain by Acupuncture at a Distance.' *LMR*, 1880, **8**, 6.

ANON. (147). 'A Summary of the Research concerning the [Physiological] Effects of Acupuncture.' Tr. of a section from Anon. (*123*) by J. O'Connor & D. Bensky. *AJCM*, 1975, **3**, 377.

ANON. (149). 'A Preliminary Investigation of the Mechanism of Anti-Pain and Counter-Injury Effects of Acupuncture Anaesthesia' (from the Acupuncture Anaesthesia Group, Dept of Biology, Peking University). *SCISA*, 1976, **19** (no. 4), 529.

ANON. (151). 'The Evaluation of Therapeutic Acupuncture' (an analysis of 661 cases treated at the Medical Acupuncture Centre, Miami, Florida, 1974–5). *SSM*, in the press.

ANON. (152). 'The Inhibition Effect and the Mode of Action of Electro-acupuncture upon Discharges from the Pain-sensitive Cells in the Spinal Trigeminal Nucleus.' *SCISA*, 1977, **20** (no. 4), 485.

ARBER, AGNES (3). *Herbals, their Origin and Evolution; a Chapter in the History of Botany, 1470 to 1670.* Cambridge, 1912. 2nd edn. greatly revised and enlarged, 1938, repr. 1953.

ASCHOFF, JÜRGEN (1) (ed.). *Circadian Clocks.* North Holland Pub. Co., Amsterdam, 1965. (Proc. Feldafing Summer School, Sept. 1964.)

AUSTIN, MARY (1). *The Textbook of Acupuncture Therapy.* ASI Publishers, New York, 1972.

AVALON, A. (ps.). See Woodroffe, Sir J. G.

AVERY, J. F. (1). *De Usu Moxae* (Inaug. Diss.). Neill, Edinburgh, 1821.

BABICH, A. M. (1). 'An Analysis of a Portable Electronic Stimulator manufactured in the People's Republic of China.' *AJCM*, 1973, **1**, 341.

BACHE, F. (1). 'Cases illustrative of the Remedial Effects of Acupuncture.' *NAMSJ*, 1825, **1**, 311.

BACHMANN, G. (1). 'Die Meridianbezeichnungen und ihre Abkürzung.' *DZA*, 1956, **5** (nos. 1–2), 18.
BACHMANN, G. (2). 'Heilung eines Subileus durch Akupunktur.' *DZA*, 1959, **8** (nos. 3–4), 39. Ch. tr. in (*108*), pp. 89 ff.
BACHMANN, G. (3). 'Leitfaden der Akupunktur.' Haug, Ulm-Donau, 1961.
[BAKER, THOMAS] (1). *Reflections upon Learning, wherein is shewn the Insufficiency Thereof, in its several Particulars; in order to evince the Usefulness and Necessity of Revelation. By a Gentleman.* Bosvile, London, 1700; Knapton & Wilkin, London, 1714, 1727.
DE BALZAC, HONORÉ (1). *Physiologie du Mariage.* Paris, 1829; often repr., e.g. Calman-Lévy, Paris, 1920; Gallimard, Paris, 1971.
BARATOUX, J. (1). *Précis Élémentaire d'Acupuncture; avec Repérage Anatomique des Points et leurs Applications Thérapeutiques.* Le François, Paris, 1942.
BARATOUX, J. & KHOUBESSERIAN, H. (1). *Thérapeutique et Acupuncture; Points à employer dans chaque Maladie.* Peyronnet, Paris, 1945.
BARBER, T. X. (1). *Hypnosis; a Scientific Approach.* Van Nostrand, New York, 1969.
BARBER, T. X. (2). 'Suggested ("Hypnotic") Behaviour; the Trance Paradigm *versus* an Alternative Paradigm.' Art. in *Hypnosis; Research Developments and Perspectives*, ed. E. Fromm & R. E. Shor (*q.v.*), pp. 115–82.
BARDE, R. (5) (tr.). 'Les Vies de Pien Chhio et de Shunyü I; *Shih Chi* ch. 105.' Unpub. MS.
BARR, M. L. (1). *The Human Nervous System; an Anatomical Viewpoint.* Harper & Row (Medical), New York, Evanston, San Francisco and London, 1972.
BARUCH, C. (1). 'La Méthode de l'Ou-Rou [*wu hu hsüeh fa*].' *RIAC*, 1959, **12**, (no. 1) no. 47, 35; (no. 2) no. 48, 56. German tr. by G. Bachmann, *DZA*, 1960, **9** (no. 5), 113. Chinese tr. in Anon. (*108*), pp. 69 ff.
BARUCH, C. (2). 'Les Applications Thérapeutiques des Points "iu" [*pei shu hsüeh*], dits "Points Assentiments" en Acupuncture.' *NRIAC*, 1969, **4** (no. 14), 307.
BASALLA, G. (1). 'William Harvey and the Heart as a Pump.' *BIHM*, 1962, **36**, 467.
BASU, B. K. (1). 'My Impression of Acupuncture and Moxibustion.' *CMJ*, 1959, **78** (no. 6), 580.
BATAILLON, E. (1). 'L'Embryogénèse complète provoquée chez les Amphibiens par piqûre de l'œuf vierge; Larves parthénogénétiques de *Rana fusca*.' *CRAS*, 1910, **150**, 996.
BATAILLON, E (2) 'La Parthénogénèse expérimentale chez *Bufo vulgaris*.' *CRAS*, 1911, **152**, 920, 1271; AS/NZ 1912 (9ᵉsér.), **16**, 249
BATE, JOHN (1). *The Mysteryes of Nature and Art: conteined in foure Severall Tretises, the first of Water Workes, the second of Fyer Workes, the third of Drawing, Colouring, Painting and Engraving, the fourth of Divers Experiments, as wel serviceable as delightful; partly collected annd partly of the author's peculiar practice and invention.* Harper, Mab, Jackson & Church, London, 1634, 1635, 1654. Bibliography in John Ferguson (2).
BAUNSCHEIDT, K. (1). *Der Baunscheidtismus.* 7th ed. Bonn, 1870.
BAYER, G. S. (2). *Museum Sinicum in quo Sinicae Linguae et Litteraturae Ratio explicatur.* Imperial Academy, 2 vols., St Petersburg, 1730.
BAYLE, A. L. J. (1) (ed.). *Bibliothèque de Therapeutique*, 4 vols. Gabon, Paris, 1828–37.
BAYLE, PIERRE (1). *Nouvelles de la République des Lettres.* 1686.
BAYON, H. P. (1). 'William Harvey, Physician and Biologist; his Precursors, Opponents and Successors.' *ANS*, 1938, **3**, 59, 83, 435; 1939, **4**, 65, 329.
BAYON, H. P. (2). 'The Significance of the Demonstration of the Harveian Circulation by Experimental Tests.' *ISIS*, 1941, **33**, 443.
BAYON, H. P. (3). 'Allusions to a "Circulation" of the Blood in MSS anterior to *De Motu Cordis*, 1628.' *PRSM*, 1939, **32**, 707.
BEAU, G. (1). *La Médecine Chinoise.* Editions du Seuil, Paris, 1965. (Le Rayon de la Science series, no. 23). Rev. *ATOM*, 1965, **20**, no. 226, 323. Eng. tr. Lowell Bair, Avon (Hearst), New York, 1972.
BECK, D. (1). *Versuche über die Acupunctur.* Wolf, Munich, 1828.
BEEBE, R. J., ANDERSEN, T. W. & PERKINS, H. M. (1). 'Preliminary Findings with Acupuncture Treatment of Pain.' Contribution to the First Bethesda Conference on Acupunture Research, in Jenerick (1), p. 1.
BEECHER H. K. (1). *The Measurement of Subjective Responses; Quantitative Effects of Drugs.* Oxford and New York, 1959.
BEECHER, H. K. (2). 'Pain in Men Wounded in Battle.' *ANTSAH*, 1946, **123**, 96.
BEECHER, H. K. (3). 'The Relationship of the Significance of a Wound to the Pain Experienced.' *JAMA*, 1956, **161**, 1609.
BEECHER, H. K. (4). 'The Measurement of Pain.' *PHREV*, 1957, **9**, 140.
BELLUZZI, J. D., GRANT, N., GARSKY, V., SARANTSKIS, D., WISE, C. D. & STEIN, L. (1). 'Analgesia Induced *in vivo* by Central Administration of Enkephalin in the Rat.' *N*, 1976, **260**, 625.
BENICHOU, A. (1). 'Techniques Pratiques d'Acupuncture.' *BSAC*, 1957, no. 23, 11.

BENJAMIN, F. B. & HELVEY, W. M. (1). 'Iontophoresis of Potassium for Experimental Determination of Pain Endurance in Man.' *PSEBM*, 1963, **113**, 566.

BENKOV, AMOS (PENN KUAN-CHIN) & PEI LUNG-TANG (1). 'Golden Remedies' [art. containing quotation from *NCSW* on the circulation of the blood]. *NN*, 1933, Jan. 11. Cited in Hogben (3), p. 800.

BENNETT, M. F. (1). *Living Clocks in the Animal World.* Thoms, Springfield, 1974. (American Lectures (Environmental Studies series,) no. 902.)

BENZER, H., MAYRHOFER, O., PAUSER, G. & THOMA, H. (1). 'Klinische und experimentelle Erfahrungen mit der Akupunktur-Analgesie.' *WKW*, 1974, **86** (no. 3), 65.

BENZER, H. & PAUSER, G. (1). 'Zur Problematik der Akupunktur-Analgesie.' *OARZ*, 1973, **28** (no. 18), 1015.

DE BERGERAC, CYRANO (1). *L'autre Monde; ou, Les États et Empires de la Lune et du Soleil.* De Sercy, Paris, 1659; collated with the MSS and ed. L. Jordan, Niemeyer, Halle and Dresden, 1910 (Veröfftl. d. Gesellsch. für romanischen Literatur, no. 23); also in *Oeuvres Libertines de Cyrano de Bergerac*, ed. F. Lachèvre, 2 vols. Champion, Paris, 1921. Abridged text in *Three Philosophical Voyages*, ed. J. E. White, Dell, New York, 1964. English translations: A. Lovell, Rhodes, London, 1687; R. Aldington, Routledge, London, n.d. [1923]; G. Strachan, Oxford, 1965 (*The Comical History of the States and Empires of the Worlds of the Moon and the Sun*).

BERITASHIVILI, J. S. (1). *Neural Mechanisms of Higher Vertebrate Behaviour*, tr. from the Russian by W. T. Liberson. Churchill, London, 1965.

BERLIN, F. S., BARTLETT, R. L. & BLACK, J. D. (1). 'Acupuncture and Placebo; Effects on Delaying the Terminating Response to a Painful Stimulus.' *ANAESTH*, 1975, **42**, 527.

BERLIOZ, L. V. J. (1). *Mémoires sur les Maladies Chroniques, les Évacuations Sanguines et l'Acupuncture.* 2 vols. Croullebois, Paris, 1816.

BERNSTEIN, JOSEPH (1). 'Über den Nutzen der Akupunktur in verschiedenen Krankheitsfällen durch mehrere Krankengeschichten erläutert, nebst einige Bemerhkungen über die Suct neue Systeme und neue Heilmittel in der Medizin aufzusuchen.' *JPHK*,1828, 67, 84. 120.

BETZ, H. (1). 'Un Succès Surprenant [de l'Acupuncture] chez un Nourrisson de 19 Jours.' *RIAC*, 1956, **9**, no. 38, 191.

BHISHAGRATNA, (KAVIRAJ) KUNJA LAL SHARMA (1) (tr.). *An English Translation of the 'Sushruta Samhita', Based on the Original Sanskrit Text.* 3 vols, with an index volume, pr. pr. Calcutta, 1907–18. Re-issued, Chowkhamba Sanskrit Series Office, Varanasi, 1963. Rev. M. D. Grmek, *A/AIHS*, 1965, **18**, 130.

BILLROTH, C. A. T. (1). *Die allgemeine chirurgische Pathologie und Therapie.* Berlin, 1863. English tr. of 8th ed. *Lectures on Surgical Pathology and Therapeutics.* 2 vols. London, 1877–8.

BIOT, E. (1) (tr.). *Le Tcheou-Li ou Rites des Tcheou* [*Chou*]. 3 vols. Imp. Nat., Paris, 1851. (Photographically reproduced, Wêntienko, Peiping, 1930.)

BISCHKO, J. (1). 'Akupunktur und Stress.' *DZA*, 1955, **4** (nos. 11–12), 124.

BISCHKO, J. (2). 'Observed Uses of Acupuncture.' Art. in *China Medicine as we saw it*, ed. J. R. Quinn. U.S. Govt. Printing Office, Washington, D.C., 1974 (DHEW Publication NIH/75-684; Fogarty International Centre China Health Studies, no. 8). Foreword by E. G. Dimond.

BISHOP, G. H. (1). 'The Relation between Nerve-Fibre Size and Sensory Modality; Phylogenetic Implications of the Afferent Innervation of the Cortex.' *JNMD*, 1959, **128**, 89.

BITTAR, E. E. (1). 'A Study of Ibn al-Nafīs.' *BIHM*, 1955, **29**, 352, 429.

BLAIR-WEST, J. R., COGHLAN, J. P., DENTON, D. A. & WRIGHT, R. D. (1). 'The Effect of Endocrines on Salivary Glands (in man).' Art. in *A Handbook of Physiology*, sect. 6, Alimentary Canal (ed. C. F. Code), vol. 2, 'Secretion', p. 633.

BLAKEMORE, C. (1). 'The Mechanics of the Mind' (Reith Lectures for 1976). *LI*, 1976, **96** (no. 2483), 594; (no. 2484), 635; (no. 2485), 666; (no. 2486), 705; (no. 2487), 743; (no. 2488), 799, and sep. pub.

BLANCARDUS STEPHANUS. See Blankaart, Stephen.

BLANKAART, STEPHEN (1). *Accurate Abhandlung v. d. Podagra und den laufenden Gicht.* Leipzig, 1692. German tr. of *Verhandeling van het Podagra en vliegenden Jicht.* Amsterdam, 1684. Contains (pp. 318 ff.) 'Der Chineser und Japaner Weise wie selbiger allerlei Krankheiten durch das Brennen mit der Moxa und dem Stechen einer guldenen Nadel völlig und gewiss courieren...', by Willem ten Rhijne.

BLANKAART, STEPHEN (2). *Opera Medica, Theoretica, Pratica et Chirurgica, quae omnia variis observationibus, experimentis, tam ex corporibus valetudinariis, cadaveribus, quam ex Mechanicis Illustrantur et Elucidantur....* Boutestein & Lugtmans, Leiden, 1701.

BLATE, M. (1). *The G-Jo* [*Chi Chiu*, quick relief] *Handbook; Finger Pressure Techniques for Paramedical Use.* Falkynor, Davie, Fla. 1976.

BODDE, D. (15). *Statesman, Patriot and General in Ancient China.* Amer. Or. Soc., New Haven, Conn., 1940. (Biographies of Lü Pu-Wei, Ching Kho and Mêng Thien.)

BOENHEIM, F. (1). 'From Huang Ti to Harvey.' *JHMAS*, 1957, **12**, 181.

DE BONDT, JACOB (1). *De Medicina Indorum, libri quatuor.* Hack, Leiden, 1642.

DE BONDT, JACOB (2). *Historiae Naturalis et Medicae Indiae Orientalis, libri sex.* Elzevir, Amsterdam, 1658. (The first four books were reprinted with only slight changes from de Bondt (1), but the last two, which are larger, were new.)

BONICA, J. J. (1). *The Management of Pain.* Lea & Febiger, Philadelphia, 1953.

BONICA, J. J. (2). 'Therapeutic Acupuncture in the People's Republic of China; Implications for American Medicine.' *JAMA*, 1974, **228**, 1544.

BONICA, J. J. (3) (ed.). *[Proceedings of the] International Symposium on Pain, [Seattle, 1973].* Raven, New York and North Holland, Amsterdam, 1974. (Advances in Neurology, vol. 4.)

BONNET, H. (1). *Real-lexikon Egyptische Religions-geschichte.* De Gruyter, Berlin, 1952.

BONTIUS, JACOBUS. See de Bondt, J.

BØRDAHL, P. E. (1). *Den Store Tradisjon; Tradisjonell Kinesisk Medisin og Akupunktur.* Venskabsforbundet Danmark-Kina, København and Århus, 1976. (Venskaps-Sambandets Kinahefter, no. 4.)

BOURDIOL, R. J. (1). 'Mon Maître Georges Soulié de Morant tel que je l'ai vu pratiquer la Médecine Chinoise.' *NRIAC*, 1970, **5**, no. 15, 23.

BOURNE, P. G. (1). 'Non-Pharmacological Approaches to the Treatment of Drug Abuse [and Withdrawal Symptoms].' *AJCM*, 1975, **3**, 235.

BOWERS, J. Z. (2). 'Acupuncture.' *PAPS*, 1973, **117** (no. 3), 143.

BOWERS, J. Z. (3). 'Engelbert Kaempfer; Physician, Explorer, Scholar and Author.' *JHMAS*, 1966, **21**, 237.

BOWERS, J. Z. & CARRUBBA, R. W. (1). 'The Doctoral Thesis of Engelbert Kaempfer: "On Tropical Diseases, Oriental Medicine and Exotic Natural Phenomena".' *JHMAS*, 1970, **25**, 270.

BOWERS, J. Z. & CARRUBBA, R. W. (2). English tr. of Engelbert Kaempfer's *Amoenitatum Exoticarum...*, pp. 582 ff., Fasc. III, Observ. XI, 'A Cure for Colic by Acupuncture employed by the Japanese'. Unpub. MS.

BOWERS, K. S. & BOWERS, P. G. (1). 'Hypnosis and Creativity; a Theoretical and Empirical Rapprochement.' Art. in *Hypnosis; Research Developments and Perspectives*, ed. E. Fromm & R. E. Shor (*q.v.*), p. 255.

BOXER, C. R. (5). *Jan Compagnie in Japan, 1600 to 1817; an Essay on the Cultural, Artistic and Scientific Influence exercised by the Hollanders in Japan from the seventeenth to the nineteenth Centuries.* Nijhoff, The Hague, 1950; OUP, Oxford and Tokyo, 1968 (Oxford in Asia Historical Reprints).

BOYLE, JAMES (1). *A Treatise on Moxa, as applicable more particularly to Stiff Joints...with some General Observations on Spinal Disease.* Callow & Wilson, London, 1825.

BOYLE, JAMES (2). *A Treatise on a Modified Application of Moxa in the Treatment of Stiff and Contracted Joints and also in Chronic Rheumatism....* Callow & Wilson, London, 1826.

[BOYM, MICHAEL] (3). Parts of Cleyer (1) dealing with prescriptions and materia medica, though the ascription is still uncertain.

[BOYM, MICHAEL] (4). *Herbarium Parvum Sinicis Vocabulis Indici Insertis Constans* (issued by Andreas Cleyer). Frankfurt, 1680. Part of part v of Cleyer (1)? It is very doubtful whether this ever appeared as a separate work; cf. Chabrié (1), p. 257; Pelliot (50), p. 139.

BOYM, MICHAEL (5). *Clavis Medica ad Chinarum Doctrinam de Pulsibus, auctore R. P. Michaele Boymo è Soc. Jesu et in China Missionario. Hujus operis ultra viginti annos jam sepulti fragmenta, hinc indè dispersa, collegit et in gratiam Medicae Facultatis in lucem Europaem produxit Cl. Dn. Andreas Cleyerus M.D. et Societatis Batavo-Orientalis Proto-Medicus. A quo nunc demum mittitur totius operis exemplar, è China recens allatum et à mendis purgatum, Procuratore R. P. Philippo Copletio. Belgâ, è Soc. Jesu, Chinensis Missionis Romam misso.* Endt, Nuremberg, 1686. Also pub. in *Misc, Curiosa sive Ephemeridum Medico-Physicarum Acad. Naturae Curiosorum.* Adnexa ad Dec. II an. iv. Nuremberg, 1686. French tr. 'Clef de la Doctrine des Chinois sur le Pouls' in Bruix, Turben & Blanc, *Le Conservateur; ou, Collection de Morceaux Rares...*, Paris, July 1758. For all subtitles see Szczesniak (6), pp. 514 ff.

BOZETTI, S. (1). *Memoria sull'Ago-puntura.* Milan, 1820.

BRADLEY, P. B., BRIGGS, I., GAYTON, R. J. & LAMBERT, L. A. (1). 'Effects of Micro-iontophoretically applied Methionine-enkephalin on Single Neurons in Rat Brainstem.' *N*, 1976, **261**, 425.

BRANDT, J. F. & RATZENBURG, J. T. C. (1). *Medizinische Zoologie.* Berlin, 1829.

BRATU, I., PRODESCU, V., GEORGESCU, A., MARIN, D., SZIFFERT, C., NITESCU, S., IONESCU, C., TOMA, C & IAREMSKI, C. (1). 'Corticalbehandlung durch Akupunktur.' *DZA*, 1965, **14** (no. 1), 14.

BRATU, I., PRODESCU, V., GEORGESCU, A., NITESCU, S., MARIN, D., CIVICA, D. & IENEI, T. (1). 'Experimentelle Akupunkturstudien im Bereiche der Immunobiologie; I, Unspezifische Immunität, Wirkung der nervösen Befehlspunkte.' *DZA*, 1963, **12** (no. 4), 99.

BRATU, J., STOICESCU, C. & PRODESCU, V. (1). 'Experimentelle Studien auf dem Gebiete der Akupunktur; Wirkung der Akupunktur auf die Nebenniere.' *DZA*, 1958, **7** (nos. 3–4), 26. Chinese tr. in Anon. (*108*), pp. 44 ff.

BRATU, I., STOICESCU, C. & PRODESCU, V. (2). 'Der Wert der Ermittlung des elektrischen Widerstandes des Hautgewebes bei der Akupunktur.' *DZA*, 1960, **9** (no. 6), 125.

BRENNAN, R. W., VELDHUIS, J. & CHU, R. (1). 'Acupuncture Anaesthesia.' *LT*, 1973, pt. 2, 849.

BRESLER, D. E. (1). 'Acupunture Analgesia in Oral Surgery.' Communication to the First Bethesda Confeience on Acupuncture Research, in Jenerick (1), p. 68.

BRIDGMAN, R. F. (2). 'La Médecine dans la Chine Antique, d'après les Biographies de Pien-ts'io [Pien Chhio] et de Chouen-yu Yi [Shunyü I], (Chapitre 105 des *Mémoires Historiques* de Sseu-ma Ts'ien [Ssuma Chhien]).' *MCB*, 1955, **10**, 1–213.

BROCKBANK, W. (1). *Ancient Therapeutic Arts.* Heinemann, London, 1954. (Fitzpatrick Lectures, Royal College of Physicians, 1950–1.)

BROOK, S. S. (1). *The East–West Titration with Chinese Pictorial Pathology at Guy's Hospital.* In the Press.

BROUJEAN, J. (1). 'L'Acupuncture Thérapeutique Fonctionelle et Lésionelle.' *BSAC*, 1959, no. 34, 15.

BROWN, F. A., HASTINGS, J. WOODLAND & PALMER, J. D. (1). *The Biological Clock; Two Views.* Academic Press, New York and London, 1975. (The exogenous view is that rhythmic geophysical forces provide organisms with informational inputs which regulate the timing of their recurrent processes. The endogenous view is that organisms possess internal autonomous biological clocks not immediately dependent on the external world and constituting a self-sufficient timing mechanism.)

BROWN, M. L., ULETT, G. A. & STERN, J. A. (1). 'Acupuncture Loci; Techniques for their Location'. *AJCM*, 1974, **2** (no. 1), 67.

BROWN, M. L., ULETT, G. A. & STERN, J. A. (2). 'The Effects of Acupuncture on White Cell Counts.' *AJCM*, 1974, **2** (no. 4), 383.

BROWN, P. E. (1). 'The Use of Acupuncture in Major Surgery.' *LT*, 1972, pt. 1, 1328.

BROWN, S. C. (1). The Caloric Theory of Heat.' *AJPY*, 1950, **18**, 367. Cf. Porkert (1); Needham & Lu (9).

BRUNET, R. (1). 'Introduction à l'Étude de l'Acupuncture.' *BSAC*, 1960, no. 37, 7.

BRUNET, R. & GRENIER, L. (1). 'Présentation d'un nouvel Instrument, le Punctomètre [for identifying acu-points by measurement of electrical impedance of skin].' *BSAC*, 1955, no. 18, 17.

BUDGE, E. A. WALLIS (2) (tr.). *The Monks of Kublai Khan, or the History of the Life and Travels of Rabban Sawma and Markos [Marqos Bayniel].* (Tr. from Syriac.) RTS, London, 1928.

BULL, G. M. (1). 'Acupuncture Anaesthesia; a Hypothesis.' *LT*, 1973, pt. 2, 417.

BURGER, H. C., NOORDERGRAAF, A. & VONKEN, H. W. L. (1). 'Physikalische Betrachtungen über Elektro-Akupunktur.' *HIP*, 1963, **34**, 861.

BURGESS, P. R., CASEY, K. L., CHAPMAN, C. R. *et al.* (1). 'Acupuncture Anaesthesia (Hypalgesia) in the People's Republic of China; a Trip Report of the American Acupuncture Anaesthesia Study Group, Submitted to the Committee on Scholarly Communication with the P.R.C.' Nat. Acad. Sci., Washington, D.C., 1976. Summary: 'Acupuncture Anaesthesia' in *NRNAW*, 1976, **26** (no. 12), 3.

BURKILL, I. H. (1). *A Dictionary of the Economic Products of the Malay Peninsula* (with contribituons by W. Birtwhistle, F. W. Foxworthy, J. B. Scrivener & J. G. Watson). 2 vols. Crown Agents for the Colonies, London, 1935.

BURN, J. H. (1). The *The Autonomic Nervous System.* 4th ed. Blackwell, Oxford and Edinburgh, 1971.

BÜSCHER, H. H., HILL, R. C., ROMER, D., CARDINAUX, F., CLOSSE, A., HAUSER, D. & PLESS, J. (1). 'Evidence for Analgesic Activity of Enkephalin in the Mouse' (and Naloxone Blockage). *N*, 1976, **261**, 423.

BUSCHOF, HERMANN (1). *Het Podagra, Nader als oyt nagevorst en uytgevonden, mitgaders des selfs sekere Genesingh of ontlastened Hulp-Middel.* Amsterdam, 1674. English tr. *A Treatise of the Gout,* London, 1676. Title-page reproduced in Brockbank (1), p. 126.

[BUSK, M. M.] (1). *Manners and Customs of the Japanese in the Nineteenth Century, from Recent Dutch Visitors of Japan, and the German of Dr. Ph. Fr. von Siebold.* Murray, London, 1841.

CAMERON, J. F. & MANT, A. K. (1). 'Fatal Subarachnoid Haemorrhage associated with Cervical Trauma.' *MSL*, 1972, **12** (no. 1), 66.

DA CAMIN, F. S. (1). *Sulla Agopuntura, con Alcuni Cenni sulla Puntura Elettrica.* Antonelli, Venice, 1834.

DA CAMIN, F. S. (2). *Dell'Agopuntura e della Galvano-puntura; Osservazioni,* Venice, 1837.

CAMPS, F. E. & CAMERON, J. F. (1). *Practical Forensic Medicine.* Hutchinson Med. Pub., London, 1971. Based on a previous text covering the same ground by F. E. Camps & W. B. Purchase (1956).

CAMPS, F. E. & HUNT, A. C. (1). 'Pressure upon the Neck.' *JOFOM*, 1959, **6**, 116.

CANAS, J. P. (1). 'Cent vingt deux Cas d'Acupunctures standardisées' *RIAC*, 1956, **9**, no. 37, 104.

CANNON, W. B. (1). *Bodily Changes in Pain, Hunger, Fear and Rage.* New York, 1915. Many times subsequently repr., e.g. Branford, Boston, 1953.

CAPON, E. & MCQUITTY, W. (1). *Princes of Jade* (a survey of Chinese archaeology following a visit to China). Nelson, London, 1973.

CAPPERAULD, I., COOPER, E. & SALTOUN, D. (1). 'Acupuncture Anaesthesia in China.' *LT*, 1972. pt. 2, 1136.

CARDWELL, D. S. L. (3). *From Watt to Clausius; the Rise of Thermodynamics in the Early Industrial Age.* Cornell Univ. Press, Ithaca, N.Y., 1971. Rev. E. E. Daub, *TCULT*, 1972, **13**, 215. Cf. Porkert (1); Needham & Lu (9).

CARRARO, ANTONIO (1). *Saggio sull'Agopuntura.* Udine, 1825.

CARRON, H., EPSTEIN, B. S. & GRAND, B. (1). 'Complications of Acupuncture.' *JAMA*, 1974, **228**, 1552

CARRUBBA, R. W. & BOWERS, J. Z. (1) (tr.). 'The Western World's First Detailed Treatise on Acupuncture; Willem ten Rhijne's *De Acupunctura*.' *JHMAS*, 1974, **29**, 371.

CASSEDY, J. H. (1). 'Early Uses of Acupuncture in the United States, with an Addendum (1826) by Franklin Bache, M.D.' *BNYAM*, 1974, (2nd ser.), **50**, 892.

CECIL, R. L., LOEB, R. F. et al. (1). *A Textbook of Medicine.* Saunders, Philadelphia and London, 1952. (1st ed. 1927, many subsequent.)

CERNEY, J. V. (1). *Acupuncture without Needles.* Parker, West Nyack, N.Y., 1974.

CHABRIÉ, R. (1). *Michel Boym, Jésuite Polonais, et la Fin des Ming en Chine (+1646 à +1662); Contribution à l'Histoire des Missions d'Extrême-Orient.* Bossuet, Paris, 1933. Crit. rev. Pelliot (50).

CHALMERS, N. R., CRAWLEY, R. & ROSE, STEVEN P. R. (1) (ed.). *The Biological Bases of Behaviour.* Open University Press (Harper & Row), London, 1971.

CHAMFRAULT, A. & UNG KANG-SAM (1), with illustrations by M. Rouhier. *Traité de Médecine Chinoise; d'après les Textes Chinois Anciens et Modernes.* Coquemard, Angoulême, 1954–.

Vol. 1. Traité, Acupuncture, Moxas, Massages, Saignées, 1954.

Vol. 2 (tr.). Les Livres Sacrés de Médecine Chinoise (*Nei Ching*, *Su Wên* and *Nei Ching*, *Ling Shu*). 1957.

Vol. 3. Pharmacopée [372 entries from the *Pên Tshao Kang Mu*]. 1959.

Vol. 4. Formules Magistrales. 1961.

Vol. 5. De l'Astronomie à la Médecine Chinoise; Le Ciel, La Terre, l'Homme. 1963.

CHAN, S. H. H. & FÊNG, S. J. (1). 'Suppression of Polysynaptic Reflexes by Electro-acupuncture, and a possible underlying Presynaptic Mechanism in the Spinal Cord of the Cat.' *EXN*, 1975, **48**, 336.

CHANG HSIANG-THUNG (1). 'Integrative Action of the Thalamus in the Process of Acupuncture Analgesia.' *SCISA*, 1973, **16** (no. 1), 25. Repr. (without acknowledgement of origin), *AJCM*, 1974, **2** (no. 1), 1.

CHANG HUNG-CHAO (5), 'On the Question of the Existence of Elephants and Rhinoceroses in North China in Historical Times.' *BCGS*, 1926, **5** (no. 1), 99.

CHANG, M. M. & LEEMAN, S. E. (1). 'Isolation of a Sialogogic Peptide from Bovine Hypothalamic Tissue, and its Characterisation as Substance-P.' *JBC*, 1970, **245**, 4784.

CHANG, M. M., LEEMAN, S. E. & NIALL, H. D. (1). 'The Amino-acid Sequence of Substance-P.' *N* (*New Biol.*), 1971, **232**, 86.

CHAPMAN, C. R. (1). 'Psychophysical Evaluation of Acupunctural Analgesia; Some Issues and Considerations.' *ANAESTH*, 1975, **43** (no. 5), 501.

CHAPMAN, C. R. & BENEDETTI, C. (1). 'Analgesia following Transcutaneous Electrical Stimulation and its Partial Reversal by a Narcotic Antagonist [Naloxone].' In the press.

CHAPMAN, C. R., CHHEN CHAO-NAN (A. C. CHEN) & BONICA, J. J. (1). 'Effects of Intrasegmental Electrical Acupuncture on Dental Pain; Evaluation by Threshold Estimation and Sensory Decision Theory.' *PAIN*, 1977 (in the press), **3**.

CHAPMAN, C. R., GEHRIG, J. D. & WILSON, M. E. (1). 'Acupuncture compared with 33% Nitrous Oxide for Dental Analgesia; a Sensory Decision Theory Evaluation.' *ANAESTH*, 1975, **42**, 532.

CHAPMAN, C. R., GEHRIG, J. D. & WILSON, M. E. (2). 'Acupuncture, Pain, and Signal Detection Theory.' *SC*, 1975. **189**, 65.

CHAPMAN, C. R., WILSON, M. E. & GEHRIG, J. D. (1). 'Signal Detection Evaluation of the Effects of Acupuncture on the Perception of Painful Dental Stimulation.' *APRT*, 1976, **1**, 775.

CHAPMAN, C. R., WILSON, M. E. & GEHRIG, J. D. (2). 'Comparative Effects of Acupuncture and Transcutaneous Stimulation on the Perception of Painful Dental Stimuli.' *PAIN*, 1976, **2**, 265.

CHÊNG, S. B. & TING (DING), L. K. (1). 'Practical Applications of Acupuncture Analgesia.' *N*, 1973, **242**, 559.

CHÊNG TÊ-KHUN (7). 'Yin Yang, Wu Hsing and Han Art.' *HJAS*, 1957, **20**, 162.

CHERTOK, L. (1). *L'Hypnose.* Payot, Paris, 1966, 2nd ed. 1972. English tr. by G. Graham, Pergamon, London, 1966.

CHEW, E. C. See Chhiu Yin-Chhing & Plummer.

CHHEN, GREGORY S. (1). 'Enkephalin, Drug Addiction and Acupuncture.' *AJCM*, 1977, **5** (no. 1), 25.

CHHEN, GREGORY S. & ERDMANN, W. (1). 'Effects of Acupuncture on Tissue Oxygenation of the Rat Brain.' *AJCM/CM*, 1977, **5** (no. 2), 147.

CHHEN, GREGORY S. & HUANG YU-CHÊNG (1). 'Therapeutic Effects of Acupuncture for Chronic Pain.' *AJCM*, 1977, **5** (no. 1), 45.

CHHEN HSIAO WÊN-CHHING. See Tan, Tan & Veith (1).

CHHEN, JAMES Y. P. (1). 'Therapeutic Effects of Acupuncture in Cases of Chronic Pain.' Contribution to the First Bethesda Conference on Acupuncture Research, in Jenerick (1), p. 3.

CHHEN KUAN-SHÊNG (6). *Buddhism in China; a Historical Survey*. Princeton Univ. Press, Princeton, N.J., 1964.

CHHEN KUO-LIANG & LI CHHUAN-CHUNG (1). 'Acupuncture in the Treatment of Pulmonary Tuberculosis.' *CMJ*, 1959, **79** (no. 1), 62. Abridged French tr., *BSAC*, 1959, no. 34, 41.

CHHEN LIANG-TAO. See Tan, Tan & Veith (1).

CHHIU YIN-CHHING & PLUMMER, J. P. (1). 'Connective Tissue, Masson's Trichrome Stain and Acupuncture Loci.' *AJCM*, 1975, **3** (Suppl.), 26.

CHHIU YIN-CHHING & PLUMMER, J. P. (2). 'Acupuncture Points; do they exist?' *AJCM*, 1975, **3** (Suppl.), 45.

CHIANG CHEN-YÜ, CHIANG CHHING-TSHAI, CHU HSIU-LING & YANG LIEN-FANG (1). 'Peripheral Afferent Pathways for Acupuncture Analgesia.' *SCISA*, 1973, **16** (no. 2), 210.

CHIANG CHEN-YÜ, LIU JEN-I, CHU TÊ-HSING, PAI YAO-HUI & CHANG SHU-CHIEH (1). 'Studies on the Spinal Ascending Pathway for the Effect of Acupuncture Analgesia in Rabbits.' *SCISA*, 1975, **18** (no. 5), 651.

CHISHOLM, N. A. (1). 'Acupuncture Analgesia.' *LT*, 1972, pt. 2, 540.

CHRISTIANSEN, J. A. (1). 'On Hyaluronate Molecules in the Labyrinth as Mechano-electrical Transducers, and as Molecular Motors acting as Resonators.' *AOL*, 1962, **57**, 33.

CHRISTIANSEN, J. A. (2). 'An Attempt to Explain the Microphonic Effect of the Inner Ear by means of Displacement Potentials.' *AOL* (Suppl.) 1963, no. 163, 76.

CHU FU-THANG (1). 'Accomplishments in Child Health since Liberation.' *CMJ*, 1959, **79** (no. 5), 384. Partial German tr. by N. Krack, *DZA*, 1961, **10** (no. 2), 42.

CHU LIEN (1). 'Chinese *Chen Chiu* Therapy (Needling and Cautery); Modernising an Ancient Medical Practice.' *PC*, 1954 (1 Dec.), 12.

CHU YANG-MING & AFFRONTI, L. F. (1). 'Preliminary Observations on the Effect of Acupuncture on Immune Responses in Sensitised Rabbits and Guinea-pigs.' *AJCM*, 1975, **3**, 151.

CHURCHILL, J. M. (1). *A Treatise on Acupuncturation; being a Description of a Surgical Operation originally peculiar to the Japonese and Chinese, and by them denominated Zin-King, now introduced into European Practice, with Directions for its Performance, and Cases illustrating its Success.* Simpkin & Marshall, London, n.d. [1821], 1823. French tr. by R. Charbonnier, Crevot, Paris, 1825. German tr. by Wagner with comments by J. B. Friedreich, Bamberg, 1824.

CHURCHILL, J. M. (2). *Cases Illustrative of the Immediate Effects of Acupuncturation in Rheumatism, Lumbago, Sciatica, Anomalous Muscular Diseases, and in Dropsy of the Cellular Tissue, selected from various sources and intended as an appendix to the Author's Treatise on the subject.* Callow & Wilson, London, 1828.

CLAPHAM, A. R., TUTIN, T. G. & WARBURG, E. F. (1). *Flora of the British Isles.* 2nd ed. Cambridge, 1962.

CLARK, G. N. (2). *History of the Royal College of Physicians of London.* 2 vols. Oxford, 1964.

CLARK, W. C. & YANG, J. C. (1). 'Acupunctural Analgesia? Evaluation by Signal Detection Theory.' *SC*, 1974, **184**, 1096.

CLARK, W. E. LE GROS & MEDAWAR, P. B. (1) (eds.). *Essays on Growth and Form presented to d'Arcy Wentworth Thompson.* Oxford, 1945.

CLARKE, E. & DEWHURST, K. (1). *An Illustrated History of Brain Function.* University of California Press, Berkeley, California, and Sandford, Oxford, 1972.

CLEYER, ANDREAS (1) (ed.). *Specimen Medicinae Sinicae, sive cpuscula medica ad mentem Sinensium, continens*

I *De Pulsibus libros quatuor è Sinico translatos*
II *Tractatus de Pulsibus ab erudito Europaeo collectos*
III *Fragmentum operis medici ibidem ab erudito Europaeo conscripti*
IV *Excerpta literis eruditi Europaei in China*
V *Schemata ad meliorem praecedentium Intelligentiam*
VI *De Indiciis morborum ex Linguae coloribus et affectionibus*

Cum Figuris aeneis et ligneis: Edidit Andreas Cleyer Hasso-Casselanus...' Zubrodt, Frankfurt, 1682. For all subtitles see Szczesniak (6), pp. 508 ff.

CLOQUET, JULES & DANTU, T. M. (1) 'Observations sur les Effets Thérapeutiques de l'Acupuncture' in Bayle, A. L. J. (ed.), *Bibliothèque de Thérapeutique*, 1828, vol. 1, pp. 436 ff. This is part of a section entitled 'Travaux Thérapeutiques sur l'Acupuncture', which contains an introduction, abstracts of the monographs of ten Rhijne and Kaempfer, an extract from Berlioz (1), an account of the work of A. Haime at Tours on rheumatism; then the article of Cloquet & Dantu (with a table of cases, 161 successes, 7 partial successes and 56 failures); then a number of anecdotal case histories due to Churchill, Lacroix, Récamier, Tweedale and others; finally (p. 503) a summary of the state of knowledge at the time.

COHN, A. E. (1). 'The Development of the Harveian Circulation.' *AMH*, 1929, **1**, 16.

COLEY, W. (1). 'A Case of Tympanites in an Infant, relieved by the Operation of the Paracentesis; with Remarks on the Case; and a critical Analysis of the Sentiments of the principal Authors who have written on the Disease. To which is subjoined an Account of the Operation of the Acupuncture, as practised by the Japanese in Diseases analogous to the Tympany.' [1797] *MPJ*, 1802, **7**, 223.

COLEY, W. (2). 'On Acupuncturation.' *MPJ*, 1802, **7**, 235.

COLLINS, J. R., JURAS, E. P., HOUTON, R. J. V. & SPRUELL, L. (1). 'Intrathecal Cold Saline Solution; a New Approach to Pain Evaluation.' *ANAL*, 1969, **48**, 816.

COPEMAN, W. S. C. (1). 'Fibro-fatty Tissue and its Relation to Certain "Rheumatic" Syndromes.' *BMJ*, 1949, pt. 2, 191.

COPEMAN, W. S. C. & ACKERMAN, W. L. (1). 'Oedema or Herniations of Fat Lobules as a Cause of Lumbar and Gluteal Fibrositis.' *AIM*, 1947, **79**, 22.

COPPOLA, E. A. (1). 'The Discovery of the Pulmonary Circulation; a New Approach.' *BIHM*, 1957, **31**, 44.

CORDIER, H. (14). 'Les Études Chinoises.' *TP*, 1898, **9** (Suppl.), 1–141.

CRACIUN, T. & TOMA, C. (1). 'Central Nervous Reactions after Acupuncture.' *AJAP*, 1973, **1**, 61.

CRACIUN, T., TOMA, C. & TURDEANU, V. (1). 'Neurohumoral Modifications after Acupuncture.' *AJAP*, 1973, **1**, 67.

CRAFFE, M. (1). 'Le Docteur Louis Berlioz, Introducteur de L'Acupuncture en France.' *RIAC*, 1955, **7**, no. 32, 327.

CRASSET, JEAN (1). *Histoire de l'Église du Japon, par M. l'Abbé de T.* 2 vols. Michallet, Paris, 1689. Italian tr. by S. Canturani, 4 vols., Baglioni, Venice, 1737. German tr., 2 vols., Heiss & Ilger, Augsberg, 1738.

LE CRON, L. M. (1). *Experimental Hypnosis*. Macmillan, London, 1956.

LE CRON, L. M. & BORDEAUX, J. (1). *Hypnotism Today*. London, 1947.

CROSS, K. W., HENSON, R. A., CRITCHLEY, McD. & BRAIN, Sir RUSSELL (1). *Henry Head Centenary Essays and Bibliography*. Macmillan, London, 1961.

CRUMP, J. I. (1) (tr.). *The* Chan Kuo Tshê. Oxford, 1970.

CUSHING, HARVEY (1). *Life of Sir William Osler*. Oxford, 1940.

CUTHBERTSON, D. P. (1). 'The Disturbance of Protein Metabolism following Physical Injury.' Contrib. to Proceedings of a Symposium on 'The Biochemical Response to Physical Injury'. Semmering, Austria, 1958.

CUTHBERTSON, D. P. (2). 'Parenteral Fluid Therapy in relation to the Metabolic Response to Injury.' *SGO*, 1960, **110**, 105.

CYRIAX, J. (1). *Textbook of Orthopaedic Medicine*. 2 vols.
Vol. 1. *Diagnosis of Soft Tissue Lesions* (8th ed.).
Vol. 2. *Treatment by Manipulation, Massage and Injection* [of Hydrocortisone] (5th ed.).
Baillière, Tindall & Cassell, London, 1969, 1971.

CYRIAX, J. (2). 'Fibrositis.' *BMJ*, 1948, pt. 2, 251.

DABRY, C. P. See de Thiersant, P. Dabry (1), and Soubeiran & de Thiersant (1).

DALÉN, PER (1). *Season of Birth; a Study of Schizophrenia and other Mental Disorders*. North Holland, Amsterdam and New York, 1975.

DANILEVSKY, A. S. (1). *Photoperiodizm i Sezonnoe Razvitie Nasekomykh Leningrad*. University of Leningrad, Leningrad, 1961. English tr., J. Johnston & N. Waloff. *Photoperiodism and Seasonal Development of Insects*. Oliver & Boyd, Edinburgh and London, 1965.

DANTU, T. M. (1). *Quelques Propositions sur l'Acupuncture*. (Inaug. Diss.) Didot, Paris, 1825.

DANTU, T. M. (2). *Traité de l'Acupuncture, d'aprés les Observations de M. Jules Cloquet, et publié sous ses yeux par*... Béchet, Paris, 1826.

DARRAS, J. C. (1). 'Hypothèses concernant le Mode d'Action de l'Acupuncture, et la Nature des Méridiens et de leurs Points.' *NRIAC*, 1971, **6**, no. 19, 11.

DEAKIN, J. F. W., DICKENSON, A. H. & DOSTROVSKY, J. O. (1). 'Morphine Effects on Rat Raphe Neurons.' *JOP*, 1976 (Proc. Physiol. Soc.), 46*P*.

DELGADO, J. M. R., OBRADOR, S. & MARTIN-RODRIGUEZ, J. (1). 'Caudate Nucleus Stimulation and Relief of Pain in Paralysed Extremities.' Proc. Internat. Congress of Psycho-surgery, Cambridge, 1972.

DERANIYAGALA, P. E. P. (1). *Some Extinct Elephants, their Relatives and the Two Living Species.* Colombo, 1955. (Ceylon National Museum Pubs.)

DESLANDES, L. (1). *Manhood; the Causes of its Premature Decline.* Otis & Broadus, Boston, 1842.

DIEFFENBACH, F. (1). *Operative Chirurgie.* Leipzig, 1845.

DIMOND, E. G. (1). 'Acupuncture Anaesthesia; Western Medicine and Chinese Traditional Medicine.' *JAMA*, 1971, **218** (no. 10), 1558.

DIMOND, E. G. (2). *More than Herbs and Acupuncture.* Norton, New York, 1975.

DING, L. K. See Chêng, S. B. & Ting, L. K. (1).

DODWELL, C. R. (1) (ed. & tr.). *Theophilus* [Presbyter]; De Diversis Artibus (*The Various Arts*), [probably by Roger of Helmarshausen, *c.* +1130]. Nelson, London, 1961.

DU HUAN-JI. See Tu Huan-Chi & Chao Yen-Fang.

DUCHEK, J. (1). *De Moxibustione.* Prague, 1836.

DUDGEON, J. (1). 'Kung-Fu, or Medical Gymnastics.' *JPOS*, 1895, **3** (no. 4), 341–565.

DUFOUR, R. (1). *Atlas d'Acupuncture Topographique en vingt-trois régions.* Le François, Paris, 1960.

DUJARDIN, F. & PEYRILHE, B. (1). *Histoire de la Chirurgie, dépuis son origine jusqu'à nos jours.* Imp .Roy., Paris, 1774–80. 2 vols., the first by Dujardin, the second by Peyrilhe. Cf. Khoubesserian (2).

DUKE, MARC (1). *L'Agopuntura; Filosofia, Tecnica e Applicazioni della Medicina Tradizionale Cinese.* Mondadori, Rome, 1972.

DURAN-REYNALS, M. L. (1). *The Fever-Bark Tree.* Allen, London, 1947.

DUYVENDAK, J. J. L. (12). 'The Last Dutch Embassy to the Chinese Court' (+1794 to +1795). *TP*, 1938, **34**, 1, 223; 1939, **35**, 329.

DUYVENDAK, J. J. L. (13). 'Early Chinese Studies in Holland.' *TP*, 1936, **32**, 293.

EBERHARD, W. (1). 'Kultur und Siedlung der Randvölker Chinas.' *TP* (Suppl.), 1924, **36**.

EBERHARD, W. (2). 'Lokalkulturen in alten China.' *TP* (Suppl.), 1943, **37**; *MS* Monograph no. 3, 1942. (Crit. H. Wilhelm, *MS*, 1944, **9**, 209.)

EBERHARD, W. (3). 'Early Chinese Cultures and their Development, a Working Hypothesis.' *ARSI*, 1937, 513. (Pub. no. 3476.)

EISLER, ROBERT (1). *The Royal Art of Astrology.* Joseph, London, 1946. (Crit. H. Chatley, *O*, 1947.)

D'ELIA, PASQUALE (15). 'Recent Discoveries and New Studies (1938–1960) on the World Map in Chinese of Father Matteo Ricci, S.J.' *MS*, 1961, **20**, 82.

ELKANA, Y. (1). *The Discovery of the Conservation of Energy.* Hutchinson, London, 1974. Cf. Porkert (1); Needham & Lu (9).

ELKANA, Y. (2). 'The Conservation of Energy; a Case of Simultaneous Discovery?' *A/AIHS*, 1970, **23**, nos. 90–1, 31. Cf. Porkert (1); Needham & Lu (9).

ELLIOTT, F. A. (1). 'Acupuncture and other Forms of Counter-Irritation.' *TCPP*, 1962, **30**, 81.

ELSHOLZ, J. S. (1). 'Von den chinesischen Moxa, ein Mittel wider das Zipperlein.' *RKANF*, 1676, **4**, 390.

EPPINGER, H. & HESS, L. (1). 'Zur Pathologie des vegetativen Nervensystems.' *ZKM*, 1909, **66**, 345; **68**, 205.

EPPINGER, H. & HESS, L. (2). *Die Vagotonie.* Berlin, 1910.

ERAUD, H. (1). 'Association de l'Acupuncture et de la Méthode de Moss dans le Traitement des Rhumatismes Chroniques.' *RIAC*, 1956, **9** no. 37, 112.

ERIKSSON, M. & SJÖLUND, B. (1). 'Acupuncture-like Electro-analgesia in TNS [Transcutaneous Nerve] Stimulation-resistant Chronic Pain.' Art. in *Sensory Functions of the Skin*, ed. Y. Zolterman. Pergamon, Oxford and New York, 1976, p. 575.

ESDAILE, J. (1). *Mesmerism in India and its Practical Application in Surgery and Medicine.* Longman, Brown, Green & Longman, London, 1846; Andrus, Hertford, 1850.

ESDAILE, J. (2). *Natural and Mesmeric Clairvoyance, with the Practical Application of Mesmerism in Surgery and Medicine*, Baillière, London, 1852.

ESDAILE, J. (3). *The Introduction of Mesmerism as an Anaesthetic and Curative Agent into the Hospitals of India.* Dewar, Perth, 1852.

ESDAILE, J. (4). *The Introduction of Mesmerism (with the Sanction of the Government) into the Public Hospitals of India.* Kent, London, 1856.

VON EULER, U. S. & GADDUM, J. H. (1). 'An Unidentified Depressor Substance in Certain Tissue Extracts.' *JOP*, 1931, **72**, 74.

EUPEN, P. J. (1). *Experimenta Quaedam de Laesione Partium Quarundam Corpori Animalis per Acupuncturam.* 1830.

EVANS, F. J. (1). 'Hypnosis and Sleep; Techniques for Exploring Cognitive Activity during Sleep.' Art. in *Hypnosis; Research Developments and Perspectives*, ed. E. Fromm & R. E. Shor (*q.v.*), p. 43.

EVANS, F. J. (2). 'The Placebo Response in Pain Reduction.' Art. in *Proc. International Pain Symposium, Seattle, 1973*, ed. Bonica (3), p. 289.

EWBANK, T. (1). *A Descriptive and Historical Account of Hydraulic and other Machines for Raising Water, Ancient and Modern...* Scribner, New York, 1842. (Best ed. the 16th, 1870.)

FANG HSIEN-CHIH, CHOU YING-CHHING, SHANG THIEN-YÜ & KU YÜN-WU (1). 'The Integration of Modern and Traditional Chinese Medicine in the Treatment of Fractures.' *CMJ*, 1963, **82**, 493; 1964, **83**, 411, 419, 425.

DE LA FARGE, M. (1). 'Traitement Acupunctural de la Maladie de Paget [osteitis deformans].' *RIAC*, 1953, **5**, no. 24, 8.

FARINA, J. M. L. (1). *De Neuralgiae Facialis Curationibus variis et notabilioribus*. Inaug. Diss. Bonn, 1823.

FEILING, A. (1). 'Sciatica; its Varieties and Treatment.' *BMJ*, 1928, pt. 1, 386.

FEINSTEIN, B., LUCE, J. C. & LANGTON, J. N. K. (1). 'The Influence of Phantom Limbs.' Art .in *Human Limbs and their Substitutes*, ed. P. E. Klopsteg & P. D. Wilson, p. 79.

FELDHAUS, F. M. (1). *Die Technik der Vorzeit, der Geschichtlichen Zeit, und der Naturvölker* [encyclopaedia]. Engelmann, Leipzig and Berlin, 1914. Photographic reprint, Liebing, Würzburg, 1965.

FÊNG YING-KHUN, CHIANG TÊ-HUA, LI TZU-HSÜEH, KUO MEI-YÜ & LI FANG-CHHEN (1). 'Immediate Effects of Acupuncture on the Electro-encephalograms of Epileptics.' *CMJ*, 1959, **79** (no. 6), 521.

FERREYROLLES, M. & DE MORANT, G. SOULIÉ (1). 'Coincidences existant entre certains Points de Weihe et certains Points d'Acupuncture Chinoise.' *HOFR*, 1929.

FEUCHT, G. (1). 'Streifzug durch die Geschichte der Akupunktur in Deutschland.' *DZA*, 1961, **10** (no. 2), 27.

FEUCHT, G. (2). 'Moxabehandlung in Europa.' *DZA*, 1963, **12** (no. 4), 104.

FEUCHT, G. (3). 'Biographische Daten zu dem Bildnis Dr Willem ten Rhyne.' *DZA*, 1964, **13** (no. 12), 59.

FEUCHT, G. (4). 'Coup d'Oeil sur l'Acupuncture dans la Médecine Européenne du 19e siècle.' *RIAC*, 1960, **13**, no. 52, 57; 1960, **13**, no. 53, 125; 1960, **13**, no. 54, 164. (The last instalment seems never to have appeared.) There are many mis-spellings of proper names in these papers, most of which may be corrected by Feucht (1) and (2).

FEUCHT, G. (5). 'Kurzer geschichtlicher Abriss der Akupunktur.' *OARZ*, 1973, **28** (no. 18), 985.

FEYJOO Y MONTENEGRO, BENITO GERONIMO (1). *Teatro Critico Universal*. 8 vols. Madrid, 1726–1739; later ed. Madrid, 1773.

FILLIOZAT, J. (1). *La Doctrine Classique de la Médécine Indienne*. Imp. Nat., CNRS and Geuthner, Paris, 1949.

FINCKH, E. (1). 'L'Acupuncture dans la Perspective des *chakras*.' *RIAC*, 1957, **10**, no. 39, 8.

FINSTERBUSCH, K. (1). *Verzeichnis u. Motivindex der Han-Darstellungen*. 2 vols. (1 register, 1 album of plates). Harrassowitz, Wiesbaden, 1971.

FLEAR, C. T. G. & CLARKE, R. (1). 'The Influence of Blood Loss and Blood Transfusion upon the Changes in the Metabolism of Water, Electrolytes and Nitrogen following Civilian Trauma' *CLS*, 1955, **14**, 575.

FLOYER, SIR JOHN (1). *The Physician's Pulse-Watch; or, an Essay to explain the Old Art of Feeling the Pulse, and to Improve it by the help of a Pulse-Watch*. In Three Parts:

I. The Old Galenic Art of Feeling the Pulse is describ'd, and many of its Errors corrected: The true Use of the Pulses, and their Causes, Differences and Prognostications by them, are fully explain'd, and Directions given for Feeling the Pulse by the Pulse-Watch or Minute-Glass.

II. A New Mechanical Method is propos'd for preserving Health, and prolonging Life, and for curing Diseases by the help of the Pulse-Watch, which shews the Pulses when they exceed or are deficient from the natural.

III. The Chinese Art of Feeling the Pulse is describ'd; and the Imitation of their Practice of Physic, which is grounded on the Observation of the Pulse, is recommended. To which is added, An Extract out of Andrew Cleyer, concerning the Chinese Art of Feeling the Pulse. Smith & Walford, London, 1707.

Vol. 2:

The Pulse Watch: or, an Essay to discover The Causes of Diseases, and a rational Method of curing them by Feeling of the Pulse. These Essays are added as an Appendix.

I. An Essay to make a new Sphygmologia, by accommodating the Chinese and European Observations about the Pulse.

II. An Inquiry into the Nature, Use, Causes and Differences of the Respirations, and the Prognostications which may be made by them in Diseases.

FLOYER, SIR JOHN (1) (*cont.*)

III. A Letter concerning the Rupture in the Lungs, which is the Cause of the Asthma in Mankind, and of the Broken-Wind in Horses, and of the Crocke in Hawks, with the palliative Cure of those several Diseases, and their Symptoms. Nicholson, Taylor & Clements, London, 1710

Italian tr. *L'Oriuolo da Polso de Medici ovvero un Saggio per ispiegare l'Arte Antica di tastare il Polso...tradotta da un Cavaliere Inglese dimorante in Toscana.* Ertz, Venice, 1715. The translator was Thomas Dercham of West Dereham, as appears from a MS. presentation in the CUL copy Hh.3.68.

FOERSTER, O. (1). *Die Leitungsbahnen des Schmerzgefühls und die chirurgische Behandlung die Schmerzzustände.* Berlin and Vienna, 1927.

FORBES, R. J. (7). 'Extracting, Smelting and Alloying' [In Early Times before the Fall of the Ancient Empires]. Art. in *A History of Technology*, ed. C. Singer, E. J. Holmyard & A. R. Hall. O.U.P. Oxford, 1954, Vol. 1, p. 572.

FORBES, R. J. (8). 'Metallurgy [in the Mediterranean Civilisations and the Middle Ages].' In *A History of Technology*, ed. C. Singer *et al.*, vol. 2, p. 41. Oxford, 1956.

FOSTER, SIR MICHAEL (1). *Lectures on the History of Physiology during the 16th, 17th and 18th Centuries.* Cambridge, 1901. Repr. 1924. (Cambridge Natural Science Manuals, Biological Series.)

FOU SI-HOUA. See Fu Hsi-Hua.

FOURNIER, ALAIN (1). 'Aspect Thermodynamique du "Livre de la Voie et de la Vertu" [*Tao Tê Ching*].' *CRIT*, 1974, 161. Cf. Porkert (1); Needham & Lu (9).

FRANKENHÄUSER, B. & LUNDERVOLD, A. (1). 'A Note on an Inhibitory Reflex from the Nose in the Rabbit.' *APSD*, 1949, **18**, 238.

FRANSISZYN, MARILYN (1). 'The Age of Acupuncture.' *OLN*, 1973, no. 13, 2.

[FRANSISZYN, MARILYN] (2) 'Osler, Peter Redpath and Acupuncture'. *ODN*, 1974, no.16, 2.

FREDERICKSON, R. C. A. & NORRIS, F. H. (1).'Enkephalin-induced Depression of Single Neurons in Brain Areas with Opiate Receptors, and its Antagonism with Naloxone.' *SC*, 1976, **194**, 440.

FREI, W. (1). 'Allgemeine pathologische Physiologie d. vegetativen Nervensystems bei Infektionskrankheiten und Immunitätsvorgängen.' *EAPPA*, 1939, **34**, 181.

FREUDE, E. & RUHEMANN, W. (1). 'Das Thermoreflektorische Verhalten von Tonus und Kinetik am Magen.' *ZGEM*, 1926, **52**, 338.

FROBENIUS, MAX (1). 'Grundzüge der altchinesischen Psychologie und deren Bedeutung für die praktische Akupunktur.' *DZA*, 1964, **13** (no. 2), 44.

FRODSHAM, J. D. (2) (tr. and ed.). *The First Chinese Embassy to the West; the Journals of Kuo Sung-Thao, Liu Hsi-Hung and Chang Tê-I.* Oxford, 1973.

FROMM, E. & SHOR, R. E. (1) (ed.). *Hypnosis; Research Developments and Perspectives.* Aldine-Atherton, New York; Elek, London, 1973. Rev. P. Morrison *SAM*, 1973, **229** (no. 2), 112.

FROST, E. & ORKIN, L. R. (1). 'The Localisation of Acupuncture Sites.' Contribution to the First Bethesda Conference on Acupuncture Research, in Jenerick (1), p. 121.

FU HSI-HUA (1) (ed.). *Corpus des Pierres Sculptées Han (Estampages).* 3 vols. Brill, Leiden, 1950-..

FU WEI-KHANG (1). *The Story of Chinese Acupuncture and Moxibustion.* Foreign Languages Press, Peking, 1975.

FUJIKAWA YU (1). *Geschichte der Medizin in Japan; Kurzgefasste Darstellung der Entwicklung der japanischen Medizin, mit besonderer Berücksichtigung der Einführung der europäischen Heilkunde in Japan.* Imper. Jap. Ministry of Education, Tokyo, 1911.

FUJITA, R. & MINAMI, S. (1). 'Experimentelle Untersuchungen über die Wirkung von Gold- und Silber-nadeln besonders hinsichtlich tonifizierende und sedierender Wirkung.' *DZA*, 1959, **8** (nos. 9-10), 97. Chinese tr. in Anon. (*108*), pp. 37 ff.

FUJITA SAIKO, PLÉE, H. & DEVÊVRE, J. (1). *Les Points Vitaux Secrets du Corps Humain; le Secret des Atémis [tang shen].* Ediprint, for Judo International, Paris, 1972.

DE LA FUYE, R. (1). 'Über die Behandlung von Blutungen und verwandten Zuständen.' *DZA*, 1959, **8** (nos. 1-2), 19. Chinese tr. in Anon. (*108*), pp. 72 ff. French version in *RIAC*, 1960, **13**, no.52, 79.

DE LA FUYE, R. (2). 'Ist die elektrische Bestimmung d. chinesischen Punkte wissenschaftlich möglich?' *DZA*, 1961, **10** (no. 1), 2. French version in *RIAC*, 1960, **13**, no. 53, 109.

DE LA FUYE, R. (3). 'Le Traitement de la Douleur par l'Acupuncture Diathermique Homéopathique.' *HOFR*, 1938, 662.

DE LA FUYE, R. (4). 'Le Traitement des Surdités par l'Acupuncture Diathermique Homéopathique.' *HOFR*, 1938, 257.

DE LA FUYE, R. (5). *Traité d'Acupuncture.* Le François, Paris, 1947.

GALDSTON, IAGO (1). 'Mesmerism.' *CIBA/S*, 1948, **9** (no. 11). 'Mesmer and animal magnetism', 832; 'Hypnosis and modern psychiatry', 845.

GALE, E. M. (1) (tr.). *Discourses on Salt and Iron* (Yen Thieh Lun), *a Debate on State Control of Commerce and Industry in Ancient China, chapters 1–19*. Brill, Leiden, 1931. (Sinica Leidensia, no. 2.). Crit. P. Pelliot, *TP*, 1932, **29**, 127.

GAMMON, G. D. & STARR, I. (1). 'Studies on the Relief of Pain by Counter-Irritation.' *JCI*, 1941, **20**, 13.

GARDNER, W. J. & LICKLIDER, J. C. R. (1). 'Auditory Analgesia in Dental Operations.' *JADA*, 1959, **59**, 1144.

A GEHEMA, ABRAHAM JANUS (1). *Die Eroberte Gicht mit der chinesischen Waffe der Moxa*. Hamburg, 1682–3.

GEILFUSS, B. W. (1). *Disputatio Inauguralis de Moxa*. Marburg, 1676.

GENT, J. P. & WOLSTENCROFT, J. H. (1). 'Effects of Methionine-enkephalin and Leucine-enkephalin compared with those of Morphine on Brainstem Neurons in the Cat.' *N*, 1976, **261**, 426.

GEORGII, A. (1). *Kinésithérapie, ou Traitement des Maladies par le Mouvement selcn la Méthode de Ling...suivi d'un Abrégé des Applicatiens de Ling á l'Éducation Physique*. Baillière, Paris, 1847.

GEORGII, A. (2). *A Biographical Sketch of the Swedish Poet and Gymnasiarch Peter Henry Ling*. Baillière, London, 1854.

GILES, H. A. (5). *Adversaria Sinica:*
1st series, no. 1, pp. 1–25. Kelly & Walsh, Shanghai, 1905.
no. 2, pp. 27–54. Kelly & Walsh, Shanghai, 1906.
no. 3, pp. 55–86. Kelly & Walsh, Shanghai, 1906.
no. 4, pp. 87–118. Kelly & Walsh, Shanghai, 1906.
no. 5, pp. 119–144. Kelly & Walsh, Shanghai, 1906.
no. 6, pp. 145–188. Kelly & Walsh, Shanghai, 1908.
no. 7, pp. 189–228. Kelly & Walsh, Shanghai, 1909.
no. 8, pp. 229–276. Kelly & Walsh, Shanghai, 1910.
no. 9, pp. 277–324. Kelly & Walsh, Shanghai, 1911.
no. 10, pp. 326–396. Kelly & Walsh, Shanghai, 1913.
no. 11, pp. 397–438 (with index). Kelly & Walsh, Shanghai, 1914.
2nd series, no. 1, pp. 1–60. Kelly & Walsh, Shanghai, 1915.

GILES, H. A. (7) (tr.). 'The *Hsi Yüan Lu* or "Instructions to Coroners" [translated from the Chinese].' *PRSM*, 1924, **17**, 59–107. First published in *CR*, 1874, **3**, 30, 92, 159, etc.

GILES, L. (13). *Descriptive Catalogue of the Chinese Manuscripts from Tunhuang in the British Museum*. British Museum, London, 1957. Rev. J. Průsek, *ARO*, 1959, **27**, 483.

GILLE, B. (14). 'Machines [in the Mediterranean Civilisations and the Middle Ages].' Art. in *A History of Technology*, ed. C. Singer *et al.*, vol. 2, p. 629, Oxford, 1956.

GILLET, J. & PINET, C. (1). 'Contrôle Expérimentale des Effets de l'Acupuncture dans l'Asthme par la Méthode Tachypneumographique.' *RAC*, 1965, no. 2, 11.

GINGRAS, G. & GEEKIE, D. A. (1) (ed.). 'China Report; Health care in the World's most Populous Country.' *CMAJ*, 1973, **109** (no. 2), 150A–N.

GOLDSTEIN, A. & HILGARD, E. R. (1). 'Failure of the Opiate Antagonist Naloxone to modify Hypnotic Analgesia.' *PNASW*, 1975, **72**, 2041.

GOOD, M. G. (1). 'The Objective Diagnosis and Curability of Non-Articular Rheumatism.' *BJPM*, 1951, **14** (no. 1), 1.

GORDON, J. E. (1) (ed.). *Handbook of Clinical and Experimental Hypnosis*. Macmillan, New York; Collier & Macmillan, London, 1967.

GRAD, B. (1). 'Diurnal and Age Changes in the Sodium and Potassium Concentration of Human Mixed Saliva.' *JGER*, 1951, **6** (Suppl.), 93; 1954, **9**, 276.

GRAF, L., SZEKELY, J. I., RONAI, A. Z., DUNAI-KOVACS, Z. & BAJUSE, S. (1). 'A Comparative Study of the Analgesic Effect of Methionine-enkephalin and related lipotropin Fragments.' *N*, 1976, **263**, 240.

GRAHAM, A. C. (6) (tr.). *The Book of Lieh Tzu*. Murray, London, 1960.

GRALL, YVON (1). 'Étude d'un Punctomètre Japonais de Manaka (type Nara Stonom).' *BSAC*, 1962, no. 44, 9.

GRAYSTONE, P. & JAMES, L. (1). *Acupuncture and Pain Theory*, 1975; *a Comprehensive Bibliography*. Biomedical Engineering Services, Vancouver, B.C. *1975*.

GREENWOOD, M. (1). 'A Short History of Medical Statistics.' *BIOM*, 1942, **32**, 101, 203.

GREGOIR, W. (1). 'Acupuncture et Appendicite.' *BSAC*, 1964, no. 53, 63.

GREGUSS, PAL (1). 'A Model for Making Acupuncture Consistent with Western Concepts of Biological Information Processing.' Contribution to the First Bethesda Conference on Acupuncture Research, in Jenerick (1), p. 95.

GRIFFIN, W. & GRIFFIN, D. (1). *Observations on Functional Affections of the Spinal Cord and Ganglionic System of Nerves, in which their Identity with Sympathetic Nervous and Imitative Diseases is Illustrated*. Burgess & Hill, London, 1834.

GRIFFIN, W. & GRIFFIN, D. (2). *Medical and Physiological Problems, being chiefly Researches for Correct Principles of Treatment in Disputed Points of Medical Practice.* Sherwood, Gilbert & Piper, London, 1843

DE GRIJS, C. F. M. (1) (tr.). 'Geregtelijke Geneeskunde, uit het Chineesch vertaald...' (the *Hsi Yuan Lu*, +1247, oldest extant work on forensic medicine). Leiden, 1862.

GRMEK, M. D. (1). 'Les Reflets de la Sphygmologie Chinoise dans la Médecine Occidentale.' Specia, for Biologie Médicale, Paris, 1962 (*LBM*, 1962, **51**, i–cxx, Numéro Hors-Série). Rev. E. Hintzsche, *A/AIHS*, 1963, **16**, 450.

GRUZANSKI, C. V. (1). *Spike and Chain; Japanese Fighting Arts.* Tuttle, Rutland, Vt. and Tokyo, 1968; repr. 1973.

GUILLAUME, M. (1). 'Les Limites d'Action de l'Acupuncture.' *RIAC*, 1953, **5**, no. 26, 23.

GUNN, C. CHAN, MILBRANDT, W. E. *et al.* (1). 'Recent Papers on Acupuncture and Related Subjects from the Workers' Compensation Board of British Columbia' (Sixteen papers). Clinical Research Unit, Rehabilitation Dept., Workers' Compensation Board, Vancouver, B.C., 1977.

HADDAD, SAMI I. & KHAIRALLAH, AMIN A. (1). 'A Forgotten Chapter in the History of the Circulation of the Blood.' *ASURG*, 1936, **104**, 1.

HAGBARTH, K. E. & KERR, D. I. B. (1). 'Central Influences on Spinal Afferent Conduction.' *JNP*, 1954, **17**, 295.

HAINES, BRUCE A. (1). *Karate; its History and Traditions.* Tuttle, Rutland, Vt. and Tokyo, 1968; repr. 1973.

HALBERG, F. (1). 'Physiological 24-Hour Periodicity; General and Procedural Considerations with reference to the Adrenal Cycle.' *ZVHFF*, 1959, **10**, 225.

HALBERG, F. (2). 'The Cycle of Adrenal Function in Man.' *CSHSQB*, 1960, **25**, 289.

HALBERG, F., HALBERG, E., BARNUM, C. P. & BITTNER, J. J. (1). 'Physiological 24-Hour Periodicity in Human Beings and Mice; the Lighting Regimen and Daily Routine.' Art. in *Photoperiodism and Related Phenomena in Plants and Animals*, ed. R. Withrow. Amer. Assoc. Adv. Sci., Washington, D.C., 1959, p. 803.

DU HALDE, J. B. (1). *Description Géographique, Historique, Chronologique, Politique et Physique de l'Empire de la Chine et de la Tartarie Chinoise...* 4 vols. le Mercier, Paris, 1735, 1739; The Hague, 1736. English tr. R. Brookes, 4 vols. Watts, London, 1736, 1741. German tr. Rostock, 1748.

HALL, MARSHALL (1). *On the Diseases and Derangements of the Nervous System, in their Primary Forms and in their Modifications by Age, Sex, Constitution, Hereditary Predisposition, Excesses, General Disorders and Organic Disease.* Baillière, London, 1841.

HALL, MARSHALL (2). *Principles of Diagnosis.* Sherwood, Gilbert & Piper, London, 1834.

HALLER, J. S (1). 'Acupuncture in Nineteenth-Century Western Medicine.' *NYSJM*, 1973, **73**, 1213.

HALLMAN, J. G. (1). *De Moxae atque Ignis in Medicina rationali Usu.* Edman, Upsala, 1788. Dissertation presided by C. P. Thunberg.

HAMILTON, S. G., BROWN, P., HOLLINGTON, M. & RUTHERFORD, K. (1). 'Anaesthesia by Acupuncture' (followed by queries and discussion involving also M. A. E. Ramsay, P. E. Pearce, I. Capperauld and D. Saltoun). *BMJ*, 1972, pt. 3, 352, 703; pt. 4, 232–3, 612.

HAN FÊNG-YEN, LIN JU-HÊNG, CHHEN KHO-CHHIN & SUN JUNG-KHUN (1). 'Electro-acupuncture for Dental Anaesthesia in Exodontia; Preliminary Report of 100 Cases.' *CMJ*, 1960, **80** (no. 2), 100.

HAN SU-YIN (1). 'Acupuncture – the Scientific Evidence.' *EHOR*, 1964, **3** (no. 4), 8.

HANSEN, K. (1). *Sensibilitätsschema; Segmentäre Innervation.* Thieme, Stuttgart, 1940, 1951. Rev. ed. 1955.

HANSEN, K. & SCHLIAK, H. (1). *Segmentale Innervation; ihre Bedeutung für Klinik und Praxis.* Thieme, Stuttgart, 1962.

HANSON, N. R. (1). 'Causal Chains.' *M*, 1955, **64**, 289. Cf. Porkert (1); Needham & Lu (9).

HARDY, J. D., WOLFF, H. G. & GOODELL, H. (1). *Pain Sensations and Reactions.* Baillière, Tindall & Cox, London, and Hafner, New York, 1967.

HARKER, JANET E. (1). *The Physiology of Diurnal Rhythms.* Cambridge, 1964. (Cambr. Monographs in Experimental Biology, no. 13.)

HARKER, JANET E. (2). 'Factors affecting the Diurnal Rhythm of Activity in *Periplaneta americana.* *JEB*, 1956, **33**, 224; 1958, **35**, 251; 1960, **37**, 164; prelim. pub. *N*, 1955, **175**, 773.

HARKER, JANET E. (3). 'Diurnal Rhythms in the Animal Kingdom.' *BR*, 1958, **33**, 1–52.

HARPER, D. J. (1). 'Ma-wang tui-Tomb Three; Documents, the Medical Texts.' *EARLC*, 1976, no. 2, 68.

HARVEY, WILLIAM (1). *Exercitatio Anatomica de Motu Cordis et Sanguinis in Animalibus.* Fitzer, Frankfurt, 1628. Facsimile edition, with English tr. (modified from that of R. Willis, 1847), and prefatory note. Moreton, Canterbury, 1894. Keynes (3), pp. 25–6.

HAVEROFF, S. R. (1). '*Chhi*, is it a Neural Hologram? Micro-tubules, Bio-holography and Acupuncture.' *AJCM*, 1974, **2** (no. 2), 163.
HAWTHORNE, J. G. & SMITH, C. S. (1) (tr.). '*On Divers Arts*'; *the Treatise of Theophilus* [Presbyter, probably by Roger of Helmarshausen, *c.* +1130], *translated from the Mediaeval Latin with Introduction and Notes*... Univ. of Chicago Press, Chicago, 1963.
HAYES, R. L., BENNETT, G. J. & MAYER, D. J. (1). 'Acupuncture, Pain, and Signal Detection Theory.' *SC*, 1975, **189**, 65.
HEAD, SIR HENRY (1). 'On Disturbances of Sensation with especial reference to the Pain of Visceral Disease;
I, [Distribution of the Segmental Areas].' *BRN*, 1893, **16**, 1–133.
II, Head and Neck.' *BRN*, 1894, **17**, 339–480.
III, Pain in Diseases of the Heart and Lungs.' *BRN*, 1896, **19**, 153–276.
HEAD, SIR HENRY (2). *Studies in Neurology*. Kegan Paul, London, 1920.
HEISTER, LORENZ (1). *Chirurgie*... Nuremberg, 1718, repr. 1731. English tr. *A General System of Surgery*. 2 vols. London, 1748.
HELLBRÜGGE, T. (1). 'The Development of Circadian Rhythms in Infants.' *CSHSQB*, 1960, **25**, 311.
HENNEMAN, P. H., DULL, T. A., AVIOLI, L. V., BASTOMSKY, C. H. & LYNCH, T. N. (1). 'Effects of Aspirin and Corticosteroids on Paget's Disease of Bone.' *TCPP*, 1963, **31**, 10.
HEROLDOVÁ, DANA (1). *Acupuncture and Moxibustion*. 2 vols., the second containing anatomical charts and other illustrations. Oriental Inst., Czechoslovak Acad. Sci., Prague, 1968. (Dissertationes Orientales, no. 13.)
HEYDEN, DORIS (1). 'Autosacrificios Prehispanicos con Puas y Punzones.' *BINAH*, 1972, **1** (no. 2), 27.
HEYFELDER, J. F. (1). 'Acupunctura', entry in J. N. Rust's *Theoretisch-Praktisches Handbuch der Chirurgie*... Berlin, 1830– . Vol. 1, p. 286.
HILL, H. E., KORNETSKY, C. H., FLANARY, H. G. & WIKLER, A. (1). 'Effects of Anxiety and Morphine on the Discrimination of Intensities of Painful Stimuli.' *JCI*, 1952, **31**, 473.
HILL, H. E., KORNETSKY, C. H., FLANARY, H. G. & WIKLER, A. (2). 'Studies on Anxiety associated with Anticipation of Pain; I, Effects of Morphine.' *ANEURP*, 1952, **67**, 612.
HITCHCOCK, E. (1). 'Hypothermic Subarachnoid Irrigation for Intractable Pain.' *LT*, 1967, pt. 1, 1133.
HO PING-YÜ (17). 'Doctors take a new look at Acupuncture.' *HEM*, 1973, **17** (no. 3), 10.
HO TSUNG-YÜ (1). 'Über die moderne wissenschaftliche Auffassung der *ching lo* Punkte in der Akupunktur.' *DZA*, 1958, **7** (nos. 7–8), 73; (nos. 9–10), 114.
HO, WAYNE Y. H. & CHHEN, JAMES, Y. P. (1). 'Acupuncture Analgesia; a Report of Two Cases.' *AJCM*, 1973, **1** (no. 1), 151.
HOGBEN, L. (3). *Science for the Citizen; a Self-Educator based on the Social Background of Scientific Discovery*. Allen & Unwin, London, 1938.
HÖKFELT, T., KELLERTH, J. O., NILSSON, G. & PERNOW, B. (1). 'Substance-P; its Localisation in the Central Nervous System and in some Primary Sensory Neurons.' *SC*, 1975, **190**, 889.
HOLLANDER, B. (1). 'Hypnosis and Anaesthesia.' *PRSM*, 1932, **25**, 597.
HOLMGREN, E. (1). 'Increase of Pain Threshold as a Function of Conditioning Electrical Stimulation; an Experimental Study with Application to Electro-acupuncture for Pain Suppression.' *AJCM*, 1975, **3**, 133.
HOLTON, G. & BRUSH, S. G. (1). *Introduction to Concepts and Theories in Physical Science*. 2nd, revised and enlarged edition. Addison-Wesley, Reading, Mass., 1973. Cf. Porkert (1); Needham & Lu (9).
HSI TSÊ-TSUNG, YEN TUN-CHIEH, PO SHU-JEN, WANG CHIEN-MIN, CHHEN CHIU-CHIN & CHHEN MEI-TUNG (1). 'The Heliocentric Theory in China.' *SCISA*, 1973, **16**, 364.
HSIN YU-LING (1). 'Acupuncture Anaesthesia with One Needle.' *CREC*, 1973, **22** (no. 3), 18.
HUANG MAN. See Huang Wên.
HUANG WÊN (1). '*Nei Ching*, the Chinese Canon of Medicine.' *CMJ*, 1950, **68**, 1 (originally M.D. Thesis, Cambridge, 1947).
HUANG WÊN-SHAN (1). *Fundamentals of Thai-chi Chhüan; an Exposition of its History, Philosophy, Technique, Practice and Application*. South Sky (Nan Thien) Book Co., Hongkong, 1973.
HUARD, P. & HUANG KUANG-MING (M. WONG) (1). 'La Notion de Cercle et la Science Chinoise.' *A/AIHS*, 1956, **9**, 111. (Mainly physiological and medical.)
HUARD, P. & HUANG KUANG-MING (M. WONG) (6). 'La Vie et l'Oeuvre du Professeur Li Thao (1901 à 1959).' *A/AIHS*, 1963, **16**, 432.
HUARD, P. & HUANG KUANG-MING (M. WONG) (7). *Soins et Techniques du Corps en Chine, au Japon et en Inde; Ouvrage précédé d'une Étude des Conceptions et des Techniques de l'Éducation Physique, des Sports et de la Kinésithérapie en Occident dépuis l'Antiquité jusqu'á l'Époque contemporaine*. Berg International, Paris, 1971.
HUARD, P. & HUANG KUANG-MING (M. WONG) (8). 'Histoire de l'Acupuncture Chinoise.' *BSEIC*, 1959, **34** (no. 4), 403.

HUARD, P. & HUANG KUANG-MING (10). *Chinese Medicine*. Tr. from *La Médecine Chinoise* by B. Fielding. Weidenfeld & Nicolson, London, 1968.

HUARD, P. & HUANG KUANG-MING (M. WONG) (13). 'Les Tendances actuelles de l'Acupuncture.' *CONCM*, 1963, **85** (no. 2), 277.

HÜBOTTER, F. (1). *Die chinesische Medizin zu Beginn des XX Jahrhunderts, und ihr historischer Entwicklungsgang*. Schindler, Leipzig, 1929. (China-Bibliothek d. Asia Major, no. 1.)

HÜBOTTER, F. (3). 'Zwei berühmte chinesische Ärzte des Altertums, Chouen Yu-J [Shunyü I] und Hoa T'ouo [Hua Tho].' *MDGNVO*, 1927, **21** (Teil A), 1–48. Enlarged from 'Berühmte chinesische Ärzte', *AGMN*, 1913, **7** (no. 2), 115. (Translation of the biography of Shunyü I from *Shih Chi*, ch. 105, and of Hua Tho from *Thu Shu Chi Chhêng, I shu tien*, ch. 525.)

HÜBOTTER, F. (4) (tr.). 'Leben des Pien Chhio [tr. of *Shih Chi*, ch. 105]. *AGMN*, 1914, **7** (no. 2), 115.

HÜBOTTER, F. (5) (tr.). 'Chia I Ching, *erstmalig aus dem chinesischen Urtext übersetzt*' (offset typescript). Pr. pr., Rothacker am Steinplatz, Charlottenberg, Berlin, n.d.

HÜBOTTER, F. (7). On the Etymology of 'Moxa'. *CIBA/MZ*, 1943, **8** (no. 94), 3132.

HUGHES, J., SMITH, T. W., KOSTERLITZ, H. W., FOTHERGILL, LINDA A., MORGAN, B. A. & MORRIS, H. R. (1). 'Identification of Two Related Pentapeptides from the Brain with Potent Opiate Agonist Activity.' *N*, 1975, **258**, 577. Cf. *NS*, 1975, **68**, no. 980, 675.

HUI WÊN & FU WEI-KHANG (1). *Acupuncture Anaesthesia*. Foreign Languages Press, Peking, 1972. Also in French tr.

HUNEKE, W. (1). *Impletol-therapie und andere Neural-therapeutische Verfahren*. Hippokrates-Verlag (Marquardt), Stuttgart, 1952.

HUSSON, R. A. (1). 'L'Electro-diagnostic dans l'Acupuncture en Extrême-Orient.' *BSAC*, 1961, no. 40, 41.

HUXLEY, SIR JULIAN (1). *Problems of Relative Growth*. Methuen, London, 1932.

HYODO, MASAYOSHI & GEGA OSAMU (1). 'Use of Acupuncture Analgesia for Normal Delivery.' *AJCM*, 1977, **5** (no. 1), 63.

INGLIS, BRIAN (1). *Fringe Medicine*. Faber & Faber, London, 1964.

IRWIN, YUKIKO & WAGENVOORD, J. (1). *Shiatzu* (Japanese pressure points). Routledge & Kegan Paul, London, 1977. Rev. M. Weinstein, *AJCM/CM*, 1977, **5**, 195.

JACQUET, Y. F. & LAJTHA, A. (1). 'Morphine Action at Central Nervous System Sites in the Rat; Analgesia or Hyperalgesia depending on Site and Dose.' *SC*, 1973, **182**, 490.

JACQUET, Y. F. & LAJTHA, A. (2). 'Paradoxical Effects after Micro-injection of Morphine in the Periaqueductal Grey Matter in the Rat.' *SC*, 1974, **185**, 1055.

JALIL, ABDUL (1). 'A Note on Acupuncture Therapy.' *HAM*, 1974, **17** (nos. 7–12), 97.

JENERICK, H. P. (1) (ed.). *Proceedings of the National Institutes of Health Acupuncture Research Conference at Bethesda, February* 1973. Bethesda, Md., 1974.

JESSELL, T., IVERSEN, L. L. & KANASAWA, I. (1). 'The Release and Metabolism of Substance-P in Rat Hypothalamus.' *N*, 1976, **264**, 81.

JEVONS, F. R. (1). 'Harvey's Quantitative Method.' *BIHM*, 1962, **36**, 462.

JOSEY, C. & MILLER, C. (1). 'Race, Sex and Class Differences in the Ability to Endure Pain.' *JSPC*, 1932, **3**, 364.

JOSHI, N. P. (1). 'Some Kuśāṅa Passages in the *Harivaṃśa*.' Art. in *Indologen-Tagung*, 1971, ed. H. Härtel & V. Moeller. Steiner, Wiesbaden, 1973.

JUNG, C. G. (2). 'Synchronicity; an Acausal Connecting Principle' [on extra-sensory perception]; essay in the collection *The Structure and Dynamics of the Psyche*. Routledge & Kegan Paul, London, 1960 (Collected Works, vol. 8). Rev. C. Allen, *N*. 1961, **191**, 1232. Cf. Porkert (1); Needham & Lu (9).

JUNG, C. G. (11). 'Über Synchronizität.' *ERJB*, 1952, **20**, 271. English tr. 'On Synchronicity'. *ERYB*, 1958, **3**, 201. Original form of the material later enlarged and published in Jung (2) and Jung & Pauli (1). Cf. Porkert (1); Needham & Lu (9).

JUNG, C. G. & PAULI, W. (1). *The Interpretation of Nature and the Psyche*.
(*a*) 'Synchronicity; an Acausal Connecting Principle', by C. G. Jung.
(*b*) 'The Influence of Archetypal Ideas on the Scientific Theories of Kepler', by W. Pauli.
Tr. R. F. C. Hull, Routledge & Kegan Paul, London, 1955. Orig. publ. in German as *Naturerklärung und Psyche*, Rascher, Zürich, 1952 (Studien aus dem C. G. Jung Institut, no. 4). Cf. Porkert (1); Needham & Lu (9).

JUNKER, JOHANN (1). *Chirurgie*... Halle, 1722.

KAADA, B. R. (1). 'Somato-motor, autonomic and Electro-corticographic Responses to Electrical Stimulation of "Rhinencephalic" and other Structures in Primates, Cat and Dog.' *APSD*, 1951, **24** (Suppl. no. 83), 1–285.

KAADA, B. R. (2). 'Neuro-physiology and Acupuncture; a Review.' Art. in *Advances in Pain Research and Therapy*, vol. 1, ed. J. J. Bonica & D. Albe-Fessard. Raven, New York, 1976, p. 733.

KAADA, B. R., HOEL, E., LESETH, K., NYGAARD-ØSTBY, B., SETEKLEIV, J. & STOVNER, J. (1). 'Acupuncture Analgesia in the People's Republic of China; with glimpses of other aspects of Chinese Medicine' (Report from a Norwegian Medical Study Group). *TNLF*, 1974, **94**, 417–42. Also issued separately. Cf. *NM*, 1974 (Oct.).

KAECH, R. (1). 'Le Mesmérisme.' *CIBA/R*, 1948, **6** (no. 67). 'Sources et précurseurs du magnétisme animal', 2318.
'La jeunesse de Mesmer et son activité à Vienne (1734–1778)', 2324.
'Mesmer à Paris; seconde partie de sa vie (1778–1815)', 2331.
'Le magnétisme animal après Mesmer', 2341.

KAEMPFER, ENGELBERT (1). *Amoenitates Exoticae*; corr. title – *Amoenitatum Exoticarum Politico-Physico-Medicarum Fasciculi V, quibus continentur Variae Relationes, Observationes et Descriptiones Rerum Persicarum et Ulterioris Asiae, multâ attentione, in peregrinationibus per universum Orientem Collectae ab*... Meyer, Lemgoviae, 1712.

KAEMPFER, ENGELBERT (2). *Geschichte und Beschreibung von Japan*. Lemgo, 1777.

KALTENMARK, M. (7). 'Les Communautés Taoistes.' Contribution to the Cini Symposium 'Sviluppi Scientifici, Prospettive Religiose, Movimenti Rivoluzionari della Cina Classica', Venice, 1973. In *Atti del Convegno Internazionale Marco Polo*, ed. L. Lanciotti, Olschki, Florence 1975, p. 89 (much abridged). (Civiltà Veneziana, Studi, no. 31.)

KAO, F. F. (1) (tr.). 'Acupuncture Therapy for Deaf-Mutism.' *AJCM*, 1973, **1** (no. 2), 361. (Translated from an appendix of a clinical manual of treatments of common recurrent diseases according to Chinese traditional medicine, unidentifiable because the Chinese title is not given.)

KAO, F. F. (2) (tr.). 'New Medical Therapy for the Common Cold, Influenza and Bronchitis.' *AJCM*, 1975, **3**, 187. (Translated from *Selected Topics in the Treatment of the Common Cold and Bronchitis*, issued by the Bronchitis Prevention and Treatment Cooperative Group, Peking Medical College, 1972.)

KAO, F. F., BAKER, R. H. & LEUNG SOON-JACK (1). 'The Efficacy of Acupuncture for the Treatment of Sensori-neural Deafness.' *AJCM*, 1973, **1** (no. 2), 283.

KAO, J. J. (1) (tr.). 'Acupuncture Therapy in the Treatment of Schizophrenia.' A translation of pp. 489–91 of the 1974 edition of Anon. (*161*). *AJCM/CM*, 1977, **5** (no. 2), 181.

KAPFERER, R. (1). 'Der Blutkreislauf im altchinesischen Lehrbuch *Huang Ti Nei Ching*.' *MMW*, 1939 (no. 18), 718.

KARLGREN, B. (14) (tr.). *The Book of Odes; Chinese Text, Transcription and Translation*. Museum of Far Eastern Antiquities, Stockholm, 1950. (A reprint of the translation only, from his papers in *BMFEA*, **16** and **17**.)

KAROFF, J. (1). 'Akupunktur Punkt-messung in China.' *NRIAC*, 1971, **6**, no. 22, 287.

KAROW, O. (3). 'Akupunktur und internationale Nomenklatur.' *DZA*, 1954, **3** (nos. 5–6), 16; (nos. 7–8), 49. Cf. Porkert (1); Needham & Lu (9).

KATZ, R. L., KAO, C. Y., SPIEGEL, H. & KATZ, G. J. (1). 'Pain Acupuncture and Hypnosis.' Art. in *Proc. International Pain Symposium, Seattle*, 1973, ed. Bonica (3), p. 819.

KEEGAN, J. J. (1). 'Dermatome Hyperalgesia associated with Herniation of the Intervertebral Disc.' *ANEURP*, 1943, **50**, 67.

KEEGAN, J. J. & GARRETT, F. D. (1). 'The Segmental Distribution of the Cutaneous Nerves in the Limbs of Man.' *ANATR*, 1948, **102**, 409.

KEELE, K. D. (1). *The Evolution of Clinical Methods in Medicine*. Pitman, London, 1963. (Fitzpatrick Lectures, Royal College of Physicians, 1960–1.)

KELLGREN, J. H. (1). 'Observations on Referred Pain arising from Muscle.' *CLS*, 1937, **3**, 175.

KELLGREN, J. H. (2). 'On the Distribution of Pain arising from Deep Somatic Structures, with Charts of Segmental Pain.' *CLS*, 1939, **4**, 35, 303.

KELLNER, G. (1). 'Bau und Funktion der Haut.' *DZA*, 1966, **15** (no. 1), 1–31. Abridged French tr. in *NRIAC*, 1967, **1**, no. 4, 17.

KELLNER, G. & FEUCHT, G. (1). 'Die Mikrowunde; Mikroskopische Studien des Nadelstiches.' *NRIAC*, 1969, **5**, no. 15, 45.

KENNARD, M. A. (1). 'The Course of Ascending Fibres in the Spinal Cord of the Cat essential to the Recognition of Painful Stimuli.' *JCN*, 1954, **100**, 511.

KENNARD, M. A. & HAUGEN, F. P. (1). 'The Relation of Subcutaneous Focal Sensitivity to Referred Pain of Cardiac Origin.' *ANAESTH*, 1955, **16**, 297.

KEYNES, SIR GEOFFREY (2). *The Life of William Harvey*. Oxford, 1966.

KEYNES, SIR GEOFFREY (3). *A Bibliography of the Writings of William Harvey M.D., Discoverer of the Circulation of the Blood*. Cambridge, 1928.

KHOUBESSERIAN, H. (1). 'Libres Propos.' *RAC*, 1965, nos. 3–4, 7. (A plea for the interpretation of acupuncture in terms of modern science, and for the abandonment of the classical theories of mediaeval Chinese medical scholasticism.)

KHOUBESSERIAN, H. (2). 'Ce que l'Europe savait de la Médecine Orientale au 18e Siècle.' *BSAC*, 1962, no. 46, 13. An edited reproduction of the chapter on Chinese and Japanese medicine in Dujardin & Peyrilhe (1), +1774.

KHOUBESSERIAN, H. (3). 'La Maladie du Révérend Père Huc à Kuen-kiang-hien [Chün-chiang Hsien].' *BSAC*, 1963 (no. 48), 55, (no. 49), 33. Description taken from Huc's *Empire Chinois* (2); including his opinions on acupuncture.

KHOUBESSERIAN, H. & MARTINY, THÉRÈSE (1). 'Trois Cas de Douleurs des Amputés et Phénomènes de Membres Fantômes Soulagés par l'Acupuncture suivant la Méthode des Docteurs Labrousse et Duron.' *BSAC*, 1954, no. 11, 5.

KIBLER, M. (1). *Segment-therapie bei Gelenk-erkrankungen und innere Krankheiten.* 2nd ed. Hippokrates-Verlag (Marquardt), Stuttgart, 1953.

KIM BONGHAN (1). 'On the Kyungrak [Ching-Lo] System.' *JKAMS*, 1963 (no. 5), 1–41. Versions in Korean and Chinese simultaneously published. Abstract in *NCNA*, 14 Dec. 1963. Repr. in hard covers, Foreign Languages Publishing House, Pyongyang, 1964. Popular account in *KTD*, 1964, nos. 92, 93. Cf. Kim Bonghan (*1*).

KLAPROTH, J. (7). *Verzeichniss der chinesischen und mandshuischen Bücher und Handschriften der königlichen Bibliothek zu Berlin.* Paris, 1822. Rev. J. P. A. Rémusat (11), vol. 2, pp. 352 ff.

KLEISER, A. (1). 'Die Gesandschaftsreise des P. Michel Boym S.J. im Auftrage einer christlichen Kaiserin in China, 1650–9.' *KM*, 1926.

KLOPSTEG, P. E. & WILSON, P. D. (1) (ed.). *Human Limbs and their Substitutes.* McGraw-Hill, New York, 1954. Repr. with additional bibliography, Hafner, New York and London, 1968.

KÖNIG, G. (1). 'Ohrakupunktur.' *OARZ*, 1973, **28** (no. 18), 1002.

KORR, I. M., THOMAS, P. E. & WRIGHT, H. M. (1). 'Symposium on the Functional Implications of Segmental Facilitation.' *JAOA*, 1955, **54**, 1.
I. The Concept of Facilitation and its Origins.
II. Sympathetic Activity in Facilitated Segments; Sudomotor Studies.
III. Sympathetic Activity in Facilitated Segments; Vasomotor Studies.
IV. Clinical Significance of the Facilitated State.

KOSAMBI, D. D. (2). 'Living Prehistory in India.' *SAM*, 1967, **216** (no. 2), 105.

KRACK, N. (1). 'Akupunktur und Appendicitis.' *DZA*, 1956, **5** (nos. 3–4), 32.

KRACMAR, F. (1). 'Die Biophysikalischen Grundlagen der Akupunktur.' *DZA*, 1961, **10** (no. 5), 104; 1962, **11** (no. 6), 131; 1963, **12** (no. 1), 1.

KRAFT, EVA S. (1). 'Christian Mentzel, Philippe Couplet, Andreas Cleyer und die chinesische Medizin; Notizen aus Handschriften des 17. Jahrhunderts.' Art. in *Fernöstliche Kultur* (Wolf Haenisch Festschrift). Marburg, 1975, p. 158.

KRAFT, EVA S. (2). 'Frühe Chinesische Studien in Berlin.' *MHJO*, 1976, **11**, 91.

KRETZSCHMAR, K. E. (1). 'Neural Therapy, with Special Reference to certain uses of Procaine for Therapeutic Purposes.' *MDT*, 1956, **84** (no. 5), 516; (no. 6), 635.

KROGER, W. S. (1). *Clinical and Experimental Hypnosis in Medicine, Dentistry and Psychology.* Lippincott, Philadelphia and Montreal, 1963.

KROGER, W. S. (2). 'Hypnotism and Acupuncture.' *JAMA*, 1972, **220**, 1012. 'Acupuntural Anaesthesia – its explanation by Conditioning Theory, Autogenic Training and Hypnosis.' *AJPSY*, 1973, **130**, 855.

KROGER, W. S. & DE LEE, S. T. (1). 'The Use of Hypno-anaesthesia for Caesarean Section and Hysterectomy.' *JAMA*, 1957, **163**, 442.

KRZYWANEK, J. (1). *De Electricitate et Acupunctura...* Prague, 1839.

KUBISTA, E., KUCERA, H. & MÜLLER-TYL, E. (1). 'Initiating Contractions of the Gravid Uterus through Electro-acupuncture.' *AJCM*, 1975, **3**, 343.

KUHAR, M. J., PERT, C. B. & SNYDER, S. H. (1). 'The Opiate Receptor in the Brain.' *N*, 1974, **245**, 447.

KUHN, T. S. (1). 'Energy Conservation as an Example of Simultaneous Discovery.' Art. in *Critical Problems in the History of Science*, ed. M. Clagett. Univ. Wisconsin Press, Madison, Wis., 1959, p. 321. With discussions by C. B. Boyer and E. Hiebert following. Cf. Porkert (1); Needham & Lu (9).

KUNTZ, A. (1). *The Autonomic Nervous System.* 3rd ed. Baillière, Tindall & Cox, London, 1946; 4th ed. Lea & Febiger, Philadelphia, 1953.

KUNTZ, A. (2). 'Anatomical and Physiological Properties of Cutaneo-visceral Vasomotor Reflex Arcs.' *JNP*, 1945, **8**, 421.

KUNTZ, A. & HAZELWOOD, L. A. (1). 'Circulatory Reactions in the Gastro-intestinal Tract elicited by Local Cutaneous Stimulation.' *AHJ*, 1940, **20**, 743.

LABROUSSE, J. L. (1). 'Fünf Jahre Akupunkturbehandlung am "Institut National des Invalides" mit besonderer Berücksichtigung der Phantomschmerzbehandlung.' *DZA*, 1956, **5** (nos. 5–6), 64. French version in *RIAC*, 1956, **9**, no. 38, 178.

LABROUSSE, J. L. & DURON, A. J. (1). 'Le Traitement des Algies des Amputés par l'Acupuncture.' *BSAC*, 1953, no. 7, 9.

LACH, D. F. (5). *Asia in the Making of Europe.*
Vol. 1 (in two parts), *The Century of Discovery.*
Vol. 2, pt. 1, *A Century of Wonder; the Visual Arts.*
Univ. Chicago Press, Chicago, 1965– .

LACROIX, A. (1). *Observations sur l'Acupuncture, recueillies à l'Hôtel-Dieu de Paris...* Paris, 1825.

LAFORET, J. (1). 'Note Clinique sur les Résultats obtenus par une seule Séance d'Acupuncture.' *BSAC*, 1960, no. 36, 64.

LALLEMAND, C. F. (1). *A Practical Treatise on the Causes, Symptoms and Treatment of Spermatorrhoea.* Tr. from the French by H. J. McDougall, Churchill, London, 1847.

LANDGREN, GUSTAF (1). 'Afhandling om Acupuncturen.' Inaug. Diss., Uppsala, 1829. Eng. tr. by H. Ågren. *AJCM/CM*, in the press.

DE LANDRESSE, E. A. X. C. (1). *Catalogue des Livres imprimés, des Manuscrits et des Ouvrages chinois, tartares et japonais, composant la Bibliothèque de feu M. Klaproth.* 2 vols. 1st vol. Merlin, Paris, 1839. 2nd vol. Pihan de la Forest, Paris, 1839, 1840.

DE LANGRE, JACQUES (1). *The First Book of Dō-in* [*Tao-yin*] and *The Second Book...*, with Wall Atlas. Happiness Press, Magalia, Calif. 1976.

LARREY, BARON D. J. (1). *On the use of the Moxa as a Therapeutical Agent.* Tr. from the French by R. Dunglison, Underwood, London, 1822. Cf. *NGNHK*, 1813, **1**, 311.

LAUFER, B. (43). *Ivory in China.* Chicago, 1925. (Field Museum of Natural History Pubs. Anthropology Leaflet no. 21.)

LAVERGNE, M. & LAVERGNE, C. (1). *Précis d'Acupuncture Pratique.* Baillière, Paris, 1947.

LAVIER, J. (1). *Les Bases Traditionnelles de l'Acuponcture Chinoise; les Définitions essentielles de la Bio-énergetique Chinoise dans la Terminologie des Acuponcteurs.* Maloine, Paris, 1964.

LAVIER, J. (2). *Points of Chinese Acupuncture.* Tr., indexed and adapted by P. M. Chancellor. Health Sci. Press, Rustington, Sussex, 1965.

LAVIER, J. (3). *Le Micro-Massage Chinois et les Techniques qui en derivent.* Maloine, Paris, 1965.

LAVIER, J. (4). 'Elektro-physiologie der Akupunkturpunkte.' *DZA*, 1960, **9** (no. 3), 49. Chinese tr. in Anon. (*108*), pp. 12 ff.

LAWSON-WOOD, D. & LAWSON-WOOD, J. (1). *Acupuncture Handbook.* Health Sci. Press, Rustington, Sussex, 1964.

LEE DOCHIL, LEE MYUNG-O & CLIFFORD, D. H. (1). 'Cardiovascular Effects of Acupuncture in Anaesthetised Dogs.' *AJCM*, 1974, **2**, 271.

LEE DOCHIL, LEE MYUNG-O & CLIFFORD, D. H. (2). 'Cardiovascular Effects of Moxibustion at the Jen-chung Acu-point (TM 25) during Halothane Anaesthesia in Dogs.' *AJCM*, 1975, **3**, 245.

LEE DOCHIL, LEE MYUNG-O & CLIFFORD, D. H. (3). 'Modification of Cardiovascular Function in Dogs by Acupuncture; a Review' (sympathomimetic, parasympathomimetic and parasympatholytic effects depending on status and locus). *AJCM*, 1976, **4** (no. 4), 333.

LEGGE, J. (7) (tr.). *The Texts of Confucianism:* Pt. III. *The 'Li Chi'*. 2 vols. Oxford, 1885; reprint, 1926. (*SBE* nos. 27 and 28.)

LEGGE, J. (8) (tr.). *The Chinese Classics etc.*: Vol. 4, pts. 1 and 2. '*Shih Ching*';*The Book of Poetry.* Lane Crawford, Hongkong, and Trübner, London 1871; repr. without notes Com. Press, Shanghai, n.d. Photolitho re-issue Hongkong, Univ. Press, Hongkong, 1960, with supplementary volume of concordance tables, etc.

LEHRNBECHER, W. (1). 'A Biophysical Model of the Initial Effects of Acupuncture.' *GMI*, 1974, 68.

LEMBECK, F. (1). 'Zur Frage der zentralen Übertragung afferenter Impulse; III, Das Vorkommen und die Bedeutung der Substanz-P in den dorsalen Wurzeln des Rückenmarks.' *AEPP*, 1953, **219**, 197.

LENZ, H. O. (2). *Botanik der alten Griechen und Römer, deutsch in Auszügen aus deren Schriften, nebst Anmerkungen.* Thienemann, Gotha, 1859.

LEONARD, K. (1). 'Eigenartige Tageschwankungen des Zustandbildes bei Parkinsonismus.' *ZGNP*, 1931, **134**, 76.

LERICHE, R. (1). *The Surgery of Pain*, tr. from the French by A. Young. Baillière, Tindall & Cox, London, 1939.

LESLIE, D. (2). 'The Problem of Action at a Distance in Early Chinese Thought' (discussion on lecture by J. Needham). *Actes du VIIe Congrès International d'Histoire des Sciences, Jerusalem 1953* (1954), p. 186. Cf. Porkert (1); Needham & Lu (9).

LESLIE, D. (7). 'Les Théories de Wang Tch'ong [Wang Chhung] sur la Causalité.' Art. in *Mélange offertes à Monsieur Paul Demiéville.* Paris, 1974, p. 179. Cf. Porkert (1); Needham & Lu (9).
LEUNG, C. Y. See Spoerel, Varkey & Liang (1).
LEUNG SOON-JACK (1). 'Acupuncture Treatment for Pain Syndromes; I, Sciatica, a Report on Ninety Cases.' *AJCM*, 1973, **1** (no. 2), 317.
LEVINE, J. D., GORDON, N. C. & FIELDS, H. L. (1). 'The Mechanism of Placebo Analgesia.' *LT*, 1978, pt. 2 (no. 8091), 654.
LEWIN, ROGER (1). 'In Search of the Biological Clock.' *NS*, 1975, **68**, 386.
LEWIN, ROGER (2). 'The Brain's Own Opiate.' *NS*, 1976, **69**, 13.
LEWIS, P. R. & LOBBAN, M. C. (1). 'Effects of Prolonged Periods of Life on Abnormal Time Routines upon Excretory Rhythms in the Human Subject.' *QJEP*, 1957, **42**, 356.
LEWIS, P. R. & LOBBAN, M. C. (2). 'Dissociation of Diurnal Rhythms in Human Subjects Living on Abnormal Time Routines.' *QJEP*, 1957, **42**, 371.
LEWIS, SIR THOMAS (1). *Pain.* Macmillan, London, 1942.
LI CHO-LU (1). 'The Neurological Basis of Pain and its Possible Relationships to Acupuncture Analgesia.' *AJCM*, 1973, **1** (no. 1), 61.
LI THAO (1). 'Achievements of Chinese Medicine in the Northern Sung Dynasty (+960 to +1127).' *CMJ*, 1954, **72**, 65.
LI THAO (2). 'Achievements of Chinese Medicine in the Southern Sung Dynasty (+1127 to +1279).' *CMJ*, 1954, **72**, 225.
LI THAO (3). 'Medical Ethics in Ancient China.' *BIHM*, 1943, **13**, 268.
LI THAO (4). 'The [Medical] Doctor in Chinese Drama.' *CMJ*, 1950, **68**, 34.
LI THAO (5). 'A Brief History of Paediatrics in China.' *CMJ*, 1959, **79**, 184.
LI THAO (6). 'Chinese Medicine during the [Jurchen] Chin (+1127 to +1234) and Yuan (+1234 to +1368) Eras.' *CMJ*, 1955, **73**, 241.
LI THAO (7). 'Achievements of Chinese Medicine in the Sui (+589 to +617) and Thang (+618 to +907) Dynasties.' *CMJ*, 1953, **71**, 301.
LI THAO (8). 'A Short History of Old Chinese Ophthalmology.' *CMJ*, 1936, **50**, 1513.
LI THAO (9). 'Achievements of Chinese Medicine in the Chhin (−221 to −207) and Han (−206 to +219) Dynasties.' *CMJ*, 1953, **71**, 380.
LI THAO (10). 'Chinese Medicine during the Ming Dynasty (+1368 to +1644).' *CMJ*, 1958, **76**, 178, 285.
LI THAO (11). 'Achievements in Materia Medica during the Ming Dynasty (+1368 to +1644).' *CMJ*, 1956, **74**, 177.
LI THAO (12). 'A Brief History of Obstetrics and Gynaecology in China from Ancient Times to before the Opium War.' *CMJ*, 1958, **77**, 477.
LI THAO (13). 'A Brief History of Endocrine Disorders in China.' *CMJ*, 1941, **59**, 379.
LI THAO (14). 'Historical Notes on Some Vitamin-Deficiency Diseases in China.' *CMJ*, 1940, **58**, 314.
LI THAO (15). 'A Short History of the Acute Infectious Diseases in China.' *CMJ*, 1936, **50**, 172.
LI THAO (16). 'The History of Tuberculosis in China.' *CMJ*, 1942, **61**, 272.
LI THAO (17). 'Ten Celebrated [Chinese] Physicians and their Temple.' *CMJ*, 1940, **58**, 267.
LI THAO (posthumous), CHHÊNG CHIH-FAN & CHANG CHHI-SHAN (1). 'Some Early Records of Nervous and Mental Diseases in Traditional Chinese Medicine.' *CMJ*, 1962, **81**, 55.
LI THAO. See Huard & Huang Kuang-Ming (6).
LI TSUN-NIN (1). 'Lidocaine Injection of Auricular [Acupuncture] Points in the Treatment of Insomnia.' *AJCM*, 1977, **5** (no. 1), 71.
LI TSUNG-YING (1). 'Eastern Diary; Medicine in China.' *EHOR*, 1973, **12** (no. 1), 2.
LIANG PO-CHHIANG (1). 'Überblick ü. d. seltenste chinesische Lehrbruch d. Medizin, *Huang Ti Nei Ching*.' *AGM*, 1938, **26**, 121.
LIBBRECHT, U. (1). *Chinese Mathematics in the Thirteenth Century; the* Shu Shu Chiu Chang *of Chhin Chiu-Shao.* M.I.T. Press, Cambridge, Mass., 1973. (M.I.T. East Asian Science Series, no. 1.)
LIEBESKIND, J. C., GUILBAUD, G., BESSON, J. M. & OLIVERAS, J. L. (1). 'Analgesia from Electrical Stimulation of the Peri-aqueductal Grey Matter in the Cat; Behavioural Observations and Inhibitory Effects on Spinal Cord Inter-neurons.' *BRNR*, 1973, **50**, 441.
LIM KAH-TI (KATIE). See Lin Chhiao-Chih.
LIN CHHIAO-CHIH (1). 'Obstetrics and Gynaecology [in China] during the Past Ten Years.' *CMJ*, 1959, **79** (no. 5), 375.
LINEBERRY, C. G. & VIERCK, C. J. (1). 'Effects of Caudate Nucleus Stimulation on Reactivity to Noxious Electro-cutaneous Stimulation,' Proc. 2nd Annual Meeting of the Society for Neuroscience, Houston, Texas, 1972. Abstract 4.9.

LINZER, M. & VAN ATTA, LOCHE (1). 'Effects of Acupuncture Stimulation on the Activity of Single Thalamic Neurons in the Cat.' Art. in *Proc. International Pain Symposium, Seattle, 1973*, ed. Bonica (3), p. 799.
LIPPERT, M. & LIPPERT, E. L. (1). 'Acupuncture [in early 19th-century England].' *N*, 1972, **240**, 578.
LISOWSKI, F. P. (1). 'Acupuncture Today.' *MMEDA*, 1976, **12** (no. 6), 14.
LIU, Y. KING, VARELA, M. & OSWALD, R. (1). 'The Correspondence between some Motor Points and Acupuncture Loci.' *AJCM*, 1975, **3**, 347.
LO, H. H., TSÊNG LIANG-FU, WEI, E. & LI CHO-HAO (1). β-Endorphin as a Potent Analgesic Agent.' *PNASW*, 1976, **73** (no. 8), 2895.
LOBBAN, M. C. (1). 'Dissociation in Human Rhythmic Functions.' Art. in *Circadian Clocks*, ed. J. Aschoff (1), 1965, p. 219.
LOEB, JACQUES (1). *Artificial Parthenogenesis and Fertilisation.* Chicago, 1913.
LOHMAYER, L. H. A. (1). 'Ein Beitrag zur Acupunctur.' *MDGHK*, 1928, **25**, 173.
LOONEY, G. L. (1). 'Acupuncture in Drug Addiction and the Possible Role of the Autonomic Nervous System.' Contribution to the First Bethesda Conference on Acupuncture Research, in Jenerick (1), p. 82.
LOONEY, G. L. (2). 'A Neurological Basis for Acupuncture; the Autonomic Theory.' *AETR*, 1975, **1**, 210.
LOWNEY, L. J., SHULTZ, K., LOWERY, P. J. & GOLDSTEIN, A. (1). 'Partial Purification of an Opiate Receptor from Mouse Brain.' *SC*, 1974, **183**, 749.
LU GWEI-DJEN (3). 'On Acupuncture in China and its History.' Contribution to the Cini Symposium in 'Sviluppi Scientifici, Prospettive Religiose e Movimenti Rivoluzionari in Cina'. Venice, 1973 ed. L. Lanciotti. Olschki, Florence, 1975. *Atti d. Convegno Internazionale Marco Polo.* p. 69 (Civiltà Veneziana, Studi, no 31)
LU GWEI-DJEN & NEEDHAM, JOSEPH (2). 'China and the Origin of (Qualifying) Examinations in Medicine.' *PRSM*, 1963, **56**, 63.
LU, HENRY C. (1), (tr). *The Chinese Versions of Modern Acupuncture.* 2nd ed. Academy of Oriental Heritage, Vancouver, B.C., 1973. (A partial translation from the Chinese of two books, one published at Shanghai in 1970, the other, Peking, 1971.)
LUNG, C. H., SUN, A. C., TSAO, C. J., CHANG, Y. L. & FAN, L. (1). 'Observation of a Humoral Factor in Acupuncture Analgesia in Rats.' Abridged translation of Kung Chhi-Hua, Sun Ai-Chên, Tshao Chi-Jen, Chang Yu-Lang & Fan Li (*1*), *q.v.* (Owing to this slip in the romanisation of the name of the first collaborator in *AJCM*, 1974, **2**, (no. 2), 203, many subsequent misquotations of this important paper are met with in bibliographies.)
LURIA, A. R. (1). *The Working Brain; an Introduction to Neuropsychology.* Tr. from the Russian by Basil Haigh. Lane (Penguin), London, 1973.

MCBURNEY, D. H. (1). 'Acupuncture, Pain, and Signal Detection Theory.' *SC*, 1975, **189**, 66.
MCCARTHY, P. S., WALKER, R. J. & WOODRUFF, J. N. (1). 'Depressant Actions of Enkephalins on Neurons in the Nucleus Accumbens.' *JOP*, 1976 (Proc. Physiol. Soc.), 42*P*.
MCDONALD, A. J. R. (1). 'Developing Medical Acupuncture.' *MIMS*, 1977 (in the press).
MCKENZIE, J. (1). 'Contributions to the Study of Sensory Symptoms associated with Visceral Disease.' *MCHR*, 1892, **16**, 293.
MCLEOD, J. G., SAINSBURY, M. J. S. & JOSEPH, D. (1). *Acupuncture; a Report to the National Health and Medical Research Council.* Australian Govt. Pub. Service, Canberra, 1974.
MCROBERT, G. R. (1). 'Acupuncture Analgesia.' *BMJ*, 1972, pt. 3, 472.
MADDEN, J., AKIL, H., PATRICK, R. L. & BARCHAS, J. D. (1). 'Stress-induced Parallel Changes in Central Opioid Levels and Pain Responsiveness in the Rat.' *N*, 1977, **265**, 358.
MAILLET, ANNIE (1) (ed.). *A propos de l'Anesthésie par Acupuncture; Textes Chinois publiés en français et Témoignages Vécus, présentés par le Dr A. M....* Centenaire, Paris, 1972.
MAJER, E. H. & BISCHKO, J. (1). 'Experiences with Acupuncture Analgesia in the Field of Ear, Nose and Throat' (especially tonsillectomies). *Proc. Xth International Congress of Otorhinolaryngology*, Venice, 1973 p. 758.
MAN, PANG L. & CHEN, CALVIN H. (1). 'Acupuncture "Anaesthesia"; a New Theory and Clinical Study.' *CUTHR*, 1972, **14**, 390.
MAN, S. C. & BARAGAR, F. D. (1). 'Local Skin Sensory Changes after Acupuncture.' *CMAJ*, 1973, **109**, 609.
MANAKA YOSHIO & URQUHART, U. A. (1). *The Layman's Guide to Acupuncture*, with foreword by Sally Reston. Weatherhill, New York and Tokyo, 1972, repr. 1975.
MANN, F. (1). *Acupuncture; the Ancient Chinese Art of Healing.* Heinemann, London, 1962 (with foreword by Aldous Huxley); revised ed., 1962, repr. 1965, 1970. Second edition, replacing the others, 1971; also Random House, New York, 1972. Revised second edition, London, 1973, repr. 1974.

MANN, F. (2). *The Treatment of Disease by Acupuncture.* Heinemann, London, 1963. 2nd ed., 1967, repr. 1972.

MANN, F. (3). *Anatomical Charts of Acupuncture Points, Meridians and Extra Meridians.* Barnet Publications, Barnet, Herts. 1962. Repr. 1971, 1972.

MANN, F. (4). *The Meridians of Acupuncture.* Heinemann, London, 1964. Repr. 1971, 1972.

MANN, F. (5). *Acupuncture, Cure of Many Diseases.* Heinemann, London, 1971. Revised repr. 1972.

MANN, F. (6). 'Acupuncture Analgesia in Dentistry.' *LT*, 1972 pt. 1 (ii,) 898

MANN, F. (7). 'Acupuncture Anaesthesia.' *LT*, 1973, pt. 2, 563.

MANN, F. (8). 'Acupuncture Analgesia; a Report of 100 Experiments.' *BJA*, 1974, **46**, 361.

MANN, F. (9). 'Acupuncture in Auditory and Related Disorders.' *BJAU*, 1974, **8**, 23.

[MANN, F.] (10). 'Acupuncture and Migraine.' *MIGN*, 1974 , no. 25.

MANN, F. (11). *Scientific Aspects of Acupuncture.* Heinemann (Medical), London, 1977.

MANN, F., BOWSHER, D., MUMFORD, J., LIPTON, S. & MILES, J. (1). 'The Treatment of Intractable Pain by Acupuncture.' *LT*, 1973, pt. 2, 57. Correspondence following (A. Taub), pt. 2, 618; (J. Miles & S. Lipton), pt. 2, 975.

MANN, F., WHITTAKER, R., PERLOW, B., GRAHAM, R., RENTOUL, J., KING, G., MARTIN, R., KOBNER, H., HYMAN, L. & BLAKE, D. (1). 'Analysis of the Treatment of One Thousand Consecutive Patients by Ten Doctors using Acupuncture.' Unpub. MS. (Nov. 1967). The statistical table reported by F. Mann in 'Acupuncture, a Two-Thousand Year Old Approach to Disease', *LD*, 1971, **2**, 100,

MARMER, M. J. (1). 'Hypno-analgesia and Hypno-anaesthesia for Cardiac Surgery.' *AMA*, 1959. **171**, 512.

MARYON, H. (2). 'Fine Metal-Work [in the Mediterranean Civilisations and the Middle Ages].' Art. in *A History of Technology*, ed. C. Singer et al., Oxford, 1956, vol. 2, p. 449.

MASON, A. A. (1). Surgery under Hypnosis [a bilateral mammaplasty] *ANAL*, 1955, **10** (no. 3), 295.

MATSUMOTO TERUO, AMBRUSO, V. & HAYES, M. F. (1). 'Effects of Acupuncture; I, Gastro-intestinal atony following Vagotomy; II, Intestinal Motility, experimental and clinical Studies.' Contribution to the First Bethesda Conference on Acupuncture Research, in Jenerick (1), p. 106.

MAUGHAM, W. S. *On a Chinese Screen.* Heinemann, London, 1922; repr. Cape, London, 1934 (Traveller's Library, no. 31). In Collected Works, Heinemann, London, 1935, repr. 1953.

MAXIMOW, A. A. & BLOOM, W. (1). *Textbook of Histology.* 7th ed. Saunders, Philadelphia and London, 1957.

MAYER, D. J. (1). 'Pain Inhibition by Electrical Brain Stimulation; a Comparison with Morphine. *NSRPB*, 1975, **13**, 94.

MAYER, D. J., PRICE, D. D. & RAFII, A. (1). 'Antagonism of Acupuncture Analgesia in Man by the Narcotic Antagonist Naloxone.' *BRNR*, 1977, **121**, 368. Prelim. pub.: 'Acupuncture Hypalgesia; Evidence for Activation of a Central Control System as a Mechanism of Action.' Proc. 1st World Congress of the Internat. Assoc. for the Study of Pain (Florence, 1975). Raven, New York, 1976, abstr. no. 276.

MAYER, D. J., WOLFLE, T. H., AKIL, H., CARDER, B. & LIEBESKIND, J. C. (1). 'Analgesia from Electrical Stimulation in the Brain-stem of the Rat.' *SC*, 1971, **174**, 1351.

MAYERS, W. F. (1). *Chinese Reader's Manual.* Presbyterian Press, Shanghai, 1874; reprinted, 1924.

MAZZEO, J. A. (1). 'Notes on John Donne's Alchemical Imagery.' *ISIS*, 1957, **48**, 103.

MEAD, MARGARET (2). *Blackberry Winter; my Earlier Years.* Morrow, New York, 1972; repr. Simon & Schuster, New York (Pocket Book ed.), 1975.

MEDAWAR, P. B. (1). 'Size, Shape and Age.' Art. in *Essays on Growth and Form*. . . (d'Arcy Thompson Presentation Volume), ed. W. E. Le Gros Clark & P. B. Medawar, 1945, p. 157.

VAN MEERDERVOORT, J. L. C. POMPE (1). *Doctor on Desima; Selected chapters from 'Vijf Jaren in Japan' (1857–63).'* Tr. E. P. Witternaus & J. Z. Bowers. Sophia University, Tokyo, 1970 (Monumenta Nipponica Monographs, no. 9.).

MELZACK, RONALD (1). *The Puzzle of Pain.* Basic Books, New York, 1973; Penguin, London, 1974. Rev. P. Morrison, *SAM*, 1974, **231** (no. 2), 115.

MELZACK, RONALD (2). 'The Perception of Pain.' *SAM*, 1961, **204** (no. 2), 41.

MELZACK, RONALD (3). 'Pain and Acupuncture.' Unpub. MS. of Lecture. Cf. Melzack & Jeans (1), a similar text.

MELZACK, RONALD (4). 'How Acupuncture can Block Pain.' *IMPAC*, 1973, **23** (no. 1), 65.

MELZACK, RONALD (5). 'Shutting the Gate on Pain.' Art. in *Science Year* (World Book Science Annual). Chicago, 1975, p. 57.

MELZACK, RONALD & JEANS, M. E. (1). 'Acupuncture Analgesia; a Psychophysiological Explanation.' *MINM*, 1974, **57**, 161. Cf. Melzack (3), a similar text.

MELZACK, RONALD & MELINKOFF, D. F. (1). 'Analgesia produced by Brain Stimulation; Evidence of a Prolonged Onset Period.' *EXN*, 1974, **43**, 369.

MELZAK, RONALD & SCOTT, T. H. (1). 'The Effects of Early Experience on the Response to Pain.' *JCPP*, 1957, **50**, 155.

MELZACK, RONALD, STOTLER, W. A. & LIVINGSTON, W. K. (1). 'Effects of Discrete Brainstem Lesions in Cats on Perception of Noxious Stimulation.' *JNP*, 1958, **21**, 353.
MELZACK, RONALD & WALL, PATRICK D. (1). 'Pain Mechanisms; a New Theory.' *SC*, 1965, 150, no. 3699, 971.
MELZACK, RONALD, WEISZ, A. Z. & SPRAGUE, L. T. (1). 'Stratagems for Controlling Pain; Contributions of Auditory Stimulation and Suggestion.' *EXN*, 1963, **8**, 239.
MERCIER, C. A. (1). *Astrology in Medicine.* Macmillan, London, 1914.
MERY, A. (1). 'Le Traitement de l'Asthme par l'Acupuncture.' *BSAC*, 1958, no. 27, 45.
MEYERHOF, M. (1). 'Ibn al-Nafīs und seine Theorie d. Lungenkreislaufs.' *QSGNM*, 1935, **4**, 37.
MEYERHOF, M. (2). 'Ibn al-Nafīs (+13th century) and his Theory of the Lesser Circulation.' *ISIS*, 1935, **23**, 100.
MILES, J. & LIPTON, S. (1). 'Acupuncture in the Treatment of Intractable Pain.' *LT*, 1973, pt. 2, 975.
MIYASHITA SABURŌ (1). 'A Link in the Westward Transmission of Chinese Anatomy in the Later Middle Ages.' *ISIS*, 1968, **58**, 486.
MORAND, S. (1). *Memoir on Acupuncturation, embracing a Series of Cases drawn up under the Inspection of M. Julius Cloquet.* Desiluer, Philadelphia, 1825.
DE MORANT, G. SOULIÉ (2). *L'Acuponcture Chinoise.* 4 vols.
I. 'L'Energie (Points, Méridiens, Circulation).'
II. 'Le Maniement de l'Energie.'
III. 'Les Points et leurs Symptômes.'
IV. 'Les Maladies et leurs Traitements.'
Mercure de France, Paris, 1939. Republished in 1 vol. text and 1 vol. plates, Maloine, Paris, 1957, repr. 1972.
I. L'Energie (Points, Méridiens, Circulation).
II. Le Maniement de l'Energie.
III. La Physiologie de l'Energie.
IV. Les Méridiens, les Points et leurs Symptômes.
V. Les Maladies et leurs Traitements.
DE MORANT, G. SOULIÉ (3). *Précis de la vraie Acuponcture Chinoise; Doctrine, Diagnostique, Thérapeutique.* Mercure de France, Paris, 1934.
DE MORANT, G. SOULIÉ. See Bourdiol (1).
MORLEY, HENRY (2). *The Life of Girolamo Cardano of Milan, Physician.* Chapman & Hall, London 1854.
MORSE, W. R. (4). 'A Memorandum on the Chinese Procedure of Acupuncture.' *JWCBRS*, 1932, **5**, 153–220.
MOSS, L. (1). *Acupuncture and You; a New Approach to Treatment based on the Ancient Method of Healing.* Elek, London, 1964.
MULLIKIN, M. A. & HOTCHKIS, A. M. (1). *The Nine Sacred Mountains of China; an illustrated Record of Pilgrimages made in the Years 1935–6.* Vetch & Lee, Hongkong, 1973.
MUMFORD, J. & BOWSHER, J. (1). 'Electro-acupuncture and Pain Threshold.' *LT*, 1973, pt. 2, 667

NAKAYAMA MASATOSHI & DRAEGER, D. F. (1). *Practical Karate.* 6 vols.
1. *Fundamentals.*
2. *Against the Unarmed Assailant.*
3. *Against Multiple Unarmed Assailants.*
4. *Against Armed Assailants.*
5. *For Women.*
6. *In Special Situations.*
Tuttle, Rutland, Vt. and Tokyo, 1966. Repr. 1972.
NAKAYAMA TADAJIKI (1). *Acuponcture et Médicine Chinoise vérifiées au Japon.* Tr. from the Japanese by T. Sakurazawa & G. Soulié de Morant. Éditions Hippocrate (le François), Paris, 1934.
NAMIKOSHI TOKUJIRO (1). *Japanese Finger-Pressure Therapy; Shiatsu.* Japan Pubs. Inc., Tokyo and San Francisco, 1972.
NASHOLD, B. S. & FRIEDMAN, H. (1). 'Dorsal Column Stimulation for Pain; a Preliminary Report on 30 Patients.' *JNS*, 1972, **36**, 590.
NATHAN, P. W. (1). *The Nervous System.* Penguin (Pelican), London, 1969.
NATHAN, P. W. (2). 'Reference of Sensation at the Spinal Level.' *JNNSP*, 1956, **19**, 88.
NATHAN, P. W. (3). 'The Gate-Control Theory of Pain; a Critical Review.' *BRN*, 1976, **99** (no. 1), 123.
NATHAN, P. W. (4). 'Acupuncture Anaesthesia.' *TRNS*, 1978.
NATHAN, P. W. (5). 'When is an Anecdote?' *LT*, 1967, pt. 2, 607.
NATHAN, P. W. (6). 'Pain.' *BMB*, 1977, **33** (no. 2), 149.

NEEDHAM, JOSEPH (2). *A History of Embryology.* Cambridge Univ. Press, 1934. 2nd ed., revised with the assistance of A. Hughes. Cambridge, 1959; Abelard-Schuman, New York, 1959.

NEEDHAM, JOSEPH (12). *Biochemistry and Morphogenesis.* Cambridge, 1942; repr. 1950, repr. 1966, with historical survey as foreword. Cf. Porkert (1); Needham & Lu (9).

NEEDHAM, JOSEPH (32). *The Development of Iron and Steel Technology in China.* (Dickinson Lecture, 1956.) Newcomen Society, London, 1958, repr. Heffer, Cambridge, 1964. Précis in *TNS*, 1960, **30**, 141. Rev. L. C. Goodrich, *ISIS*, 1960, **51**, 108. French tr. (unrevised, with some illustrations omitted and others added by the editors), *RHSID*, 1961, **2**, 187, 235; 1962, **3**, 1, 62.

NEEDHAM, JOSEPH (56). 'Time and Eastern Man.' *RAI/OP*, 1964. ((Henry Myers Lecture.)

NEEDHAM, JOSEPH (64). *Clerks and Craftsmen in China and the West* (Collected Lectures and Addresses). Cambridge, 1970. Based largely on collaborative work with Wang Ling, Lu Gwei-Djen & Ho Ping-Yü. Cf. Porkert (1); Needham & Lu (9).

NEEDHAM, JOSEPH (72). 'The Evolution of Iron and Steel Technology in East and South-east Asia.' Contribution to the Cyril Stanley Smith Presentation Volume, 1978.

NEEDHAM, JOSEPH (78). 'History and Human Values; a Chinese Perspective for World Science and Technology.' *CR/MSU*, 1976, **20**, 1.

NEEDHAM, JOSEPH & LU GWEI-DJEN (1). 'Hygiene and Preventive Medicine in Ancient China.' *JHMAS*, 1962, **17**, 429; abridged in *HEJ*, 1959, **17**, 170.

NEEDHAM, JOSEPH & LU GWEI-DJEN (8). 'Medicine and Culture in China.' Art. in *Medicine and Culture.* Symposium of the Wellcome Historical Medical Museum and Library and the Wenner-Gren Foundation, London, 1966.

NEEDHAM, JOSEPH & LU GWEI-DJEN (9). 'Manfred Porkert's Interpretations of Terms in Ancient and Mediaeval Chinese Natural and Medical Philosophy.' *ANS*, 1975, **32**, 491.

NEEDHAM, JOSEPH, WANG LING & PRICE, DEREK J. DE S. (1). *Heavenly Clockwork; the Great Astronomical Clocks of Medieval China.* Cambridge, 1960. (Antiquarian Horological Society Monographs, no. 1). Prelim. pub. *AHOR*, 1956, **1**, 153.

NG, LORENZ K. Y., NGUYEN B. THOA, DOUTHITT, T. C. & ALBERT, CHALOM A. (1). 'Experimental "Auricular Electro-acupuncture" in Morphine-Dependent Rats; Behavioural and Biochemical Observations.' *AJCM*, 1975, **3**, 335.

NG, LORENZ K. Y., NGUYEN B. THOA, DOUTHITT, T. C., ALBERT, CHALOM A. & ALBERT, SOLOMON N. (1). 'Attenuation of Morphine Withdrawal Syndrome in Rats following Pre-treatment with Electro-acupuncture.' *Proc. 2nd World Symposium on Acupuncture and Chinese Medicine*, p. 334.

NGUYỄN TRẦN-HUÂN (3). 'Biographie de Pien Tsio [Pien Chhio; in *Shih Chi*, cf. 105].' *BSEIC*, 1957, **32** (no. 1), 59.

NGUYEN VAN NGHI (1). 'Acupuncture Analgesia; the first Fifty Surgical Cases in France.' *AJCM* 1973, 1 (no. 1), 135.

NGUYEN VAN NGHI (2). 'Ictères et Médecine Chinoise.' *NRIAC*, 1971, **6**, no. 20, 115.

NGUYEN VAN NGHI (3), (tr.). *Hoang Ti Nei King So Ouenn* [*Huang Ti Nei Ching, Su Wên*]. Facsimile of the first 14 Chapters, with French tr., pr. pr. 1973 (Socedim, Marseille).

NGUYEN VAN NGHI, MAI VAN DONG & LANZA, ULDERICO (1). *Théorie et Pratique de l'Analgésie par Acupuncture.* Socedin, Marseilles, 1974.

NIBOYET, J. E. H. (2) (with the assistance of M. Borsarello & M. Dumortier). 'Étude sur la Moindre Résistance Cutanée à l'Électricité de certains Points de la Peau dits "Points Chinois".' *BSAC*, 1961, no. 39, 16–88.

NIBOYET, J. E. H. (3). 'Nouvelles Constatations sur les Propriétés Électriques des Points Chinois.' *BSAC*, 1958, no. 30, 7.

NIBOYET, J. E. H. & BOURDIOL, R. J. (1). *Traité d' Acupuncture.* 3 vols. Paris, 1970, repr. 1971.

NIBOYET, J. E. H. & MERY, A. (1). 'Experimentelle Studien über den Meridianverlauf.' *DZA*, 1958, **7** (nos. 11–12), 140.

NICHOLSON, A. N. (1). 'The Adaptation of Man to World-wide Air Travel.' *JRSA*, 1975, **123**, 175.

NOGIER, P. F. M. (1). 'Nouveaux Aperçus concernant les Points Réflexes portés portés par le Pavillon de l'Oreille.' *BSAC*, 1956, no. 20, 51; 1957, no. 25, 25; 1958, no. 29, 7. 'Über die Akupunktur der Ohrmuskel', etc. *DZA*, 1957, **6** (nos. 3–4), 25; (nos. 5–6), 58; (nos. 7–8), 87; 1961, **10** (no. 3), 52; 1963, **12** (no. 1), 14; 1967, **16** (no. 4), 115, 121, 125. The first three of these instalments, all translated by G. Bachmann, were further translated into Chinese in Yeh Hsiao-Lin (*1*).

NOGIER, P. F. M. (2). 'L'Auriculothérapie.' *NRIAC*, 1970, **5**, no. 15, 15.

NOGIER, P. F. M. (3). *Treatise of Auriculotherapy.* Maisonneuve, Paris, 1972. Also in French.

NOORDENBOS, W. (1). *Pain.* Elsevier, Amsterdam, 1959.

NOORDERGRAAF, A. & SILAGE, D. (1). 'Electro-Acupuncture.' *IEEET/BME*, 1973, **20** (no. 5), 364.

NOWAK, G. D. (1). *National Library of Medicine, Literature Search no. 72-1; Acupuncture* (*Jan. 1969 to end Feb. 1972*).' [69 entries.] U.S. Dept. of Health, Education and Welfare, Public Health Service, National Institutes of Health, Bethesda, Md., 1972.

O'MALLEY, C. D. (1). 'A Latin Translation (+1547) of Ibn al-Nafīs, related to the Problem of the Circulation of the Blood.' *JHMAS*, 1957, **12**, 248. Abstract in *Actes du VIIIe Congrès International d'Histoire des Sciences*, p. 716. Florence, 1956.

O'MALLEY, C. D., POYNTER, F. N. L. & RUSSELL, K. F. (1) (tr.). 'Lectures on the Whole of Anatomy', by William Harvey; an annotated translation of the *Praelectiones Anatomiae Universalis* [Lumleian Lectures at the Royal College of Physicians, +1616 onwards, with later interpolations by the lecturer].' Univ. Calif. Press, Berkeley and Los Angeles, 1961. Rev. W. Pagel, *HOSC*, 1963, **2**, 114.

OHASHI WATARU (1). *Do it Yourself Shiatsu; how to perform the Ancient Japanese Art of 'Acupuncture without Needles'*. Allen & Unwin (Mandala), London., 1977.

OHSAWA, GEORGES (ps.). See Sakurazawa, Nyoichi.

OLDS, J. (1). 'Self -stimulation of the Brain; its Use to Study Local Effects of Hunger, Sex and Drugs [pleasure and aversion centres in the mammalian brain]'. *SC*, 1958, **127**, 315.

OLDS, J. (2). 'Emotional Centres in the Brain.' Art. in *The Biological Bases of Behaviour*, ed. Chalmers, Crawley & Rose (*q.v.*), p. 171.

OLIVERAS, J. L., REDJEMI, F., GUILBAUD, G. & BESSON, M. (1). 'Analgesia induced by Electrical Stimulation of the Inferior Centralis Nucleus of the Raphe in the Cat.' *PAIN*, 1975, **1**, 139.

OLSCHKI, L. (11). 'Medical Matters in Marco Polo's "Description of the World".' *BIHM*, 1944, Suppl. no. 3, 237.

OMURA YOSHIAKI (1). 'The Patho-physiology of Acupuncture Treatment; Effects of Acupuncture on the Cardio-vascular and Nervous Systems.' *AETR*, 1975, **1**, 51–140.

OSLER, SIR WILLIAM (1). *The Principles and Practice of Medicine.* 8th ed., London, 1912.

OSTRANDER, S. & SCHROEDER, L. (1). *Psychic Discoveries behind the Iron Curtain.* Bantam, Toronto and New York, 1968; Abacus (Sphere), London, 1973.

OTSUKA, M. & KONISHI, S. (1). 'Substance-P an Excitatory Transmitter of Primary Sensory Neurons.' *CSHSQB*, 1976, **40**, 135.

OTSUKA, M. & KONISHI, S. (2). 'Release of Substance-P-like Immunoreactivity from Isolated Spinal Cord of the Newborn Rat.' *N*, 1976, **264**, 83.

OWEN-FLOOD, A. (1). 'Appendectomy under Hypno-anaesthesia.' *BJA*, 1955, **27**, 398.

PAGEL, W. (1). 'Religious Motives in the Medical Biology of the Seventeenth Century.' *BIHM*, 1935, **3**, 97.

PAGEL, W. (4). 'William Harvey; Some Neglected Aspects of Medical History.' *JWCI*, 1944, **7**, 144.

PAGEL, W. (6). 'A Background Study to Harvey.' *MBH*, 1948, **2**, 407.

PAGEL, W. (9). 'Giordano Bruno; the Philosophy of Circles and the Circular Movement of the Blood.' *JHMAS*, 1951, **6**, 116. 'The Circular Motion of the Blood and Giordano Bruno's Philosophy of the Circle.' *BIHM*, 1950, **24**, 398. 'Giordano Bruno and the Circular Motion of the Blood.' *BMJ*, 1950, pt. 2, 621.

PAGEL, W. (10). *Paracelsus; an Introduction to Philosophical Medicine in the Era of the Renaissance.* Karger, Basel and New York, 1958. Rev. D. G[eoghegan], *AX*, 1959, **7**, 169.

PAGEL, W. (19). 'William Harvey and the Purpose of the Circulation.' *ISIS*, 1951, **42**, 22.

PAGEL, W. (20). 'Harvey's Role in the History of Medicine.' *BIHM*, 1950, **24**, 70.

PAGEL, W. (21). 'Keynes on William Harvey' (review of Sir Geoffrey Keynes' *Life of William Harvey*, Oxford, 1966). *MH*, 1967, **11**, 201.

PAGEL, W. (22). 'A Harveian Prelude to Harvey' (review of O'Malley, Poynter & Russell, 1). *HOSC*, 1963, **2**, 114.

PAGEL, W. (23). 'Vesalius and the Pulmonary Transit of Venous Blood.' *JHMAS*, 1964, **19**, 327.

PAGEL, W. (24). 'William Harvey Revisited.' *HOSC*, 1969, **8**, 1; 1970, **9**, 1.

PAGEL, W. (25). 'The Philosophy of Circles – Cesalpino–Harvey; a Penultimate Assessment.' *JHMAS*, 1957, **12**, 140.

PAGEL, W. (26). *William Harvey's Biological Ideas; Selected Aspects and Historical Background.* Karger, Basel and New York, 1967.

PÁLOS, S. (1). *Chinesische Heilkunst; Rückbesinnung auf eine grosse Tradition*, tr. from the Hungarian by W. Kronfuss. Delp, München, 1963.

PAPPENHEIMER, J. R., KOSKI, G., FENCL, F., KARNOVSKY, M. L. & KRUEGER, J. (1). 'The Extraction of Sleep-promoting Factor S from Cerebrospinal Fluid and from Brains of Sleep-deprived Animals.' *JNP*, 1975, **38**, 1299.

PARMENTER, C. L. (1). 'Haploid, Diploid, Triploid and Tetraploid Chromosome Numbers, and their Origin in Parthenogenetically Developed Larvae and Frogs of *Rana pipiens* and *Rana palustris*.' *JEZ*, 1933, **66**, 409.

PARSONS, C. M. & GOETZL, F. R. (1). 'The Effect of Induced Pain on Pain Threshold.' *PSEBM*, 1945, **60**, 327.

PATTERSON, MARGARET A. (1). *Addictions can be Cured; the Treatment of Drug Addiction by Neuro-electric Stimulaion [especially Acupuncture]—an Interim Report.* Lion, Berkhamsted, 1975.

PATTERSON, MARGARET A. (2). 'Electro-Acupuncture in Alcohol and Drug Addictions.' *CLIME*, 1974. **81**, 9.

PAVLOV, I. P. (1). *Conditioned Reflexes.* Oxford, 1927.

PAVLOV, I. P. (2). *Lectures on Conditioned Reflexes.* International Pub., London, 1928.

PEACHER, W. G. (1). 'Adverse Reactions, Contra-indications and Complications of Acupuncture and Moxibustion.' *AJCM*, 1975, **3** (no. 1), 35.

PEARSON, MARGARET J. (1). 'Symptoms of Decay in the Later Han Dynasty (+23 to +220) described by Wang Fu, a Chinese Recluse of the +2nd Century.' In the press.

PELLER, S. (1). 'The Role of Harvey and of Cesalpino in the History of Medicine.' *BIHM*, 1949, **23**, 213.

PELLETAN, PIERRE (1). 'Über die Wirkung des Acupunctur.' *NGNHK*, 1824, **9**, 295.

PELLETAN, PIERRE (2). *Notice sur l'Acupuncture.* Gabon, Paris, 1825.

PELLIOT, P. (3). 'Notes sur Quelques Artistes des Six Dynasties et des Thang.' *TP*, 1923, **22**, 214. (On the Bodhidharma legend and the founding of Shao-Lin Ssu on Sung Shan, pp. 248 ff., 252 ff.)

PELLIOT, P. (50). 'Michel Boym' (a critique of Chabrié (1), *q.v.*). *TP*, 1934, **31**, 95.

PENFIELD, W. & RASMUSSEN, T. (1). *The Cerebral Cortex of Man; a Clinical Study of Localisation of Function.* Macmillan, New York, 1957.

PENGELLEY, E. (1) (ed.). *Circannual Clocks; Annual Biological Rhythms.* Academic Press, New York and London, 1975.

PENN KUAN-CHIN. See Benkov, Amos.

PERRIN, M. W. See Poynter, F. N. L. (3).

PERT, AGU & YAKSH, T. L. (1). 'The Neuro-anatomical and Neuro-chemical Substrates underlying Morphine-induced Analgesia in the Rhesus Monkey.' Communication to the 34th Meeting of the Committee on Problems of Drug Addiction (National Research Council), Mexico City, 1974.

PERT, AGU & YAKSH, T. L. (2). 'Sites of Morphine-induced Analgesia in the Primate Brain; their Relation to Pain Pathways.' *BRNR*, 1974, **80**, 135.

PERT, C. B. & SNYDER, S. H. (1). 'The Opiate Receptor in the Brain.' *SC*, 1973, **179**, 1011.

PETREN, K. & THORLING, I. (1). 'Untersuchungen ü. d. Vorkommen von Vagotonus und Sympathikotonus.' *ZKM*, 1911, **73**, 27.

PETRICEK, E. (1). 'Möglichkeiten der Akupunktur in der Zahnheilkunde.' *OARZ*, 1973, **28** (no. 18), 1033.

PFISTER, L. (1). *Notices Biographiques et Bibliographiques sur les Jésuites de l'Ancienne Mission de Chine (+1552 to +1773).* 2 vols. Mission Press, Shanghai, 1932 (*VS.* 59).

PHÊNG KUAN-CHIN. See Benkov, Amos & Pei Lung-Tang (1).

PICAZA, J. A., CANNON, B. W., HUNTER, S. E., BOYD, A. S., GAMA, J. & MAURER, D. (1). 'Pain Suppression by Peripheral Nerve Trunk Stimulation; I, Observations with Transcutaneous Stimuli.' Unpub. MS.

PINTO, FERNAÕ MENDES (1). *The Voyages and Adventures of Fernand Mendez Pinto, a Portugal: During his Travels for the Space of one and twenty years in the Kingdoms of Ethiopia, China, Tartaria, Cauchin-china, Calaminham, Siam, Pegu, Japan, and a great part of the East-Indiaes. With a Relation and Description of most of the Places thereof; their Religion, Laws, Riches customs and Government in time of Peace and War. Where he five times suffered Shipwrack, was sixteen times sold, and thirteen times made a Slave. Written Originally by himself in the Portugal Tongue, and Dedicated to the Majesty of Philip King of Spain. Done into English by H. C[ogan], Gent.* Macock, Cripps & Lloyd, London, 1653; facsimile edition, Dawson, London, 1969.

PIOLLET, P. (1). *Du Moxa, et de son Application au Traitement de la Carie qui Attaque les Os du Tronc...* (Inaug. Diss.) Didot, Paris, 1817.

PLEDGE, H. T. (1). *Science since 1500; a Short History of Mathematics, Physics, Chemistry and Biology.* HMSO, London, 1939; 2nd ed. 1966, with new prefatory note and added subject index. Cf. Porkert (1); Needham & Lu (9).

PLUMMER, J. P. (1). 'Acupuncture in China in the Seventies.' Unpub. review, Hongkong, 1977.

POMERANZ, B. (1). 'Brain's Opiates at work in Acupuncture?' *NS*, 1977, **73** (no. 1033), 12.

POMERANZ, B. & CHIU, D. (1). 'Naloxone Blockade of Acupuncture Analgesia; Endorphin Implicated.' *LS*, 1976, **19**, 1757.

PORKERT, MANFRED (1). *The Theoretical Foundations of Chinese Medicine; Systems of Correspondence.* M.I.T. Press, Cambridge, Mass. 1974 (M.I.T. East Asian Science Series, no. 3). English tr. of *Die theoretischen Grundlagen der chinesischen Medizin; Das Entsprechungssystem.* Steiner, Wiesbaden, 1973 (Münchener Ostasiatische Studien, no. 5). Cf. Needham & Lu (9).

PORKERT, MANFRED (2). 'Untersuchungen einiger philosophisch-wissenschaftlicher Grundbegriffe und Beziehungen im Chinesischen.' *ZDMG*, 1961, **110**, 422. Cf. Porkert (1); Needham & Lu (9).

PORKERT, MANFRED (3). 'Wissenschaftliches Denken im alten China – das System der energetischen Beziehungen.' *ANT*, 1961, **2**, 532. Cf. Porkert (1); Needham & Lu (9).

PORKERT, MANFRED (4). 'Farbemblematik in China.' *ANT*, 1962, **4**, 154.

PORKERT, MANFRED (5). 'Die energetische Terminologie in den chinesischen Medizinklassikern.' *S*, 1965, **8**, 184. Cf. Porkert (1); Needham & Lu (9).

POUILLET, M. (1). 'Bemerkungen ü. die electro-magnetischen Phänomene die bei der Acupunctur sich offenbaren.' *NGNHK*, 1825, **11**, 209.

POYNTER, F. N. L. (3) (ed.). *The History and Philosophy of Knowledge of the Brain and its Functions.* Foreword by M. W. Perrin. Israel, Amsterdam, 1973. Repr. from the first ed. of the Proceedings of an Anglo-American Symposium preluding the First International Congress of Neurological Sciences, 1957; Blackwell, Oxford, 1958.

PREMUDA, L. (1). 'L'Agopuntura tra la Cina e il Veneto.' Contribution to the Cini Symposium 'Sviluppi Scientifici, Prospettive Religiose e Movimenti Rivoluzionari in Cina.' Venice, 1973 ed. L. Lanciotti. Olschki, Florence, 1975. *Atti d. Convegno Internazionale Marco Polo*, p. 73 (Civiltà Veneziana, Studi, no. 31.)

PRESCOTT, F. (1). *The Control of Pain.* English Universities Press, London, 1964. (New Science Series, no. 2.)

PRINZING, G. (1). 'Über die unterschiedliche Wirkung der Gold- und Silber-nadels in der Akupunktur.' *DZA*, 1960, **9** (no. 2), 29. Chinese tr. in Anon. (*108*), pp. 28 ff.

PRODESCU, V., STOICESCU, C. & BRATU, I. (1). 'Die Wirkung auf die Gallenabsonderung und der komparative Effekt von Silber- und Gold-nadeln auf die Cholerese.' *DZA*, 1959, **8** (nos. 3–4), 25. Chinese tr. in Anon. (*108*), pp. 42 ff.

PRUNIER, M. (1). 'Les Convulsions dans la première Enfance.' *RIAC*, 1953, **5**, no. 25, 4.

PRUNIER, M. (2). 'Les Ulcères Variqueux traités par l'Acupuncture.' *RIAC*, 1955, **7**, no. 31, 225.

PURCELL, V. (4). *The Boxer Uprising; a Background Study.* Cambridge, 1963.

PURMANN, M. G. (1). *Chirugia Curiosa.* London, 1706.

PUTENSEN, O. (1). 'Heilung eines völligen Geruchsverlust durch eine einzige Akupunkturbehandlung.' *DZA*, 1955, **4** (nos. 11–12), 127.

QUAGLIA-SENTA, A. (1). 'Les Points "Hérauts" [*mu hsüeh*]; ou, le Parasympathique en Acupuncture.' *NRIAC*, 1971, **6**, no. 20, 87.

RALL, JUTTA, (3). 'Tradition aus Zweieinhalb Jahrtausenden; die traditionelle chinesische Medizin und ihre Bedeutung heute.' *DAAM*, 1965, **62**, 1956.

RALL, JUTTA (4). 'Wissenschaftliche Grundlagen der Akupunktur entdeckt.' *DAAM*, 1964, **61**, 2688.

RALL, JUTTA (5). 'Das Bonghan-System.' *ASKL*, 1965, **6** (no. 11), 1.

RATNAVALE, D. N. (1). 'Psychiatry in Shanghai.' *CNOW*, 1975, no. 52, 7; more fully in *AJPSY*, 1973, **130** (no. 10), 1082.

RATNER, S. C. (1). 'Comparative Aspects of Hypnosis', in J. E. Gordon (1), *Handbook of Clinical and Experimental Hypnosis*, pp. 530–87.

VON REICHERT, K. R. (1). 'Geschichte der Moxa.' *DAGM*, 1879, **2**, 45.

REICHMANIS, M., MARINO, A. A. & BECKER, R. O. (1). 'D.C. Skin Conductance Variation at Acupuncture Loci.' *AJCM*, 1976, **4**, 69.

REICHMANIS, M., MARINO, A. A. & BECKER, R. O. (2). 'Electrical Correlates of Acupuncture Points.' *IEEET/BME*, 1975, **22**, 533.

REINBERG, A. (1). 'Hours of Changing Responsiveness in relation to Allergy and the Circadian Adrenal Cycle.' Art. in *Circadian Clocks*, ed. J. Aschoff (1), 1965, p. 214.

RÉMUSAT, J. P. A. (11). *Mélanges Asiatiques; ou, Choix de Morceaux de Critique et de Mémoires relatifs aux Religions, aux Sciences, aux Coutumes, à l'Histoire et à la Géographie des Nations Orientales.* 2 vols. Dondey-Dupré, Paris, 1825–6.

RÉMUSAT, J. P. A. (12). *Nouveaux Mélanges Asiatiques; ou, Recueil de Morceaux de Critique et de Mémoires relatifs aux Religions, aux Sciences, aux Coutumes, à l'Histoire et à la Géographie des Nations Orientales.* 2 vols. Schubart & Heideloff and Dondey-Dupré, Paris, 1829.

RÉMUSAT, J. P. A. (13). *Mélanges Posthumes d'Histoire et de Littérature Orientales.* Imp. Roy., Paris 1843.

RÉMUSAT, J. P. A. (14). 'Sur l'Acupuncture' [1825]. Art. in Rémusat (12), pp. 358–80.

RÉMUSAT, J. P. A. (15). 'Sur une Collection d'Ouvrages relatif au Japon formée par Titsingh.' Art. in Rémusat (12), pp. 266 ff.

REYNOLDS, D. V. (1). 'Surgery in the Rat during Electrical Analgesia induced by Focal Brain Stimulation,' *SC*, 1969, **164**, 444.

TEN RHIJNE, WILLEM (1). *Dissertatio de Arthritide; Mantissa Schematica; de Acupunctura; et Orationes Tres, I. De Chymiae et Botaniae Antiquitate et Dignitate, II. De Physionomia, III. de Monstris.* Chiswell, London; Leers, The Hague, and Leipzig, 1683. German tr., E. W. Stiefvater (2). English tr., Carubba, R. W. & Bowers, J. Z. (1). Rev. Anon., *PTRS*, 1683, **13**, no. 148, 222.

RICE, F. M. & ROWLAND, B. (1). *Art in Afghanistan; Objects from the Kabul Museum.* Lane, London, 1971.

RICHINS, C. A. & BRIZZEE, K. (1). 'The Effect of Localised Cutaneous Stimulation on Circulation in Duodenal Arterioles and Capillary Beds.' *JNP*, 1949, **12**, 131.

RICHTER, C. P. (1). 'Biological Clocks in Medicine and Psychiatry; the Shock-Phase Hypothesis.' *PNASW*, 1960, **46**, 1506. Cf. Porkert (1); Needham & Lu (9).

RICHTER, J. A., BAUM, M., KUNKEL, R., BAUERLE, A., HEIMISCH, W., AMERELLER, H., SCHUMACHER, F., ERDMANN, K. & VON BOHUSZEWICZ, U. (1). 'Clinical Experience with Electrical Acupuncture Analgesia in 125 Patients undergoing Open-Heart Surgery.' *AETR*, 1975, **1**, 143.

RIEDERER, P., TENK, H., WERNER, H., BISCHKO, J., RETT, A. & KRISPER, H. (1). 'Manipulation of Neuro-transmitter [Substances] by Acupuncture; a preliminary communication.' *JNT*, 1975, **37**, 81.

RINTZLER, W. (2). 'Les Points de Moss et l'Acupuncture; Essai d'Interprétation du Mécanisme de son Action.' *RIAC*, 1956, **9**, no. 37, 121.

DE ROBERTIS, E. D. P., NOWINSKI, W. W. & SAEZ, F. A. (1). *General Cytology.* Saunders, Philadelphia and London, 1948. Cf. Porkert (1); Needham & Lu (9).

ROBERTS, S. K. (1). 'The Significance of the Endocrine Glands and the Central Nervous System in Circadian Rhythms (in Man).' Art. in *Circadian Clocks*, ed. J. Aschoff (1), 1965, p. 198.

ROLLER, D. E. (1). *The Early Development of the Concepts of Temperature and Heat; Rise and Decline of the Caloric Theory.* Harvard Univ. Press, Cambridge, Mass., 1960 (Harvard Case Histories in Exper. Sci., no. 3). Cf. Porkert (1); Needham & Lu (9).

ROLLINS, C. P. (1). 'Illustration in Printed Medical Books.' *CIBA/S*, 1949, **10** (no. 6), 1072.

ROSE, STEVEN P. R. (1). *The Conscious Brain.* Weidenfeld & Nicolson, London, 1973.

ROSEN, G. (1). 'From Mesmerism to Hypnotism.' *CIBA/S*, 1948, **9** (no. 11), 838.

DE ROSNY, L. (1) (tr.). *'Chan-Hai-King [Shan Hai Ching]'; Antique Géographie Chinoise.* Maisonneuve, Paris, 1891.

ROSSI, G. F. & ZANCHETTI, A. (1). 'The Brain Stem Reticular Formation; Anatomy and Physiology.' *AIB*, 1957, **95**, 199.

ROSTAND, JEAN (1). *La Parthénogénèse des Vertébrés.* Hermann, Paris, 1938.

ROUGEMONT, C. J. (1). *Versuche über die Zugmittel in der Heilkunde.* Tr. from the French by H. Wegeler, Frankfurt, 1798.

ROUSSEAU, M. (1). 'L'Origine des Points de Weihe et de l'Homéosiniatrie.' *RIAC*, 1953, **5**, no. 24, 4.

RUBIN, M. (1). *Manuel d'Acuponcture Fondamentale; Pratique Moderne en République Populaire de Chine* (on title-page, different sub-title: 'd'après les Publications de l'Institut National de Médecine Traditionelle de Pékin'). Mercure de France, Paris, 1974.

RUCH, T. C. & FULTON, J. F. (1). *Medical Physiology and Biophysics* (18th ed. of Howell's *Textbook of Physiology*). Saunders, Philadelphia and London, 1961.

RUDOLPH, R. C. & WÊN YU (1). *Han Tomb Art of West China; a Collection of First and Second Century Reliefs.* Univ. of Calif. Press, Berkeley and Los Angeles, 1951 (rev. W. P. Yetts, *JRAS*, 1953, 72).

RYAN, T. J. & BOWERS, E. F. (1). *Teeth and Health.* Putnam, New York, 1921.

SAID, HAKIM MUHAMMAD (1). *Medicine in China.* Hamdard Academy, Karachi, Pakistan, 1965.

SAINSON, C. (1) (tr.). *Histoire particulière du Nan Tchao;* Nan Tchao Ye Che [*Nan Chao Yeh Shih*]; *Traduction d'une Histoire de l'Ancien Yun-nan; accompagnée d'une Carte et d'un Lexique Géographique et Historique.* Imp. Nat. Leroux, Paris, 1904. (Pub. Ec. Lang. Or. Viv. (5e sér.), no. 4.)

ST GIRONS, M. C. (1). 'On the Persistence of Circadian Rhythms in Hibernating Mammals.' Art. in *Circadian Clocks*, ed. J. Aschoff (1), 1965, p. 321.

SAKURAZAWA, NYOICHI (1). *L'Acuponcture et la Médecine d'Extrême Orient.* Vrin, Paris, 1969.

SARLANDIÈRE, LE CHEVALIER J. B. (1). *Mèmoires sur l'Electro-Puncture, considérée comme moyen nouveau de traiter efficacement la Goutte, les Rhumatismes, et les Affections Nerveuses, et sur l'emploi du Moxa Japonais en France. Suivis d'un Traité de l'Acupuncture et du Moxa, principaux moyens curatifs chez les Peuples de la Chine, de la Corée et du Japon, orné de Figures Japonaises...* Priv. pub., Paris, 1825. Cf. Vergier (1).

SATO, M. & TAKAGI, H. (1). 'Enhancement by Morphine of the Central Descending Inhibitory Influence on Spinal Sensory Transmission.' *EJPH*, 1971, **14**, 60.

SATO TORU & NAKATANI YOSHIO (1). 'Acupuncture for Chronic Pain in Japan.' Art. in *Proc. International Pain Symposium, Seattle*, 1973, ed. Bonica (3), p. 813.

SAUERBRUCH, F. & WENKE, H. (1). *Pain, its Meaning and Significance*, tr. from the German by E. Fitzgerald. Allen & Unwin, London, 1963. First German ed., 1936.

SAXÉN, L. & TOIVONEN, S. (1). *Primary Embryonic Induction.* Academic Press (Logos) & Elek, London, 1962. Cf. Porkert (1); Needham & Lu (9).

SCHACHT, J. (1). 'Ibn al-Nafīs, Servetus and Colombo.' *AAND*, 1957, **22**, 317.

SCHATZ, J., LARRE, C. & DE LA VALLÉE, E. ROCHAT (1). *Structures de L'Acupuncture Traditionelle*. Vol. 1. *Notions d'Energétique Fondamentale*. Sénart-Typo, for Ecole Européenne d'Acupuncture, Paris, 1978.

SCHEIDER, C. A. L. (1). *De Acupunctura*. Berlin, 1825.

SCHEVING, L. E. (1). 'The Dimension of Time in Biology and Medicine – Chronobiology.' *END*, 1976, **35**, 66.

SCHMIDT, P. (1). 'Die grosse Nadelung; la Grande Piqûre' (immediate relief of pain by acupuncture). *DZA*, 1958, **7** (nos. 9–10), 108. Chinese tr. in Anon. (*108*), pp. 25 ff.

SCHMITT, C. B. & WEBSTER, C. (1). 'Harvey and M. A. Severino [1580 to 1656], a Neglected Medical Relationship.' *BIHM*, 1971, **45**, 49.

SCHOELER, H. (1). *Die Weihe'schen Druckpunkte, ihre Beziehung zur Akupunktur, Neuraltherapie und Homöopathie*. Haug, Ulm (Donau), 1954. French abstract in *RIAC*, 1954, **6**, no. 30, 182; 1955, **7**, no. 31, 229. With comments by R. de la Fuye, pp. 231 ff.; continued 1955, **7**, no. 32, 304, **7**, no. 33, 390, **7**, no. 34, 438.

SCHULDT, H. (1). 'Condensations of Field Force in Biological Systems; an Interpretation of the Acupuncture Lines.' *AJAP*, 1976, **4** (no. 4), 344.

SEIDEL, A. (1). 'A Taoist Immortal of the Ming Dynasty; Chang San-Fêng.' Art. in *Self and Society in Ming Thought*, ed. W. T. de Bary. Columbia Univ. Press, New York, 1970, p. 483.

SELYE, H. (1). *The Physiology and Pathology of Exposure to Systemic Stress*, Acta Inc. Med. Pub., Montreal, 1950.

SELYE, H. (2). 'The Adaptation Syndrome in Clinical Medicine.' *PRACT*, 1954, **172**, 5.

SELYE, H. (3). 'The General Adaptation Syndrome and Gastro-enterology.' *RGE*, 1953, **20** (no. 3), 185.

SELYE, H. (4). *Stress without Distress*. Lippincott, Philadelphia and New York, 1974.

SHEALY, C. N., MORTIMER, J. T. & HAGFORS, N. R. (1). 'Dorsal Column Electro-analgesia.' *JNS*, 1970, **32** (no. 5), 560.

SHEN Ê, TSHAI THI-TAO & LAN CHHING (1). 'Supraspinal Participation in the Inhibitory Effect of Acupuncture on Viscero-Somatic Reflex Discharges.' *CMJ*, 1975 (N.S.), **1**, 431.

SHÊNG LÜ-CHHIEN & CHANG TAO-HSIEH (1). 'Electro-acupuncture Anaesthesia in Oral Surgery; a Preliminary Report [248 Cases].' *CMJ*, 1960, **80** (no. 2), 97. Earlier publication in *JMPC*, 1959, no. 8, 729.

SHIBUTANI KIN-ICHI (1). 'Evaluation of the Therapeutic Effect of Acupuncture; Attitudes of Patients with Chronic Pain, Psychological and Hypnotic Profiles, and Circulatory Changes during Treatment.' Contribution to the First Bethesda Conference on Acupuncture, in Jenerick (1), p. 28.

SHIFMAN, A. C. (1). 'The Clinical Response of 328 Private Patients to Acupuncture Therapy.' *AJCM*, 1975, **3**, 165.

SHIH LIU & SSU CHI (1). 'Achievement of Mao Tsê-Tung's Thought Propaganda Team of Medical Workers From the P.L.A. 3016 Unit's Health Section' (on the treatment of deaf-mutism with acupuncture). *CMJ*, 1968, no. 11, 641.

SHIRAI, MITSUTARŌ (1). 'A Brief History of Botany in Old Japan.' Art. in *Scientific Japan, Past and Present*, ed. Shinjo Shinzo. Kyoto, 1926. (Commemoration Volume of the 3rd Pan-Pacific Science Congress.)

SHUAIB, M. (1). 'Acupuncture Treatment of Drug Dependence in Pakistan' (opium addicts). *AJCM*, 1976, **4** (no. 4), 403.

SICARD, J. A. (1). *Traité de Pathologie Médicale et Thérapeutique Appliquée*, ed. E. Sargent, L. Ribadeau-Dumas & L. Babonneix, 33 vols. Paris, 1920–25.

VON SIEBOLD, P. F. (1). 'Beiträge zur Kenntnis d. japanischen Akupunktur.' *MBG*, 1832. Repr. in von Siebold (2), p. 78.

VON SIEBOLD, P. F. (2). *Nippon*, 2nd ed. 1897.

SIGNER, E. & GALSTON, A. W. (1). 'Education and Science in China.' *SC*, 1972, **175**, 15. Abstr. in *NSW*, 1971 (7 June), 48.

SILVERSTEIN, M. E., CHANG I-LO & MACON, N. (1) (tr.). *Acupuncture and Moxibustion; a Handbook for the Barefoot Doctors of China*. A translation of *Chen Chiu* (Jen-min Wei-Shêng, Peking, 1965, repr. 1970), a manual for paramedical personnel prepared by the Health Department of Hopei province (Anon. *200*). Schocken, New York, 1975, repr. 1976.

SINCLAIR, D. C., WEDDELL, G. & FEINDEL, W. (1). 'Referred Pain and Associated Phenomena.' *BRN*, 1948, **71**, 184.

SINGER, C. (3). 'The Scientific Views and Visions of St Hildegard.' Art. in *Studies in the History and Method of Science*, ed. C. Singer, Vol. 1, p. 1. Oxford, 1917. Repr. Arno, New York, 1975

SINGER, C. (4). *From Magic to Science; Essays on the Scientific Twilight*. Benn, London, 1928.

SINGER, C. (16). 'The Visions of Hildegard of Bingen.' Art. in Singer (4), p. 199.

SINGER, D. W. (1). *Giordano Bruno; His Life and Thought, with an annotated Translation of his Work 'On the Infinite Universe and Worlds'*. Schuman, New York, 1950.

SIVIN, N. (11). 'Copernicus in China' in *Studia Copernicana*, VI, Polish Acad. Sci., Division of Hist. of Sci. & Tech. Warsaw, 1973. (= *Colloquia Copernicana*, II, 'Études sur l'Audience de la Théorie Héliocentrique', Conférence du Symposium IUHPS, Toruń, 1973.)

SJÖLUND, B. & ERIKSSON, M. (1). 'Electro-acupuncture and Endogenous Morphines.' *LT*, 1976, pt. 2 (13 Nov.), 1085.

SJÖLUND, B., TERENIUS, L. & ERIKSSON, M. (1). 'Increased Cerebrospinal Fluid Levels of Endorphins after Electro-Acupuncture.' *APSD*, 1977. **100**, 382.

SMITH, G. M., CHIANG, H. T., KITZ, R. J. & ANTOON, A. (1). 'Acupuncture and Experimentally Induced Ischaemic Pain.' Art. in *Proc. International Pain Symposium, Seattle*, 1973, ed. Bonica (3), p. 827.

SMITH, I. D. & SHEARMAN, R. P. (1). 'Circadian Aspects of Prostaglandin F_{2a}–induced Termination of Pregnancy' (Intra-amniotic effectiveness for abortion greatest at 6 p.m. in a diurnal rhythm.) *JOGBC*, 1974, **81**, 841. Cf. editorial in *BMJ*, 1975, pt. 2 (5 Apr.), 3.

SMITH, L. A., CHRISTENSEN, N. A., HANSON, N. O., RALSTON, D. E., ACHOR, R. W. P., BERGE, K. G., MORROW, G. W. & BULBULIAN, A. H. (1). *An Atlas of Pain Patterns; Sites and Behaviour of Pain in Certain Common Diseases of the Upper Abdomen*. Thomas, Springfield, Ill., 1961.

SMITH, R. W. (1). *Secrets of Shao-Lin Temple Boxing*. Tuttle, Rutland, Vt. and Tokyo, 1964; repr. 1973.

SMITH, V. A. (3). *The Jain Stupa; Antiquities of Mathura*. Archaeological Survey of India, Allahabad, 1901, (New Imperial Series, no. 20.)

SMITHERS. SIR DAVID, ALEXANDER, P., HAMILTON-FAIRLEY, G., ADEY, E., WILLIAMS, P. O., GOODWIN, J. F., CLELAND, W. P., MCDONALD, E. LAWSON & WALL, PATRICK D. (1). Report of the British Medical Delegation to China, Apr.–May 1974. Unpub. documents, Medical Research Council, London.

SNYDER, S. H. & SIMANTOV, R. (1). 'The Opiate Receptor and Opioid Peptides.' *JNC*, 1977, **28**, 13.

SONG TE-SUCK. See Sung Tê-Su.

SOUBEIRAN, J. L. & DE THIERSANT, P. DABRY (1). *La Matière Médicale chez les Chinois*. Paris, 1874.

SPOEREL, W. E. (1). 'Acupuncture Analgesia in China.' *AJCM*, 1975, **3**, 359.

SPOEREL, W. E., VARKEY, M. & LIANG, C. Y. (1). 'Acupuncture in Chronic Pain.' *AJCM*, 1976, **4** (no. 3), 267.

STACHER, G., WANCURA, I., BAUER, P., LAHODA, R. & SCHULZE, D. (1). 'The Effect of Acupuncture on Pain Threshold and Pain Tolerance determined by Electrical Stimulation of the Skin; a Controlled Study.' *AJCM*, 1975, **3**, 143.

STARLING, E. H. (1). *Principles of Human Physiology*. 6th ed., rev. by C. Lovatt Evans & H. Hartridge. Churchill, London, 1933.

STERMAN, LÉON (1). 'Une Médecine specifiquement Orientale-Vietnamienne, le "Bat-Gio".' *RIAC*, 1953, **5**, no. 25, 29.

STERNBACH, R. A. (1). *Pain; a Psycho-physiological Analysis*. Academic Press, New York and London, 1968.

STEWART, D., THOMSON, J. & OSWALD, I. (1). 'Acupuncture Analgesia; an Experimental Investigation.' *BMJ*, 1977, pt. 1 (no. 6053), 67.

STIEFVATER, E. W. (1). *Akupunktur als Neural-therapie*. 2nd ed. Haug, Ulm-Donau, 1956. Rev. G. Bachmann, *DZA*, 1957, **6** (nos. 3–4), 47.

STIEFVATER, E. W. (2). *Die Akupunktur des ten Rhyne*. Haug, Ulm, 1955. German tr. of Willem ten Rhijne's *De Arthritide*... omitting all the copious footnotes. Rev. [H.] Schmidt, *DZA*, 1956, **5** (nos. 1–2), 20.

ŠTOVIČKOVÃ, A. (1). 'What is Acupuncture?' *EHOR*, 1961, **1** (no. 8), 11.

SUN JEN I-TU & SUN HSÜEH-CHUAN (1) (tr.). *'Thien Kung Khai Wu', Chinese Technology in the Seventeenth Century, by Sung Ying-Hsing*. Pennsylvania State Univ. Press; University Park & London, Penn. 1966.

SUNG TÊ-SU (1). 'Über die verschiedene Wirkung der Gold- und der Silber-nadel.' *DZA*, 1959, **8** (nos. 7–8), 84. Chinese tr. in Anon. (*108*), pp. 39 ff.

VAN SWIETEN, G. (1). *Erläuterungen zu den Boerhaaveschen Lehrsätzen*. Vienna, 1755.

SWIFT, JONATHAN (1) (ed.). *Letters written by Sir William Temple and other Ministers of State, both at Home and Abroad, containing an Account of the Most Important Transactions that pass'd in Christendom from 1665 to 1672*. 2 vols. Tonson, Churchill & Simpson, London, 1700.

SYDENHAM, THOMAS (1). *The Works of Thomas Sydenham MD [+1624 to +1689], translated from the Latin edition of Dr Greenhill, with a life of the author, by R. G. Latham M.D. etc.* 2 vols. Sydenham Society, London, 1850.

SZCZESNIAK, B. (6). 'The Writings of Michael Boym.' *MS*, 1955, **14**, 481.
SZCZESNIAK, B. (11). 'John Floyer and Chinese Medicine.' *OSIS*, 1954, **11**, 127. (The reader should beware of sinological errors in this otherwise valuable paper.)

TAKESHIGE *et al.* (1). Pain-threshold Increases in Cross-circulation Experiments with Acupuncture Analgesia. Art. in *Advances in Pain Research and Therapy*, vol. 1, ed. J. J. Bonica & D. Albe-Fessard. Raven, New York, 1976.
TAM KWONG-CHUEN & YIU HEUNG-HUNG (1). 'The Effect of Acupuncture on Essential Hypertension.' *AJCM*, 1975, **3**, 369.
TAN, LEONG T., TAN, MARGARET Y. C. & VEITH, I. (1). *Acupuncture Therapy; Current Chinese Practice.* Temple Univ. Press, Philadelphia, 1973.
TANG. See Thang.
AL-ṬAṬĀWĪ, M. (1). 'Der Lungenkreislauf nach al-Korachie [Ibn al-Qarashi al-Nafīs].' Inaug. Diss. Freiburg i/Breisgau, 1924.
TAYLOR, D. (1). 'In Search of New Leeches?' (Blood viscosity in diagnosis and therapy). *NS*, 1977, **73** (no. 1033), 32.
TEBOUL, G. & TEBOUL-WIART, H. (1). 'Sur l'Amélioration d'une Maladie de Parkinson.' *RIAC*, 1959, **12**, no. 47, 8.
TEMKIN, O. (2). 'Was Servetus influenced by Ibn al-Nafīs?' *BIHM*, 1940, **8**, 731.
TEMPLE, SIR WILLIAM (2). *Miscellanea* [collected essays, in several editions].
Pt. I. *A Survey of the Constitutions..., Upon the Original and Nature of Government, Upon the Advancement of Trade in Ireland, Upon the Conjuncture of Affairs in Oct. 1673, Upon the Excesses of Grief, and Upon the Cure of the Gout by Moxa.* Tonson & Churchill, London, 1693; fourth ed. 1705.
Pt. II. *Upon Ancient and Modern Learning, Upon the Gardens of Epicurus, Upon Heroick Virtue, Upon Poetry.* Simpson, London, 1692; fifth edition, 1705.
Pt. III. *On Popular Discontents, Upon Health and Long Life, and a Defence of the Essay Upon Ancient and Modern Learning.* Tooke, London, 1701.
TEN RHYNE. See ten Rhijne.
TERENIUS, L. (1). 'Opiate Receptors and their Ligands.' Proc. 6th Internat. Congress of Pharmacology, Helsinki, 1975, ed. J. Tuomisto & M. K. Paasonen, Vol. 1, p. 153.
TERENIUS, L. & WAHLSTRÖM, A. (1). 'Studies in Endorphins on Man.' Proc. 10th Colleguim Internationale Neuro-pharmacologicum, Quebec, 1976.
TERENIUS, L. & WAHLSTRÖM, A. (2). 'A Method for Site Selectivity Analysis applied to Opiate Receptors.' *EJPH*, 1976, **40** (no 2), 241.
THAN PO-FU, WÊN KUNG-WÊN, HSIAO KUNG-CHÜAN & MAVERICK, L. A. (tr.). *Economic Dialogues in Ancient China; Selections from the 'Kuan Tzu' (Book)...* pr. pr. Carbondale, Illinois and Yael Univ. Hall of Graduate Studies, New Haven, Conn., 1954. (Rev. A. W. Burks, *JAOS*, 1956, **76**, 198.)
THANG PEI-CHIN (1). 'Possible Humoral Mechanisms of Electro-acupuncture Anaesthesia.' Contribution to the First Bethesda Conference on Acupuncture Research, in Jenerick (1), p. 65.
THEOBALD, D. W. (1). *The Concept of Energy.* Spon, London, 1966. Cf. Porkert (1); Needham & Lu (9).
[DE THIERSANT], P. DABRY (1). *La Médecine chez les Chinois.* Plon, Paris, 1863. Ed. J. L. Soubeiran.
DE THIERSANT, P. DABRY. See Cordier (14), pp. 28 ff.
THOMPSON, D'ARCY W. (2). *Growth and Form.* Cambridge, 1917; 2nd ed., 1942.
THOMPSON, F. C. (1). 'The Early History of Wire.' *WI*, 1935, **2**, 159.
THORET, F. (1). 'Peut-on Provoquer le Dégout du Tabac par les Aiguilles Chinoises?' *RIAC*, 1959, **12**, no. 47, 14.
THUNBERG, C. P. (1). *Travels in Europe, Africa and Asia, made between the Years 1770 and 1779.* 4 vols.
Vol. 1. *A Voyage to the Southern Parts of Europe, and to the Cape of Good Hope in Africa, in the Years 1770–3.*
Vol. 2. *Two Expeditions to the Interior Parts of the Country adjacent to the Cape of Good Hope, and a Voyage to the Island of Java, performed in the Years 1773–5.*
Vol. 3. *A Voyage to Japan, and Travels in Different Parts of that Empire, in the Years 1775 and 1776.*
Vol. 4. *Travels in the Empire of Japan, and in the Islands of Java and Ceylon, together with the Voyage Home.*
2nd ed. Rivington, London, 1795. Tr. from the German edition of 1792–4 (Berlin).
THUNG SHANG-THAI & CHOU TÊ-I (1). 'Acupuncture combined with the Traditional Drug *wu mei thang* in the Treatment of Biliary Ascariasis.' *CMJ*, 1959, **78** (no. 6), 542. Abridged French tr. *BSAC*, 1959, no. 34, 47.
TIEDEMANN, H. (1). 'Extrinsic and Intrinsic Information Transfer in Early Differentiation of Amphibian Embryos.' *SSEB*, 1971, **25**, 223. Cf. Porkert (1); Needham & Lu (9).
TIERS, M. (1). 'Mode d'Action Générale de l'Acupuncture.' *RIAC*, 1956, **9**, no. 38, 188.

TITSINGH, ISAAC (1). *Cérémonies usitées au Japon pour les Mariages et les Funérailles, suivies de Détails sur la Poudre Dosia* [a plant drug alleged to reverse *rigor mortis*], *et de la Préface d'un Livre de Confoutzée* [*Confucius*] *sur la Piété Filiale*... Nepveu, Paris, 1819.

The preface or Avertissement contains a 'Notice des Livres et des Manuscrits Japonais, Français, Anglais et Hollandais, ainsi que des Peintures, Gravures, Cartes, Rouleaux, Dessins et Monnaies du Japon, réunis par feu M. Titsingh.'

TITSINGH, ISAAC (2). *Illustrations of Japan, consisting of Private Memoirs and Anecdotes of the Reigning Dynasty of the Djogouns* [Shoguns] *or Sovereigns of Japan, a Description of the Feasts and Ceremonies observed throughout the year at their Court; and of the Ceremonies and Funerals; to which are subjoined, Observations on the Legal Suicide of the Japanese, Remarks on their Poetry, an Explanation of their Mode of Reckoning Time, Particulars respecting the Dosia Powder, the Preface of a Work by Confoutzee on Filial Piety, etc.* Tr. from French by F. Schoberl. Ackermann, London, 1822.

TOBIMATSU, G. et al. (1). 'Akupunktur-anestesi i Kina; Observationer under en Studieresa 1972.' *LTD*, 1973, **70**, 709. Trans. from *JMJ*, 1972, no. 2523, 29.

TORGASHEV, B. P. (1). *The Mineral Industry of the Far East.* Chali, Shanghai, 1930.

TOYAMA, P. N. & NISHIZAWA, M. (1). 'Traditional Oriental Medicine and Acupuncture.' *JMSMA*, 1973, **14** (no. 11), 488.

TRAVELL, J. & RINZLER, S. H. (1). 'Relief of Cardiac Pain by Local Block of Somatic Trigger Areas.' *PSEBM*, 1946, **63**, 480.

TRAVELL, J. & RINZLER, S. H. (2). 'The Myofascial Genesis of Pain.' *PGMED*, 1952, **11**, 425.

TRUBERT, E. A. (1). 'Les Points Hérauts, ou Système des "Mou" [*mu hsüeh*].' *NRIAC*, 1969, **4**, no. 13, 231.

TRUMAN, D. E. S. (1). *The Biochemistry of Cytodifferentiation.* Blackwell, Oxford, 1974. Cf. Porkert (1); Needham & Lu (9).

TSÊNG LIANG-FU, LO, H. H. & LI CHO-HAO (1). 'β-Endorphin as a Potent Analgesic by Intravenous Injection.' *N*, 1976, **263**, 239.

TU HUAN-CHI & CHAO YEN-FANG (1). 'The Localisation of Central Structures involved in Descending Inhibitory Effects of Acupuncture on Viscero-Somatic Reflex Discharges.' *SCISA*, 1976, **19**, 137.

VACCA, G. (11). 'Osservazioni sopre alcune Stampe anatomiche Cinesi del Gabinetto delle Stampe della Accademia dei Lincei.' *RAL/MSF*, 1948 (ser. 8), **3**, 41. (The originals of the plates in Cleyer's *Specimen Medicinae Sinicae*.)

VALENTIN, LOUIS (1). *Mémoire et Observations Concernant les Bons Effets du Cautère Actuel, appliqué sur la Tête, ou sur la Nuque, dans Plusieurs Maladies des Yeux, des Enveloppes du Crâne, du Cerveau et du Système Nerveux.* Hissette, Nancy, 1815.

VALENTINI, M. B. (1). *Historia Moxae cum adjunctis medicationibus Podagrae.* Leiden, 1686.

VALORY, F. A. (1). 'L'Acupuncture et les Maladies Veineuses.' *NRIAC*, 1969, **4**, no. 12, 97.

VEITH, I. (1) (tr.) *'Huang Ti Nei Ching Su Wên'; the Yellow Emperor's Classic of Internal Medicine, chs. 1–34, translated from the Chinese, with an Introductory Study.* Williams & Wilkins, Baltimores 1949. (Revs. J. R. H[ightower], *HJAS*, 1951, **14**, 306; J. R. Ware, *BIHM*, 1950, **24**, 487; author's reply, *BIHM*, 1951, **25**, 86; see also W. Hartner, *ISIS*, 1951, **42**, 265.) Circumspection must be exercised in the use of this translation, done before the appearance of the modern *pai hua* versions. Cf. Chamfrault & Ung Kang-Sam (1).

VEITH, I. (2). 'Government Control and Medicine in +11th-Century China.' *BIHM*, 1943, **14**, 159.

VEITH, I. (4). 'Acupuncture; Ancient Enigma to East and West.' *AJPSY*, 1972, **129** (no. 3), 333.

VEITH, I. (5). 'Medicine in Japan.' *CIBA/S*, 1950, **11** (no. 4). 'Ancient Japanese Medicine', 1190. 'Introduction of Chinese Medicine to Japan', 1193. 'The Revival of Chinese Medicine and the Introduction of Western Medicine', 1202. 'Modern Japanese Medicine', 1218. Bibliography, 1220.

VEITH, I. See Tan, Tan & Veith (1).

VERGIER, M. (1). 'l'Acupuncture et l'Electro-acupuncture au début du 19e Siècle' (on the Chevalier Sarlandière, *q.v.*). *BSAC*, 1952, no. 6, 29.

VICQ-D'AZYR, FÉLIX (1). *Oeuvres, recueillies et publiées avec des Notes et un Discours sur sa vie et ses Ouvrages*, ed. J. L. Moreau de la Sarthe. 6 vols. Duprat-Duverger, Paris, 1805.

DI VILLA, E. M. (1). *The Examination of Mines in China.* North China Daily Mail, Tientsin, 1919.

VILSTRUP, T. & JENSEN, C. E. (1). 'On the Displacement Potential in Acid Muco-Polysaccharides.' *AOL* (Suppl.), 1963 **58**, no. 163, 42.

VAN VLOTEN, H. VORTISCH (1). *Chinesische Patienten und ihre Ärzte; Erlebrisse eines deutschen Ärztes.* Bertelsmann, Gütersloh, 1914.

VOGRALIK, V. G. (1). *Osnovy Kitaiskogo Letchevnogo Metoda Chen-Chiu* (Basis of the Chinese Therapy by Needles and Moxa) (In Russian). Gorki Press, Gorki, 1961.

VOGRALIK, V. G. (2). 'Die Klinisch-physiologischen Grundlagen der Nadelungstherapie und der Moxa bei inneren Erkrankungen.' *DZA*, 1960, **9** (no. 5), 97. Chinese tr. in Anon. (*108*), pp. 1 ff.

VOGRALIK, V. G. (3). 'Die Summe der Ergebnisse der wissenschaftlichen Forschung und Anwendung der chinesischen Methode *tschen-zsiu* [*chen chiu*, acupuncture and moxibustion] in der UdSSR [Soviet Union]'. *DZA*, 1962, **11** (no. 4), 73. (German tr. by H. Dolgoi & G. Bachmann.)

VOGRALIK, V. G. (4), (ed.). *Chen-Chiu Terapia; Materialvi Konferencii po Voprosam Physiologischeskogo Odosmovanyia i Prakticheskogo Primenniya Metoda Igloukalvivaniyia i Prischiganiyia* (*Chen-Chiu*). Gorki Press, Gorki, 1959.

VOS, ISAAC (1). *Variarum Observationum Liber.* Scott, London, 1685. (Contains, *inter alia, De Artibus et Scientiis Sinarum*, p. 69; *De Origine et Progressu Pulveris Bellici apud Europaeos*, p. 86; *De Triremium et Liburnicarum Constructione*, p. 95.) Cf. Duyvendak (13).

VOSSIUS. See Vos, Isaac.

WADDINGTON, C. H. (3). 'Concepts and Theories of Growth, Development, Differentiation and Morphogenesis' in *Towards a Theoretical Biology*, Edinburgh Univ. Press, Edinburgh, 1970, vol. 3, p. 177. Cf. Porkert (1); Needham & Lu (9).

WADDINGTON, C. H. (4). *Biological Development.* EB (15th ed.), 1974, p. 643. Cf. Porkert (1); Needham & Lu (9).

WAGMAN, I. H., DONG, W. K. & MCMILLAN, J. A. (1). 'Possible Physiological Bases for Acupuncture Analgesia.' *AJCM*, 1976, **4** (no. 4), 313. A paper at the Symposium on Pain and Acupuncture, Philadelphia, 1974.

WAGMAN, I. H. & PRICE, D. D. (1). 'Responses of Dorsal Horn Cells of *M. mulatta* to Cutaneous and Sural Nerve A- and C-fibre Stimuli.' *JNP*, 1969, **32**, 803.

WALEY, A. (1) (tr.). *The Way and its Power; a Study of the 'Tao Tê Ching' and its Place in Chinese Thought.* Allen & Unwin, London, 1934. (Crit. Wu Ching-Hsiung, *TH*, 1935, **1**, 225.)

WALL, PATRICK D. (1). 'Acupuncture – an Eye on the Needle.' *NS*, 1972, **55** (20 July), 129; also in *NTIM*, 1972 (24 Aug.), 1661.

WALL, PATRICK D. (2). 'Acupuncture Revisited.' *NS*, 1974, **64** (No. 917), 31.

WALL, PATRICK D. (3). 'Feeling no Pain.' Unpub. MS. lecture.

WALL, PATRICK D. See Melzack & Wall (1).

WALL, PATRICK D. & SWEET, W. H. (1). 'The Temporary Abolition of Pain.' *SC*, 1967, **155**, 108.

WALLACE, WM. (1). *Moxa; A Physiological Enquiry respecting the action of Moxa, and its Utility in inveterate Cases of Sciatica, Lumbago, Paraplegia, Epilepsy and some Other Painful, Paralytic and Spasmodic Diseases of the Nerves and Muscles.* Hodges & M'Arthur, Dublin, 1827.

WALLNÖFER, H. & VON ROTTAUSCHER, ANNA (1). *Der Goldene Schatz der Chinesischen Medizin.* Schuler, Stuttgart, 1959. Eng. tr. by M. Palmedo, *Chinese Folk Medicine and Acupuncture*, Crown (Bell), New York, 1965; Signet, New York, 1972; White Lion, London, 1975.

WANG CHI-MIN & FU WEI-KHANG (1) (=*1*). *Catalogue of Publications on Chinese Medicine in Foreign Languages, 1656 to 1962.* Museum of the History of Medicine, Shanghai Academy of Chinese Medicine, Shanghai, 1963.

WANG CHI-MIN & WU LIEN-TÊ (1). *History of Chinese Medicine.* National Quarantine Service, Shanghai, 1932. 2nd ed., 1936.

WANSBOROUGH, D. (1). 'Acupuncturation,' *LT*, 1826, **10**, 847.

WARE, J. R. (6) (tr.). *The Sayings of Mencius.* Mentor, New York, 1960.

WATERFIELD, A., HUGHES, J. & KOSTERLITZ, H. W. (1). 'Cross Tolerance between Morphine and Methionine-enkephalin.' *N*, 1976, **260**, 624.

WEBSTER, C. (2). 'William Harvey's Conception of the Heart as a Pump.' *BIHM*, 1965, **39**, 508.

WÊN HSIANG-LAI (1). 'Acupuncture Anaesthesia for Neurosurgery.' *AJM*, 1974, **10**, 157.

WÊN HSIANG-LAI & CHAU, K. (1). 'Status asthmaticus treated by Acupuncture and Electro-stimulation.' *AJM*, 1973, **9**, 191.

WÊN HSIANG-LAI & CHEUNG, S. Y. C. (1). 'The Treatment of Drug Addiction by Acupuncture and Electrical Stimulation.' *AJM*, 1973, **9**, 138; *DRS*, 1973, **2** (no. 8), 18. Cf. G. Patterson, *SPECT*, 1973 (1 Dec.), 697.

WÊN HSIANG-LAI, CHEUNG, S.Y.C. & METHAL, Z. D. (1). 'Acupuncture Anaesthesia in Surgery for Trigeminal Neuralgia.' *AJM*, 1973, **9**, 167.

WENGER, M. A. (1). 'The Measurement of Individual Differences in Autonomic Balance.' *PSM*, 1941, **3**, 427; 1942, **4**, 94; 1943, **5**, 148.

WERNØE, T. B. (1). 'Viscero-Cutane Reflexe.' *AFDGP*, 1925, **210**, 1–34. Also pub. Springer, Berlin, 1925 in *Collected Papers of the August Krogh Institute* (Zoophysiological Laboratory A), University of Copenhagen.

WESTERBLAD, C. A. (3). *[Pehr Hendrik] Ling, the Founder of Swedish Gymnastics; his life, his Work and his Importance.* Norstedt, Stockholm, 1909.

WHITE, J. C. & SWEET, W. H. (1). *Pain and the Neuro-Surgeon.* Thomas, New York, 1969.

WHITTERIDGE, G. (1) (tr.). *The Anatomical Lectures of William Harvey* [Praelectiones Anatomiae Universalis, *Lumleian Lectures at the Royal College of Physicians, +1616 onwards, with later interpolations by the lecturer*]. Livingstone, Edinburgh, 1964.

WISSLER, C. (1). 'The Sun Dance of the Blackfoot Indians.' *AMNH/AP*, 1921, **16**, 223.

WITHROW, R. (1) (ed.). *Photoperiodism and Related Phenomena in Plants and Animals.* Amer. Assoc. Adv. Sci., Washington, D.C., 1959.

WOGRALIK. See Vogralik.

WOODLEY, JOHN (1). 'Journey into China; September and October, 1972, a Diary.' Unpub. MS.

WOODROFFE, SIR J. G. (ps. A. Avalon) (1). *Śakti and Śakta; Essays and Addresses on the Śakta Tantra Śāstra.* 3rd edn Ganesh, Madras, Luzac, London, 1929.

WOODROFFE, SIR J. G. (ps. A. Avalon) (2). *The Serpent Power* [Kuṇḍalinī Yoga], *being the* Śat-cakra-nirūpana [i.e. ch. 6 of Pūrnānanda's *Tathra-chintāmani*, +1577] *and* Pādukā-panohaka, *two Works on Laya Yoga...* Ganesh, Madras, Luzac, London, 1919, repr. 1931.

WOODVILLE, W. (1). *Medical Botany, containing Systematic and General Descriptions, with Plates of all the Medicinal Plants, Indigenous and Exotic, comprehended in the Catalogues of the Materia Medica as published by the Royal Colleges of Physicians of London and Edinburgh; accompanied with a circumstantial Detail of their Medicinal Effects, and of the Diseases in which they have been most successfully Employed.* 3 vols. Phillips, London, 1790–3. With supplementary volume of the *Principal Medicinal Plants not included in the...Collegiate Pharmacopoeias.* Phillips, London, 1794.

WOOST, G. E. (1). *Quaedam de Acupunctura Orientalium ex oblivionis Tenebris ab Europaeis Medicis nuper revocata.* (Inaug. Diss.) Leipzig, 1826.

WOTTON, WILLIAM (1). *Reflections upon Ancient and Modern Learning.* Prefaces of 1694 and 1697. 2nd ed., Leake & Buck, London, 1697. Printed 'With a Dissertation upon the Epistles of Phalaris, Themistocles, Socrates, Euripides and Aesop's Fables' by Richard Bentley [in a letter addressed to Wotton]. 3rd ed., Goodwin, London, 1705. 'To which is added a Defence thereof in Answer to the Objections of Sir William Temple and Others...'

WRIGHT, SAMSON (1). *Applied Physiology.* 7th ed. Oxford, 1942.

WU CHIEN-PHING, CHAO CHIH-CHHI & WEI JEN-YÜ (1). 'The Inhibitory Effect produced by Stimulation of Afferent Nerves on the Responses of Dorsolateral Fasciculus Fibres in the Cat to Nocuous Stimuli; its relation to Acupuncture Analgesia.' *SCISA*, 1974, **17** (no. 5), 688.

WU HUI-PHING (1). *Chinese Acupuncture.* French tr. from the Chinese, with added comments, by J. Lavier. English tr. by P. M. Chancellor. Health Science Press, Rustington, Sussex, 1962.

WU HUI-PHING (2). *Formulaire d'Acuponcture; la Science des Aiguilles et des Cautérisations Chinoises.* Tr. from Chinese (Thaipei ed.) and abridged by J. Lavier. Maloine, Paris, 1959.

WU WEI-PING. See Wu Hui-Phing.

YI CHHING-CHHÊNG, LU TA-HSIEN, WU SHIH-HSIANG & TSOU KANG (1). 'A Study on the Release of H^3-5-Hydroxytryptamine [Tritium-labelled Serotonin] from the Brain during Acupuncture and Morphine Analgesia.' *SCISA*, 1977, **20** (no. 1), 113.

YIN, Y. C. (1). 'A Wire Needle in the Abdominal Cavity; an Accident in Acupuncture.' *CMJ*, 1937, **52** (no. 1), 107.

YIP, S. K., PANG, J. C. K. & SUNG, M. L. (1). 'Induction of Labour by Acupuncture Electro-Stimulation.' *AJCM*, 1976, **4**, (no. 3), 257.

YIU HEUNG-HUNG & TAM KWONG-CHUEN. See Yü Hsiung-Hung & Than Kuang-Chüan (1).

YÜ HSIUNG-HUNG & THAN KUANG-CHÜAN (1). 'Acupuncture for Several Functional Disorders.' *AJCM*, 1976, **4** (no. 3), 281.

YULE, SIR HENRY (1) (ed.). *The Book of Ser Marco Polo the Venetian, concerning the Kingdoms and Marvels of the East, translated and edited, with Notes, by H. Y....*, 1st ed. 1871, repr. 1875. 2 vols. ed. H. Cordier. Murray, London, 1903 (reprinted 1921). 3rd ed. also issued, Scribners, New York, 1929. With a third volume, *Notes and Addenda to Sir Henry Yule's Edition of Ser Marco Polo*, by H. Cordier. Murray, London, 1920.

YULE, SIR HENRY (2). *Cathay and the Way Thither; being a Collection of Mediaeval Notices of China.* 2 vols. Hakluyt Society Pubs. (2nd ser.), London, 1913–15. (1st ed. 1866.) Revised by H. Cordier, 4 vols. Vol. 1 (no. 38), *Introduction; Preliminary Essay on the Intercourse between China and the Western Nations previous to the Discovery of the Cape Route.* Vol. 2 (no. 33), *Odoric of Pordenone.* Vol. 3 (no. 37), *John of Monte Corvino and others.* Vol. 4 (no. 41), *Ibn Baṭṭuṭah and Benedict of Goes.* (Photolitho reprint, Peiping, 1942.)

ZARETSKY, H. H., LEE, M. H. M. & RUBIN, M. (1). 'Psychological Factors and Clinical Observations in Acupuncture Analgesia and Pain Abatement.' *JPS*, 1976, **93**, 113.

ZBOROWSKI, M. (1). 'Cultural Components in Responses to Pain.' *JSIS*, 1952, **8**, 16.

ZOTTERMAN, YNGVE (1). 'Touch, Pain and Tickling; an Electro-physiological Investigation on Cutaneous Sensory Nerves.' *JOP*, 1939, **95**, 1.
ZOTTERMAN, YNGVE (2) (ed.). *Sensory Functions of the Skin. Proceedings of a Symposium held in Jan. 1976.* Stockholm, 1976.
ZOTTERMAN, Y. (3). 'Studies in the Peripheral Nervous Mechanism of Pain.' *AMSD*, 1933, **80** (no. 3), 185.

GENERAL INDEX

by Muriel Moyle

Notes

(1) Articles (such as 'the', 'al-', etc.) occurring at the beginning of an entry, and prefixes (such as 'de', 'van', etc.) are ignored in the alphabetical sequence. Saints appear among all letters of the alphabet according to their proper names. Styles such as Mr, Dr, if occurring in book titles or phrases, are ignored; if with proper names, printed following them.

(2) The various parts of hyphenated words are treated as separate words in the alphabetical sequence. It should be remembered that, in accordance with the conventions adopted, some Chinese proper names are written as separate syllables while others are written as one word.

(3) In the arrangement of Chinese words, Chh- and Hs- follow normal alphabetical sequence, and *ü* is treated as equivalent to *u*.

(4) References to footnotes are not given except for certain special subjects with which the text does not deal. They are indicated by brackets containing the superscript letter of the footnote.

(5) Explanatory words in brackets indicating fields of work are added for Chinese scientific and technologial persons (and occasionally for some of other cultures), but not for political or military figures (except kings and princes).

	夏	Hsia kingdom (legendary?)		c. −2000 to c. −1520
	商	Shang (Yin) kingdom		c. −1520 to c. −1030
	周	Chou dynasty (Feudal Age)	Early Chou period	c. −1030 to −722
			Chhun Chhiu period 春秋	−722 to −480
			Warring States (Chan Kuo) period 戰國	−480 to −221
First Unification	秦	Chhin dynasty		−221 to −207
	漢	Han dynasty	Chhien Han (Earlier or Western)	−202 to +9
			Hsin interregnum	+9 to +23
			Hou Han (Later or Eastern)	+25 to +220
	三國	San Kuo (Three Kingdoms period)		+221 to +265
First Partition	蜀	Shu (Han)	+221 to +264	
	魏	Wei	+220 to +265	
	吳	Wu	+222 to +280	
Second Unification	晉	Chin dynasty: Western		+265 to +317
		Eastern		+317 to +420
	劉宋	(Liu) Sung dynasty		+420 to +479
Second Partition		Northern and Southern Dynasties (Nan Pei chhao)		
	齊	Chhi dynasty		+479 to +502
	梁	Liang dynasty		+502 to +557
	陳	Chhen dynasty		+557 to +589
	魏		Northern (Thopa) Wei dynasty	+386 to +535
			Western (Thopa) Wei dynasty	+535 to +556
			Eastern (Thopa) Wei dynasty	+534 to +550
	北齊	Northern Chhi dynasty		+550 to +577
	北周	Northern Chou (Hsienpi) dynasty		+557 to +581
Third Unification	隋	Sui dynasty		+581 to +618
	唐	Thang dynasty		+618 to +906
Third Partition	五代	Wu Tai (Five Dynasty period) (Later Liang, Later Thang (Turkic), Later Chin (Turkic), Later Han (Turkic) and Later Chou)		+907 to +960
	遼	Liao (Chhitan Tartar) dynasty		+907 to +1124
		West Liao dynasty (Qarā-Khiṭāi)		+1124 to +1211
	西夏	Hsi Hsia (Tangut Tibetan) state		+986 to +1227
Fourth Unification	宋	Northern Sung dynasty		+960 to +1126
	宋	Southern Sung dynasty		+1127 to +1279
	金	Chin (Jurchen Tartar) dynasty		+1115 to +1234
	元	Yuan (Mongol) dynasty		+1260 to +1368
	明	Ming dynasty		+1368 to +1644
	清	Chhing (Manchu) dynasty		+1644 to +1911
	民國	Republic		+1912

N.B. When no modifying term in brackets is given, the dynasty was purely Chinese. Where the overlapping of dynasties and independent states becomes particularly confused, the tables of Wieger (1) will be found useful. For such periods, especially the Second and Third Partitions, the best guide is Eberhard (9). During the Eastern Chin period there were no less than eighteen independent States (Hunnish, Tibetan, Hsienpi, Turkic, etc.) in the north. The term 'Liu chhao' (Six Dynasties) is often used by historians of literature. It refers to the south and covers the period from the beginning of the +3rd to the end of the +6th centuries, including (San Kuo) Wu, Chin, (Liu) Sung, Chhi, Liang and Chhen. For all details of reigns and rulers see Moule & Yetts (1).

ROMANISATION CONVERSION TABLES

BY ROBIN BRILLIANT

PINYIN/MODIFIED WADE-GILES

Pinyin	Modified Wade–Giles	Pinyin	Modified Wade–Giles
a	a	chou	chhou
ai	ai	chu	chhu
an	an	chuai	chhuai
ang	ang	chuan	chhuan
ao	ao	chuang	chhuang
ba	pa	chui	chhui
bai	pai	chun	chhun
ban	pan	chuo	chho
bang	pang	ci	tzhu
bao	pao	cong	tshung
bei	pei	cou	tshou
ben	pên	cu	tshu
beng	pêng	cuan	tshuan
bi	pi	cui	tshui
bian	pien	cun	tshun
biao	piao	cuo	tsho
bie	pieh	da	ta
bin	pin	dai	tai
bing	ping	dan	tan
bo	po	dang	tang
bu	pu	dao	tao
ca	tsha	de	tê
cai	tshai	dei	tei
can	tshan	den	tên
cang	tshang	deng	têng
cao	tshao	di	ti
ce	tshê	dian	tien
cen	tshên	diao	tiao
ceng	tshêng	die	dieh
cha	chha	ding	ting
chai	chhai	diu	tiu
chan	chhan	dong	tung
chang	chhang	dou	tou
chao	chhao	du	tu
che	chhê	duan	tuan
chen	chhên	dui	tui
cheng	chhêng	dun	tun
chi	chhih	duo	to
chong	chhung	e	ê, o

Pinyin	Modified Wade–Giles	Pinyin	Modified Wade–Giles
en	ên	jia	chia
eng	êng	jian	chien
er	êrh	jiang	chiang
fa	fa	jiao	chiao
fan	fan	jie	chieh
fang	fang	jin	chin
fei	fei	jing	ching
fen	fên	jiong	chiung
feng	fêng	jiu	chiu
fo	fo	ju	chü
fou	fou	juan	chüan
fu	fu	jue	chüeh, chio
ga	ka	jun	chün
gai	kai	ka	kha
gan	kan	kai	khai
gang	kang	kan	khan
gao	kao	kang	khang
ge	ko	kao	khao
gei	kei	ke	kho
gen	kên	kei	khei
geng	kêng	ken	khên
gong	kung	keng	khêng
gou	kou	kong	khung
gu	ku	kou	khou
gua	kua	ku	khu
guai	kuai	kua	khua
guan	kuan	kuai	khuai
guang	kuang	kuan	khuan
gui	kuei	kuang	khuang
gun	kun	kui	khuei
guo	kuo	kun	khun
ha	ha	kuo	khuo
hai	hai	la	la
han	han	lai	lai
hang	hang	lan	lan
hao	hao	lang	lang
he	ho	lao	lao
hei	hei	le	lê
hen	hên	lei	lei
heng	hêng	leng	lêng
hong	hung	li	li
hou	hou	lia	lia
hu	hu	lian	lien
hua	hua	liang	liang
huai	huai	liao	liao
huan	huan	lie	lieh
huang	huang	lin	lin
hui	hui	ling	ling
hun	hun	liu	liu
huo	huo	lo	lo
ji	chi	long	lung

Pinyin	Modified Wade–Giles	Pinyin	Modified Wade–Giles
lou	lou	pa	pha
lu	lu	pai	phai
lü	lü	pan	phan
luan	luan	pang	phang
lüe	lüeh	pao	phao
lun	lun	pei	phei
luo	lo	pen	phên
ma	ma	peng	phêng
mai	mai	pi	phi
man	man	pian	phien
mang	mang	piao	phiao
mao	mao	pie	phieh
mei	mei	pin	phin
men	mên	ping	phing
meng	mêng	po	pho
mi	mi	pou	phou
mian	mien	pu	phu
miao	miao	qi	chhi
mie	mieh	qia	chhia
min	min	qian	chhien
ming	ming	qiang	chhiang
miu	miu	qiao	chhiao
mo	mo	qie	chhieh
mou	mou	qin	chhin
mu	mu	qing	chhing
na	na	qiong	chhiung
nai	nai	qiu	chhiu
nan	nan	qu	chhü
nang	nang	quan	chhüan
nao	nao	que	chhüeh, chhio
nei	nei	qun	chhün
nen	nên	ran	jan
neng	nêng	rang	jang
ng	ng	rao	jao
ni	ni	re	jê
nian	nien	ren	jên
niang	niang	reng	jêng
niao	niao	ri	jih
nie	nieh	rong	jung
nin	nin	rou	jou
ning	ning	ru	ju
niu	niu	rua	jua
nong	nung	ruan	juan
nou	nou	rui	jui
nu	nu	run	jun
nü	nü	ruo	jo
nuan	nuan	sa	sa
nüe	nio	sai	sai
nuo	no	san	san
o	o, ê	sang	sang
ou	ou	sao	sao

Pinyin	Modified Wade–Giles	Pinyin	Modified Wade–Giles
se	sê	wan	wan
sen	sên	wang	wang
seng	sêng	wei	wei
sha	sha	wen	wên
shai	shai	weng	ong
shan	shan	wo	wo
shang	shang	wu	wu
shao	shao	xi	hsi
she	shê	xia	hsia
shei	shei	xian	hsien
shen	shen	xiang	hsiang
sheng	shêng, sêng	xiao	hsiao
shi	shih	xie	hsieh
shou	shou	xin	hsin
shu	shu	xing	hsing
shua	shua	xiong	hsiung
shuai	shuai	xiu	hsiu
shuan	shuan	xu	hsü
shuang	shuang	xuan	hsüan
shui	shui	xue	hsüeh, hsio
shun	shun	xun	hsün
shuo	shuo	ya	ya
si	ssu	yan	yen
song	sung	yang	yang
sou	sou	yao	yao
su	su	ye	yeh
suan	suan	yi	i
sui	sui	yin	yin
sun	sun	ying	ying
suo	so	yo	yo
ta	tha	yong	yung
tai	thai	you	yu
tan	than	yu	yü
tang	thang	yuan	yüan
tao	thao	yue	yüeh, yo
te	thê	yun	yün
teng	thêng	za	tsa
ti	thi	zai	tsai
tian	thien	zan	tsan
tiao	thiao	zang	tsang
tie	thieh	zao	tsao
ting	thing	ze	tsê
tong	thung	zei	tsei
tou	thou	zen	tsên
tu	thu	zeng	tsêng
tuan	thuan	zha	cha
tui	thui	zhai	chai
tun	thun	zhan	chan
tuo	tho	zhang	chang
wa	wa	zhao	chao
wai	wai	zhe	chê

Pinyin	Modified Wade–Giles	Pinyin	Modified Wade–Giles
zhei	chei	zhui	chui
zhen	chên	zhun	chun
zheng	chêng	zhuo	cho
zhi	chih	zi	tzu
zhong	chung	zong	tsung
zhou	chou	zou	tsou
zhu	chu	zu	tsu
zhua	chua	zuan	tsuan
zhuai	chuai	zui	tsui
zhuan	chuan	zun	tsun
zhuang	chuang	zuo	tso

MODIFIED WADE–GILES/PINYIN

Modified Wade–Giles	Pinyin	Modified Wade–Giles	Pinyin
a	a	chhio	que
ai	ai	chhiu	qiu
an	an	chhiung	qiong
ang	ang	chho	chuo
ao	ao	chhou	chou
cha	zha	chhu	chu
chai	chai	chhuai	chuai
chan	zhan	chhuan	chuan
chang	zhang	chhuang	chuang
chao	zhao	chhui	chui
chê	zhe	chhun	chun
chei	zhei	chhung	chong
chên	zhen	chhü	qu
chêng	zheng	chhüan	quan
chha	cha	chhüeh	que
chhai	chai	chhün	qun
chhan	chan	chi	ji
chhang	chang	chia	jia
chhao	chao	chiang	jiang
chhê	che	chiao	jiao
chhên	chen	chieh	jie
chhêng	cheng	chien	jian
chhi	qi	chih	zhi
chhia	qia	chin	jin
chhiang	qiang	ching	jing
chhiao	qiao	chio	jue
chhieh	qie	chiu	jiu
chhien	qian	chiung	jiong
chhih	chi	cho	zhuo
chhin	qin	chou	zhou
chhing	qing	chu	zhu

Modified Wade–Giles	Pinyin	Modified Wade–Giles	Pinyin
chua	zhua	huan	huan
chuai	zhuai	huang	huang
chuan	zhuan	hui	hui
chuang	zhuang	hun	hun
chui	zhui	hung	hong
chun	zhun	huo	huo
chung	zhong	i	yi
chü	ju	jan	ran
chüan	juan	jang	rang
chüeh	jue	jao	rao
chün	jun	jê	re
ê	e, o	jên	ren
ên	en	jêng	reng
êng	eng	jih	ri
êrh	er	jo	ruo
fa	fa	jou	rou
fan	fan	ju	ru
fang	fang	jua	rua
fei	fei	juan	ruan
fên	fen	jui	rui
fêng	feng	jun	run
fo	fo	jung	rong
fou	fou	ka	ga
fu	fu	kai	gai
ha	ha	kan	gan
hai	hai	kang	gang
han	han	kao	gao
hang	hang	kei	gei
hao	hao	kên	gen
hên	hen	kêng	geng
hêng	heng	kha	ka
ho	he	khai	kai
hou	hou	khan	kan
hsi	xi	khang	kang
hsia	xia	khao	kao
hsiang	xiang	khei	kei
hsiao	xiao	khên	ken
hsieh	xie	khêng	keng
hsien	xian	kho	ke
hsin	xin	khou	kou
hsing	xing	khu	ku
hsio	xue	khua	kua
hsiu	xiu	khuai	kuai
hsiung	xiong	khuan	kuan
hsü	xu	khuang	kuang
hsüan	xuan	khuei	kui
hsüeh	xue	khun	kun
hsün	xun	khung	kong
hu	hu	khuo	kuo
hua	hua	ko	ge
huai	huai	kou	gou

Modified Wade–Giles	Pinyin	Modified Wade–Giles	Pinyin
ku	gu	mu	mu
kua	gua	na	na
kuai	guai	nai	nai
kuan	guan	nan	nan
kuang	guang	nang	nang
kuei	gui	nao	nao
kun	gun	nei	nei
kung	gong	nên	nen
kuo	guo	nêng	neng
la	la	ni	ni
lai	lai	niang	niang
lan	lan	niao	niao
lang	lang	nieh	nie
lao	lao	nien	nian
lê	le	nin	nin
lei	lei	ning	ning
lêng	leng	niu	nüe
li	li	niu	niu
lia	lia	no	nuo
liang	liang	nou	nou
liao	liao	nu	nu
lieh	lie	nuan	nuan
lien	lian	nung	nong
lin	lin	nü	nü
ling	ling	o	e, o
liu	liu	ong	weng
lo	luo, lo	ou	ou
lou	lou	pa	ba
lu	lu	pai	bai
luan	luan	pan	ban
lun	lun	pang	bang
lung	long	pao	bao
lü	lü	pei	bei
lüeh	lüe	pên	ben
ma	ma	pêng	beng
mai	mai	pha	pa
man	man	phai	pai
mang	mang	phan	pan
mao	mao	phang	pang
mei	mei	phao	pao
mên	men	phei	pei
mêng	meng	phên	pen
mi	mi	phêng	peng
miao	miao	phi	pi
mieh	mie	phiao	piao
mien	mian	phieh	pie
min	min	phien	pian
ming	ming	phin	pin
miu	miu	phing	ping
mo	mo	pho	po
mou	mou	phou	pou

Modified Wade–Giles	Pinyin	Modified Wade–Giles	Pinyin
phu	pu	tên	den
pi	bi	têng	deng
piao	biao	tha	ta
pieh	bie	thai	tai
pien	bian	than	tan
pin	bin	thang	tang
ping	bing	thao	tao
po	bo	thê	te
pu	bu	thêng	teng
sa	sa	thi	ti
sai	sai	thiao	tiao
san	san	thieh	tie
sang	sang	thien	tian
sao	sao	thing	ting
sê	se	tho	tuo
sên	sen	thou	tou
sêng	seng, sheng	thu	tu
sha	sha	thuan	tuan
shai	shai	thui	tui
shan	shan	thun	tun
shang	shang	thung	tong
shao	shao	ti	di
shê	she	tiao	diao
shei	shei	tieh	die
shên	shen	tien	dian
shêng	sheng	ting	ding
shih	shi	tiu	diu
shou	shou	to	duo
shu	shu	tou	dou
shua	shua	tsa	za
shuai	shuai	tsai	zai
shuan	shuan	tsan	zan
shuang	shuang	tsang	zang
shui	shui	tsao	zao
shun	shun	tsê	ze
shuo	shuo	tsei	zei
so	suo	tsên	zen
sou	sou	tsêng	zeng
ssu	si	tsha	ca
su	su	tshai	cai
suan	suan	tshan	can
sui	sui	tshang	cang
sun	sun	tshao	cao
sung	song	tshê	ce
ta	da	tshên	cen
tai	dai	tshêng	ceng
tan	dan	tsho	cuo
tang	dang	tshou	cou
tao	dao	tshu	cu
tê	de	tshuan	cuan
tei	dei	tshui	cui

Modified Wade–Giles	Pinyin	Modified Wade–Giles	Pinyin
tshun	cun	wang	wang
tshung	cong	wei	wei
tso	zuo	wên	wen
tsou	zou	wo	wo
tsu	zu	wu	wu
tsuan	zuan	ya	ya
tsui	zui	yang	yang
tsun	zun	yao	yao
tsung	zong	yeh	ye
tu	du	yen	yan
tuan	duan	yin	yin
tui	dui	ying	ying
tun	dun	yo	yue, yo
tung	dong	yu	you
tzhu	ci	yung	yong
tzu	zi	yü	yu
wa	wa	yüan	yuan
wai	wai	yüeh	yue
wan	wan	yün	yun